Frontiers in CNS Drug Discovery

Volume 2

Editor

Prof. Atta-ur-Rahman, *FRS*

Honorary Life Fellow

Kings College

University of Cambridge

UK

Co-Editor

Prof. M. Iqbal Choudhary

H.E.J. Research Institute of Chemistry

International Center for Chemical and Biological Sciences

University of Karachi

Pakistan

CONTENTS

Contd.....

PREFACE

The present volume 2 of *Frontiers in CNS Drug Discovery* brings you the latest medical researches on the human Central Nervous System (CNS). Special themes of the 11 chapters in this volume are animal models, natural medicine, mental disorders, and particularly neurodegeneration. Neurodegenerative disorders such as Parkinson's disease (PD), Alzheimer's disease (AD), Huntington's disease (HD) and amyotrophic lateral sclerosis (ALS) have huge personal, social and economic impacts.

Brian Appleby's review examines possible treatment targets for protein misfolding disorders, utilizing the knowledge obtained in the field of prion disease. Prion diseases are rapidly progressing neurodegenerative maladies caused by an abnormal conformer of the native prion protein. Even though prion diseases are relatively rare in humans, other neurodegenerative protein misfolding disorders such as Alzheimer's and Parkinson's disease are now known to exhibit prion-like behavior and they are likely to benefit from treatments originally designed to deal with prion disease.

Candace Lewis and Foster Olive discuss the relevant epigenetic mechanisms that modulate gene transcription. They review and summarize the existing literature on epigenetic changes that occur after acute and chronic exposure to or self-administration of alcohol, psychostimulants, opiates, and nicotine, and studies examining the effects of manipulation of epigenetic processes in reward-related brain regions on addiction-like behaviors. The authors also discuss the possible implications of epigenetic factors as predictors of addiction vulnerability prior to drug exposure. Finally, they review findings from preclinical studies on the effects of pharmacological modifiers of epigenetic processes on addiction-related behaviors, and discuss the advantages and disadvantages of developing novel epigenetic-based CNS therapeutics for the treatment of addiction.

The mammalian brain has the capacity to generate new neurons throughout adulthood through a process referred to as adult neurogenesis. Joana M. Gil-Mohapel *et al.* review the results obtained in rodent models of AD, PD, and HD with regard to therapies aimed at restoring adult neurogenesis and discuss whether such therapies might have therapeutic relevance for the treatment of these devastating neurodegenerative disorders.

HIV-1 is largely impervious to highly active anti-retroviral therapeutic drugs (HAART). Jean-Pierre Louboutin discuss that since curing CNS HIV-1 is currently not possible, limiting the damage caused by the virus may be a useful approach to treatment. The chapter presents models which offer a better understanding of the pathogenesis of HIV-1 in the brain as well as provide new therapeutic avenues.

Transient receptor potential (TRP) ion channels have been extensively studied over the past few years and they are being ardently explored as targets for drug discovery. Recent findings in the field of pain have established a subset of TRP channels that are activated by temperature and are able to initiate sensory nerve impulses following the detection of thermal, as well as mechanical and chemical irritant stimuli. The review by Merab Tsagareli focuses on the latest developments in the TRP ion channel-related area and highlights evidence supporting TRP channels as promising targets for new analgesic drugs at the periphery and central levels and opportunities for therapeutic intervention.

Antipsychotics (APs) have been used for treating schizophrenia and other severe mental disorders for more than fifty years. The aim of the review by Alessandro De Risio and Davide Carlino is to address the boundaries of polypharmacy with APs, from epidemiological features to clinical significance. The chapter looks at prescription patterns, compares the theoretical rationale of monotheraphy and the pharmacokinetic and pharmachodynamic properties of the combined selective associations of two APs. The reasons for using polypharmacy in routine practice are also discussed in the chapter.

The search for new effective chemical entities, capable of acting in diverse biochemical targets, with new mechanisms of action and low toxicity continues to benefit from modern natural products chemistry that can provide active, sophisticated and complex new lead molecules to drug discovery and development. Claudio Viegas-Jr. *et al.* discuss in their chapter some contributions of natural products chemistry for the discovery of active constituents in plants, herbs and extracts to treat senile neurodegenerative disorders, especially for AD and PD, in the period after the 2000s.

Flavonoids are the most abundant plant polyphenolic substances, and they are found in fruits, vegetables and plant-derived beverages. Quite a few natural flavonoids with potential antioxidants and signaling properties are being investigated to identify preventive neuroprotective compounds to stop the progression of PD. The chapter by Elena González-Burgos' and Pilar Gómez-Serranillos concentrates on the multiple neuroprotection mechanisms of natural flavonoids in PD, covering the latest preclinical *in vitro* and *in vivo* PD animal model studies and clinical trials. It provides an overview and the current challenges that may be helpful for future research.

Inflammation plays an important part in the onset and progress of neurodegenerative diseases. Among new products, omega (n)-3 fatty acids have anti-inflammatory and neuroprotective benefits with few side effects. The chapter by Cai Song reviews the new findings from studies in relationship between inflammation and neurodegenerative disease. It also presents the important role of polyunsaturated fatty acids (PUFA) in the brain and the immune system.

Monoterpenoids and their derivatives are important starting materials for the development of new bioactive substances, including drugs. Many of these compounds exhibit feature substantial CNS activities such as antinociceptive, neuroprotective and anticonvulsant. Konstantin Volcho *et al.* cover the recent literature on monoterpenoids and their derivatives, exhibiting various types of CNS activity in their review.

Use of zebrafish to identify new CNS drugs by high throughput screening is discussed by Thomas Boyd. Many behavioral assays developed in other animals are available in zebrafish, including assays for locomotion, avoidance behaviors, learning, and conditioned place preference. Zebrafish offer an exciting assays for identification of new medicines to treat disorders due to nicotinic cholinergic and dopaminergic dysregulation including nicotine addiction, schizophrenia, Alzheimer's disease and Parkinson's disease.

I am grateful for the timely efforts made by the editorial personnel, especially **Mr. Mahmood Alam** (Director Publications) and **Mrs. Sana Mokarram** at Bentham Science Publishers.

Prof. Atta-ur-Rahman, *FRS*
Honorary Life Fellow
Kings College
University of Cambridge
UK

LIST OF CONTRIBUTORS

Brian S. Appleby
Cleveland Clinic Foundation, Lou Ruvo Center for Brain Health, 9500 Euclid Avenue/U10, Cleveland, OH 44195, USA

Robert T. Boyd
Department of Neuroscience, The Ohio State University College of Medicine, Wexner Medical Center, 333 West Tenth Avenue, Columbus Ohio 43210, USA

Flávia P.D. Viegas
LFQM – Laboratório de Fitoquímica e Química Medicinal, Instituto de Química, Universidade Federal de Alfenas (UNIFAL-MG), 37130-000, Alfenas, MG, Brazil

Rodolfo do C. Maia
LASSBio–Laboratório de Avaliação e Síntese de Substâncias Bioativas, Faculdade de Farmácia, Universidade Federal do Rio de Janeiro (UFRJ), 21941-902, Rio de Janeiro, RJ, Brazil

Roberta Tesch
LASSBio–Laboratório de Avaliação e Síntese de Substâncias Bioativas, Faculdade de Farmácia, Universidade Federal do Rio de Janeiro (UFRJ), 21941-902, Rio de Janeiro, RJ, Brazil

Carlos A.M. Fraga
Programa de Pós-Graduação em Farmacologia e Química Medicinal, Instituto de Ciências Biomédicas, Universidade Federal do Rio de Janeiro (UFRJ), 21941-902, Rio de Janeiro, RJ, Brazil

Claudio Viegas-Jr.
Programa de Pós-Graduação em Química, Universidade Federal de Alfenas (UNIFAL-MG), 37130-000, Alfenas, MG, Brazil

Cai Song
Research Institute for Marine Nutrition and Drugs, Guangdong Ocean University, China; Department of Psychology and Neurosciences, Dalhousie University, Canada

Candace R. Lewis
Arizona State University, Tempe, AZ 930 S McAllister Ave., Tempe, AZ 85287, USA

Michael F. Olive
Arizona State University, Tempe, AZ 930 S McAllister Ave., Tempe, AZ 85287, USA

Anna Patten
Division of Medical Sciences, Island Medical Program, University of Victoria, Victoria, British Columbia, Canada

Patricia S. Brocardo
Neuroscience Program, Federal University of Santa Catarina, Florianópolis, Santa Catarina, Brazil

Joana M. Gil-Mohapel
Division of Medical Sciences, Island Medical Program, University of Victoria, Victoria, British Columbia, Canada

Jean-Pierre Louboutin
Department of Pathology, Anatomy and Cell Biology, Thomas Jefferson University, Philadelphia, PA 19107, USA

David S. Strayer
Department of Pathology, Anatomy and Cell Biology, Thomas Jefferson University, Philadelphia, PA 19107, USA

Merab G. Tsagareli
Pain Research Group, Department of Neurophysiology, Ivane Beritashvili Center for Experimental Biomedicine, Tbilisi, Georgia

Elena González-Burgos
Department of Pharmacology, Faculty of Pharmacy, University Complutense, Madrid, Spain

Maria P. Gómez-Serranillos
Department of Pharmacology, Faculty of Pharmacy, University Complutense, Madrid, Spain

Alla V. Pavlova
Novosibirsk Institute of Organic Chemistry, Siberian Branch of the Russia Academy of Science, Novosibirsk, Russia

Konstantin P. Volcho
Novosibirsk Institute of Organic Chemistry, Siberian Branch of the Russia Academy of Science, Novosibirsk, Russia

Tatyana G. Tolstikova
Novosibirsk Institute of Organic Chemistry, Siberian Branch of the Russia Academy of Science, Novosibirsk, Russia

Alessandro De Risio
NSH Health Trust No. 10 "Veneto Orientale", Unit of Psychiatry of Portogruaro, Via Forlanini, 2, 30026 Portogruaro, Venezia, Italia

Davide Carlino
Department of Morphological, Technological and Clinical Science, Clinic of Psychiatry, University of Trieste, Via De Ralli, 5 34128 Trieste, Italia

CHAPTER 1

Developing Treatments for Prion Diseases and Implications for Other Protein Misfolding Disorders

Brian S. Appleby*

Cleveland Clinic Foundation, Lou Ruvo Center for Brain Health, 9500 Euclid Avenue/U10, Cleveland, OH 44195, USA

Abstract: Prion diseases are rapidly progressive neurodegenerative illnesses caused by an abnormal conformer of the native prion protein. Human prion diseases include Creutzfeldt-Jakob disease, variant Creutzfeldt-Jakob disease, fatal familial insomnia, Gerstmann-Sträussler-Scheinker disease, and variable protease sensitive prionopathy for which there are no available treatments. Several treatments have been investigated, mostly focusing on inhibiting the conversion of the native prion protein to its pathological form. Although *in vitro* and animal model studies have been encouraging, success has yet to be translated to clinical trials. In addition to prion protein conversion inhibitors, other avenues of research have focused on blocking the expression of the normal prion protein, hence removing the substrate required for further disease propagation. This technique is complicated by the elusive physiological role(s) of the native prion protein in humans and the unknown complications that could arise with this type of treatment. Although prion diseases are relatively rare in humans, other neurodegenerative protein misfolding disorders such as Alzheimer's and Parkinson's disease are now known to exhibit prion-like behavior and will also benefit from treatments originally designed to combat prion disease. The goal of this review is to examine possible treatment targets for protein misfolding disorders utilizing knowledge obtained from the field of prion disease.

Keywords: Prion disease, protein misfolding, Creutzfeldt-Jakob disease, treatment, Alzheimer's disease, frontotemporal dementia, Parkinson's disease.

INTRODUCTION

Many neurodegenerative disorders are associated with the accumulation of abnormal proteins that are thought to be neurotoxic. For example, Alzheimer's disease (AD) is associated with amyloid plaques composed of aggregated a-beta

***Address correspondence to Brian S. Appleby:** Cleveland Clinic Foundation, Lou Ruvo Center for Brain Health, 9500 Euclid Avenue/U10, Cleveland, OH 44195, USA; Tel: 216-636-9467; Fax: 216-445-7013; E-mail: applebb@ccf.org

Atta-ur-Rahman & M. Iqbal Choudhary (Eds.)

peptides and neurofibrillary tangles composed of hyperphosphorylated tau. Similarly, Parkinson's disease (PD) is associated with Lewy bodies composed of accumulated alpha-synuclein. Such neurodegenerative disorders are usually differented from each other based on the type of accumulated protein, neuropathologic characteristics, and clinical phenomenology. Neurodegenerative diseases associated with protein aggregates are often referred to as protein misfolding disorders (PMD).

PMDs are characterized by aggregates of abnormal proteins. Proteins are composed of an amino acid sequence (primary structure) that then assumes secondary and tertiary structures based on different molecular interactions. Most PMDs are caused by changes in protein conformation commencing at the level of the secondary structure. A normative physiologically active protein may be composed primarily of alpha-helices whereas the pathologic protein conformer assumes a structure composed primarily of beta-sheets as in the example of the prion protein. These proteins contain the same sequence of amino acids, but their shape differs. This change in shape affects its functioning and can result in loss of normal function or even a gain of a pathological function.

Cells have a complex protein quality control system that usually prevents the aggregation of pathologic proteins. Through the use of molecular chaperones and the proteasome, abnormal proteins are degraded and cleared from the cell. However, sometimes the quality control systems may become dysfunctional or the amount of abnormal protein requiring clearance and degradation exceeds its abilities. These abnormal conformers then aggregate and are typically deposited within the brain in the form of amyloid deposits. Neurotoxicity of PMDs is likely related to distinct neurotoxic oligomers as opposed to the aggregates themselves.

Many human diseases are caused by PMDs, a concept that largely arose from prion disease research. Alzheimer's disease, Parkinson's disease, prion disease, and diabetes mellitus are all associated with aggregates of pathologic protein conformers. Many experimental treatments of these diseases focus on pathologic protein misfolding or the conseqeuces thereof. Prion diseases are often seen as the achetype of PMDs and can be a useful platform to use when discussing the pathophysiology and treatment approaches for other PMDs. This chapter reviews basic prion disease pathophysiology and uses information from prion disease research as a model from which PMD therapeutics may be derived.

PRION DISEASES

Human prion diseases are a group of transmissible neurodegenerative conditions characterized by the presence of a pathologic form of the native prion protein (PrP^{Sc}) [1]. Also referred to as transmissible spongiform encephalopathies (TSEs) because of the extensive vacuolization of the brain parenchyma demonstrated in these diseases, there are well described prion diseases in other animals including scrapie in sheep and goats, bovine spongiform encephalopathy (BSE) in cows, and chronic wasting disease (CWD) in cervids. All prion diseases are fatal neurodegenerative illnesses that are usually characterized by a rapid clinical decline.

There are three etiologies of human prion diseases: sporadic, genetic, and acquired (Fig. **1**). The majority of cases (85%) are sporadic in origin with no overt

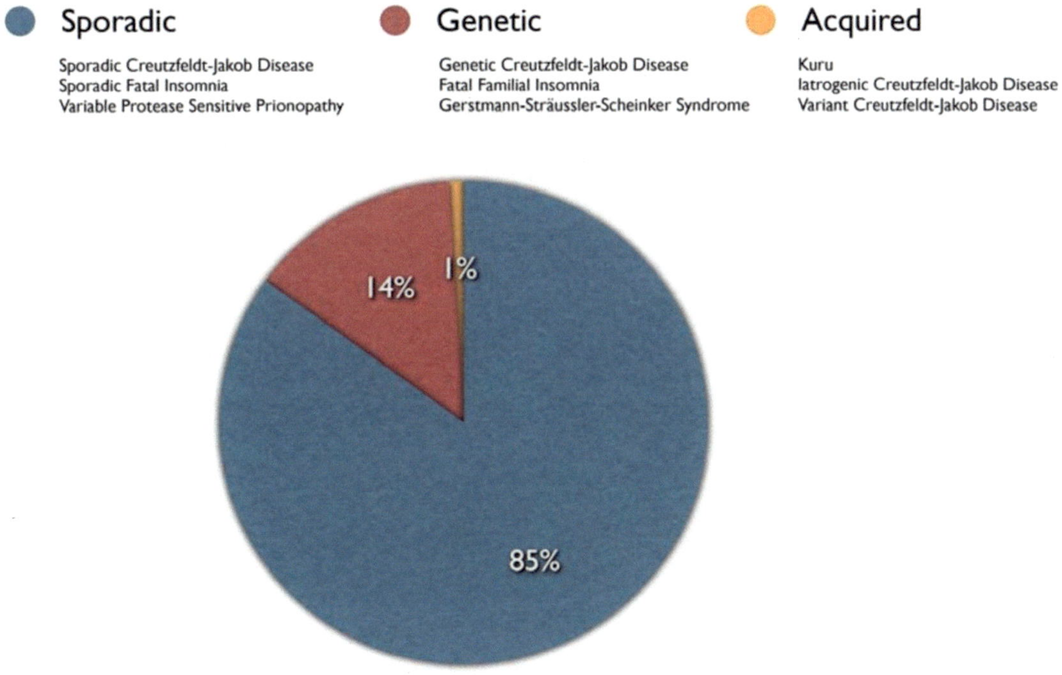

Fig. (1). Etiologies of human prion diseases.

cause or precipitating factor. 10-15% of cases are caused by genetic mutations in the prion protein gene (*PRNP*) and the remainder of cases are acquired *via* iatrogenic or dietary means. The mean age at onset of sporadic Creutzfeldt-Jakob disease (sCJD) is approximately the early 60s [2] and although reported mean survival times often differ by country, most reports fall between 6 and 12 months following disease onset [3]. sCJD is characterized by a rapid neurodegenerative decline that is often manifested by cerebellar and visual impairments, pyramidal and extrapyramidal symptoms, dementia, myoclonus, and akinetic mutism. CJD is characterized neuropathologically by the presence of spongiform changes, neuronal loss, and astrogliosis [4]. Immunocytochemistry is used to demonstrate the presence of PrP^{Sc} (Fig. **2**). Although definitive diagnosis can only be made by neuropathological inspection, a diagnosis of probable sCJD can be made antemortem. Diagnostic criteria for probable and possible sCJD combine the presence of clinical symptoms with diagnostic test results [5] (Table **1**). Diagnostic findings suggestive of sCJD are periodic sharp wave complexes on

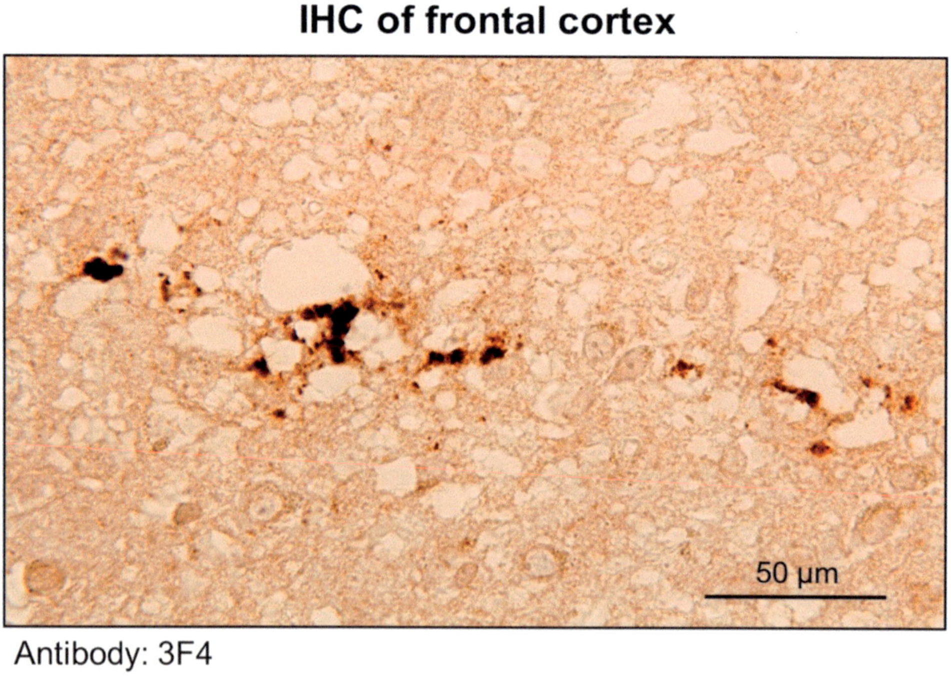

Fig. (2). Immunohistochemistry (IHC) staining for prion protein in the brain of a prion disease patient.

Table 1. MRI-CJD Consortium Diagnostic Criteria for Probable and Possible Sporadic Creutzfeldt-Jakob Disease[a]

Clinical Symptoms	Diagnostic Test Results
Visual or Cerebellar	EEG: Presence of PSWCs
Pyramidal or Extrapyramidal	CSF: Presence of 14-3-3 protein and illness duration < 2 years
Dementia	Brain MRI: High signal intensity in caudate and putamen or ≥ 2 cortical regions (excluding frontal lobes) on DWI or FLAIR
Akinetic Mutism	

Probable sCJD: ≥ 2 clinical symptoms and ≥ 1 diagnostic test result(s)
Possible sCJD: ≥ 2 clinical symptoms and illness duration < 2 years
[a]Reference [5].
EEG=electroencephalogram, PSWC=periodic sharp wave complexes, CSF=cerebrospinal fluid, MRI=magnetic resonance imaging, DWI=diffusion weighted imaging, FLAIR=fluid attenuated inversion recovery, sCJD=sporadic Creutzfeldt-Jakob disease.

electroencephalogram (EEG) and the presence of elevated 14-3-3 protein levels in cerebrospinal fluid (CSF). Recently CSF tau levels have been used in the diagnosis of sCJD and have higher specificity compared to 14-3-3 protein detection [6]. Negative CSF tau and neuron specific enolase levels are the most specific to a non-prion disease diagnosis (88%) compared to other CSF biomarkers (*e.g.*, 14-3-3 and S100b) [7]. Interpretation of CSF biomarkers within the clinical context is essential. For example, elevated CSF 14-3-3 protein levels are much less specific in more acute neurological disorders (*i.e.*, epilepsy, inflammatory disorders) (82-87%) compared to other neurodegenerative diseases (95-97%) [8]. Brain magnetic resonance imaging (MRI) is also useful for clinical diagnosis and diagnostic consensus criteria have been changed to reflect its utility [5]. Found characteristics of CJD are observed on diffusion weighted imaging (DWI) and fluid attenuated inversion recovery (FLAIR) sequences that include hyperintensity in the temporal, parietal, or occipital cortices and/or in the basal ganglia (Fig. **3**).

Similar to other neurodegenerative diseases, genetics play a causal and disease modifying role in prion disease. Over 30 pathological mutations have been described to result in genetic prion disease, all of which occur in the prion protein gene (*PRNP*) [9]. Most mutations are point mutations, though octapeptide repeat insertion and deletion mutations have also been described. Most mutations cause

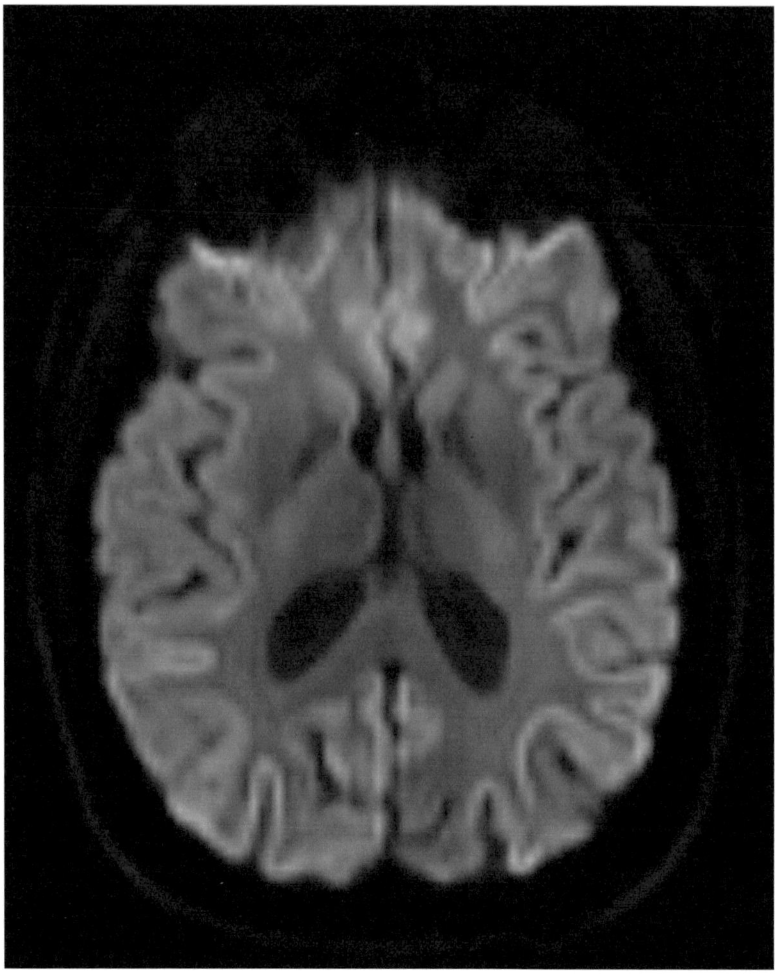

Fig. (3). Brain MRI using DWI of a prion disease patient. Observe the characteristic hyperintensity of the caudate nucleus and throughout the cortex in a "cortical ribbon" pattern.

diseases that phenotypically resemble sCJD and are generally termed genetic CJD (gCJD) (*e.g.*, E200K mutation). Other mutations demonstrate specific clinical and neuropathological phenotypes that differ from the classic CJD phenotype. Gerstmann-Sträussler-Scheinker syndrome (GSS) is a prion disease caused by several different mutations resulting in an illness of several years duration, prominent cerebellar symptoms, and kuru plaques in the cerebellum [9]. Fatal familial insomnia (FFI) is a genetic prion disease caused by a very specific haplotype. The D178N mutation coupled with valine at codon 129 of *PRNP* on the mutated allele results in a gCJD phenotype, whereas the same mutation coupled with methionine at codon 129 produces the FFI phenotype [10]. FFI is characterized by persistent and progressive insomnia, lost of normal sleep architecture on polysomnography, autonomic instability, and lack of dementia for the majority of the disease course [11]. Neuropathological changes are also mostly confined to the thalamus. Codon 129 also has important effects on the risk of all types of prion disease as well as clinical symptoms and disease duration [12-14].

PATHOPHYSIOLOGY OF PRION DISEASE

Our understanding of prion diseases began to coalesce following the description of kuru by Carlton Gajdusek [15]. Kuru was an endemic illness among the Fore tribe of Papua New Guinea that resulted in rapidly progressive neurological decline that mainly affected women and young children and was transmitted through ritualistic cannabilism. Neuropathologic examination of kuru cases revealed profound neuronal loss and astrogliosis [16] that were later commented on by William Hadlow to be reminiscent of neuropathological findings of scrapie affected animals [17]. As scrapie had been experimentally transmitted to goats *via* intracerebral inoculation, Hadlow suggested intracerebrally inoculating primates with brain homogenate from kuru patients [18]. Following an incubation period of approximately 1.5 years, chimpanzees that were intracerebrally inoculated with brain homogenate from kuru patients became fatally ill and exhibited similar clinical characteristics to kuru patients [19]. Subsequently similar experiments were conducted using human brains of patients affected by another spongiform encephalopathy, Creutzfeldt-Jakob disease (CJD), which was initially described by Hans Creutzfeldt and Alfons Jakob in the early 1920s [20-22]. One year after intracerebral inoculation with brain homogenate from CJD patients, chimpanzees developed a similar illness marking this unique category of diseases as transmissible spongiform encephalopathies (TSEs) [23].

Although transmission was well documented in TSEs, the etiological agent was somewhat of an enigma. Early studies performed by Tikvah Alper cast significant doubt on the possibility of the causative agent containing nucleic acid, excluding known bacteria and viruses as culprits [24,25]. Around this time, a mathematician named James Griffith published a theoretical model of scrapie transmission that considered an aberrant protein to be the transmissible agent [26]. Building on this prior work, Stanley Prusiner published a manuscript coining the term "prion" as the infectious agent in TSEs, demarcating its *pro*-teinacious and infectious (*-ion*) nature [1]. The pathologic form of the prion protein (PrP^{Sc}) was purified and isolated two years later [27]. Replication without the use of nucleic acids brought a new paradigm to biology and sparked controversy. However, there now exists multiple lines of evidence in favor of the "protein only" hypothesis (Table **2**) and most researchers agree that PrP^{Sc} is the major if not sole determinant of prion diseases. Although spontaneous conversion of PrP^{Sc} without mammalian cofactors has been performed within a laboratory setting [28], various cofactors may modulate the conversion process [29]. The prion conversion process can best be described as template directed protein misfolding as illustrated in Fig. (**4**).

Table 2. Evidence Supporting the "Protein Only" Prion Hypothesis

Agent is smaller than conventional microorganisms
Agent is resistant to ribonucleases and dexyribonucleases
Agent is resistant to ultraviolet irradiation at 254nm
Nucleic acid has not been consistently associated with the agent
PrP^{Sc} is required for transmission and infectivity is dose-related
Inactivation of PrP^{Sc} reduces or eliminates infectivity
All inherited forms of human prion disease are caused by mutations in the prion protein gene (*PRNP*)
PRNP $^{-/-}$ knockout mice are resistant to prion transmission
Transgenic animal models that over-express *PRNP* spontaneously develop prion disease
PrP^{Sc} causes template directed protein misfolding of PrP^{c} to PrP^{Sc} *in vitro*
PrP^{Sc} can be produced without mammalian cofactors present

The neurotoxicity underlying prion diseases is poorly understood, though the majority is likely due to a pathological gain of function of PrP^{Sc} as opposed to a biological loss of PrP^{c} function. The exact functions of PrP^{c} are not well defined but generally include cell signaling, immune functions, neuroprotective effects, and binding of various metals [30]. *PRNP* -/- knockout mice do not demonstrate any clear or consistent phenotypic changes compared to non-genetically modified mice [31]. However, subtle differences have been observed in some studies using *PRNP*-/- knockout mice including changes in the peripheral nervous system, depressive-like behavior, and alteration of excitatory neurotransmitters [32-34]. PrP^c is required for prion disease to occur, acting as a substrate for further PrP^{Sc} generation and potentially as a signal transducer or modulator of PrP^{Sc} activity. *PRNP-/-* knockout mice are resistant to scrapie infection [31] and when PrP^c is present, it must be bound to the cell membrane by a glycosylphosphatidylinositol (GPI) anchor for prion infection to occur [35]. Other potential neurotoxic mechanisms of prion diseases are described later in this chapter in relation to other PMDs.

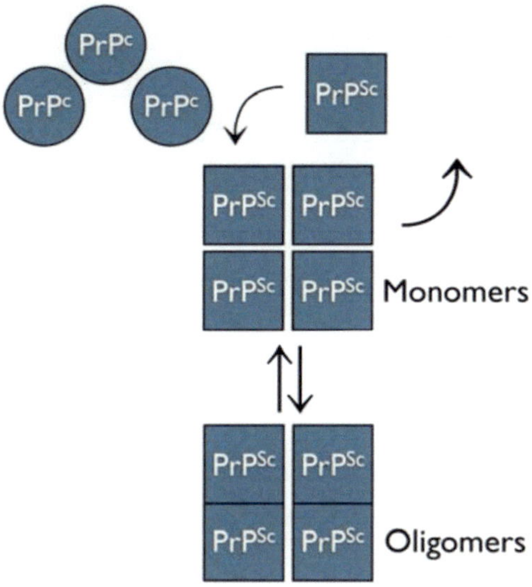

Fig. (4). Depiction of template directed protein misfolding in prion diseases. PrP^c = native "cellular" prion protein; PrP^{Sc} = pathological "scrapie" prion protein.

Recent research has determined that prion infectivity can be uncoupled from prion neurotoxicity. There are certain conditions in which PrP^{Sc} accumulation occurs without neurotoxic effects including non-GPI anchored PrP^c cell models and extraneuronal PrP^{Sc} replication [36]. Excellent work performed by Mallucci and colleagues has demonstrated that depleting PrP^c during active prion infection reverses neuropathological and clinical changes and prevents further neurotoxicity despite continued PrP^{Sc} accumulation [37,38]. Hence PrP^{Sc}, at least by itself, is not directly or solely responsible for neurotoxicity in prion diseases. It is possible that PrP^{Sc} requires PrP^c as a signaling molecule to trigger neurotoxicity. Research examining various PrP mutants also demonstrate that neurodegenerative phenotypes can be produced by altering the amino acid sequence of PrP^c without PrP^{Sc} formation [39]. Despite our current knowledge of prion disease, many questions remain unanswered (Table **3**).

Table 3. Unresolved Issues in the Field of Prion Disease

Neurotoxic mechanism(s) underlying prion disease
Determinants of prion disease toxicity *versus* transmissibility
Role of protease sensitive prion proteins in prion disease
Role of cofactors in mediating prion protein conversion
Mediators of strain differentiation depending on environmental context
Determinants of different prion protein strains
Physiologic role of native prion protein (PrP^c)
Second passage transmission of prion disease from prion protein knockout mice
Determinants of "species barrier" in prion disease
Determinants of prion protein gene mutation penetrance

TREATMENT OF PRION DISEASE

Human prion diseases are invariably fatal illnesses, with no currently available treatments proven to reverse or halt the disease course. Several clinical trials examining potential treatments have been conducted in humans with prion disease (Table **4**). Most of the compounds studied were thought to be beneficial in prion diseases by inhibiting the conversion of PrP^c to PrP^{Sc}. A United States randomized, double blind, placebo controlled trial using quinacrine has been completed, though final results have not been reported. Mid-point survival analyses of this study did not demonstrate any differences between the treatment and placebo group [40] replicating the results from two other quinacrine trials [41,42]. Three other studies examining doxycycline 100mg/day orally in prion disease patients have also concluded in Germany, Italy, and France [43-45]. Mid-point analyses of the German study revealed statistically significant prolongation of survival times in those treated with doxycycline with patients having methionine homozygosity at codon 129 of the *PRNP* gene receiving statistically significant greater benefit than other codon 129 genotypes [46]. An Italian study of doxycycline in FFI mutation carriers has also been initiated to assess possible prophylactic effects of doxycycline on disease onset [44].

Table 4. Clinical Treatment Trials in Human Prion Diseases

Study	Compound	MoA	Trial Design	Results
Terzano MG, Arch Neurol 1983	Amantadine	Antiviral	Comparative	-increased alertness -no difference in survival time
Neri G, Riv Neurobiol 1984	Amantadine	Antiviral	Comparative	-less cognitive decline -no difference in survival time
Otto M, Neurology 2004	Flupirtine	Neuroprotective	Double Blind	-less cognitive decline -no difference in survival time
Bone I, Eur J Neurol 2008	Pentosan polysulphate	Conversion inhibitor	Observational	-possibly extends survival time
Tsuboi Y, Neuropathology 2009	Pentosan polysulphate	Conversion inhibitor	Observational	-possibly extends survival time
Haik S, Neurology 2004	Quinacrine	Conversion inhibitor	Case-control	-no difference in survival time
Collinge J, Lancet Neurol 2009	Quinacrine	Conversion inhibitor	Observational	-no difference in survival time

Lessons Learned

Although the results of clinical treatment trials in prion diseases have been disappointing, the field has learned a lot about conducting trials in this population. Given the rarity of the disease and its usual rapid progression, lessons learned from conducting trials even if they have negative outcomes are quite valuable. The first lesson can be gleaned from the discovery of quinacrine as an anti-prion compound *in vitro* [47]. This exciting finding led the authors of the study manuscript to call for immediate clinical trials in human prion diseases on the grounds of "compassionate treatment." Without verifying the anti-prion effects of quinacrine in animal models, three negative studies of quinacrine in humans were conducted [40-42] consuming time, money, and patient contributions that may have been spent in other ways had animal models been conducted first.

Despite the negative outcomes of the quinacrine clinical trials, much can be learned about the challenges of conducting clinical trials in prion diseases from the UK's PRION-1 study [42]. PRION-1 was a placebo controlled trial in which patients could choose randomization, quinacrine, or placebo. The study results make it clear that patients and families had distinct preferences on whether or not treatment was received. Only 2 of 107 (1.8%) subjects chose to be randomized. Subjects that were less cognitively and functionally impaired chose quinacrine treatment whereas those that were more cognitively and functionally impaired actively declined quinacrine treatment. Though various conclusions may be made from this observation, one factor frequently considered by patients and families is quality of life. If a treatment were to prolong survival with no quality of life benefit, many choose to forego treatment. Hence quality of life measures are an important endpoint to include in future clinical trials of prion diseases.

Further information regarding recruitment strategies for future clinical trials in prion diseases can be gathered from the United States' quinacrine trial [40]. One of the purported goals of this study was to assess the feasibility of a randomized, double-blind, placebo-controlled treatment trial in prion diseases. Of the initial referrals, a third of cases were excluded because they were not thought to be prion diseases or because of insufficient records. Surprising, only 16% of the initial referrals consented to participate in the study and only 12% were ultimately enrolled. Aside from the usual screening failures common in clinical trials, the second major decrement in the potential sample size of the study occurred at the consent level. One possible reason consent was declined in many of these patients may be related to the PRION-1 study's findings that patients and families have a strong preference whether or not they receive a potential treatment and hence do not want the decision chosen for them *via* randomization. In a comparison between the PRION-1 and U.S. quinacrine studies, 72% of eligible participants were enrolled over a 28 month period in PRION-1 compared to an enrollment of 30% of eligible participants over 46 months in the U.S. study. Although feasible, these statistics suggest that a randomized clinical trial in prion diseases may not be entirely practical as currently envisioned.

The most promising clinical reports in human prion disease have been the pentosan polysulphate (PPS) studies [48,49]. Although these studies are severely hampered by methodological issues, PPS does demonstrate some promise in prolonging survival times, especially in vCJD [48]. Unfortunately, PPS does not cross the blood-brain barrier (BBB) and most be administered directly into the cerebral ventricles. There are multiple problems with this approach such as prion contamination risks to others and risk of neurosurgical complications to the patients. Many patients sustained subdural hematomas and although survival may have been prolonged in some cases, quality of life certainly was not preserved [49]. Less invasive methods of administering compounds that cannot cross the BBB may need to be explored [50,51].

Finally, it is well recognized that genetic factors may influence treatment response in various diseases. An example of this can be found in experimental treatment trials of Alzheimer's disease patients, in which APOE4 carriers frequently experience different treatment effects compared to non-APOE4 carriers [52]. Similar treatment effects have been observed in the German doxycycline study in which *PRNP* codon 129 methionine homozygotes experience a statistically significant different effect from treatment [46]. As is often done in Alzheimer's disease clinical trials with APOE4 carriers, future trials in prion disease may also choose to control for *PRNP* codon 129 genotype to examine potential differences in treatment effects in more detail.

Treatment Targets

Most prion disease treatments have been aimed at preventing the conversion of PrP^{c} to PrP^{Sc} likely because of the large focus on the prion hypothesis in relation to these illnesses. As observed in the case of quinacrine, *in vitro* anti-prion activity does not always translate into treatment effectiveness in humans with prion diseases. With the possible exception of PPS, no prion protein conversion inhibitors have demonstrated a treatment effect in human prion diseases. There are several possibilities for this observation including greater disease severity at the time of treatment in humans and other possible neurotoxic mechanisms involved in prion diseases as described above. Another possibility may be due to the adaptability and natural selection of different PrP^{Sc} strains caused by selected treatments. Although prion diseases do not require nucleic acids, it appears that they nonetheless undergo strain mutations, adaptation, and natural selection depending on the environment. When PrP^{Sc} is subjected to the prion protein conversion inhibitor swainsonine, a swainsonine-resistant substrain becomes the dominant species [53]. Selection of treatment-resistant strains could pose a problem for treatments that just target prion protein conversion. Such a treatment approach may require the simultaneous administration of multiple different prion protein conversion inhibitors to prevent disease adaptability to treatment as is seen with antiretroviral treatment in human immunodeficiency virus (HIV) infection.

A different treatment approach involves clearing PrP^{Sc} from infected cells. Several compounds are known to induce autophagy and clear cells of pathologic proteins. Two such compounds, lithium and rapamycin, have been shown to clear PrP^{Sc} from infected cells *in vitro* [54]. Antibodies specifically targeting PrP^{Sc} could also be used to clear infected cells, however, results have not been satisfactory thus far in animal models [55].

According to the prion hypothesis and work done in *PRNP-/-* knockout mice, PrP^c is necessary for prion infection. Treatments blocking PrP^c remove potential substrate for prion protein conversion as well as possible neurotoxic signaling mechanism employed by PrP^c. Clinical and neuropathological effects of early stage prion disease were successfully reversed following the depletion of neuronal PrP^c [38]. In a mouse model, prion disease onset was delayed following administration of the prion antagonist PrP-Fc_2 *via* lentiviral gene transfer [56]. Survival time was extended, clinical symptoms improved, and neuropathological characteristics of prion disease were also reduced in mice with late stage prion disease that received intracerebral anti-prion PrPQ167R virions injections [57]. Similar results have been described using RNA interference (RNAi) techniques against PrP^c [58]. Instead of blocking PrP^c, an alternate approach is to screen for compounds that decrease PrP^c expression. Such an approach has recently been reported in a "proof of concept" study using a high throughput assay that screened for compounds associated with decreased PrP^c expression [59]. Two promising compounds were discovered (astemizole and tacrolimus) using this approach and will be further studied as potential treatment options. Unfortunately, we do not completely understand the physiological functions of PrP^c in humans and whereas mice devoid of PrP^c are largely phenotypically normal, targeting PrP^c in humans may result in psychiatric, immunological, or other disturbances that we currently cannot predict.

Other treatment targets for prion diseases are not directed towards the prion protein itself, but towards downstream neurotoxic pathways. One study using cell based screening assays examining PrP^{Sc} reduction in infected cells found several anti-prion compounds, none of which showed affinity for PrP [60]. These results suggest that the majority of potential prion disease therapeutics do not actually target the prion protein. Examples of non-prion protein directed therapeutics include targeting pathways associated with neuroinflammation or the unfolded protein response (UPR) [61,62].

An exhaustive review of research into prion disease therapeutics is beyond the scope of this chapter. For further information on investigative prion disease treatments, the reader is referred elsewhere [43,63-66].

BORROWING FROM THE PRION PARADIGM

The prion hypothesis has since expanded beyond the realm of prion disease into other PMDs. The possibility of template directed protein misfolding in Parkinson's disease (PD) and other synucleinopathies occurred following treatment of PD patients with embryonic stem cells (ESC). Upon autopsy, Lewy bodies were discovered within the ESC implants, implying the spread of disease from the host's diseased brain to the transplant tissue [67]. Similar transmissible properties have been described in other PMDs including Alzheimer's disease, frontotemporal lobar degeneration, and Huntington's disease [68]. Template directed protein misfolding has also been observed in the absence of disease in yeast and may even be a mechanism behind non-genetic inheritance patterns of certain types of cancers [69]. Yeast prions are formed by the, "structural conversion of certain cellular proteins to amyloid prions," in relation to environmental stressors resulting in an epigenetic phenomena that may be useful in understanding the increased incidence of neurodegenerative diseases in patients with a history of traumatic brain injury and depression [69].

Therapeutic targets for prion disease are likely relevant to other protein misfolding disorders. As mentioned earlier, if most prion disease therapeutic compounds are unrelated to the prion protein, their mechanism of action may target pathways shared with other neurodegenerative diseases. One example is targeting one of the pathways in the UPR that decreases translation. As all protein misfolding disorders invoke this response, addressing this common pathway across seemingly disparate illnesses may have a much higher yield compared to prion protein conversion inhibitors.

NEUROTOXIC MECHANISMS ACROSS PROTEIN MISFOLDING DISORDERS

In addition to sharing template-directed protein misfolding behavior, many PMDs share similar toxic mechanisms. PMDs likely cause neurotoxicity *via* several different mechanisms as opposed to one neurotoxic pathway. These "down stream" effects of PMDs can also be targeted for treatment. Early work looking at the neurotoxic effects of amyloid deposits has demonstrated oxidative stress as a common neurotoxic pathway, regardless of the amyloid protein constituents [70]. This is likely related to consequences of beta-sheet structures common to all amyloid deposits.

Synaptic dysfunction is an early event seen across PMDs [71]. Inhibition of long term potentiation and enchanced long-term depression in addition to decreased pre- and post-synaptic markers are common in PMDs. Neurotransmitter disruption is often an early sign and has been targeted in the treatment of AD and PD by ameliorating cholinergic deficit with cholinesterase inhibitors and dopamine depletion with levodopa respectively. Most importantly, synaptotoxicity appears to precede neuronal death and may be a "down stream" treatment target that is still capable of curing clinical disease as shown in prion disease models [72].

Another common pathophysiologic occurrence observed across PMDs is calcium homeostasis dysregulation. There are two possible explainations for calcium dysregulation in PMDs that are not mutually exclusive of each other; activation of preexisting ion channels and the formation of calcium-permeable amyloid pores [71]. Excitotoxicity, another common feature of PMDs, may result in overstimulation of N-methyl-D-aspartate (NMDA) receptors that could then cause increased calcium influx. The putative action of the NMDA receptor antagonist memantine, a treatment for moderate to severe Alzheimer's disease, is attenuating this response. Alternatively, PMDs may directly or indirectly initiate the formation of calicium-permeable pores much like a bacterial toxin. Excessive intracellular calcium levels may result in cellular dysfunction through a variety of pathways including changes in gene expression, oxidative damage, and/or apoptosis.

PMDs can also affect the homeostasis of other cellular constituents besides calcium leading to cellular dysfunction and neurotoxicity. The prion protein binds metals such as copper in its normal conformation and altering its structure may prevent this function from occuring properly resulting in biometal homeostasis dysregulation. The disruption of biometal homeostasis and possible consequent increase in oxidative stress has been raised as a possible treatment target for prion disease [73] and metal protein attenuating compounds have been investigated in the treatment of AD as well [74].

The formation of amyloid deposits in PMDs also begs the question of what role protein quality control systems play in these disorders. Chaperones clear soluble misfolded proteins and their dysfunction or an increasing amount of substrate requiring clearance may overload their capabilities resulting in protein aggregate deposition [75]. A dysfunctional proteasome may also underlie PMDs, inhibiting proper protein degradation. Other pathways of protein clearance aside from the proteasome may be targeted across PMDs including inducing autophagy with compounds such as trehalose or lithium [76,77]. Manipulating cellular pathways that occur in response to PMDs, such as the UPR, is another option to maintain protein homeostasis.

Some may argue that treating downstream events in PMDs is not an effective or efficient treatment strategy. Clearly, eliminating toxic protein components that form the core of PMDs is the most intuitive treatment target. However, as demonstrated above, there may be downstream neurotoxic pathways that are shared among PMDs that could result in cure or prevention of clinical disease. The two most promising downstream treatment targets to date are addressing synaptotoxicity and the unfolded protein response. As these pathophysiologic effects are indistinguishable regardless of the causative pathologic protein, researchers can focus on treatments aimed at PMDs in general, as opposed to an individual PMD. Research concentrating on neurotoxic mechanisms shared by all PMDs may actually be the most efficient research strategy in the long term given the potential for developing treatments for multiple diseases compared to one illness across the population.

SUMMARY

Prion diseases are rapidly progressive neurodegenerative illnesses that are invariably fatal. Prion diseases are transmissible illnesses based on an abnormal isoform of the native prion protein. Without the aid of nucleic acids, the abnormal prion protein uses template directed protein misfolding resulting in autocatalytic replication of itself. There is no current treatment for prion diseases and most investigational treatments have been aimed at inhibiting the conversion of PrP^c to PrP^{Sc}. Although several treatments showed promising results *in vitro*, anticipated results did not translate to human trials. Other challenges in conducting clinical trials in human prion disease include overcoming the BBB for some compounds, accurate and early diagnosis of disease, and patient preferences on whether or not to receive treatment complicating the gold standard of randomized, double-blind, placebo-controlled trials. Other outcome measures besides survival time need to be incorporated into prion disease trials. There exist several other avenues for potential treatments of prion diseases. The majority of potential treatment targets are not related to the prion protein and likely share biological pathways with other PMDs suggesting that focusing on common neurodegenerative pathways of protein misfolding disorders in general may be a more efficient avenue for treatment development.

ACKNOWLEDGEMENTS

None declared.

CONFLICT OF INTEREST

The author states that there is no conflict of interest.

REFERENCES

[1] Prusiner SB. Novel proteinaceous infectious particles cause scrapie. Science. 1982; 216(4542): 136-44.

[2] Appleby BS, Appleby KK, Rabins PV. Does the presentation of Creutzfeldt-Jakob disease vary by age or presumed etiology? A meta-analysis of the past 10 years. J Neuropsychiatry Clin Neurosci. 2007; 19(4): 428-35.

[3] Appleby BS, Rincon-Beardsley TD, Appleby KK, Wallin MT. Racial and ethnic differences in individuals with sporadic Creutzfeldt-Jakob disease in the United States of america. PloS One. 2012; 7(6): e38884.

[4] World Health Organization. WHO manual for surveillance of human transmissible spongiform encephalopathies including variant Creutzfeldt-Jakob disease. World Health Organization; 2003.

[5] Zerr I, Kallenberg K, Summers DM, Romero C, Taratuto A, Heinemann U, *et al.* Updated clinical diagnostic criteria for sporadic Creutzfeldt Jakob disease. Brain. 2009; 132(Pt 10): 2659-68.

[6] Hamlin C, Puoti G, Berri S, Sting E, Harris C, Cohen M, *et al.* A comparison of tau and 14-3-3 protein in the diagnosis of Creutzfeldt-Jakob disease. Neurology. 2012 Aug 7; 79(6): 547-52.

[7] Sanchez-Juan P, Green A, Ladogana A, Cuadrado-Corrales N, Saanchez-Valle R, Mitrovaa E, *et al.* CSF tests in the differential diagnosis of Creutzfeldt-Jakob disease. Neurology. 2006 Aug 22; 67(4): 637-43.

[8] Stoeck K, Sanchez-Juan P, Gawinecka J, Green A, Ladogana A, Pocchiari M, *et al.* Cerebrospinal fluid biomarker supported diagnosis of Creutzfeldt-Jakob disease and rapid dementias: a longitudinal multicentre study over 10 years. Brain. 2012 Oct; 135(Pt 10): 3051-61.

[9] Kong Q. Inherited prion diseases. In: Prusiner SB, Ed. Prion Biology and Diseases, 2nd ed. Cold Spring Harbor, New York: Cold Spring Harbor Laboratory Press; 2004. pp. 673-775.

[10] Goldfarb LG, Petersen RB, Tabaton M, Brown P, LeBlanc AC, Montagna P, *et al.* Fatal familial insomnia and familial Creutzfeldt-Jakob disease: disease phenotype determined by a DNA polymorphism. Science. 1992; 258(5083): 806-8.

[11] Lugaresi E, Medori R, Montagna P, Baruzzi A, Cortelli P, Lugaresi A, *et al.* Fatal familial insomnia and dysautonomia with selective degeneration of thalamic nuclei. The New England Journal of Medicine. 1986; 315(16): 997-1003.

[12] Deslys JP, Jaegly A, d'Aignaux JH, Mouthon F, de Villemeur TB, Dormont D. Genotype at codon 129 and susceptibility to Creutzfeldt-Jakob disease. The Lancet. 1998; 351(9111): 1251.

[13] Parchi P, Castellani R, Capellari S, Ghetti B, Young K, Chen SG, *et al.* Molecular basis of phenotypic variability in sporadic Creutzfeldt-Jakob disease. Annals of Neurology. 1996; 39(6): 767-78.

[14] Pocchiari M, Puopolo M, Croes EA, Budka H, Gelpi E, Collins S, *et al.* Predictors of survival in sporadic Creutzfeldt-Jakob disease and other human transmissible spongiform encephalopathies. Brain. 2004; 127(10): 2348-59.

[15] Gajdusek D, Zigas V. Degenerative disease of the central nervous system in New Guinea; the endemic occurrence of kuru in the native population. The New England Journal of Medicine. 1957; 257(20): 974-8.

[16] Gajdusek DC, Zigas von. Kuru; clinical, pathological and epidemiological study of an acute progressive degenerative disease of the central nervous system among natives of the Eastern Highlands of New Guinea. The American Journal of Medicine. 1959; 26(3): 442-69.

[17] Hadlow WJ. Scrapie and kuru. The Lancet. 1959; 274(7097): 289-90.

[18] Gordon W, Pattison I. The experimental production of scrapie in goats. The Veterinary Record. 1957; 69: 1444.

[19] Gajdusek DC, Gibbs CJ, Alpers M. Experimental transmission of a Kuru-like syndrome to chimpanzees. Nature. 1966; 209(5025): 794-6.

[20] Creutzfeldt H. Uber eine eigenartige herdformige Erkrankung des Zentralnervensystems. Vorlaufige Mitteilung. Z Ges Neurol Psychiatr. 1920; 57: 1-18.

[21] Jakob A. Uber eigenartige Erkrankungen des Zentralnervensystems mit bemerkenswerten anatomischen Befunden (spastische Pseudosklerose-Encephalomyelopathie mit disseminierten Degenerationsherden). Z Ges Neurol Psychiatr. 1921; 64: 147-228.

[22] Jakob A. Uber eine der multiplen Sklerose klinisch nahestehende Erkrankung des Zentralnervensystems (spastische Pseudosklerose) mit bemerkenswertem anatomischem Befunde. Mitteilung eines vierten Falles. Med Klin. 1921; 17: 372-6.

[23] Gibbs CJ, Gajdusek DC, Asher DM, Alpers MP, Beck E, Daniel PM, *et al.* Creutzfeldt-Jakob disease (spongiform encephalopathy): transmission to the chimpanzee. Science. 1968; 161(839): 388-9.

[24] Alper T, Haig DA, Clarke MC. The exceptionally small size of the scrapie agent. Biochemical and Biophysical Research Communications. 1966; 22(3): 278-84.

[25] Alper T, Cramp WA, Haig DA, Clarke MC. Does the agent of scrapie replicate without nucleic acid? Nature. 1967; 214(5090): 764-6.

[26] Griffith JS. Nature of the Scrapie Agent: Self-replication and Scrapie. Nature. 1967; 215(5105): 1043-4.

[27] Prusiner SB, Groth DF, Bolton DC, Kent SB, Hood LE. Purification and structural studies of a major scrapie prion protein. Cell. 1984; 38(1): 127-34.

[28] Kim J, Cali I, Surewicz K, Kong Q, Raymond G, Atarashi R, *et al.* Mammalian prions generated from bacterially expressed prion protein in the absence of any mammalian cofactors. Journal of Biological Chemistry. 2010; 285(19): 14083-7.

[29] Deleault NR, Walsh DJ, Piro JR, Wang F, Wang X, Ma J, *et al.* Cofactor molecules maintain infectious conformation and restrict strain properties in purified prions. Proceedings of the National Academy of Sciences. 2012 Jul 10; 109(28): E1938-46.

[30] Linden R, Martins VR, Prado MAM, Cammarota MIN, Izquierdo IAN, Brentani RR. Physiology of the prion protein. Physiological Reviews. 2008; 88(2): 673-728.

[31] Bueler H, Aguzzi A, Sailer A, Greiner RA, Autenried P, Aguet M, *et al.* Mice devoid of PrP are resistant to scrapie. Cell. 1993; 73(7): 1339-47.

[32] Benvegnù S, Gasperini L, Legname G. Aged PrP null mice show defective processing of neuregulins in the peripheral nervous system. Molecular and cellular neurosciences. 2011 May; 47(1): 28-35.

[33] Gadotti VM, Bonfield SP, Zamponi GW. Depressive-like behaviour of mice lacking cellular prion protein. Behav Brain Res. 2012 Feb 14; 227(2): 319-23.

[34] Pathmajeyan MS, Patel SA, Carroll JA, Seib T, Striebel JF, Bridges RJ, *et al.* Increased excitatory amino acid transport into murine prion protein knockout astrocytes cultured *in vitro*. Glia. 2011 Jul 15; 59(11): 1684-94.

[35] McNally KL, Ward AE, Priola SA. Cells Expressing Anchorless Prion Protein Are Resistant to Scrapie Infection. J. Virol. 2009; 83(9): 4469-75.

[36] Chesebro B, Trifilo M, Race R, Meade-White K, Teng C, LaCasse R, *et al.* Anchorless prion protein results in infectious amyloid disease without clinical scrapie. Science. 2005 Jun 3; 308(5727): 1435-9.
[37] Mallucci G, Dickinson A, Linehan J, Klohn P-C, Brandner S, Collinge J. Depleting Neuronal PrP in Prion Infection Prevents Disease and Reverses Spongiosis. Science. 2003; 302(5646): 871-4.
[38] Mallucci GR, White MD, Farmer M, Dickinson A, Khatun H, Powell AD, *et al.* Targeting cellular prion protein reverses early cognitive deficits and neurophysiological dysfunction in prion-infected mice. Neuron. 2007; 53(3): 325-35.
[39] Solomon IH, Schepker JA, Harris DA. Prion Neurotoxicity: Insights from Prion Protein Mutants. In: Tatzelt J, editor. The Prion Protein. U.K.: Savanna Press; 2010. pp. 1-12.
[40] Geschwind M, Kuo A, Raudabaugh B, Haman A, Devereux G, Johnson D, *et al.* P.2.62 A randomized, double-blind, controlled study of the efficacy of quinacrine in the treatment of sporadic CJD. Prion 2009, Thessaloniki-Chalkidiki; 2009.
[41] Haik S, Brandel JP, Salomon D, Sazdovitch von, Delasnerie-Laupretre N, Laplanche JL, *et al.* Compassionate use of quinacrine in Creutzfeldt-Jakob disease fails to show significant effects. Neurology. 2004; 63(12): 2413-5.
[42] Collinge J, Gorham M, Hudson F, Kennedy A, Keogh G, Pal S, *et al.* Safety and efficacy of quinacrine in human prion disease (PRION-1 study): a patient-preference trial. Lancet Neurology. 2009; 8(4): 334-344.
[43] Zerr I. Therapeutic trials in human transmissible spongiform encephalo-pathies: recent advances and problems to address. Infectious Disorders Drug Targets. 2009; 9(1): 92-9.
[44] Forloni G. Doxycycline trials in CJD and FFI. CJD 2011, Washington, DC; 2011.
[45] Brandel JP, Haik S. [Doxycycline *versus* placebo trial in human prion diseases: a therapeutic challenge]. Revue neurologique. 2010; 166(3): 266-8.
[46] Zerr I. Clinical diagnosis of CJD: are there predictors of treatment response? Prion 2009, Chalkidiki, Greece; 2009.
[47] Korth C, May BC, Cohen FE, Prusiner SB. Acridine and phenothiazine derivatives as pharmacotherapeutics for prion disease. Proceedings of the National Academy of Sciences of the United States of America. 2001; 98(17): 9836-41.
[48] Bone I, Belton L, Walker AS, Darbyshire J. Intraventricular pentosan polysulphate in human prion diseases: an observational study in the UK. European Journal of Neurology. 2008; 15(5): 458-64.
[49] Tsuboi Y, Doh-ura K, Yamada T. Continuous intraventricular infusion of pentosan polysulfate: Clinical trial against prion diseases. Neuropathology. 2009; 29(5): 632-6.
[50] Rassu G, Gavini E, Jonassen H, Zambito Y, Fogli S, Breschi MC, *et al.* New chitosan derivatives for the preparation of rokitamycin loaded microspheres designed for ocular or nasal administration. J Pharm Sci. 2009 Dec; 98(12): 4852-65.
[51] Pocchiari M. Pentosan polysulphate: A friendly delivery system for therapy in prion diseases. CJD 2009, Washington, DC; 2009.
[52] Kennelly S, Abdullah L, Kenny RA, Mathura V, Luis CA, Mouzon B, *et al.* Apolipoprotein E genotype-specific short-term cognitive benefits of treatment with the antihypertensive nilvadipine in Alzheimer's patients--an open-label trial. Int J Geriatr Psychiatry. 2012 Apr; 27(4): 415-22.
[53] Li J, Browning S, Mahal SP, Oelschlegel AM, Weissmann C. Darwinian evolution of prions in cell culture. Science. 2010 Feb 12; 327(5967): 869-72.

[54] Heiseke A, Aguib Y, Riemer C, Baier M, Schatzl HM. Lithium induces clearance of protease resistant prion protein in prion-infected cells by induction of autophagy. Journal of Neurochemistry. 2009 Apr; 109(1): 25-34.

[55] Sakaguchi S, Ishibashi D, Matsuda H. Antibody-based immunotherapeutic attempts in experimental animal models of prion diseases. Expert Opinion on Therapeutic Patents. 2009; 19(7): 907-17.

[56] Genoud N, Ott D, Braun N, Prinz M, Schwarz P, Suter U, *et al.* Antiprion prophylaxis by gene transfer of a soluble prion antagonist. The American Journal of Pathology. 2008; 172(5): 1287-96.

[57] Toupet K, Compan V, Crozet C, Mourton-Gilles C, Mestre-Frances N, Ibos F, *et al.* Effective gene therapy in a mouse model of prion diseases. PloS One. 2008; 3(7): e2773.

[58] White MD, Mallucci GR. RNAi for the treatment of prion disease: a window for intervention in neurodegeneration? CNS Neurol Disord Drug Targets. 2009; 8(5): 342-52.

[59] Karapetyan YE, Sferrazza GF, Zhou M, Ottenberg G, Spicer T, Chase P, *et al.* Unique drug screening approach for prion diseases identifies tacrolimus and astemizole as antiprion agents. Proceedings of the National Academy of Sciences. 2013 Apr 23; 110(17): 7044-9.

[60] Poncet-Montange G, St Martin SJ, Bogatova OV, Prusiner SB, Shoichet BK, Ghaemmaghami S. A survey of antiprion compounds reveals the prevalence of non-PrP molecular targets. Journal of Biological Chemistry. 2011 Aug 5; 286(31): 27718-28.

[61] Riemer C, Guitner S, Heise I, Holtkamp N, Baier M. Neuroinflammation in prion diseases: concepts and targets for therapeutic intervention. CNS Neurol Disord Drug Targets. 2009; 8(5): 329-41.

[62] Moreno JA, Radford H, Peretti D, Steinert JR, Verity N, Martin MG, *et al.* Sustained translational repression by eIF2α-P mediates prion neurodegeneration. Nature. 2012 May 24; 485(7399): 507-11.

[63] Trevitt CR, Collinge J. A systematic review of prion therapeutics in experimental models. Brain. 2006; 129(Pt 9): 2241-65.

[64] Stewart L, Rydzewska L, Keogh G, Knight R. Systematic review of therapeutic interventions in human prion disease. Neurology. 2008; 70(15): 1272-81.

[65] Brown P. An historical perspective on efforts to treat transmissible spongiform encephalopathy. CNS Neurol Disord Drug Targets. 2009; 8: 316-22.

[66] Appleby BS, Lyketsos CG. Rapidly progressive dementias and the treatment of human prion diseases. Expert Opin Pharmacother. 2011 Jan; 12(1): 1-12.

[67] Kordower JH, Chu Y, Hauser RA, Freeman TB, Olanow CW. Lewy body-like pathology in long-term embryonic nigral transplants in Parkinson's disease. Nature Medicine. 2008; 14(5): 504-6.

[68] Aguzzi A, Rajendran L. The transcellular spread of cytosolic amyloids, prions, and prionoids. Neuron. 2009; 64(6): 783-90.

[69] Antony H, Wiegmans AP, Wei MQ, Chernoff YO, Khanna KK, Munn AL. Potential roles for prions and protein-only inheritance in cancer. Cancer Metastasis Rev. 2012 Jun; 31(1-2): 1-19.

[70] Schubert D, Behl C, Lesley R, Brack A, Dargusch R, Sagara Y, *et al.* Amyloid peptides are toxic *via* a common oxidative mechanism. Proceedings of the National Academy of Sciences of the United States of America. 1995 Mar 14; 92(6): 1989-93.

[71] Malchiodi-Albedi F, Paradisi S, Matteucci A, Frank C, Diociaiuti M. Amyloid oligomer neurotoxicity, calcium dysregulation, and lipid rafts. Int J Alzheimers Dis. 2011; 2011: 906964.

[72] Moreno JA, Mallucci GR. Dysfunction and recovery of synapses in prion disease: implications for neurodegeneration. Biochemical Society Transactions. 2010 Apr; 38(2): 482-7.

[73] Brown DR. Metal toxicity and therapeutic intervention. Biochemical Society Transactions. University of Bath; 2002; 30(part 4): 742-45.

[74] Sampson E, Jenagaratnam L, McShane R. Metal protein attenuating compounds for the treatment of Alzheimer's disease. Cochrane Database Syst Rev. 2008; (1): CD005380.

[75] Dabbs RA, Wyatt AR, Yerbury JJ, Ecroyd H, Wilson MR. Extracellular Chaperones. Top Curr Chem. 2011; 328: 241-68.

[76] Casarejos MJ, Solano RM, Gómez A, Perucho J, de Yébenes JG, Mena MA. The accumulation of neurotoxic proteins, induced by proteasome inhibition, is reverted by trehalose, an enhancer of autophagy, in human neuroblastoma cells. Neurochem. Int. 2011 Mar; 58(4): 512-20.

[77] Appleby BS. Psychotropic medications and the treatment of human prion diseases. CNS Neurol Disord Drug Targets. 2009 Nov; 8(5): 353-62.

Frontiers in CNS Drug Discovery, 2013, *2*, 26-42

CHAPTER 2

Epigenetic Modifications as Novel Targets for Drug Addiction

Candace R. Lewis* **and Michael F. Olive**

Arizona State University, Tempe, AZ 930 S McAllister Ave., Tempe, AZ 85287, USA

Abstract: Drug addiction is a chronic relapsing disorder characterized by maladaptive patterns of cognition and behavior related to drug use, which are thought to arise from long term changes in the neural circuitries underlying reward, motivation, affect, learning and memory, and executive function. Recently, a large body of evidence has been accumulated showing that epigenetic mechanisms such as DNA methylation and histone modification are involved in drug-induced maladaptive neural plasticity. Epigenetics not only provides a novel avenue for examining the molecular mechanisms underlying interactions between inheritable vulnerabilities and environmental factors that contribute to addiction and relapse, but also provides novel potential pharmacological targets for the treatment of addiction. In this chapter, we begin by introducing relevant epigenetic mechanisms that modulate gene transcription. We then review and summarize the existing literature on epigenetic changes that occur after acute and chronic exposure to or self-administration of alcohol, psychostimulants, opiates, and nicotine, and studies examining the effects of manipulation of epigenetic processes in reward-related brain regions on addiction-like behaviors. We also discuss the possible implications of epigenetic factors as predictors of addiction vulnerability prior to drug exposure. Finally, we will review findings from preclinical studies on the effects of pharmacological modifiers of epigenetic processes on addiction-related behaviors, and discuss the advantages and disadvantages of developing novel epigenetic-based CNS therapeutics for the treatment of addiction.

Keywords: Drug addiction, epigenetics, gene expression, psychostimulants, alcohol, nicotine, opiates.

INTRODUCTION

Decades ago, studies of embryonic development concluded that various cell types with differing phenotypes were all derived from an identical genome contained within the mother cell. Although all cells of an organism contain an identical

***Address correspondence to Candace R. Lewis:** Arizona State University, Tempe, AZ 950 S McAllister Ave., Tempe, AZ 85287, USA; Tel: (480) 965-7598; E-mail: Candace.lewis@asu.edu

Atta-ur-Rahman & M. Iqbal Choudhary (Eds.)

DNA code, they exhibit the ability to differentiate into numerous cellular phenotypes and populations with varying functions. Since DNA is considered to be the blueprint for cellular functioning, a significant unanswered question is - how can cells containing an identical blueprint produce divergent cell types with unique cellular processes, functions, and tissue types? Perhaps a question more relevant for CNS disorders is: environmental factors aside, how is it possible that monozygotic twins that share identical DNA differ widely in their vulnerability to CNS disorders with known genetic components such as schizophrenia, Alzheimer's disease, and drug addiction?

The term *epigenetics* (derived from the Greek word '*epi*', which can be translated to meaning above, upon, over, near, or in addition to) was first termed in 1942 by Conrad Waddington [1]. The most widely accepted definition of epigenetics is the process by which regulation of the genome, such as activation or repression of gene transcription, is modulated by extra-genomic factors. Such factors that alter gene function without changing the underlying nucleotide sequence include chromatin modification or remodeling. Epigenetic regulation not only occurs in developing cells, but also in mature post-mitotic cells such as neurons.

Neurons exhibit changes in gene expression that can be triggered by factors such as nutritional status, psychological and physiological stress, emotional states, early life experiences, education, exposure to environmental toxins, and the topic that will be the focus of this chapter, drugs of abuse. The mechanisms of epigenetic regulation of gene transcription are numerous and complex. They include activation and inhibition of DNA-binding transcription factors and co-factors, alterations in chromatin 3D structure such as chromatin looping, chemical modification of DNA and histones, nucleosome repositioning and excision, and interactions of non-coding RNAs with chromatin.

EPIGENETIC REGULATION OF GENE EXPRESSION

Chromatin is composed of nucleosomes that are made up of 147 base pairs of genomic DNA that is coiled, or wrapped, around a spherical histone octameric protein complex (see Fig. **1**). The octameric protein complex is generally composed of 8 histones, two copies each of H2A, H2B, H3, and H4 [2]. The DNA and histone octamer interact to form a tightly bound unit in which meters of DNA can be compactly organized. When the structure is compact and tightly wound it is referred to as *heterochromatin*. When the structure is in a looser, less compact form it is referred to as *euchromatin*. Due to the compact structure of heterochromatin, transcription factors are prevented from accessing the regulatory regions of genes, and as a result expression of the gene is suppressed or silenced. In contrast, the relaxed structure of euchromatin is easily more accessible to transcription factors to facilitate gene transcription [3].

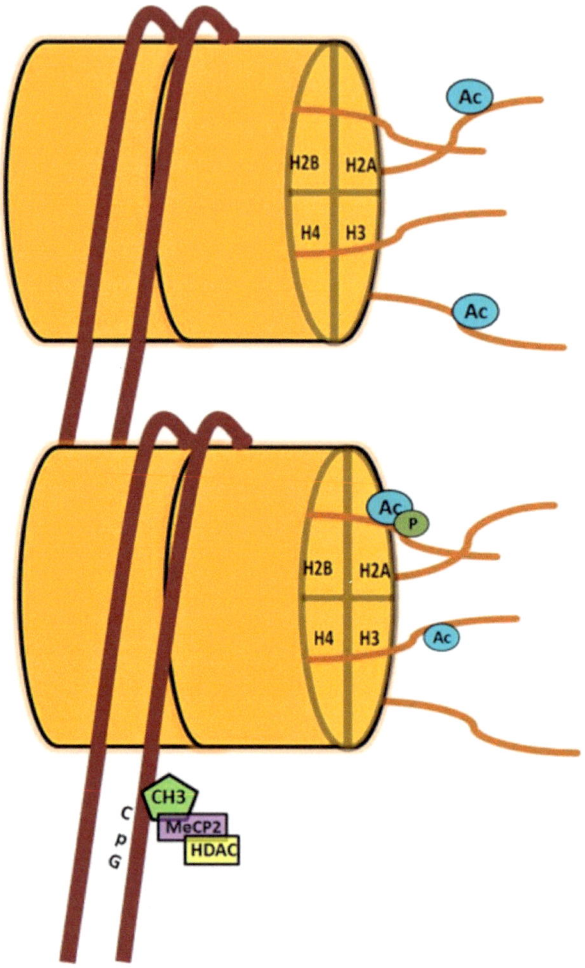

Fig. (1). Schematic of DNA wrapped around two histone octamers demonstrating common epigenetic modifications including histone tail acetylation and phospho-acetylation, DNA methylation at a CpG island, and bound MeCP2 and HDAC.

The core histones possess "unstructured", "undefined", or "loose" amino terminal tails that can range from 16 (H2A) to 44 (H3) amino acids in length [4]. The tails are positioned at the N-terminal position of the histone proteins with the exception of H2A where it is at the C-terminal end [5]. Theses tails serve as the site for multiple posttranslational covalent modifications such as acetylation, phosphorylation, methylation (which also includes di- and tri-methylation), ubiquitination, and several others. Histone tail acetylation is of particular interest as it neutralizes the previously positive charge on specific amino acid residues, such as lysine, in turn reducing the electrostatic attraction of the negatively charged DNA backbone which results in changing chromatin structure from heterochromatin to euchromatin, thus allowing more gene expression (Fig. **1**). Acetylation on specific residues of the H3 tail in particular has been considered a marker for chromatin in an active state. These acetylation and deacetylation processes are mediated *via* histone acetyltransferases (HATs) and histone deacetylases (HDACs), respectively [6]. Additionally, phosphorylation of H3 is associated with the induction of immediate early genes (IEGs) [7] and may play a role in signaling subsequent acetylation of lysine residues [4].

While the general effects of histone acetylation and deacetylation on gene expression are fairly well understood, the effects of histone methylation, which occurs on arginine or lysine residues, are more complex. Histone methylation has been implicated in both gene transcription and repression. As with acetylated histones, methylated histones can exist in three different states: mono, di, or tri-methylated, and methylation processes are regulated *via* histone methyltransferases (HMTs) and histone demethylases (HDMs) [8]. Another major epigenetic mechanism modifying gene expression is the methylation of cytosine nucleotides at the 5′ position of the cytosine ring in cytosine-phosphate-guanine (CpG) dinucleotide sites on a single strand of DNA. In a very general sense, methylation of CpG sites in gene promoter regions leads to decreased gene expression. DNA methylation hinders gene transcription due to the chemical blockade it creates for the binding of transcription factors, as well as 3D modifications in chromatin structure [9]. Additionally, methylated DNA attracts co-repressor complexes (for example, HDACs) that also block transcriptional machinery or decrease histone acetylation. One of these methyl-CpG-binding complexes is methyl CpG binding protein 2 (MeCP2), which has been implicated in drug addiction (see below) [10].

In addition to DNA methylation and histone modifications, there are numerous other epigenetic phenomena that regulate chromatin accessibility and gene expression which have been implicated in various psychiatric disorders including drug addiction [11]. Other epigenetic modifiers include: changes in chromatin looping and other aspects of 3D chromatin structure, ATP-dependent chromatin remodeling complexes that can excise or reposition nucleosomes along a gene sequence, and the binding of non-coding RNAs to regulatory gene sequences. Unfortunately, to date, very little is known about the effects of drug of abuse on these particular epigenetic processes or how they contribute to addiction-related behaviors and associated maladaptive neuroplasticity. The studies that have been conducted thus far have almost exclusively focused on DNA methylation and histone modifications. Therefore, in this chapter, we will primarily focus on reviewing the existing literature on these epigenetic processes in the context of drug addiction.

DRUG-INDUCED EPIGENETIC MODIFICATIONS

The American Psychiatric Association characterizes substance dependence, or drug addiction, as a condition in which an individual has difficulty limiting drug intake, exhibits high motivation to obtain and consume the drug, continues drug use despite negative consequences, and experiences negative emotional and physiological states when the drug is withheld [12]. Drug addiction is a chronic relapsing disorder involving long term adaptations in behavior and central reward pathways. For decades, the popular thought on the mechanisms of addiction has centered on the notion of drugs ‘hijacking’ of the brain’s natural reward system. The reward circuitry mainly consists of dopaminergic outputs from the ventral tegmental area (VTA) in the midbrain to various forebrain regions such as the nucleus accumbens (NAc)/ventral striatum and prefrontal cortex (PFC). Other basal ganglia and limbic structures such as the dorsal striatum (DS), hippocampus (HPC), and amygdala (AMG) are also intricately connected to the mesolimbic dopamine reward pathway [13,14]. From an evolutionary perspective, the reward circuitry developed to encourage life sustaining behaviors such as eating nutrient rich food, pursuing sex for procreation, and obtaining and maintaining social networks. However, it is apparent that drugs of abuse activate this system more strongly than natural rewards. Therefore, after chronic drug use, it is not surprising that the addicted individual may lose the ability to feel adequate reinforcement from natural rewards. Indeed, one of the defining characteristics of drug addiction is the narrowing of the behavioral repertoire towards the procurement and use of drugs of abuse, and away from proper social, occupational, or academic functioning [12].

Although drugs of abuse may have different anatomical sites of action and affect various neurotransmitter and receptor systems, their chronic use leads to specific alterations in gene expression. These changes in gene expression are thought to lead to the changes in behavior, brain structure, and neuronal function that underlie impaired cognition and maladaptive behaviors that are characteristic of addiction. Rodent and human research has established that multiple mechanisms of epigenetic regulation are directly affected by drugs of abuse [15-17]. These epigenetic changes may be the primary process by which drugs induce highly stable changes in the expression of genes in multiple brain regions that mediate the transition for casual intermittent drug use to compulsive habitual drug use in addiction [18,19].

Histone Acetylation

As described previously, histone modification in the form of acetylation is considered to represent activation of gene expression. This is thought to occur *via* two separate mechanisms. First, an acetyl group is attached to a lysine residue of the histone tail, which neutralizes the positive charge and therefore reduces the electrostatic attraction to the negative charge of the DNA phosphate backbone [20,21]. This creates a more relaxed nucleosome structure that allows transcription factors access to the promoter regions of specific genes. Secondly, the acetylated histones serve as a docking site for proteins that attract and recruit transcription factors and co-factors, as well as enzymes such as RNA polymerase that actively participate in gene transcription. Additionally, H3 acetylation in some genes is commonly coupled with the phosphorylation of neighboring serine residues [4,22].

Cocaine and Amphetamines

Acute exposure to cocaine and amphetamine induces the IEGs *c-fos* and *fosB* in the NAc [23]. The increase in these IEGs corresponds with histone H4 acetylation and phosphoacetylation of H3 in *c-fos* and *fosB* promoter regions [7,24]. The time course of the histone modification after cocaine exposure is consistent with induction of these IEGs [7].

Furthermore, repeated or chronic exposure to cocaine and amphetamine attenuates the induction of these IEGs, which is correlated with hypoacetylation of histone H4 in the *c-fos* promoter region [7,25]. Chronic cocaine exposure also induces the expression of cyclin-dependent kinase 5 (*cdk5*) and brain derived neurotrophic factor (*bdnf*) in the NAc, which remains stable for long periods after the last drug exposure [7]. In conjunction with this, histone H3 acetylation in the promoter regions of both *cdk5* and *bdnf* remains stable for up to 7 days after the last exposure to cocaine [7].

Some studies suggest that there is a switch from H4 hyperacetylation to H3 hyperacetylation of IEG promoters following acute *vs* chronic exposure to cocaine [16]. A small number of genes are hypoacetylated on H3 or H4 after chronic cocaine [7]. Both experimenter and self-administered cocaine down-regulate the expression of two histone methyltranferases in the NAc - G9a and GLP, which specifically methylate H3 and lysine residue 9 (H3K9me1 and H3K9me2) [26]. This may be indicative that cocaine regulated gene expression in the NAc is mediated *via* acetylation *in combination with* inhibition of histone methylation [16,27]. Such epigenetic changes from drug exposure may be the driving force behind observed behavioral changes characteristic of the transition from recreational to habitual drug use. For example, co-administration of a D1 receptor agonist and an HDAC inhibitor has been shown to enhance the rewarding effects of cocaine in mice [28].

Histone acetylation and altered expression of certain genes have also been shown to be correlated in the PFC after cocaine exposure. The PFC is an area not only interconnected with the brain reward circuitry, but also thought to mediate numerous cognitive deficits in addiction such as behavioral perseveration, loss of inhibitory control, and executive dysfunction [29]. For example, increased neuropeptide Y (NPY) expression and hyperacetylation of its promoter region in the PFC can last up to 2 weeks post cocaine exposure [30-32]. Cocaine also down-regulates the expression of the early growth response 1 (*egr-1*) gene and hypoacetylation of its promoter region in the PFC.

Ethanol

Exposure to ethanol alters acetylation patterns of multiple genes, such as *npy* and *grin2a/grin2b* (which encode the NR2A and NR2B subunits of the NMDA receptor respectively), both of which are highly implicated in alcohol consumption, intoxication, and withdrawal [33-35]. For example, an increase in acetylation of the promoter region of the *grin2a* promoter region with an accompanying increase in expression of the gene in cortical neurons was found after chronic ethanol treatment and withdrawal in rodents [36]. Pandey *et al.* [36] investigated the effects of acute ethanol withdrawal in rats on HDAC activity and *npy* mRNA levels in the amygdala. They found that 1 hour after acute ethanol injection, HDAC activity was inhibited in the amygdala along with increases in H3 and H4 acetylation. Also, mRNA and protein levels of *npy* were increased in the amygdala. These changes were accompanied by a decrease in anxiety as measured on the elevated plus maze paradigm [37]. The decrease in HDAC activity and increase in acetylation therefore potentially mediates ethanol-induced increases in *npy* expression in the amygdala.

Pandey and colleagues [36] also investigated the effects of chronic ethanol exposure and withdrawal on epigenetic regulation of *npy* expression. They found that H3 and H4 acetylation was decreased, as was mRNA and peptide levels of *npy*. Concurrent treatment with trichostatin A (TSA), an HDAC inhibitor, restored these reductions and TSA-treated rats did not develop ethanol withdrawal-induced anxiety [37]. These data suggests that the epigenetic mechanisms mediating the expression of *npy* may be involved in anxiolytic effects of ethanol and the anxiogenic effects of ethanol withdrawal.

Nicotine

Very few studies to date have been conducted on the effects of nicotine on histone modification processes. Despite this, it has been shown that chronic exposure (7 days) of rats to nicotine increased acetylation of both histones H3 and H4 in the whole striatum and specifically at the *FosB* promoter [38]. Chronic nicotine treatment was also found to reduce striatum HDAC activity [38]. Certainly, much more work needs to be done to elucidate the effects of acute and chronic nicotine on histone modifications, particularly in brain reward-related regions.

DNA Methylation

Cocaine and Amphetamines

MeCP2 is a commonly studied methyl-CpG-binding protein involved in gene transcription regulation. MeCP2 binds to methylated DNA where it then acts as a physical barrier to transcription factors and attracts HDACs. Cocaine self-administration increases MeCP2 mRNA in the anterior cingulate cortex, DS, and NAc [39]. Consistent with this, 10 days of cocaine injections in mice increased MeCP2 levels in the dentate gyrus, frontal cortex, and DS [40]. Im *et al.* [40] showed that a lentiviral knockdown of MeCP2 in the dorsal striatum decreases drug intake under extended access conditions [41]. MeCP2 appears to up-regulate the expression of *bdnf via* homeostatic interactions with microRNA-212 [41].

In contrast, Deng *et al.* [41] demonstrated that a viral knockdown of MeCP2 in the NAc of mice enhanced amphetamine-induced conditioned place preference, and overexpression of MeCP2 in the NAc reduced cocaine place preference [42]. It is interesting that the findings by Im *et al.* demonstrated a positive relationship between MeCP2 levels in the DS with cocaine SA, while Deng *et al.* showed a negative relationship between MeCP2 levels in the NAc and amphetamine reward. These opposite findings may be a result of different psychostimulants administered (cocaine *vs* amphetamine), species tested (rats *vs* mice), and brain region analyzed (DS *vs* NAc).

Deng *et al.* also demonstrated that MeCP2 in the NAc is involved with amphetamine-induced increases in dendritic spine density and increases in the number of GABAergic synapses in this region [42]. Aside from MeCP2, there is also evidence that DNA cytosine-5-methyltransferase 3A (DNMT3A) plays a role in addiction. It has been demonstrated that inhibition of DNA methylation in the NAc potentiates cocaine reward, whereas NAc-specific DNMT3A overexpression attenuates cocaine reward. The same study found that 24 hours after cocaine self-administration, DNMT3A mRNA levels in the NAc were reduced, yet they were increased 4 hours after self-administration [43]. Further studies on the role of DNMT3A in addictive behaviors are clearly warranted.

Ethanol

As mentioned previously, *grin2A* is implicated in alcohol consumption, intoxication, and withdrawal [34]. Both acute and long-term ethanol exposure produce changes in DNA methylation of multiple genes. Chronic ethanol exposure causes demethylation of CpG islands in the NMDA receptor NR2B subunit gene *grin2b* in cortical neurons of mice, with a corresponding increase in NR2B expression [44].

Although DNA methylation is generally associated with silencing of gene transcription, occasionally opposite results have been observed. For example, in a post-mortem study, human alcoholics had higher *prodynorphin* gene expression in the dorsolateral PFC as compared with controls, and elevated methylation of three CpGs in the same gene compared to controls, indicating increased expression when methylated [45]. This group later showed that CpG methylation sites affect the conformational flexibility of prodynorphin fragments, which may alter subsequent DNA-protein or DNA-DNA recognitions and alter gene gene transcription in non-traditional manners [46]. Global DNA hypermethylation in lymphocytes was also increased in alcoholic patients, although DNMT3b expression was reduced compared to controls [47]. Methylation of the *MAOA* gene promoter has been associated with alcohol use in women, but not in men [48]. Multiple other genes have been associated with changes in methylation in studies involving human participants including α-synuclein gene *snca* [49], the vasopressin *avp* gene [50], the nerve growth factor *ngf* gene [51], and the *dlk1* gene [52].

Nicotine

Cigarette smoking has been implicated in DNA methylation of multiple genes in the human genome [53]. Altered methylation of the *MAOA* gene promoter in lymphoblasts is associated with nicotine dependence in women but not in men [48]. Satta *et al.* [53] found that 4 days of nicotine exposure decreased the level of methylation on the GAD67 promoter region in the mouse frontal cortex [54]. Additionally, the same group found that an acetylcholine receptor agonist decreased DNMT1 mRNA and increased GAD67 mRNA levels in the cerebral cortex [55]. These data implicate a role for methylation of components of the GABAergic system in nicotine dependence.

Opiates

As with nicotine, very few studies have examined epigenetic changes in opiate addiction. One study found that methylation in the promoter region of the opioid receptor mu-1 (*OPRM1*) gene was increased in methadone-maintained former heroin addicts [56]. Since OPRM1 is the major target of many abused opiates, these findings suggest that chronic opiate use may alter the expression of this receptor *via* epigenetic mechanisms. On the other hand, it remains to be determined if OPRM1 methylation is a predisposing factor towards the development of opiate addiction.

SUMMARY OF FINDINGS AND THE FUTURE OF EPIGENETICS AS A NOVEL TARGETS FOR THE TREATMENT OF ADDICTION

The ability of drugs of abuse to alter neuronal plasticity and gene expression is one of the major biological mechanisms that contribute to the development of drug addiction and relapse. Many drugs of abuse, including psychostimulants, alcohol, and nicotine, induce the expression of various IEGs that belong to the *fos* family of transcription factors [57]. These transcription factors, in turn, alter the expression of numerous genes and their protein products implicated in addiction such as *npy* and *bdnf*. Drugs of abuse also alter the expression and/or activity of proteins involved in epigenetic processes such as MeCP2 and various histone chemical modifiers, which further alter gene expression.

So how can epigenetic phenomena be targeted pharmacologically so as to combat the maladaptive plasticity and gene expression alterations that are observed in addiction? It turns out that some psychopharmacological agents that have been in clinical use for decades are actually epigenetic modifiers. For example, the mood stabilizer valproic acid, which affects GABAergic transmission as well as voltage-gated sodium and calcium channels, is also an HDAC1 inhibitor [58]. Studies in mice have revealed that valproic acid attenuates the expression of behavioral sensitization to amphetamine [59,60]. Clinical trials of valproic acid in the treatment of cocaine dependence have shown mixed effects [61], although there is a possibility that substance use disorders that are co-morbid with bipolar disorder might benefit from treatment with valproic acid [62]. Future work may investigate the effects of other more selective HDAC inhibitors such as vorinostat and romidepsin that are currently approved for the treatment of lymphoma. Conversely, animals studies have also shown that decreasing histone deacetylase activity, pharmacologically or genetically, can increase cocaine reward [7,24] while overexpressing HDACs or histone acetyltransferases ablation may attenuate cocaine reward [7,63]. Thus, pharmacological manipulation of histone acetylation in either direction for the treatment of addiction begs further investigation.

Additional pharmacological inhibitors of epigenetic phenomenon such as histone or DNA methyltransferases have only recently been developed, primarily as anticancer agents [64,65]. Thus, studies on the effects of such compounds on addictive behaviors in rodents or in human clinical trials are virtually non-existent. However, given the critical role of proteins such as DNMT3A and MeCP2 in addictive behaviors in rodents as summarized in this chapter, behavioral studies on these compounds in established animal models of addiction are clearly needed.

A note of caution should be made, however, over any enthusiasm for rapidly translating the studies reviewed here into the clinic. We are only beginning to unravel the epigenome and its involvement in neuropsychiatric disorders such as drug addiction. As a complex disorder with numerous developmental, environmental, and biological factors, our knowledge of the role of epigenetics in addiction has only begun to be explored. Much more research is needed on the epigenetic phenomena that underlie the pathological brain adaptations that develop with chronic drug use, as well as potential transgenerational effects of drug exposure on the offspring of drug users [66]. In addition, medicinal chemists and geneticists alike are faced with the daunting task of developing epigenetic modifiers that are selective for their targets. For example, thus far, at least 11 HDACs have been identified [38], and subtype specific HDAC inhibition *via* pharmacological mechanisms is only in its infancy, as is our knowledge of the precise genes with which they interact. To target epigenetics as a novel CNS target for the treatment of addiction is an exciting and open field of exploration, one that is likely to continue to unravel for many generations.

ACKNOWLEDGEMENTS

The authors wish to acknowledge the financial support of NIH grants AA013852, DA025606, and DA024355.

CONFLICT OF INTEREST

The authors state that there is no conflict of interest.

REFERENCES

[1] Waddington CH. The epigenotype. Endeavour. 1942;1(1):18-20.
[2] Morales V, Giamarchi C, Chailleux C, Moro F, Marsaud V, Le Ricousse S, *et al.* Chromatin structure and dynamics: functional implications. Biochimie 2001;83(11-12):1029-39.
[3] Tamaru H. Confining euchromatin/heterochromatin territory: jumonji crosses the line. Genes & Development 2010; 24(14):1465-78.
[4] Bode AM, Dong Z. Inducible covalent posttranslational modification of histone H3. Science STKE 2005;281:re4.
[5] Zheng C, Hayes JJ. Structures and interactions of the core histone tail domains. Biopolymers 2003; 68(4):539-46.
[6] Peserico A, Simone C. Physical and functional HAT/HDAC interplay regulates protein acetylation balance. Journal of Biomedicine & Biotechnology 2011; 2011:371832.
[7] Kumar A, Choi K-H, Renthal W, Tsankova NM, Theobald DEH, Truong H-T, *et al.* Chromatin remodeling is a key mechanism underlying cocaine-induced plasticity in striatum. Neuron 2005; 48(2):303-14.
[8] Zhang Y, Reinberg D. Transcription regulation by histone methylation: interplay between different covalent modifications of the core histone tails. Genes & Development 2001; 15(18):2343-60.
[9] Bird A. DNA methylation patterns and epigenetic memory. Genes & Development 2002; 16(1):6-21.
[10] Feng J, Nestler EJ. MeCP2 and drug addiction. Nature Neuroscience 2010; 13(9):1039-42.
[11] Tsankova N, Renthal W, Kumar A, Nestler EJ. Epigenetic regulation in psychiatric disorders. Nature Reviews Neuroscience 2007;8(5):355-67.

[12] American Psychiatric Association. Diagnostic and Statistical Manual of Mental Disorders, Fourth Edition, Text Revision. American Psychiatric Association Publishing 2000, p. 943.
[13] Kelley AE. Memory and addiction: shared neural circuitry and molecular mechanisms. Neuron 2004;44(1):161-79.
[14] Taylor SB, Lewis CR, Olive MF. The neurocircuitry of illicit psychostimulant addiction: acute and chronic effects in humans. Substance Abuse and Rehabilitation. 2013; 2013:29-43.
[15] Wong CCY, Mill J, Fernandes C. Drugs and addiction: an introduction to epigenetics. Addiction 2011; 106(3):480-9.
[16] Maze I, Nestler EJ. The epigenetic landscape of addiction. Annals of the New York Academy of Sciences 2011; 1216:99-113.
[17] Robison AJ, Nestler EJ. Transcriptional and epigenetic mechanisms of addiction. Nature Reviews Neuroscience 2011; 12(11):623-37.
[18] Nielsen DA, Utrankar A, Reyes JA, Simons DD, Kosten TR. Epigenetics of drug abuse: predisposition or response. Pharmacogenomics 2012; 13(10):1149-60.
[19] Schmidt HD, McGinty JF, West AE, Sadri-Vakili G. Epigenetics and psychostimulant addiction. Cold Spring Harbor Perspectives in Medicine 2013; 3(3):a012047.
[20] Hong L, Schrothp GP, Matthew HR, Yaus P, Bradburysliii EM. Studies of the DNA binding properties of histone H4 amino terminus. Thermal denaturation studies reveal that acetylation markedly reduces the binding constant of the H4 "tail" to DNA. Journal of Biological Chemistry 1993; 268(1):305-14.
[21] Struhl K. Histone acetylation and transcriptional regulatory mechanisms. Genes & Development 1998; 12(5):599-606.
[22] Brami-Cherrier K, Roze E, Girault J-A, Betuing S, Caboche J. Role of the ERK/MSK1 signaling pathway in chromatin remodeling and brain responses to drugs of abuse. Journal of Neurochemistry 2009; 108(6):1323-35.
[23] Graybiel AM, Moratalla R, Robertson HA. Amphetamine and cocaine induce drug-specific activation of the c-fos gene in striosome-matrix compartments and limbic subdivisions of the striatum. Proceedings of the National Academy of Sciences of the United States of America 1990; 87(17):6912-6.
[24] Renthal W, Maze I, Krishnan V, Covington HE, Xiao G, Kumar A, *et al.* Histone deacetylase 5 epigenetically controls behavioral adaptations to chronic emotional stimuli. Neuron 2007; 56(3):517-29.
[25] Renthal W, Carle TL, Maze I, Covington HE, Truong H-T, Alibhai I, *et al.* Delta FosB mediates epigenetic desensitization of the c-fos gene after chronic amphetamine exposure. Journal of Neuroscience2008; 28(29):7344-9.
[26] Maze I, Iii HEC, Dietz DM, Laplant Q, Renthal W, Russo SJ, *et al.* Essential role of the histone methyltransferase G9a in cocaine induced plasticity. Science 2010; 327(5962): 213-6.
[27] Renthal W, Kumar A, Xiao G, Wilkinson M, Covington HE, Maze I, *et al.* Genome-wide analysis of chromatin regulation by cocaine reveals a role for sirtuins. Neuron 2009; 62(3):335-48.
[28] Schroeder FA, Penta KL, Matevossian A, Jones SR, Konradi C, Tapper AR, *et al.* Drug-induced activation of dopamine D1 receptor signaling and inhibition of class I/II histone deacetylase induces chromatin remodeling in reward circuitry and modulates cocaine-related behaviors. Neuropsychopharmacology 2008; 33(12):2981-92.

[29] Bibb JA, Chen J, Taylor JR, Svenningsson P, Nishi A, Snyder GL, *et al.* Effects of chronic exposure to cocaine are regulated by the neuronal protein Cdk5. Nature 2001; 410(6826):376-80.

[30] Grimm JW, Lu L, Hayashi T, Hope BT, Su T-P, Shaham Y. Time-dependent increases in brain-derived neurotrophic factor protein levels within the mesolimbic dopamine system after withdrawal from cocaine: implications for incubation of cocaine craving. Journal of Neuroscience 2003;23(3):742-7.

[31] Freeman WM, Patel KM, Brucklacher RM, Lull ME, Erwin M, Morgan D, Roberts DCS, Vrana K. Persistent alterations in mesolimbic gene expression with abstinence from cocaine self-administration. Neuropsychopharmacology 2008; 33(8):1807-17.

[32] Thiele T, Marsh DML, Bernstein IL, Palmiter RD. Ethanol consumption and resistance are inversely related to neuropeptide Y levels. Nature 1998; 396:366-9.

[33] Wang J, Carnicella S, Phamluong K, Jeanblanc J, Ronesi JA, Chaudhri N, *et al.* Ethanol induces long-term facilitation of NR2B-NMDA receptor activity in the dorsal striatum: implications for alcohol drinking behavior. Journal of Neuroscience 2007; 27(13):3593-602.

[34] Thorsell A. Neuropeptide Y (NPY) in alcohol intake and dependence. Peptides 2007; 28(2):480-3.

[35] Qiang M, Denny A, Lieu M, Carreon S, Li J. Histone H3K9 modifications are a local chromatin event involved in ethanol-induced neuroadaptation of the NR2B gene. Epigenetics 2011; 6(9):1095-104.

[36] Pandey SC, Ugale R, Zhang H, Tang L, Prakash A. Brain chromatin remodeling: a novel mechanism of alcoholism. Journal of Neuroscience 2008; 28(14):3729-37.

[37] Levine A, Huang Y, Drisaldi B, Griffin EA Jr, Pollak DD, Xu S, Yin D, Schaffran C, Kandel DB, Kandel ER. Molecular mechanism for a gateway drug: epigenetic changes initiated by nicotine prime gene expression by cocaine. Science Translational Medicine 2011; 3(107):107ra109.

[38] Host L, Dietrich J-B, Carouge D, Aunis D, Zwiller J. Cocaine self-administration alters the expression of chromatin-remodeling proteins; modulation by histone deacetylase inhibition. Journal of Psychopharmacology 2011; 25(2):222-9.

[39] Cassel S, Carouge D, Gensburger C, Anglard P, Burgun C, Dietrich J, *et al.* Fluoxetine and cocaine induce the epigenetic factors MeCP2 and MBD1 in adult rat brain. Molecular Pharmacology 2006; 70(2):487-92.

[40] Im H-I, Hollander JA, Bali P, Kenny PJ. MeCP2 controls BDNF expression and cocaine intake through homeostatic interactions with microRNA-212. Nature Neuroscience 2010; 13(9):1120-7.

[41] Deng J V, Rodriguiz RM, Hutchinson AN, Kim I-H, Wetsel WC, West AE. MeCP2 in the nucleus accumbens contributes to neural and behavioral responses to psychostimulants. Nature Neuroscience 2010;13(9):1128-36.

[42] LaPlant Q, Vialou V, Covington HE, Dumitriu D, Feng J, Warren BL, *et al.* Dnmt3a regulates emotional behavior and spine plasticity in the nucleus accumbens. Nature Neuroscience 2010; 13(9):1137-43.

[43] Marutha Ravindran CR, Ticku MK. Role of CpG islands in the up-regulation of NMDA receptor NR2B gene expression following chronic ethanol treatment of cultured cortical neurons of mice. Neurochemistry International 2005; 46(4):313-27.

[44] Taqi MM, Bazov I, Watanabe H, Sheedy D, Harper C, Alkass K, *et al.* Prodynorphin CpG-SNPs associated with alcohol dependence: elevated methylation in the brain of human alcoholics. Addiction Biology 2011; 16(3):499-509.

[45] Taqi MM, Wärmländer SKTS, Yamskova O, Madani F, Bazov I, Luo J, *et al.* Conformation effects of CpG methylation on single-stranded DNA oligonucleotides: analysis of the opioid peptide dynorphin-coding sequences. PloS One 2012; 7(6):e39605.

[46] Bönsch D, Lenz B, Fiszer R, Frieling H, Kornhuber J, Bleich S. Lowered DNA methyltransferase (DNMT-3b) mRNA expression is associated with genomic DNA hypermethylation in patients with chronic alcoholism. Journal of Neural Transmission 1996; 113(9):1299-304.

[47] Philibert RA, Gunter TD, Beach SRH, Brody GH, Madan A. MAOA methylation is associated with nicotine and alcohol dependence in women. American Journal of Medical Genetics B Neuropsychiatric Genetics 2008;147B(5):565-70.

[48] Bönsch D, Lenz B, Kornhuber J, Bleich S. DNA hypermethylation of the alpha synuclein promoter in patients with alcoholism. Neuroreport 2005; 16(2):167-70.

[49] Hillemacher T, Frieling H, Luber K, Yazici A, Muschler MAN, Lenz B, *et al.* Epigenetic regulation and gene expression of vasopressin and atrial natriuretic peptide in alcohol withdrawal. Psychoneuroendocrinology 2009; 34(4):555-60.

[50] Heberlein A, Muschler M, Frieling H, Behr M, Eberlein C, Wilhelm J, *et al.* Epigenetic down regulation of nerve growth factor during alcohol withdrawal. Addiction Biology 2013; 18(3):508-10.

[51] Ouko LA, Shantikumar K, Knezovich J, Haycock P, Schnugh DJ, Ramsay M. Effect of alcohol consumption on CpG methylation in the differentially methylated regions of H19 and IG-DMR in male gametes: implications for fetal alcohol spectrum disorders. Alcoholism Clinical Experimental Research 2009; 33(9):1615-27.

[52] Wan ES, Qiu W, Baccarelli A, Carey VJ, Bacherman H, Rennard SI, *et al.* Cigarette smoking behaviors and time since quitting are associated with differential DNA methylation across the human genome. Human Molecular Genetics 2012; 21(13):3073-82.

[53] Satta R, Maloku E, Zhubi A, Pibiri F, Hajos M, Costa E, *et al.* Nicotine decreases DNA methyltransferase 1 expression and glutamic acid decarboxylase 67 promoter methylation in GABAergic interneurons. Proceedings of the National Academy of Sciences of the United States of America 2008; 105(42):16356-61.

[54] Maloku E, Kadriu B, Zhubi A, Dong E, Pibiri F, Satta R, *et al.* Selective α4β2 nicotinic acetylcholine receptor agonists target epigenetic mechanisms in cortical GABAergic neurons. Neuropsychopharmacology 2011;36(7):1366-74.

[55] Nielsen DA, Yuferov V, Hamon S, Jackson C, Ho A, Ott J, *et al.* Increased OPRM1 in lymphocytes of methadone-maintained former heroin addicts. Neuropsychopharmacology 2009; 34(4):867-73.

[56] McClung CA, Nestler EJ. Neuroplasticity mediated by altered gene expression. Neuropsychopharmacology 2008; 33(1):3-17.

[57] Rosenberg G. The mechanisms of action of valproate in neuropsychiatric disorders: can we see the forest for the trees? Cellular and Molecular Life Sciences 2007; 64(16):2090-103.

[58] Kalda A, Heidmets L-T, Shen H-Y, Zharkovsky A, Chen J-F. Histone deacetylase inhibitors modulates the induction and expression of amphetamine-induced behavioral sensitization partially through an associated learning of the environment in mice. Behavioural Brain Research 2007; 181(1):76-84.

[59] Reid MS, Casadonte P, Baker S, Sanfilipo M, Braunstein D, Hitzemann R, *et al.* A placebo-controlled screening trial of olanzapine, valproate, and coenzyme Q10/L-carnitine for the treatment of cocaine dependence. Addiction 2005;100 Suppl 1:43-57.
[60] Myrick H, Henderson S, Brady KT, Malcom R, Carolina S. Divalproex loading in the treatment of cocaine dependence. Journal of Psychoactive Drugs 2001; 3:283-7.
[61] Albanese MJ, Clodfelter RC, Khantzian EJ. Divalproex sodium in substance abusers with mood disorder. Journal of Clinical Psychiatry 2000; 61(12):916-21.
[62] Levine AA, Guan Z, Barco A, Xu S, Kandel ER, Schwartz JH. CREB-binding protein controls response to cocaine by acetylating histones at the fosB promoter in the mouse striatum. Proceedings of the National Academy of Sciences of the United States of America 2005; 102(52):19186-91.
[63] Travers J, Blagg J, Workman P. Epigenetics: targeting leukemia on the DOT. Nature Chemical Biology 2011;7(10):663-5.
[64] Popovic R, Licht JD. Emerging epigenetic targets and therapies in cancer medicine. Cancer Discovery 2012; 2(5):405-13.
[65] Vassoler FM, White SL, Schmidt HD, Sadri-Vakili G, Pierce RC. Epigenetic inheritance of a cocaine resistant phenotype. Nature Neuroscience 2013; 16(1):42-7.
[66] Renthal W, Nestler EJ. Histone acetylation in drug addiction. Seminars in Cell & Developmental Biology 2009; 20(4):387-94.

CHAPTER 3

Manipulation of Endogenous Neural Stem Cells as a Therapeutic Strategy for Neurodegenerative Diseases: Insights from Animal Models

Anna Patten[1,2], Patricia S. Brocardo[1,3] and Joana M. Gil-Mohapel[*,1]

[1]Division of Medical Sciences, Island Medical Program, University of Victoria, Victoria, British Columbia, Canada; [2]Department of Biology and Graduate Program in Neuroscience, University of Victoria, Victoria, British Columbia, Canada; [3]Neuroscience Program, Federal University of Santa Catarina, Florianópolis, Santa Catarina, Brazil

Abstract: The mammalian brain retains the capacity to generate new neurons throughout adulthood through a process referred to as adult neurogenesis. This capacity is restricted to well-defined brain regions, namely the sub-ventricular zone (SVZ) adjacent to the lateral ventricles, and the sub-granular zone (SGZ) of the hippocampal dentate gyrus (DG). Adult neurogenesis and each one of its phases are tightly regulated and can be influenced by multiple behavioral, physiological, and pathological factors. Indeed, mounting evidence from animal models has indicated that neurodegenerative conditions such as Alzheimer's disease (AD), Parkinson's disease (PD), and Huntington's disease (HD) may be associated with altered neurogenic function. Importantly, alterations in adult hippocampal neurogenesis may be responsible, at least in part, for some of the cognitive deficits observed in animal models of these neurodegenerative conditions as well as individuals afflicted with these disorders. On the other hand, since adult neural progenitors have been proposed as an endogenous source of healthy neurons, it has been suggested that harnessing the endogenous neurogenic capacity in the diseased brain might be of therapeutic value for these neurodegenerative conditions. In this chapter we review the results obtained in rodent models of AD, PD, and HD with regards to therapies aimed at restoring adult neurogenesis and discuss whether such therapies might have therapeutic relevance for the treatment of these devastating neurodegenerative disorders.

Keywords: Adult neurogenesis; Alzheimer's disease, environmental enrichment, Huntington's disease, Parkinson's disease, pharmacological strategy, physical exercise, therapy.

***Address correspondence to Joana M. Gil-Mohapel:** Division of Medical Sciences, Island Medical Program, University of Victoria, Victoria, B.C., V8W 2Y2, Canada; Tel: +1.250-721-6586; Fax: +1.250-472-5505; E-mail: jgil@uvic.ca

Atta-ur-Rahman & M. Iqbal Choudhary (Eds.)

INTRODUCTION

Adult Neurogenesis

It is now well established that the mammalian brain retains the capacity to generate new neurons into adulthood. However, this neurogenic capacity appears to be restricted to a few limited brain regions, the subventricular zone (SVZ) adjacent to the lateral ventricles and the subgranular zone (SGZ) in the hippocampal dentate gyrus (DG) [1-4].

Neural stem cells located in the SVZ give rise to committed progenitor cells. These migrate through the rostral migratory stream (RMS) into the olfactory bulb (OB) where they differentiate into granule and periglomerular neurons (for review see [5]). On the other hand, immature neurons originated in the SGZ of the hippocampal DG migrate from the SGZ to the granule cell layer, where they integrate into the existing circuitry (for review see [5]). Each progenitor cell divides into daughter cells that differentiate into granule neurons. These project dendrites to the DG molecular layer and axons to the *cornu ammonis* (CA) 3 region of the hippocampus [6]. This maturation process takes about four weeks. Approximately 9000 new cells are generated each day in the rodent hippocampus (hundreds of thousands of cells each month; *i.e.* 6% of the total granule cell population), and the vast majority (*i.e.*, 80-90%) of these new cells differentiate into neurons [7].

Adult neurogenesis is a tightly regulated process that can be up- or down-regulated by many different factors. Thus, multiple genetic, behavioural, physiological, and pathological conditions can modulate the proliferation, differentiation, and ultimately the survival of new neurons in the adult brain. For example, stress [8], glucocorticoids [9], inflammation [10], and aging [11-13] can down-regulate adult neurogenesis. On the other hand, estrogen [14,15], antidepressant agents [16-18], growth factors such as brain-derived neurotrophic factor (BDNF) [19] and insulin growth factor 1 (IGF-1) [20], learning [21], physical exercise [22,23], and environmental enrichment [24] are known to up-regulate the neurogenic capacity in the adult mammalian brain.

Adult Hippocampal Neurogenesis and Cognition

The hippocampus is critical for certain aspects of cognition such as spatial learning and memory and it is now believed that newly generated neurons play a role in these hippocampal-mediated behaviors. In agreement with this hypothesis, numerous correlative studies have shown that hippocampal neurogenesis can be modulated by learning and behavioural experience, and that loss of hippocampal neurogenic function can have consequences on memory formation (for review see [25-27]). Indeed, several studies have shown that behavioral tasks that require the involvement of the hippocampus can enhance the survival of newborn neurons in the DG of adult rats, whereas learning tasks that do not involve the hippocampus have no effect on neurogenesis [21,28,29]. Similarly, disrupting or ablating adult hippocampal neurogenesis has been shown to impair hippocampal-dependent learning and memory without affecting hippocampal-independent behaviors [30-33]. Furthermore, it was recently shown that new neurons are indeed recruited into neuronal circuits involved in spatial learning and memory in the hippocampus [34]. Thus, it is currently believed that hippocampal new neurons are required for the separation of events based on their spatial and temporal characteristics (a process that preserves the uniqueness of a memory representation), as well as space representation, long-term memory retention, and flexible inferential memory expression (for review see [27]).

Neurodegenerative Diseases

Neurodegenerative diseases constitute a heterogeneous group of disorders of the nervous system that share the common characteristic of progressive structural and functional loss of specific populations of neurons and/or glial cells in the central nervous system (CNS) [35]. These include cortical and hippocampal cholinergic neurons in the case of Alzheimer's disease (AD) [36], nigral dopamine (DA)-producing neurons in the case of Parkinson's disease (PD) [37], and striatal medium-sized gamma-aminobutyric acid (GABA)ergic spiny neurons in the case of Huntington's Disease (HD) (for review see [38]). Clinically, neurodegenerative diseases are characterized by an insidious adult onset and chronic progression. Their incidence, particularly in the case of AD and PD, is continuously increasing due to the overall aging of the population.

There are many similarities between different neurodegenerative disorders such as atypical protein assemblies and oligomerization, as well as cell death of specific neuronal populations. Moreover, during the late phases of neurodegeneration, protein aggregation and neuronal cell death are no longer restricted to specific brain regions (for review see [39]). Interestingly, all these neurodegenerative diseases are characterized by a more or less severe loss of certain cognitive functions such as learning and memory. This cognitive impairment progresses over the course of the disease, often resulting in dementia [40,41]. Given that adult hippocampal neurogenesis is thought to play a role in learning and memory (Section 1.2), it is reasonable to speculate that a reduction in this endogenous neurogenic capacity might underlie, at least in part, the cognitive abnormalities seem in animal models of these disorders as well as patients afflicted with these neurodegenerative diseases. Additionally, the generation of new neurons in the adult brain (both in the DG of the hippocampus and in the SVZ) makes the manipulation of the endogenous neuronal restorative capacity a possible therapeutic avenue for the treatment of these neurodegenerative diseases (for review see [42,43]).

ALZHEIMER'S DISEASE

Altered Adult Neurogenesis in AD

AD is an age-related, progressive and irreversible neurodegenerative disease, being the most common cause of dementia. The most affected brain regions are the neocortex and the hippocampus. At the neuropathological level the disease is characterized by the formation of senile plaques [extracellular deposits of amyloid-β (Aβ) peptide, which derives from the proteolysis of the amyloid precursor protein (APP) by β- and γ-secretases] and neurofibrillary tangles (intraneuronal aggregations of hyperphosphorylated microtubule-associated protein tau) (for review see [44]). Most cases of AD are sporadic but there are also a few cases of familial AD that are inherited in an autosomal dominant manner. These cases are associated with mutations in the genes that codify the proteins APP, presenilin 1 (PS1) and presenilin 2 (PS2). On the other hand, polymorphisms in the apolipoprotein E (APOE) gene, particularly in its ε*4* allele, were shown to increase the risk of sporadic AD (for review see [45]).

Although the cases of AD that are associated with genetic mutations are rare, various AD transgenic mouse models have been generated (for review see [46]). Adult hippocampal neurogenesis has been investigated in several of these models and contradictory results have been obtained (reviewed by us elsewhere; [47,48]). Briefly, while a decrease in neurogenic function has been reported in transgenic or knock-in mice carrying the Swedish mutation in the APP gene [49-52] the PDAPP mutation [53], mutations in the PS1 gene [51,52,54-56], as well as in double-transgenic mice for APP and PS1 [51,52] and in triple-transgenic mice for APP, PS1, and tau protein [57], others have found increased hippocampal neurogenesis in transgenic mice that express APP with the Swedish and the Indiana mutations [58,59], or with the Swedish, Dutch, and London mutations [60]. Differences among the various transgenic mouse models used, the stage of disease progression when neurogenesis was evaluated, and differences in the protocols used to evaluate neurogenesis are factors that might have contributed to the discrepancies reported in the literature (for a more detailed discussion see [47]).

In human AD patients, the expression of several immature neuronal markers [doublecortin (DCX), polysialylated nerve cell adhesion molecule (PSA-NCAM), neurogenic differentiation factor (NeuroD), and βIII-tubulin] appears to be increased [61], while the expression of the mature neuronal marker microtubule-associated protein (MAP) was found to be dramatically decreased [62] in the DG of the hippocampus. These results suggest that, regardless of an increase in proliferation, the later stages of differentiation and maturation of the neurogenic process might be compromised in the human AD brain.

Harnessing Endogenous Neurogenesis as a Therapeutic Strategy for AD

It is still uncertain whether regions of the brain that have been damaged by AD can incorporate newly generated neurons into existing circuits. However, the use of endogenous neural precursor cells (NPCs) holds promise for future therapies.

Studies in animals have shown that endogenous cell proliferation and neurogenesis can be increased in the aged hippocampus using manipulations such as exercise or exposure to environmental enrichment [22-24,63-66], suggesting that a neurogenic niche is retained in this brain region despite aging and/or disease. In the next sections we will focus on three of the main therapeutic strategies that have been utilized in AD rodent models to stimulate adult neurogenesis: physical exercise, environmental enrichment, and the use of pharmacological agents. For a wider overview of therapeutic strategies that have been used to increase the neurogenic capacity of the AD brain, including the use of exogenous stem cells, please see the excellent reviews [67-71].

Physical Exercise

Exercise is a known inducer of hippocampal proliferation and neurogenesis and can benefit both the normal and the aging brain [22,23,63,72]. In a study utilizing the APP23 mouse model of AD, mice were allowed access to a running wheel for 10 days at the ages of 6 and 18 months. In the 6 month-old cohort, proliferation was decreased as compared to control animals and no effect of running was observed. However, at the 18 month time point, a running-induced increase in proliferation was detected and no differences were observed between wild-type and APP23 runners [73]. A similar increase in neuronal differentiation (as assessed with the immature neuronal markers calretinin and DCX) was also detected with voluntary wheel running [73], indicating that the AD brain still retains the ability to up-regulate cell proliferation and neuronal differentiation in response to physical exercise.

In a different study, APP23 transgenic mice were given access to a running wheel for 11 months starting at 10 weeks of age. The exogenous mitotic marker bromodeoxyuridine (BrdU) was injected for five consecutive days four weeks before sacrifice at 17 months of age. However, this study failed to detect an increase in BrdU incorporation or DCX and calretinin expression in the running group [74]. It is possible that by the time of analysis the disease progression was already too advanced to allow for detection of any changes in endogenous neurogenesis and further neuropathological analyses are thus warranted. Alternatively, these findings might also be a consequence of the well known age-induced decrease in adult hippocampal neurogenesis [11,13]. However, previous studies have shown that voluntary physical exercise can still increase hippocampal neurogenesis in wild-type aged mice [75].

Environmental Enrichment

Environmental enrichment is a known stimulator of adult hippocampal neurogenesis in both the normal and aging brain [24,64]. In the laboratory setting, an enriched environment includes multiple sources of external stimulation that allow for increased social interaction, enhanced learning and exploration, and offer opportunities to exercise. In the AD brain however, the effect of enrichment on neurogenesis is not yet fully elucidated.

In a PS1 mouse model of AD, basal levels of neurogenesis were not altered at 2 months of age. However, exposure to an enriched environment for one month had no effect on the neurogenic capacity of these mice [76]. Similar findings were also observed in PS1 knock-out animals at 9 months of age [77]. A possible explanation for the lack of effect of environmental enrichment on hippocampal neurogenesis in these AD mouse models could be related with an increase in microglia in the vicinity of the neurogenic niche, which in turn can release soluble factors that may interfere with the neurogenic process [76].

However, in a double mutation model of AD (APP_{Swe}/PS1ΔE9) one month of environmental enrichment was able to rescue the deficits in neurogenesis that were detected at 2-3 months of age [78]. Interestingly, the increase in neurogenesis was also accompanied by a reduction in the levels of hyperphosphorylated tau and oligomeric Aβ [78], indicating that this regime of environmental enrichment may also impact the neuropathological changes associated with the progression of the disease. In agreement with this study, environmental enrichment was also shown to increase cell proliferation and neurogenesis in the APP23 transgenic mouse model both at 6 and 18 months of age [73].

Pharmacological Agents

Numerous different pharmacological agents have been examined in rodent models for their benefits in treating neurodegeneration associated with AD. This section will highlight some of the most common pharmacological therapies used to enhance the endogenous neurogenic capacity in animal models of AD, including trophic factors, antidepressants, hormones, and steroids.

Trophic Factors and Peptides. It is well established that several neurotrophins and growth factors possess neuroprotective and neurogenic functions. As such, several studies have tested whether trophic factors have the potential to promote cell proliferation and the migration of new neurons into affected brain regions in rodent models of neurodegenerative diseases including AD (for review see [43]). Peptide 6 is an 11-mer that forms the active region of the neurotrophic factor ciliary neurotrophic factor (CNTF). This peptide has been tested for its potential neurogenic properties in the 3xTg-AD mouse model [79]. When peripherally administered to 6-7 month-old 3xTg-AD mice during a 6-week period, this peptide was able to enhance cell proliferation and neurogenesis to wild-type levels. Additionally, treatment with peptide 6 was able to increase hippocampal neuronal plasticity and improve cognitive function without significant side effects [79]. Given these promising results, additional research is currently being conducted in order to test the potential beneficial effects of this peptide in human AD patients.

Cerebrolysin is a nootropic agent formed by a mixture of peptides and amino acids derived from porcine brain and it has been shown to have neurogenic properties in the APP751 mouse model of AD [80]. At 3 months of age these animals already present Aβ plaques, a phenomenon that is accompanied by a significant reduction in cell proliferation and neurogenesis. However, cerebrolysin treatment (for either 1 or 3 months) was able to reverse these deficits in neurogenesis [80]. Interestingly, while cerebrolysin treatment did not alter the ratio of newly generated cells that differentiated into neurons and glial cells [as assessed by the proportion of BrdU-positive cells that express either the mature neuronal marker neuronal nuclei (NeuN) or the glial marker glial fibrillary acid protein (GFAP)], it reduced the number of apoptotic cells, indicating that cerebrolysin promotes the survival of newly generated cells [80]. Importantly, earlier studies had already shown that cerebrolysin can improve memory in cognitively impaired patients [81] and enhance neurotrophic activity *in vitro* [82], making it a promising therapeutic candidate for clinical trials with AD patients.

Antidepressants. A reduction in adult hippocampal neurogenesis has been correlated with the occurrence of depressive-like symptoms in rodents [8] (reviewed in [83]), while antidepressants have been shown to possess neurogenic properties [16-18]. As such, the tricyclic antidepressant amitriptyline has been examined for its ability to promote neurogenesis in the 3xTgAD mouse model of AD [84]. Amitriptyline was administered through the drinking water over a period of four months starting at 14 months of age and BrdU was injected after two months of treatment during nine consecutive days. Immunohistochemistry analysis revealed a significant increase in BrdU-labelled cells in amitriptyline-treated mice as compared with vehicle-treated controls, whereas co-labelling with the mature neuronal marker NeuN indicated that these newly generated cells adopted a neuronal phenotype [84]. Importantly, this enrichment-induced increase in adult hippocampal neurogenesis was accompanied by an increase in BDNF levels as well as short- and long-term memory retention [84].

Hormones. Leptin is an adipose derived hormone that can promote hippocampal neurogenesis in healthy individuals [85]. A recent study examined whether leptin could also be beneficial in promoting neurogenesis in AD using an APP/PS1 mouse model [86]. Using a lentiviral vector, leptin was administered intracerebroventricularly for a period of three months. Following treatment, a significant increase in the number of BrdU-positive cells and neuronal precursors was observed in the DG of leptin-treated APP/PS1 mice [86]. These results indicate that leptin may be a suitable agent to up-regulate neurogenesis in the AD brain and further behavioural and neurochemical analyses are needed in order to determine the functional relevance of this increase.

Steroids. Allopregnanolone is a metabolite of progesterone that is synthesised in both the embryonic and adult CNS, and can be found in pluripotent progenitor cells [87,88]. Allopregnanolone levels are known to decline with aging and AD [89,90]. The 3xTg mouse model of AD has been used to study the effects of treatment with this neurosteroid on neurogenesis [91,92]. Three-month old 3xTg AD mice exhibit reduced hippocampal cell proliferation as well as learning and memory deficits despite a lack of noticeable plaque formation. Remarkably, a single subcutaneous injection of allopregnanolone was enough to reverse these deficits [92]. A subsequent study by the same group examined the effect of allopregnanolone treatment at later time points (6, 9 and 12 months) in this AD transgenic mouse model. While at 6 months of age Aβ accumulation is apparent but plaques are not yet formed, at 9 months of age intraneuronal Aβ is abundant and plaques can already be detected. By 12 months of age plaques are widespread and Aβ accumulation is maximal [91]. Allopregnanolone administration was able to reverse the deficits in neurogenesis and learning and memory in 6- and 9-month old 3xTg mice, but failed to show beneficial effects in 12-month old mice [91], indicating that at this late stage the disease processes may already be too advanced to be rescued by allopregnanolone treatment.

Conclusions

To conclude, the potential beneficial effects of environmental enrichment, physical activity, and pharmacological interventions on the endogenous neurogenic capacity as well as on the neuropathology and cognition of AD transgenic mouse models appear to be highly dependent on the type of genetic mutation these models carry. Furthermore, factors such as the timing of the intervention with regards to the stage of disease progression, as well as differences in the protocols of environmental stimulation and treatment paradigms might account for the confounding results that have been reported in the literature. Nevertheless, the studies reviewed here highlight the potential for these strategies to treat AD-related symptoms and future preclinical studies and clinical trials are warranted in order to determine the exact situations and time windows during which such therapies are likely to have the highest beneficial impact.

PARKINSON'S DISEASE

Altered Adult Neurogenesis in PD

PD is caused by the degeneration of DA-producing neurons that project from the substantia nigra (SN) pars compacta to the striatum of the basal ganglia. The progressive loss of DAergic input causes a severe motor dysfunction characterized by akinesia, rigidity and tremor. PD is also associated with non-motor symptoms such as hyposmia, anhedonia, lack of novelty seeking behavior, depression, and anxiety that are not directly associated with neurodegenerative processes in the SN. This vast spectrum of non-motor symptoms may partly rely on proper olfactorial processing and hippocampal function (for review see [93]). Therefore, it is conceivable that some non-motor deficits in PD are related to defective adult neurogenesis.

Various genetic defects associated with cases of familial PD have been identified (*e.g.*, α-synuclein, parkin-1), but environmental factors, including physical trauma, toxic insults and infections, have long been thought to play a more prominent role in the etiology of PD (for review see [94]). Although there are some PD transgenic mouse models available (for review see [95]), the animal models that have been most widely used in PD research are the unilateral 6-hydroxydopamine (6-OHDA) lesion rat model and the bilateral 1-methyl-4-phenyl-1,2,3,6-tetrahydropyridine (MPTP) lesion mouse model, which develop PD-like symptoms (for review see [96]).

Experimental depletion of dopamine in rodents (as a model of PD) decreases precursor cell proliferation in both the SGZ of the DG and the SVZ, whereas a selective agonist of D2-like DA receptors is enough to completely restore proliferation [97], supporting the idea that the DAergic depletion observed in PD brains might result in impaired neurogenesis. Moreover, the number of epidermal growth factor receptor (EGFR)-positive cells is decreased in the adult SVZ in human PD, which may reflect a reduction in SVZ/OB neurogenesis [98]. Decreased epidermal growth factor (EGF) levels have also been observed both in the striatum and the prefrontal cortex of PD patients, and this may be related to DAergic nigral deafferentation [99].

Several *in vivo* studies have also evaluated how hippocampal neurogenesis is altered by the expression of α-synuclein. Transgenic mice over-expressing human wild-type α-synuclein showed significantly fewer neurons both in the OB as well as in the DG of the hippocampus as compared to their control littermates, an effect that seems to result from a decrease in neuronal precursor survival [100], whereas transgenic mice expressing mutant α-synuclein were shown to have impaired hippocampal neurogenesis due to a decrease in proliferation and survival of neural precursor cells [101]. In a different study, Nuber and collaborators (2008) [102] also showed reduced hippocampal neurogenesis and cognitive deficits in a conditional α-synuclein mouse model. Turning off the transgene expression did halt the progression of these symptoms, although no regression was observed [102].

Collectively, these results from rodent PD models suggest that α-synuclein can affect survival and proliferation of precursor cells in the SGZ of the DG and that adult neurogenesis may be compromised with PD. For a more in depth overview of the evidence suggesting a dysregulation of the neurogenic capacity in the PD brain, please refer to our recent reviews published elsewhere [47,48].

Harnessing Endogenous Neurogenesis as a Therapeutic Strategy for PD

Some *in vivo* studies have shown that the SN contains a small population of resident neural stem cells and that DAergic neurons continue being generated at a low rate throughout adulthood in the SN pars reticulata, adjacent to the site of degeneration in PD (*i.e.*, the SN pars compacta) [103-105]. These findings raised the attractive possibility of recruiting endogenous stem cells from the SN pars reticulata to the SN pars compacta in order to replace the DAergic neurons that are lost in PD. However, others have failed to replicate these results and found no evidence of adult nigral neurogenesis [106] and no consensus has yet been reached with regards to the endogenous neurogenic capacity of the SN. Nevertheless, studies have shown that exogenous factors can stimulate DAergic neurogenesis in animal models of PD [107,108] and the enhancement of progenitor cell proliferation may represent a potential new source of cells for replacement therapy in PD.

The following sections will discuss the various treatments that have been tested in order to enhance endogenous neurogenesis in PD models.

Physical Exercise

Various studies have shown that physical exercise can be beneficial in ameliorating some of the neuropathological and behavioural deficits characteristic of various PD rodent models [109-112]. However, to date only a single study has evaluated how physical exercise modulates the endogenous neurogenic capacity in PD by submitting 6-OHDA-lesioned rats to a regime of treadmill exercise (30 min/day, 5 days/week for 4 weeks) [113]. Forced exercise resulted in the upregulation of the trophic factors BDNF and glial cell-derived neurotrophic factor (GDNF) in the striatum as well as an increase in cell proliferation and the migration of neural stem cells towards the lesion site. Additionally, exercise promoted the preservation of tyrosine hydroxylase (TH; the rate-limiting enzyme during the synthesis of DA) positive fibres in the striatum and TH-positive neurons in the SN [113]. These results suggest that exercise can be a promising non-invasive therapeutic intervention to minimize neuronal degeneration in the PD brain.

Environmental Enrichment

Similar to exercise, exposure to an enriched environment was also shown to promote the differentiation of endogenous neural stem cells into neurons in the SN of 6-OHDA-lesioned rats [107]. Moreover, a combination of both physical exercise and exposure to enriched conditions resulted in increased cell proliferation in this PD model. Furthermore, these non-invasive strategies also led to the alleviation of Parkinsonian-like symptoms (*e.g.*, rotational behaviour) in 6-OHDA-lesioned rats [107].

Pharmacological Agents

Neurotrophic Factors. NPCs respond to several neurotrophic factors that affect cell proliferation, migration and maturation. In the case of PD, GDNF is the most potent neurotrophic factor that can be used to promote the generation and differentiation of DAergic neurons [114-116]. In agreement, various studies have shown that continuous infusion of GDNF is able to confer an almost complete protection against the loss of DAergic neurons in the 6-OHDA rat model of PD [117-120]. Moreover, other growth factors have also shown to be effective in promoting endogenous neurogenesis in PD rodent models. For example, fibroblast growth factor 2 (FGF2) was able to increase neurogenesis in the striatum and SN in the acute MPTP model of PD [121].

Despite these promising results, a subsequent study found no evidence for the generation of new DAergic neurons (BrdU/TH-positive) after chronic infusion of GDNF into the striatum of adult rats. However, the number of TH-positive neurons present in the SN increased by 32%, suggesting that GDNF stimulated pre-existing neurons to assume a DAergic phenotype [122]. Additionally, no TH/BrdU-positive double-labelled new neurons were observed in either the lesioned or the unleasioned SN of 6-OHDA-treated rats following four weeks of intra-striatal infusion of a different trophic factor, transforming-growth factor-α (TGFα) [123]. Intraventricular infusion of either BDNF or platelet-derived neurotrophic factor (PDGF) for 10 days also failed to generate BrdU/TH-positive new neurons in the SN of adult 6-OHDA-lesioned rats and their respective non-lesioned controls [106,124]. Similar results were also obtained with the intrastriatal infusion of liver growth factor (LGF) [125].

The promising results obtained with GDNF with regards to restoring the DAergic neuronal population in experimental models of PD resulted in the implementation of clinical trials with this particular trophic factor in PD patients. An initial clinical trial reported the occurrence of some side effects including altered somatosensory perception following monthly intraventricular injections of GDNF [126]. However, when this trophic factor was directly injected into the putamen of PD patients, a reduction of motor deficits was observed, an effect that was accompanied by the partial restoration of the nigrostriatal pathway [127,128]. However, in 2006 the first double-blind placebo-controlled study showed that direct infusion of GDNF did not cause a significant improvement of the motor symptoms in GDNF-treated PD patients [129]. Therefore, it is still unclear whether the use of trophic factors such as GDNF can be beneficial in the clinical setting and future clinical trials using different neurotrophin cocktails are warranted to further elucidate this issue.

Dopamine Agonists. Stimulation of the dopaminergic system has been shown to impact neurogenic function in the adult brain. Indeed, various studies have demonstrated that activation of the DA D3 receptor can induce cell proliferation both in the SVZ [130] and the SN [108] of adult rats. In agreement, treatment of 6-OHDA-lesioned rats with a DA D3 receptor agonist was shown to induce cell proliferation and DAergic neuronal differentiation in the SN of this PD rat model [131]. In a different study, oral administration of the DA receptor agonist pramipexole (PPX) was shown to selectively enhance adult neurogenesis (*i.e.*, cell proliferation and neuronal survival) in the SVZ/OB of adult rats. Additionally, *in vitro* experiments demonstrated that both D2 and D3 DA receptors are present in adult rat SVZ-derived neural progenitors and treatment with PPX specifically increased the mRNA levels of EGFR and the paired box gene 6 (Pax6) in these neural progenitors [132]. Furthermore, the D2-like agonists ropinirole and 7-hydroxy-N,N-di-n-propyl-2-amino-tetralin (7-OH-DPAT) were both shown to significantly enhance precursor cell proliferation in the SVZ of both normal and DA-depleted rats when administered systemically [97,130]. However, various studies have demonstrated that DA antagonists (such as certain antipsychotic drugs) can also enhance the endogenous neurogenic capacity of the adult brain [133] and a study by Milosevic *et al.* (2007) failed to detect an increase in DAergic neurogenesis upon treatment of murine and human midbrain-derived neural precursor cells with DA D2 and D3 receptor agonists [134]. Therefore, the effects of specific DA receptor agonists and antagonists on adult neurogenesis is still under debate and future studies are thus warranted in order to establish the clinical relevance of using DA agonists/antagonists to stimulate DAergic neurogenesis in the SN of PD patients.

Conclusions

Overall, the studies outlined above highlight the possibility of using endogenous stem cells to treat some of the symptoms associated with PD. While many challenges still need to be overcome before this strategy can be brought into the clinic (as indicated by the less encouraging results from the few clinical trials discussed above), endogenous stem cells offer several unique advantages over other cell replacement therapies that have been used in the past to treat PD (for review see [135,136]). Namely, these strategies prevent the occurrence of undesirable immunological reactions, constitute a less invasive procedure when compared to cell transplantation, and bypass several ethical issues associated with the use of embryonic stem cells. Therefore, the continuous testing of therapeutic strategies that can enhance the endogenous neurogenic capacity of the PD brain through preclinical studies and clinical trials is highly encouraged.

HUNTINGTON'S DISEASE

Altered Adult Neurogenesis in HD

HD is a genetic neurodegenerative disease that is caused by the occurrence of an unstable expansion of cytosine-adenine-guanine (CAG) repeats in the *HD* gene, which codifies the protein huntingtin [137]. This mutation results in neuronal loss in certain brain regions, particularly the striatum and certain layers of the cerebral cortex, as well as the formation and accumulation of ubiquitinated neuronal intranuclear inclusions (NIIs) of the mutant protein. The disease is classically characterized by a severe motor impairment that leads to loss of voluntary movement coordination. Additionally, HD patients also present with cognitive impairments that can be detected years before the onset of the motor symptoms and progressively deteriorate over the course of the disease (for review see [138]).

Since the discovery of the mutation that underlies HD in 1993 [137], various genetic rodent models have been devised to mimic this neurodegenerative disorder. While presenting several similarities, the phenotypes and characteristics of these models vary as a result of differences in the size of the huntingtin fragment that is expressed, the number of CAG repeats carried, the promoter driving the expresssion of transgene, the expression level of the mutant protein, and the background strain used to create the model (for review see [139-142]).

The first studies that analyzed how adult hippocampal neurogenesis is altered in HD used the R6 transgenic lines, which express exon 1 of the human *HD* gene with either 145 (R6/2) or 115 (R6/1) CAG repeats, and in both cases a dramatic reduction in neurogenesis that is specific to the DG of the hippocampal formation was found [143-146]. Subsequent studies have also indicated that adult hippocampal neurogenesis is compromised in yeast artificial chromosome (YAC) 128 mice, which express the full-length human *HD* gene with 128 CAG repeats [147] and in a transgenic rat model for HD that expresses a 1962 bp cDNA fragment of the human *HD* gene with 51 CAG repeats [148]. Importantly, in most cases this decrease in the endogenous neurogenic capacity of the hippocampus was observed at a very early stage, prior to the development of the characteristic motor phenotype and striatal neurodegeneration [146,147]. However, studies in post-mortem human HD brains have shown no changes in hippocampal cell proliferation [149] and an actual increase in SVZ neurogenesis [150-153]. Methodological considerations and differences in the numbers of CAG repeats and the levels of expression of the mutant gene might account for the discrepancies observed between the human and the mouse studies (for review see [47,154].

Harnessing Endogenous Neurogenesis as a Therapeutic Strategy for HD

Strategies that can promote the endogenous neurogenic capacity have the potential to be of therapeutic value for the treatment of some of the symptoms associated with HD and various studies have evaluated the effectiveness of such strategies in altering disease progression in genetic models of this disease (for review see [154]). The following sections will present a brief overview of these therapeutic strategies.

Physical Exercise

The use of voluntary physical exercise as a means to promote adult neurogenesis was initially tested in 5 week-old R6/2 HD mice [155]. However, access to a running wheel during an uninterrupted period of 4 weeks was unable to induce an increase in neurogenesis (*i.e.*, cell proliferation and neuronal survival) in these HD transgenic mice. Although it is feasible that the cellular pathways underlying the pro-neurogenic effects of physical exercise might be altered by mutant huntingtin, it is also possible that the development of motor deficits that occurs around this age [156] might have incapacitated these mice to actually engage in physical activity during this four-week period. In agreement with this later hypothesis, other authors have found that exposure of R6/1 mice (which show a slower disease progression when compared to their R6/2 counterparts; [156]) to physical exercise delayed the onset of rear-paw clasping and reduced cognition in adulthood [157], and delayed the onset of locomotor deficits that can be detected in the juvenile period [158]. In addition, although Pang and collaborators (2006) [157] observed that running did not alter the protein levels of the neurotrophin BDNF both in the striatum and the hippocampus of R6/1 HD mice [157], a subsequent study by Zajac and colleagues (2010) [159] reported a running-induced increase in *bdnf* gene expression that was specifically observed in R6/1 females but not in their male counterparts [159]. Sex-specific differences in the amount of running the animals engaged in might underlie, at least in part, the dichotic effect that physical exercise had on *bdnf* expression levels in R6/1 females *versus* males. Of note, it is reasonable to speculate that the inability of physical exercise to consistently upregulate *bdnf* gene expression and protein levels in the hippocampus of R6 mice [157,159] may be responsible for the lack of pro-neurogenic effects in the hippocampus of these mice upon exercise [155].

Environmental Enrichment

Several studies using various transgenic HD mouse models have shown that exposure to an enriched environment can be beneficial in slowing the onset and progression of the disease [146,160-164] (reviewed in [165]). As such, Lazic and colleagues (2006) [146] investigated whether exposure to an enriched environment could also mitigate the deficits in hippocampal neurogenesis observed in R6/1 HD transgenic mice [146]. These authors found that environmental enrichment was enough to enhance neuronal differentiation and survival in the hippocampal DG (but not the SVZ) of symptomatic R6/1 mice [146]. These results raise the interesting hypothesis that an increase in the endogenous hippocampal neurogenic capacity may be responsible for some of the benefits that enriched environments have on the R6 lines, particularly the development of cognitive deficits [166]. Additionally, environmental enrichment was also shown to rescue striatal BDNF protein deficits in these HD transgenic mice. Since BDNF is not produced in the striatum and instead has to be imported to this brain region from the anterior cortex *via* the corticostriatal projections, it is possible that this increase in BDNF striatal levels resulted from an increase in the anterograde transport of this trophic factor induced by environmental enrichment [163]. Of note, although this study also reported an up-regulation of BDNF protein levels in the hippocampus of R6/1 HD mice housed in enriched conditions [163], a subsequent report by the same group failed to detect any enrichment-induced changes in R6/1 hippocampal levels of BDNF mRNA [159]. Nevertheless, although no changes in the mRNA levels of this neurotrophin were detected in this brain region [159], the reported increase in the protein levels of this growth factor [163] may contribute, at least in part, to the pro-neurogenic effects of environmental enrichment that were observed in these transgenic HD mice [146].

Importantly, environmental stimulation was shown to be beneficial in the clinical setting, and HD patients (including those in the late-stages of the disease) that are exposed to more enriched and stimulating conditions demonstrate improved physical, mental, and social functioning [167]. Whether these benefits are mediated, at least in part, by an increase in adult hippocampal neurogenesis is an interesting hypothesis that remains to be elucidated.

Pharmacological Agents

Trophic Factors and Peptides. Early studies have demonstrated that FGF2 can have neuroprotective and trophic effects in striatal neurons both *in vitro* [168] and *in vivo* [169]. Additionally, this neurotrophin was also shown to induce proliferation of striatal neural stem cells [170]. In agreement, subcutaneous administration of FGF2 to R6/2 mice starting at 8 weeks of age remarkably increased SVZ cell proliferation by 150%. Furthermore, this massive increase in cell proliferation was accompanied by a significant increase in neuronal migration from the SVZ to the cortex and striatum, where neuronal differentiation occurred, resulting in an increase in the number of DA and cyclic-AMP regulated phosphoprotein with a molecular weight of 32 kDa (DARPP-32)-expressing medium-sized spiny neurons. Importantly, FGF2 treatment had additional beneficial effects by reducing the inclusion load (*i.e.*, the number of NIIs) and the motor deficits, and by enhancing the average survival rate of R6/2 mice by 20% [171]. These remarkable results suggest that potentiation of the endogenous neurogenic capacity of the SVZ may be of therapeutic value in HD. Of note, since FGF2 has been shown to readily cross the blood-brain barrier upon systemic administration [172,173], it is reasonable to assume that the observed beneficial effects of FGF2 resulted from an increase in the levels of this neurotrophin in the R6/2 brain.

Over-expression of BDNF in ependymal cells results in an increase in SVZ neurogenesis and subsequent migration and integration of new neurons into the striatal neuronal architecture. Additionally, this process can be enhanced in the presence of noggin, which can suppress subependymal gliogenesis and therefore increase the pool of progenitor cells (for references see [174]). Given this background, Cho and colleagues (2007) [174] administered a combination of adenoviral BDNF (AdBDNF) and adenoviral noggin (AdNoggin) to 4- and 6-week old R6/2 mice *via* intrastriatal injections of these adenoviral vectors. Expression of AdBDNF/AdNoggin enhanced the number of ßIII-tubulin- and

DCX-positive immature neurons in the R6/2 striatum and resulted in a subsequent increase in the number of mature DARPP-32-positive GABAergic medium-sized spiny neurons that co-expressed either enkephalin or substance P as co-neurotransmitters and projected to the globus pallidus. Additionally, the combination of AdBDNF and AdNoggin also improved motor function and the survival of these mice by 16.8% [174]. Future studies are warranted in order to evaluate the efficacy of both FGF2 and BDNF/Noggin in enhancing the endogenous neurogenic capacity in the hippocampus of HD transgenic mouse models.

Recently, Decressac and colleagues (2010) [175] determined whether treatment with neuropeptide Y (NPY) could modulate the endogenous neurogenic capacity of the SVZ and the hippocampal DG in the R6/2 transgenic HD mouse model. Surprisingly, a single intracerebroventricular injection of this peptide was shown to have profound beneficial effects in this HD mouse model, increasing the survival, reducing the loss in body weight, ameliorating the locomotor impairments, and reducing brain and striatal atrophy when R6/2 mice reached 2 months of age. However, although an increase in the number of proliferating cells was detected in the SVZ of NPY-treated R6/2 mice, this enhancement of SVZ cell proliferation did not translate into a similar increase in the number of striatal new neurons. Thus, it is unlikely that the NPY-induced increase in SVZ cell proliferation underlied the alleviation of the neuropathological and behavioural abnormalities observed in NPY-treated R6/2 mice. Of note, the same regime of NPY (known to induce neurogenesis in the DG of wild-type mice) also failed to increase hippocampal neurogenesis in R6/2 mice [176]. Since the number of NPY- and Y1 receptor-expressing neurons is significantly decreased in the hippocampal DG of these HD transgenic mice [175], it is possible that a dysregulation of the NPY system might contribute, at least in part, to the impairment of the endogenous hippocampal neurogenic function observed in this HD mouse model. Future studies are thus warranted in order to test this hypothesis.

Antidepressants. Similarly to what is observed in HD afflicted individuals [177-182], the occurrence of depressive-like symptoms is one of the phenotypic characteristics of several transgenic HD mouse models [183-185]. Since antidepressants such as selective serotonin reuptake inhibitors (SSRIs) are known to possess neurogenic properties [16-18], various studies have evaluated whether treatment with SSRIs could ameliorate the neurogenic deficits observed in HD transgenic mice. In an initial report, treatment of R6/1 mice with fluoxetine was shown to abolish the impairment in adult hippocampal neurogenesis that is observed in these mice. Importantly, this neurogenic effect of fluoxetine treatment was accompanied by an increase in cognitive performance (namely hippocampal-dependent spatial learning and memory). However, this antidepressant drug was unable to rescue the motor abnormalities and the decrease in body weigh characteristic of these HD mice [183]. Nevertheless, these preclinical findings highlight the fact that increasing hippocampal neurogenic capacity in the HD brain might result in improved cognition.

More recently, daily treatment of R6/2 HD mice with sertraline from six weeks of age onwards failed to prevent the loss of body weight and the increase in the number of huntingtin aggregates (*i.e.*, NIIs). Nevertheless, sertraline treatment resulted in improved motor coordination (as assessed with the rotarod test), attenuated striatal atrophy, and most importantly, increased survival. Additionally, treatment with this SSRI also increased striatal and hippocampal BDNF levels as well as the levels of hippocampal neurogenesis [186]. Of note, the levels of sertraline achieved both in the serum and brain of R6/2 mice [186] are comparable to those used in the clinical setting [182], and therefore sertraline might be an attractive candidate for clinical trials in HD patients. Finally, treatment of N171-82Q HD transgenic mice (which expresses a cDNA encoding a 171 amino acid N-terminal fragment of human huntingtin with 82 CAG repeats) with the SSRI paroxetine resulted in similar beneficial effects [187].

Cytokines. The cytokine asialoerythropoietin (asialoEPO) is a potent derivative of the kidney-produced erythropoietin and has been shown to possess potent neuroprotective and neurogenic effects (for references see [143]). Based on these properties, one study has investigated whether treatment of R6/2 mice with this cytokine could have beneficial effects in halting the progression of the disease in this HD transgenic mouse model. However, treatment with asialoEPO from 5 weeks of age onwards was ineffective in rescuing the locomotor deficits as well as the neuropathological abnormalities (including the formation of NIIs, the striatal and neuronal atrophy, and the reduction in adult hippocampal neurogenesis) characteristic of these mice [143]. These disappointing results might indicate that while being extremely potent in acute conditions associated with the occurrence of massive cell death, asialoEPO might not be as neuroprotective in situations of chronic neurodegeneration that are characterized by limited cell death, as is the case of the R6/2 HD mouse model.

Conclusions

The preclinical studies described above indicate that therapies aimed at enhancing adult neurogenesis in the HD brain may have beneficial effects in restoring not only cognitive function, but also some aspects of the neuropathology and motor deficits characteristic of this neurodegenerative disorder. The optimization of therapeutic regimes involving non-invasive strategies such as environmental enrichment and physical exercise in combination with the development of non-toxic and stable synthetic molecules with neurogenic and neuroprotective properties that can be administered orally and easily cross the blood-brain barrier, provide interesting therapeutic options to increase neurogenesis in HD. Additionally, restorative therapeutic approaches that can enhance the endogenous neurogenic function in the HD brain may lead to the migration of new neurons into degenerated areas of the brain.

FINAL CONCLUSIONS

Adult neurogenesis is a complex and tightly regulated phenomenon that occurs in restricted areas of the adult mammalian brain particularly in the SVZ and the SGZ of the hippocampal DG. The multi-factorial nature of adult neurogenesis implies that this complex process can also be compromised by a variety of disease conditions and mounting evidence from rodent models over the last two decades suggest that alterations in the normal neurogenic capacity can either contribute to or be a consequence of a wide range of neurological disorders including AD, PD and HD. Despite some inconsistencies in the literature, there seems to be an overall trend towards a decrease in neurogenesis with neurodegeneration. However, in some cases an up-regulation of the endogenous neurogenic function has also been found, which can reflect an intrinsic attempt of the brain to regenerate itself and replace the neurons lost during the degenerative process. Furthermore, discrepancies between studies performed in animal models and post-mortem human brains are also present in the literature and may reflect differences in the quantity of progenitor cell proliferation in human diseased brains and the respective rodent models (for review see [188]).

Nevertheless, the discovery that adult neurogenesis is altered in these chronic neurodegenerative conditions raises the possibility that some of the cognitive deficits associated with these disorders can be caused, at least in part, by these alterations and that therapies aimed at restoring or improving the endogenous neurogenic capacity might be of therapeutic value. As such, various studies have now used rodent models of these disorders to test the potential beneficial effects of therapeutic strategies that are known to promote neurogenesis. In particular, environmental stimulation and physical activity are two non-invasive and relatively inexpensive strategies that have been repeatedly shown to up-regulate adult neurogenesis. In agreement, several preclinical studies have now demonstrated that these strategies have the potential to mitigate several aspects of the neuropathology and behavioural abnormalities characteristic of various animal models of these disorders while also promoting neurogenesis. Furthermore, numerous pharmacological agents including growth factors and antidepressants among others, have also proven to be efficacious in promoting endogenous neurogenesis in animal models of AD, PD, and HD. Whether these therapies are equally beneficial in heterogeneous human populations is still a question that needs to be addressed.

ABBREVIATIONS

AD = Alzheimer's disease

AdBDNF = Adenoviral BDNF

AdNoggin = Adenoviral noggin

APOE = Apolipoprotein E

APP = Amyloid precursor protein

asialoEPO	=	Asialoerythropoietin
Aβ	=	Amyloid β
BDNF	=	Brain-derived neurotrophic factor
BrdU	=	Bromodeoxyuridine
CA	=	*Cornu ammonis*
CAG	=	Cytosine-adenine-guanine
CNS	=	Central nervous system
CNTF	=	Ciliary neurotrophic factor
DA	=	Dopamine
DARPP-32	=	Dopamine and cyclic-AMP regulated phosphoprotein with a molecular weight of 32 kDa
DCX	=	Doublecortin
DG	=	Dentate gyrus
EGF	=	Epidermal growth factor
EGFR	=	EGF receptor
FGF2	=	Fibroblast growth factor 2
GABA	=	Gamma-aminobutyric acid
GDNF	=	Glial cell-derived neurotrophic factor
GFAP	=	Glial fibrillary acid protein
HD	=	Huntington's disease

IGF-1	=	Insulin growth factor 1
LGF	=	Liver growth factor
MAP	=	Microtubule associated protein
MPTP	=	1-Methyl-4-phenyl-1,2,3,6-tetrahydropyridine
NeuN	=	Neuronal nuclei
NeuroD	=	Neurogenic differentiation factor
NIIs	=	Neuronal intranuclear inclusions
NPCs	=	Neural precursor cells
NPY	=	Neuropeptide Y
OB	=	Olfactory bulb
PD	=	Parkinson's disease
PDGF	=	Platelet-derived neurotrophic factor
PPX	=	Pramipexole
PS	=	Presenilin
PSA-NCAM	=	Polysialylated nerve cell adhesion molecule
RMS	=	Rostral migratory stream
SGZ	=	Subgranular zone
SN	=	Substantia nigra
SSRIs	=	Selective serotonin reuptake inhibitors
SVZ	=	Subventricular zone

TGFα	=	Transforming-growth factor-α
TH	=	Tyrosine hydroxylase
YAC	=	Yeast artificial chromosome
6-OHDA	=	6-Hydroxydopamine
7-OH-DPAT	=	7-Hydroxy-N,N-di-n-propyl-2-amino-tetralin.

ACKNOWLEDGEMENTS

A.P. was the recipient of a doctoral scholarship from NeuroDevNet, Canada. P.S.B. and J.G.M. acknowledge funding from the *Ciência Sem Fronteiras* funding program (Science Without Borders, Brazil).

CONFLICT OF INTEREST

The authors state that there is no conflict of interest.

REFERENCES

[1] Altman J, Das GD. Autoradiographic and histological evidence of postnatal hippocampal neurogenesis in rats. J Comp Neurol 1965; 124(3): 319-35.

[2] Cameron HA, Woolley CS, McEwen BS, Gould E. Differentiation of newly born neurons and glia in the dentate gyrus of the adult rat. Neuroscience 1993; 56(2): 337-44.

[3] Eriksson PS, Perfilieva E, Bjork-Eriksson T, *et al.* Neurogenesis in the adult human hippocampus. Nat Med 1998; 4(11): 1313-7.

[4] Kaplan MS, Hinds JW. Neurogenesis in the adult rat: electron microscopic analysis of light radioautographs. Science 1977; 197(4308): 1092-4.

[5] Lie DC, Song H, Colamarino SA, Ming GL, Gage FH. Neurogenesis in the adult brain: new strategies for central nervous system diseases. Annu Rev Pharmacol Toxicol 2004; 44: 399-421.

[6] Kempermann G, Wiskott L, Gage FH. Functional significance of adult neurogenesis. Curr Opin Neurobiol 2004; 14(2): 186-91.

[7] Cameron HA, McKay RD. Adult neurogenesis produces a large pool of new granule cells in the dentate gyrus. J Comp Neurol 2001; 435(4): 406-17.

[8] Gould E, Tanapat P, McEwen BS, Flugge G, Fuchs E. Proliferation of granule cell precursors in the dentate gyrus of adult monkeys is diminished by stress. Proc Natl Acad Sci 1998; 95(6): 3168-71.

[9] Gould E, Daniels DC, Cameron HA, McEwen BS. Expression of adrenal steroid receptors by newly born cells and pyknotic cells in the dentate gyrus of the postnatal rat. Mol Cell Neurosci 1992; 3(1): 44-8.

[10] Ekdahl CT, Claasen JH, Bonde S, Kokaia Z, Lindvall O. Inflammation is detrimental for neurogenesis in adult brain. Proc Natl Acad Sci 2003; 100(23): 13632-7.

[11] Ben Abdallah NM, Slomianka L, Vyssotski AL, Lipp HP. Early age-related changes in adult hippocampal neurogenesis in C57 mice. Neurobiol Aging 2010; 31(1): 151-61.

[12] Kuhn HG, Dickinson-Anson H, Gage FH. Neurogenesis in the dentate gyrus of the adult rat: age-related decrease of neuronal progenitor proliferation. J Neurosci 1996; 16(6): 2027-33.

[13] Olariu A, Cleaver KM, Cameron HA. Decreased neurogenesis in aged rats results from loss of granule cell precursors without lengthening of the cell cycle. J Comp Neurol 2007; 501(4): 659-67.

[14] Brannvall K, Korhonen L, Lindholm D. Estrogen-receptor-dependent regulation of neural stem cell proliferation and differentiation. Mol Cell Neurosci 2002; 21(3): 512-20.

[15] Pérez-Martin M, Cifuentes M, Grondona JM, *et al.* Neurogenesis in explants from the walls of the lateral ventricle of adult bovine brain: role of endogenous IGF-1 as a survival factor. Eur J Neurosci 2003; 17(2): 205-11.

[16] Malberg JE, Eisch AJ, Nestler EJ, Duman RS. Chronic antidepressant treatment increases neurogenesis in adult rat hippocampus. J Neurosci 2000; 20(24): 9104-10.

[17] Manev H, Uz T, Smalheiser NR, Manev R. Antidepressants alter cell proliferation in the adult brain *in vivo* and in neural cultures *in vitro*. Eur J Pharmacol 2001; 411(1-2): 67-70.

[18] Manev R, Uz T, Manev H. Fluoxetine increases the content of neurotrophic protein S100beta in the rat hippocampus. Eur J Pharmacol 2001; 420(2-3): R1-2.

[19] Zigova T, Pencea V, Wiegand SJ, Luskin MB. Intraventricular administration of BDNF increases the number of newly generated neurons in the adult olfactory bulb. Mol Cell Neurosci 1998; 11(4): 234-45.

[20] Aberg MA, Aberg ND, Hedbacker H, Oscarsson J, Eriksson PS. Peripheral infusion of IGF-I selectively induces neurogenesis in the adult rat hippocampus. J Neurosci 2000; 20(8): 2896-903.

[21] Gould E, Beylin A, Tanapat P, Reeves A, Shors TJ. Learning enhances adult neurogenesis in the hippocampal formation. Nat Neurosci 1999; 2(3): 260-5.

[22] van Praag H, Christie BR, Sejnowski TJ, Gage FH. Running enhances neurogenesis, learning, and long-term potentiation in mice. Proc Natl Acad Sci USA 1999; 96(23): 13427-13431.

[23] van Praag H, Kempermann G, Gage FH. Running increases cell proliferation and neurogenesis in the adult mouse dentate gyrus. Nat Neurosci 1999; 2(3): 266-70.

[24] Kempermann G, Kuhn HG, Gage FH. More hippocampal neurons in adult mice living in an enriched environment. Nature 1997; 386(6624): 493-5.

[25] Brocardo PS, Gil-Mohapel J. Studying learning and memory in animals: A look into cognitive function. In: Lee SA, Edget DM, Eds. Cognitive Behavioral Therapy: Applications, Methods and Outcomes. New York: Nova Science Publishers 2012; pp. 37-70.

[26] Bruel-Jungerman E, Rampon C, Laroche S. Adult hippocampal neurogenesis, synaptic plasticity and memory: facts and hypotheses. Rev Neurosci 2007; 18(2): 93-114.

[27] Koehl M, Abrous DN. A new chapter in the field of memory: adult hippocampal neurogenesis. Eur J Neurosci 2011; 33(6): 1101-14.

[28] Lemaire V, Koehl M, Le Moal M, Abrous DN. Prenatal stress produces learning deficits associated with an inhibition of neurogenesis in the hippocampus. Proc Natl Acad Sci USA 2000; 97(20): 11032-7.

[29] Leuner B, Mendolia-Loffredo S, Kozorovitskiy Y, Samburg D, Gould E, Shors TJ. Learning enhances the survival of new neurons beyond the time when the hippocampus is required for memory. J Neurosci 2004; 24(34): 7477-81.

[30] Madsen TM, Kristjansen PE, Bolwig TG, Wortwein G. Arrested neuronal proliferation and impaired hippocampal function following fractionated brain irradiation in the adult rat. Neuroscience 2003; 119(3): 635-42.

[31] Saxe MD, Battaglia F, Wang JW, *et al.* Ablation of hippocampal neurogenesis impairs contextual fear conditioning and synaptic plasticity in the dentate gyrus. Proc Natl Acad Sci 2006; 103(46): 17501-6.

[32] Shors TJ, Miesegaes G, Beylin A, Zhao M, Rydel T, Gould E. Neurogenesis in the adult is involved in the formation of trace memories. Nature 2001; 410(6826): 372-6.

[33] Winocur G, Wojtowicz JM, Sekeres M, Snyder JS, Wang S. Inhibition of neurogenesis interferes with hippocampus-dependent memory function. Hippocampus 2006; 16(3): 296-304.

[34] Kee N, Teixeira CM, Wang AH, Frankland PW. Preferential incorporation of adult-generated granule cells into spatial memory networks in the dentate gyrus. Nat Neurosci 2007; 10(3): 355-62.

[35] Patten DA, Germain M, Kelly MA, Slack RS. Reactive oxygen species: stuck in the middle of neurodegeneration. J Alzheimers Dis 2010; 20 (Suppl 2):S357-67.

[36] Hardy J, Duff K, Hardy KG, Perez-Tur J, Hutton M. Genetic dissection of Alzheimer's disease and related dementias: amyloid and its relationship to tau. Nat Neurosci 1998; 1(5): 355-8

[37] Shulman JM, De Jager PL, Feany MB. Parkinson's disease: genetics and pathogenesis. Annu Rev Pathol 2011; 6: 193-222.

[38] Vonsattel JP, DiFiglia M. Huntington disease. J Neuropathol Exp Neurol 1998; 57(5): 369-84.

[39] Gorman AM. Neuronal cell death in neurodegenerative diseases: recurring themes around protein handling. J Cell Mol Med 2008; 12(6A): 2263-80.

[40] Pillon B, Dubois B, Agid Y. Severity and specificity of cognitive impairment in Alzheimer's, Huntington's, and Parkinson's diseases and progressive supranuclear palsy. Ann N Y Acad Sci 1991a; 640: 224-7.

[41] Pillon B, Dubois B, Ploska A, Agid Y. Severity and specificity of cognitive impairment in Alzheimer's, Huntington's, and Parkinson's diseases and progressive supranuclear palsy. Neurology 1991b; 41(5): 634-43.

[42] Lindvall O, Kokaia Z. Stem cells for the treatment of neurological disorders. Nature 2006; 441(7097): 1094-6.

[43] Mohapel P, Brundin P. Harnessing endogenous stem cells to treat neurodegenerative disorders of the basal ganglia. Parkinsonism Relat Disord 2004; 10(5): 259-64.

[44] Perl DP. Neuropathology of Alzheimer's disease. Mt Sinai J Med 2010; 77(1): 32-42.

[45] Bird TD. Genetic aspects of Alzheimer disease. Genet Med 2008; 10(4): 231-9.

[46] Dodart JC, May P. Overview on rodent models of Alzheimer's disease. Curr Protoc Neurosci 2005; 9: 9.22.
[47] Brocardo PS, Patten A, Gil-Mohapel J. Altered adult neurogenesis in neurodegenerative diseases. In: Clark GJ, Anderson WT, Eds. Neurogenesis Research: New Developments. New York: Nova Science Publishers 2012; pp. 1-54.
[48] Gil-Mohapel J, Simpson J, Christie BR. Modulation of adult neurogenesis by physical exercise and environmental enrichment: Insights for the treatment of neurological disorders. In: Jin K, Ed. Adult Neurogenesis and CNS Diseases. Kerala: Research Signpost, Transworld Research Network 2009; pp. 125-50.
[49] Haughey NJ, Nath A, Chan SL, Borchard AC, Rao MS, Mattson MP. Disruption of neurogenesis by amyloid beta-peptide, and perturbed neural progenitor cell homeostasis, in models of Alzheimer's disease. J Neurochem 2002; 83(6): 1509-24.
[50] Dong H, Goico B, Martin M, Csernansky CA, Bertchume A, Csernansky JG. Modulation of hippocampal cell proliferation, memory, and amyloid plaque deposition in APPsw (Tg2576) mutant mice by isolation stress. Neuroscience 2004; 127(3): 601-9.
[51] Verret L, Jankowsky JL, Xu GM, Borchelt DR, Rampon C. Alzheimer's-type amyloidosis in transgenic mice impairs survival of newborn neurons derived from adult hippocampal neurogenesis. J Neurosci 2007; 27(25): 6771-80.
[52] Zhang C, McNeil E, Dressler L, Siman R. Long-lasting impairment in hippocampal neurogenesis associated with amyloid deposition in a knock-in mouse model of familial Alzheimer's disease. Exp Neurol 2007; 204(1): 77-87.
[53] Donovan MH, Yazdani U, Norris RD, Games D, German DC, Eisch AJ. Decreased adult hippocampal neurogenesis in the PDAPP mouse model of Alzheimer's disease. J Comp Neurol 2006; 495(1): 70-83.
[54] Wen PH, De Gasperi R, Gama Sosa MA, Elder GA. Neural progenitor cells do not differentiate prematurely in presenilin-1 null mutant mice. Neurosci Lett 2004; 371(2-3): 249-54.
[55] Wen PH, Hof PR, Chen X, *et al.* The presenilin-1 familial Alzheimer disease mutant P117L impairs neurogenesis in the hippocampus of adult mice. Exp Neurol 2004; 188(2): 224-37.
[56] Chevallier NL, Soriano S, Kang DE, Masliah E, Hu G, Koo EH. Perturbed neurogenesis in the adult hippocampus associated with presenilin-1 A246E mutation. Am J Pathol 2005; 167(1): 151-9.
[57] Rodriguez JJ, Jones VC, Tabuchi M, *et al.* Impaired adult neurogenesis in the dentate gyrus of a triple transgenic mouse model of Alzheimer's disease. PLoS One 2008; 3(8): e2935.
[58] Jin K, Galvan V, Xie L, *et al.* Enhanced neurogenesis in Alzheimer's disease transgenic (PDGF-APPSw, Ind) mice. Proc Natl Acad Sci USA 2004; 101(36): 13363-7.
[59] López-Toledano MA, Shelanski ML. Increased neurogenesis in young transgenic mice overexpressing human APP(Sw, Ind). J Alzheimers Dis 2007; 12(3): 229-40.
[60] Kolecki R, Lafauci G, Rubenstein R, Mazur-Kolecka B, Kaczmarski W, Frackowiak J. The effect of amyloidosis-beta and ageing on proliferation of neuronal progenitor cells in APP-transgenic mouse hippocampus and in culture. Acta Neuropathol 2008; 116(4): 419-24.
[61] Jin K, Peel AL, Mao XO, *et al.* Increased hippocampal neurogenesis in Alzheimer's disease. Proc Natl Acad Sci USA 2004; 101(1): 343-7.
[62] Li B, Yamamori H, Tatebayashi Y, *et al.* Failure of neuronal maturation in Alzheimer disease dentate gyrus. J Neuropathol Exp Neurol 2008; 67(1): 78-84.

[63] Fabel K, Kempermann G. Physical activity and the regulation of neurogenesis in the adult and aging brain. Neuromolecular Med 2008; 10(2): 59-66.

[64] Kempermann G, Gast D, Gage FH. Neuroplasticity in old age: sustained fivefold induction of hippocampal neurogenesis by long-term environmental enrichment. Ann Neurol 2002; 52(2): 135-43.

[65] van Praag H, Shubert T, Zhao C, Gage FH. Exercise enhances learning and hippocampal neurogenesis in aged mice. J Neurosci 2005; 25(38): 8680-5.

[66] Wu CW, Chang YT, Yu L, *et al.* Exercise enhances the proliferation of neural stem cells and neurite growth and survival of neuronal progenitor cells in dentate gyrus of middle-aged mice. J Appl Physiol 2008; 105(5): 1585-94.

[67] Brinton RD, Wang JM. Therapeutic potential of neurogenesis for prevention and recovery from Alzheimer's disease: allopregnanolone as a proof of concept neurogenic agent. Curr Alzheimer Res 2006; 3(3): 185-90.

[68] Briones TL. Environment, physical activity, and neurogenesis: implications for prevention and treatment of Alzhemier's disease. Curr Alzheimer Res 2006; 3(1): 49-54.

[69] Kelleher-Andersson J. Discovery of neurogenic, Alzheimer's disease therapeutics. Curr Alzheimer Res 2006; 3(1): 55-62.

[70] Schaeffer EL, Novaes BA, da Silva ER, Skaf HD, Mendes-Neto AG. Strategies to promote differentiation of newborn neurons into mature functional cells in Alzheimer brain. Prog Neuropsychopharmacol Biol Psychiatry 2009; 33(7): 1087-102.

[71] Sugaya K, Alvarez A, Marutle A, Kwak YD, Choumkina E. Stem cell strategies for Alzheimer's disease therapy. Panminerva Med 2006; 48(2): 87-96.

[72] Redila VA, Christie BR. Exercise-induced changes in dendritic structure and complexity in the adult hippocampal dentate gyrus. Neuroscience 2006; 137(4): 1299-307.

[73] Mirochnic S, Wolf S, Staufenbiel M, Kempermann G. Age effects on the regulation of adult hippocampal neurogenesis by physical activity and environmental enrichment in the APP23 mouse model of Alzheimer disease. Hippocampus 2009; 19(10): 1008-18.

[74] Wolf SA, Kronenberg G, Lehmann K, *et al.* Cognitive and physical activity differently modulate disease progression in the amyloid precursor protein (APP)-23 model of Alzheimer's disease. Biol Psychiatry 2006; 60(12): 1314-23.

[75] Kannangara TS, Lucero MJ, Gil-Mohapel J, *et al.* Running reduces stress and enhances cell genesis in aged mice. Neurobiol Aging 2011; 32(12): 2279-86.

[76] Choi SH, Veeraraghavalu K, Lazarov O, *et al.* Non-cell-autonomous effects of presenilin 1 variants on enrichment-mediated hippocampal progenitor cell proliferation and differentiation. Neuron 2008; 59(4): 568-80.

[77] Feng R, Rampon C, Tang YP, *et al.* Deficient neurogenesis in forebrain-specific presenilin-1 knockout mice is associated with reduced clearance of hippocampal memory traces. Neuron 2001; 32(5): 911-26.

[78] Hu YS, Xu P, Pigino G, Brady ST, Larson J, Lazarov O. Complex environment experience rescues impaired neurogenesis, enhances synaptic plasticity, and attenuates neuropathology in familial Alzheimer's disease-linked APPswe/PS1DeltaE9 mice. FASEB J 2010; 24(6): 1667-81.

[79] Blanchard J, Wanka L, Tung YC, *et al.* Pharmacologic reversal of neurogenic and neuroplastic abnormalities and cognitive impairments without affecting Abeta and tau pathologies in 3xTg-AD mice. Acta Neuropathol 2010; 120(5): 605-21.

[80] Rockenstein E, Mante M, Adame A, Crews L, Moessler H, Masliah E. Effects of Cerebrolysin on neurogenesis in an APP transgenic model of Alzheimer's disease. Acta Neuropathol 2007; 113(3): 265-75.

[81] Ruther E, Ritter R, Apecechea M, Freytag S, Windisch M. Efficacy of the peptidergic nootropic drug cerebrolysin in patients with senile dementia of the Alzheimer type (SDAT). Pharmacopsychiatry 1994; 27(1): 32-40.

[82] Mallory M, Honer W, Hsu L, Johnson R, Rockenstein E, Masliah E. *In vitro* synaptotrophic effects of Cerebrolysin in NT2N cells. Acta Neuropathol 1999; 97(5): 437-46.

[83] Mirescu C, Gould E. Stress and adult neurogenesis. Hippocampus 2006; 16(3): 233-8.

[84] Chadwick W, Mitchell N, Caroll J, *et al.* Amitriptyline-mediated cognitive enhancement in aged 3xTg Alzheimer's disease mice is associated with neurogenesis and neurotrophic activity. PLoS One 2011; 6(6): e21660.

[85] Garza JC, Guo M, Zhang W, Lu X-Y. Leptin increases adult hippocampal neurogenesis *in vivo* and *in vitro*. J Biol Chem 2008; 283(26): 18238-47.

[86] Perez-Gonzalez R, Antequera D, Vargas T, Spuch C, Bolos M, Carro E. Leptin induces proliferation of neuronal progenitors and neuroprotection in a mouse model of Alzheimer's disease. J Alzheimers Dis 2011; 24 (Suppl 2): 17-25.

[87] Baulieu EE, Robel P, Schumacher M. Neurosteroids: beginning of the story. Int Rev Neurobiol 2001; 46: 1-32.

[88] Gago N, El-Etr M, Sananes N, *et al.* 3alpha,5alpha-Tetrahydroprogesterone (allopregnanolone) and gamma-aminobutyric acid: autocrine/paracrine interactions in the control of neonatal PSA-NCAM+ progenitor proliferation. J Neurosci Res 2004; 78(6): 770-83.

[89] Bernardi F, Salvestroni C, Casarosa E, *et al.* Aging is associated with changes in allopregnanolone concentrations in brain, endocrine glands and serum in male rats. Eur J Endocrinol 1998; 138(3): 316-21.

[90] Marx CE, Trost WT, Shampine LJ, *et al.* The neurosteroid allopregnanolone is reduced in prefrontal cortex in Alzheimer's disease. Biol Psychiatry 2006; 60(12): 1287-94.

[91] Singh C, Liu L, Wang JM, *et al.* Allopregnanolone restores hippocampal-dependent learning and memory and neural progenitor survival in aging 3xTgAD and nonTg mice. Neurobiol Aging 2012; 33(8): 1493-506.

[92] Wang JM, Irwin RW, Liu L, Chen S, Brinton RD. Regeneration in a degenerating brain: potential of allopregnanolone as a neuroregenerative agent. Curr Alzheimer Res 2007; 4(5): 510-7.

[93] Marxreiter F, Regensburger M, Winkler J. Adult neurogenesis in Parkinson's disease. Cell Mol Life Sci 2013; 70(3): 459-73.

[94] Padovani A, Costanzi C, Gilberti N, Borroni B. Parkinson's disease and dementia. Neurol Sci 2006; 27 (Suppl 1): S40-3.

[95] Crabtree DM, Zhang J. Genetically engineered mouse models of Parkinson's disease. Brain Res Bull 2012; 88(1): 13-32.

[96] Melrose HL, Lincoln SJ, Tyndall GM, Farrer MJ. Parkinson's disease: a rethink of rodent models. Exp Brain Res. 2006; 173(2): 196-204.

[97] Hoglinger GU, Rizk P, Muriel MP, *et al.* Dopamine depletion impairs precursor cell proliferation in Parkinson disease. Nat Neurosci 2004; 7(7): 726-35.

[98] O'Keeffe GC, Tyers P, Aarsland D, Dalley JW, Barker RA, Caldwell MA. Dopamine-induced proliferation of adult neural precursor cells in the mammalian subventricular zone is mediated through EGF. Proc Natl Acad Sci USA 2009; 106(21): 8754–59.

[99] Iwakura Y, Piao Y-S, Mizuno M, *et al.* Influences of dopaminergic lesion on epidermal growth factor-ErbB signals in Parkinson's disease and its model: neurotrophic implication in nigrostriatal neurons. J Neurochem 2005; 93(4): 974-83.

[100] Winner B, Lie DCH, Rockenstein E, *et al.* Human wild-type alpha-synuclein impairs neurogenesis. J Neuropath Exp Neur 2004; 63(11): 1155-66.

[101] Crews L, Mizuno H, Desplats P, *et al.* Alpha-synuclein alters notch-1 expression and neurogenesis in mouse embryonic stem cells and in the hippocampus of transgenic mice. J Neurosci 2008; 28(16): 4250-60.

[102] Nuber S, Petrasch-Parwez E, Winner B, *et al.* Neurodegeneration and motor dysfunction in a conditional model of Parkinson's disease. J Neurosci 2008; 28(10): 2471-84.

[103] Zhao M, Momma S, Delfani K, *et al.* Evidence for neurogenesis in the adult mammalian substantia nigra. Proc Natl Acad Sci USA 2003; 100(13): 7925-30.

[104] Geraerts M, Krylyshkina O, Debyser Z, Baekelandt V. Concise review: Therapeutic strategies for Parkinson disease based on the modulation of adult meurogenesis. Stem Cells 2007; 25(2): 263-70.

[105] Yoshimi K, Ren YR, Seki T, *et al.* Possibility for neurogenesis in substantia nigra of parkinsonian brain. Ann Neurol 2005; 58(1): 31-40.

[106] Frielingsdorf H, Schwarz K, Brundin P, Mohapel P. No evidence for new dopaminergic neurons in the adult mammalian substantia nigra. Proc Natl Acad Sci USA 2004; 101(27): 10177-82.

[107] Steiner B, Winter C, Hosman K, *et al.* Enriched environment induces cellular plasticity in the adult substantia nigra and improves motor behavior function in the 6-OHDA rat model of Parkinson's disease. Exp Neurol 2006; 199(2): 291-300.

[108] Van Kampen JM, Robertson HA. A possible role for dopamine D3 receptor stimulation in the induction of neurogenesis in the adult rat substantia nigra. Neuroscience 2005; 136(2): 381-6.

[109] Fisher BE, Petzinger GM, Nixon K, *et al.* Exercise-induced behavioral recovery and neuroplasticity in the 1-methyl-4-phenyl-1,2,3,6-tetrahydropyridine-lesioned mouse basal ganglia. J Neurosci Res 2004; 77(3): 378–90.

[110] O'Dell SJ, Gross NB, Fricks AN, Casiano BD, Nguyen TB, Marshall JF. Running wheel exercise enhances recovery from nigrostriatal dopamine injury without inducing neuroprotection. Neuroscience 2007; 144(3): 1141-51.

[111] Tillerson JL, Caudle WM, Reverón ME, Miller GW. Exercise induces behavioral recovery and attenuates neurochemical deficits in rodent models of Parkinson's disease. Neuroscience 2003; 119(3): 899-911.

[112] Zigmond MJ, Cameron JL, Leak RK, *et al.* Triggering endogenous neuroprotective processes through exercise in models of dopamine deficiency. Parkinsonism Relat Disord 2009; 15(Suppl 3): S42-5.

[113] Tajiri N, Yasuhara T, Shingo T, *et al.* Exercise exerts neuroprotective effects on Parkinson's disease model of rats. Brain Res 2010; 1310: 200-7.

[114] Alexi T, Borlongan CV, Faull RL, *et al.* Neuroprotective strategies for basal ganglia degeneration: Parkinson's and Huntington's diseases. Prog Neurobiol 2000; 60(5): 409-70.

[115] Gash DM, Gerhardt GA, Hoffer BJ. Effects of glial cell line-derived neurotrophic factor on the nigrostriatal dopamine system in rodents and nonhuman primates. Adv Pharmacol 1998; 42: 911-5.
[116] Gash DM, Zhang Z, Ovadia A, *et al.* Functional recovery in parkinsonian monkeys treated with GDNF. Nature 1996; 380(6571):252-5.
[117] Rosenblad C, Kirik D, Bjorklund A. Sequential administration of GDNF into the substantia nigra and striatum promotes dopamine neuron survival and axonal sprouting but not striatal reinnervation or functional recovery in the partial 6-OHDA lesion model. Exp Neurol 2000; 161(2): 503-16.
[118] Rosenblad C, Kirik D, Devaux B, Moffat B, Phillips HS, Bjorklund A. Protection and regeneration of nigral dopaminergic neurons by neurturin or GDNF in a partial lesion model of Parkinson's disease after administration into the striatum or the lateral ventricle. Eur J Neurosci 1999; 11(5): 1554-66.
[119] Sauer H, Rosenblad C, Bjorklund A. Glial cell line-derived neurotrophic factor but not transforming growth factor beta 3 prevents delayed degeneration of nigral dopaminergic neurons following striatal 6-hydroxydopamine lesion. Proc Natl Acad Sci USA 1995; 92(19): 8935-9.
[120] Winkler C, Sauer H, Lee CS, Bjorklund A. Short-term GDNF treatment provides long-term rescue of lesioned nigral dopaminergic neurons in a rat model of Parkinson's disease. J Neurosci 1996; 16(22): 7206-15.
[121] Peng J, Xie L, Jin K, Greenberg DA, Andersen JK. Fibroblast growth factor 2 enhances striatal and nigral neurogenesis in the acute 1-methyl-4-phenyl-1,2,3,6-tetrahydropyridine model of Parkinson's disease. Neuroscience 2008; 153(3): 664-70.
[122] Chen Y, Ai Y, Slevin JR, Maley BE, Gash DM. Progenitor proliferation in the adult hippocampus and substantia nigra induced by glial cell line-derived neurotrophic factor. Exp Neurol 2005; 196(1): 87-95.
[123] Cooper O, Isacson O. Intrastriatal transforming growth factor alpha delivery to a model of Parkinson's disease induces proliferation and migration of endogenous adult neural progenitor cells without differentiation into dopaminergic neurons. J Neurosci 2004; 24(41): 8924-31.
[124] Mohapel P, Frielingsdorf H, Haggblad J, Zachrisson O, Brundin P. Platelet-derived growth factor (PDGF-BB) and brain-derived neurotrophic factor (BDNF) induce striatal neurogenesis in adult rats with 6-hydroxydopamine lesions. Neuroscience 2005; 132(3): 767-76.
[125] Reimers D, Herranz AS, Diaz-Gil JJ, *et al.* Intrastriatal infusion of liver growth factor stimulates dopamine terminal sprouting and partially restores motor function in 6-hydroxydopamine-lesioned rats. J Histochem Cytochem 2006; 54(4): 457-65.
[126] Nutt JG, Burchiel KJ, Comella CL, *et al.* Randomized, double-blind trial of glial cell line-derived neurotrophic factor (GDNF) in PD. Neurology 2003; 60(1): 69-73.
[127] Gill SS, Patel NK, Hotton GR, *et al.* Direct brain infusion of glial cell line-derived neurotrophic factor in Parkinson disease. Nat Med 2003; 9(5): 589-95.
[128] Slevin JT, Gerhardt GA, Smith CD, Gash DM, Kryscio R, Young B. Improvement of bilateral motor functions in patients with Parkinson disease through the unilateral intraputaminal infusion of glial cell line-derived neurotrophic factor. J Neurosurg 2005; 102(2): 216-22.

[129] Lang AE, Gill S, Patel NK, *et al.* Randomized controlled trial of intraputamenal glial cell line-derived neurotrophic factor infusion in Parkinson disease. Ann Neurol 2006; 59(3): 459-66.

[130] Van Kampen JM, Hagg T, Robertson HA. Induction of neurogenesis in the adult rat subventricular zone and neostriatum following dopamine D3 receptor stimulation. Eur J Neurosci 2004; 19(9): 2377-87.

[131] Van Kampen JM, Eckman CB. Dopamine D3 receptor agonist delivery to a model of Parkinson's disease restores the nigrostriatal pathway and improves locomotor behavior. J Neurosci 2006; 26(27): 7272-80.

[132] Winner B, Desplats P, Hagl C, *et al.* Dopamine receptor activation promotes adult neurogenesis in an acute Parkinson model. Exp Neurol 2009; 219(2): 543-52.

[133] Kippin TE, Kapur S, van der Kooy D. Dopamine specifically inhibits forebrain neural stem cell proliferation, suggesting a novel effect of antipsychotic drugs. J Neurosci 2005; 25(24): 5815-23.

[134] Milosevic J, Schwarz SC, Maisel M, *et al.* Dopamine D2/D3 receptor stimulation fails to promote dopaminergic neurogenesis of murine and human midbrain-derived neural precursor cells *in vitro*. Stem Cells Dev 2007; 16(4): 625-35.

[135] Nishimura K, Takahashi J. Therapeutic Application of Stem Cell Technology toward the Treatment of Parkinson's Disease. *Biol Pharm Bull* 2013; 36(2): 171-5.

[136] Pan-Montojo F, Funk RH. Implications of Parkinson's disease pathophysiology for the development of cell replacement strategies and drug discovery in neurodegenerative diseases. CNS Neurol Disord Drug Targets 2012; 11(7): 907-20.

[137] The Huntington's Disease Collaborative Research Group. A novel gene containing a trinucleotide repeat that is expanded and unstable on Huntington's disease chromosomes. Cell 1993; 72(6): 971-83.

[138] Gil JM, Rego AC. Mechanisms of neurodegeneration in Huntington's disease. Eur J Neurosci 2008; 27(11): 2803-20.

[139] Gil-Mohapel J. Transgenic Models of Huntington's Disease: Differences, Similarities, and Applications. In: Recent Developments in Brain Research. Kerala: Research Signpost 2012; vol.1, pp. 45-76.

[140] Hickey MA, Chesselet MF. The use of transgenic and knock-in mice to study Huntington's disease. Cytogenet Genome Res 2003; 100(1-4): 276-86.

[141] Levine MS, Cepeda C, Hickey MA, Fleming SM, Chesselet MF. Genetic mouse models of Huntington's and Parkinson's diseases: illuminating but imperfect. Trends Neurosci 2004; 27(11): 691-7.

[142] Menalled LB, Chesselet MF. Mouse models of Huntington's disease. Trends Pharmacol Sci 2002; 23(1): 32-9.

[143] Gil JM, Leist M, Popovic N, Brundin P, Petersen A. Asialoerythropoietin is not effective in the R6/2 line of Huntington's disease mice. BMC Neurosci 2004; 5: 17.

[144] Gil JM, Mohapel P, Araujo IM, *et al.* Reduced hippocampal neurogenesis in R6/2 transgenic Huntington's disease mice. Neurobiol Dis 2005; 20(3): 744-51.

[145] Lazic SE, Grote H, Armstrong RJ, *et al.* Decreased hippocampal cell proliferation in R6/1 Huntington's mice. Neuroreport 2004; 15(5): 811-3.

[146] Lazic SE, Grote HE, Blakemore C, *et al.* Neurogenesis in the R6/1 transgenic mouse model of Huntington's disease: effects of environmental enrichment. Eur J Neurosci 2006; 23(7): 1829-38.

[147] Simpson JM, Gil-Mohapel J, Pouladi MA, *et al.* Altered adult hippocampal neurogenesis in the YAC128 transgenic mouse model of Huntington disease. Neurobiol Dis 2011; 41(2): 249-60.
[148] Kandasamy M, Couillard-Despres S, Raber KA, *et al.* Stem cell quiescence in the hippocampal neurogenic niche is associated with elevated transforming growth factor-beta signaling in an animal model of Huntington disease. J Neuropath Exp Neur 2010; 69(7): 717-28.
[149] Low VF, Dragunow M, Tippett LJ, Faull RL, Curtis MA. No change in progenitor cell proliferation in the hippocampus in Huntington's disease. Neuroscience 2011; 199: 577-88.
[150] Curtis MA, Penney EB, Pearson AG, *et al.* Increased cell proliferation and neurogenesis in the adult human Huntington's disease brain. Proc Natl Acad Sci USA 2003; 100(15): 9023-7.
[151] Curtis MA, Penney EB, Pearson J, Dragunow M, Connor B, Faull RL. The distribution of progenitor cells in the subependymal layer of the lateral ventricle in the normal and Huntington's disease human brain. Neuroscience 2005; 132(3): 777-88.
[152] Curtis MA, Waldvogel HJ, Synek B, Faull RL. A histochemical and immunohistochemical analysis of the subependymal layer in the normal and Huntington's disease brain. J Chem Neuroanat 2005; 30(1): 55-66.
[153] Curtis MA, Faull RL, Glass M. A novel population of progenitor cells expressing cannabinoid receptors in the subependymal layer of the adult normal and Huntington's disease human brain. J Chem Neuroanat 2006; 31(3): 210-5.
[154] Gil-Mohapel J, Simpson JM, Ghilan M, Christie BR. Neurogenesis in Huntington's disease: can studying adult neurogenesis lead to the development of new therapeutic strategies? Brain Res 2011; 1406: 84-105.
[155] Kohl Z, Kandasamy M, Winner B, *et al.* Physical activity fails to rescue hippocampal neurogenesis deficits in the R6/2 mouse model of Huntington's disease. Brain Res 2007; 1155: 24-33.
[156] Mangiarini L, Sathasivam K, Seller M, *et al.* Exon 1 of the HD gene with an expanded CAG repeat is sufficient to cause a progressive neurological phenotype in transgenic mice. Cell 1996; 87(3): 493-506.
[157] Pang TY, Stam NC, Nithianantharajah J, Howard ML, Hannan AJ. Differential effects of voluntary physical exercise on behavioral and brain-derived neurotrophic factor expression deficits in Huntington's disease transgenic mice. Neuroscience 2006; 141(2): 569-84.
[158] van Dellen A, Cordery PM, Spires TL, Blakemore C, Hannan AJ. Wheel running from a juvenile age delays onset of specific motor deficits but does not alter protein aggregate density in a mouse model of Huntington's disease. BMC Neurosci 2008; 9: 34.
[159] Zajac MS, Pang TY, Wong N, *et al.* Wheel running and environmental enrichment differentially modify exon-specific BDNF expression in the hippocampus of wild-type and pre-motor symptomatic male and female Huntington's disease mice. Hippocampus 2010; 20(5): 621-36.
[160] Carter RJ, Hunt MJ, Morton AJ. Environmental stimulation increases survival in mice transgenic for exon 1 of the Huntington's disease gene. Mov Disord 2000; 15(5): 925-37.
[161] Hockly E, Cordery PM, Woodman B, *et al.* Environmental enrichment slows disease progression in R6/2 Huntington's disease mice. Ann Neurol 2002; 51(2): 235-42.

[162] Schilling G, Savonenko AV, Coonfield ML, *et al.* Environmental, pharmacological, and genetic modulation of the HD phenotype in transgenic mice. Exp Neurol 2004; 187(1): 137-49.

[163] Spires TL, Grote HE, Varshney NK, *et al.* Environmental enrichment rescues protein deficits in a mouse model of Huntington's disease, indicating a possible disease mechanism. J Neurosci 2004; 24(9): 2270-6.

[164] van Dellen A, Blakemore C, Deacon R, York D, Hannan AJ. Delaying the onset of Huntington's in mice. Nature 2000; 404(6779): 721-2.

[165] Gil JM, Rego AC. The R6 lines of transgenic mice: a model for screening new therapies for Huntington's disease. Brain Res Rev 2009; 59(2): 410-31.

[166] Nithianantharajah J, Barkus C, Vijiaratnam N, Clement O, Hannan AJ. Modeling brain reserve: experience-dependent neuronal plasticity in healthy and Huntington's disease transgenic mice. Am J Geriatr Psychiatry 2009; 17(3): 196-209.

[167] Sullivan FR, Bird ED, Alpay M, Cha JH. Remotivation therapy and Huntington's disease. J Neurosci Nurs 2001; 33(3): 136-42.

[168] Zhou D, DiFiglia M. Basic fibroblast growth factor enhances the growth of postnatal neostriatal GABAergic neurons *in vitro*. Exp Neurol 1993; 122(2): 171-88.

[169] Bjugstad KB, Zawada WM, Goodman S, Freed CR. IGF-1 and bFGF reduce glutaric acid and 3-hydroxyglutaric acid toxicity in striatal cultures. J Inherit Metab Dis 2001; 24(6): 631-47.

[170] 172. Palmer TD, Ray J, Gage FH. FGF-2-responsive neuronal progenitors reside in proliferative and quiescent regions of the adult rodent brain. Mol Cell Neurosci 1995; 6(5): 474-86.

[171] Jin K, LaFevre-Bernt M, Sun Y, *et al.* FGF-2 promotes neurogenesis and neuroprotection and prolongs survival in a transgenic mouse model of Huntington's disease. Proc Natl Acad Sci USA 2005; 102(50): 18189-94.

[172] Jin K, Xie L, Childs J, *et al.* Cerebral neurogenesis is induced by intranasal administration of growth factors. Ann Neurol 2003; 53(3): 405-9.

[173] Wagner JP, Black IB, DiCicco-Bloom E. Stimulation of neonatal and adult brain neurogenesis by subcutaneous injection of basic fibroblast growth factor. J Neurosci 1999; 19(14): 6006-16.

[174] Cho SR, Benraiss A, Chmielnicki E, Samdani A, Economides A, Goldman SA. Induction of neostriatal neurogenesis slows disease progression in a transgenic murine model of Huntington disease. J Clin Invest 2007; 117(10): 2889-902.

[175] Decressac M, Wright B, Tyers P, Gaillard A, Barker RA. Neuropeptide Y modifies the disease course in the R6/2 transgenic model of Huntington's disease. Exp Neurol 2010; 226(1): 24-32.

[176] Decressac M, Wright B, David B, *et al.* Exogenous neuropeptide Y promotes *in vivo* hippocampal neurogenesis. Hippocampus 2011; 21(3): 233-8.

[177] Duff K, Paulsen JS, Beglinger LJ, Langbehn DR, Stout JC, Predict HDIotHSG. Psychiatric symptoms in Huntington's disease before diagnosis: the predict-HD study. Biol Psychiatry 2007; 62(12): 1341-6.

[178] Folstein SE, Folstein MF. Psychiatric features of Huntington's disease: recent approaches and findings. Psychiatr Dev 1983; 1(2): 193-205.

[179] Folstein S, Abbott MH, Chase GA, Jensen BA, Folstein MF. The association of affective disorder with Huntington's disease in a case series and in families. Psychol Med 1983; 13(3): 537-42.

[180] Kirkwood SC, Su JL, Conneally P, Foroud T. Progression of symptoms in the early and middle stages of Huntington disease. Arch Neurol 2001; 58(2): 273-8.

[181] Pflanz S, Besson JA, Ebmeier KP, Simpson S. The clinical manifestation of mental disorder in Huntington's disease: a retrospective case record study of disease progression. Acta Psychiatr Scand 1991; 83(1): 53-60.

[182] Slaughter JR, Martens MP, Slaughter KA. Depression and Huntington's disease: prevalence, clinical manifestations, etiology, and treatment. CNS Spectr 2001; 6(4): 306-26.

[183] Grote HE, Bull ND, Howard ML, *et al.* Cognitive disorders and neurogenesis deficits in Huntington's disease mice are rescued by fluoxetine. Eur J Neurosci 2005; 22: 2081-8.

[184] Pang TY, Du X, Zajac MS, Howard ML, Hannan AJ. Altered serotonin receptor expression is associated with depression-related behavior in the R6/1 transgenic mouse model of Huntington's disease. Hum Mol Genet 2009; 18(4): 753-66.

[185] Pouladi MA, Graham RK, Karasinska JM, *et al.* Prevention of depressive behaviour in the YAC128 mouse model of Huntington disease by mutation at residue 586 of huntingtin. Brain 2009; 132(Pt 4): 919-32.

[186] Peng Q, Masuda N, Jiang M, *et al.* The antidepressant sertraline improves the phenotype, promotes neurogenesis and increases BDNF levels in the R6/2 Huntington's disease mouse model. Exp Neurol 2008; 210(1): 154-63.

[187] Duan W, Guo Z, Jiang H, *et al.* Paroxetine retards disease onset and progression in Huntingtin mutant mice. Ann Neurol 2004; 55(4): 590-4.

[188] Curtis MA, Low VF, Faull RL. Neurogenesis and progenitor cells in the adult human brain: a comparison between hippocampal and subventricular progenitor proliferation. Dev Neurobiol 2012; 72(7): 990-1005.

80 *Frontiers in CNS Drug Discovery*, 2013, *2*, 80-117

CHAPTER 4

New Therapies for HIV-1-Associated Neurocognitive Disorder (HAND): Animal Models and Gene Delivery of Antioxidant Enzymes by rSV40

Jean-Pierre Louboutin* **and David S. Strayer**

Department of Pathology, Anatomy and Cell Biology, Thomas Jefferson University, Philadelphia, PA 19107, USA

Abstract: HIV encephalopathy covers a range of HIV-related brain dysfunctions. HIV-1 enters the Central Nervous System (CNS) soon after it enters the body. In the CNS, it is largely impervious to highly active anti-retroviral therapeutic drugs (HAART). As survival with chronic HIV-1 infection improves, the number of people harboring the virus in their CNS increases. The prevalence of HIV-associated neurocognitive disorder (HAND) therefore continues to rise. It is also becoming clear that the brain is an important reservoir for the virus, and neurodegenerative and neuroinflammatory changes may continue despite the use of HAART.

Neurons themselves are rarely infected by HIV-1, and neuronal damage is felt to be mainly indirect. HIV-1 infects resident microglia, periventricular macrophages, leading to increased production of cytokines and to release of HIV-1 proteins, the most likely neurotoxins, among which are the envelope glycoprotein gp120 and HIV-1 *trans*-acting protein Tat. Animal model systems in which recombinant gp120, or Tat, proteins are directly injected into the striatum have been developed and recapitulate some of the features seen in HAND.

As HIV-1 infection of the brain lasts the lifetime of affected individuals, and as eradication of CNS HIV-1 is currently not possible, control of the damage caused by the virus may represent a useful approach to treatment. One way to limit the final damage could be by limiting oxidative stress-related neurotoxicity. We used SV40 vectors for long-term gene delivery of transgenes to the brain. Intracerebral injection of SV(SOD1) or SV(GPx1) carrying the antioxidant enzymes, Cu/Zn superoxide dismutase (SOD1) or glutathione peroxidase (GPx1) respectively, into the rat caudate putamen (CP), significantly protects neurons from apoptosis caused by subsequent inoculation of recombinant gp120 and Tat. Vector administration into the lateral ventricle or cisterna magna, particularly if preceded by intraperitoneal mannitol, protects from intra-CP gp120-induced neurotoxicity comparably to intra-CP vector administration. The safety of SV(SOD1) and SV(GPx1) delivered intra-CP has been demonstrated in rats and in Rhesus macaques monkeys, and resulting transgene expression is very durable. These

***Address correspondence to Jean-Pierre Louboutin:** Department of Pathology, Anatomy and Cell Biology, Thomas Jefferson University, Philadelphia, PA 19107, USA; Tel: 1-215-983-0457, 1-876-368-0554; E-mail: jplouboutin@hotmail.com models should provide a better understanding of the pathogenesis of HIV-1 in the brain as well as offer new therapeutic avenues.

Keywords: HIV-1, Central Nervous System, antioxidant enzymes, gene therapy, oxidative stress.

INTRODUCTION

Human immunodeficiency virus (HIV)-1 enters the Central Nervous System (CNS) soon after it enters the body. Advances in the treatment of HIV-1 have dramatically improved survival rates over the past 10 years, but HIV-associated neurocognitive disorders (HAND) remain highly prevalent and continue to represent a significant public health problem, partly because HIV-1 is largely impervious to highly active anti-retroviral therapeutic drugs (HAART) in the CNS. In 1991, the neurologic complications of HIV infection were classified into two levels of disturbance: 1) HIV-associated dementia (HAD) with motor, behavioral/psychosocial, or combined features; and 2) minor cognitive motor disorder (MCMD). HAD was considered as the most common cause of dementia in adults under 40 [1] and was estimated to affect as many as 30% of patients with advanced AIDS [2], but has become less common since HAART was introduced [3]. This reduction probably reflects better control of HIV in the periphery, since antiretroviral drugs penetrate the CNS poorly. Before the introduction of HAART, most neuroAIDS patients showed subcortical dementia, with predominant basal ganglia involvement, manifesting as psychomotor slowing, Parkinsonism, behavioral abnormalities and cognitive difficulties [4]. MCMD described a less severe presentation of HIV-associated neurocognitive impairment that did not meet criteria for HAD. More recently, in light of the changing epidemiology of HIV infection, the need to update and further structure the diagnostic criteria for HAND has been recognized [5]. There are several reasons for this update. First, the applicability of the old criteria appears limited in the present age of HAART. Prior to the advent of HAART, a diagnosis of HAD was associated strongly with high viral loads, low T-cell counts, and opportunistic infections. With HAART limiting viral severity, patients with HIV typically live longer with milder medical symptoms. Secondly, guidelines regarding possible neurocognitive impairment due to comorbid conditions with CNS effects (*e.g.*, substance use disorders) were not precisely described in the previous diagnostic scheme. This limitation is particularly important in the era of HAART as those infected with HIV-1 live longer with a host of CNS risk factors, including substance use disorders (*e.g.*, methamphetamine dependence), medical conditions associated with HAART treatment (*e.g.*, hyperlipidemia) and comorbid infectious diseases (*e.g.*, hepatitis C virus) [6]. Thus, the newly redefined criteria allow for three possible research diagnoses: 1) asymptomatic neurocognitive impairment (ANI); 2) HIV-associated mild neurocognitive disorder (MND); and 3) HAD. In this classification, the diagnosis of HAND must be determined by assessing at least five areas of neurocognitive functioning known to be affected by HIV infection (*e.g.*, attention/working memory, executive functions, speed of information processing, episodic memory, motor skills, language, and sensoriperception) [5]. Considered as a mild neurocognitive impairment in the absence of declines in everyday functioning, ANI is now estimated to represent the majority of cases of HAND (*i.e.*, about 50% of diagnosed cases) and 21-30% of the asymptomatic HIV-infected individuals. Detecting patients with mild, yet demonstrable, neurocognitive impairment may help in the effort to pre-identify those at risk for more significant cognitive as well as functional decline, before cognitive deficits contribute to a decline in everyday functioning with serious medical consequences [6]. As effective treatments for neurologic complications are developed, intervention at this earliest stage of HAND might offer the best opportunity to obtain remission, or at least, prevent progression. Formerly referred to as MCMD, mild neurocognitive disorder (MND) requires mild-to-moderate neurocognitive impairment in at least two cognitive domains in addition to mild everyday functioning impairment [5]. Approximately 30-50% of persons with a HAND diagnosis experience some degree of functional impairment and it is estimated that 20-40% of HAND diagnoses are of MND, which comprises 5-20% of the HIV population overall [6]. The most severe form of HAND, HIV-associated dementia (HAD) is marked by at least moderate-to-severe cognitive impairment in at least two cognitive domains along with marked ADL declines that are not fully attributable to comorbidities or delirium [5,6]. Furthermore, HAD represents the most severe form of HAND in terms of its functional impact. After the advent of HAART in the late 1990's, estimates appeared to shift downward with approximately 4% to 7% of persons with AIDS, with more recent appraisals suggesting that as few as 1% to 2% of HIV+ patients meet criteria for HAD [6].

As survival with chronic HIV-1 infection improves, the number of people harboring the virus in their CNS increases, leading to new HIV-1-related neurological manifestations. The prevalence of HAND therefore continues to rise, and less fulminant forms of HAND have become more common than their more severe predecessors [5,6]. HAND remains a significant independent risk factor for AIDS mortality [1,2,5,7-9]. Incident cases of HAND are accelerating fastest among drug users, ethnic minorities, and women [7-9]. The number of HIV-infected individuals over 50 years of age is rapidly growing, including patients taking HAART [9]. It has been suggested that in 10 years, 50% of AIDS patients in the United States will be over the age of 50. Moreover, it is becoming clear that the brain is an important reservoir for the virus, and neurodegenerative and neuroinflammatory changes may continue despite HAART [8].

PATHOGENESIS OF HAND

The principal manifestations of HIV-1 infection in CNS result from neuronal injury and loss, as well as from extensive damage to the dendritic and synaptic structures in the absence of neuronal loss. Neurons themselves are rarely infected by HIV-1, and neuronal damage is felt to be mainly indirect. In fact, the pathogenesis of HAND largely reflects the neurotoxicity of HIV-1 proteins [10]. HIV-1 infects resident microglia, periventricular macrophages and some astrocytes [11], leading to increased production of cytokines and to release of HIV-1 proteins, the most likely neurotoxins, among which are the envelope (Env) proteins gp120 and gp41 and the nonstructural proteins Nef, Rev, Vpr and Tat [1, 12-14]. Pathogenesis of HAND is summarized on Fig. (**1**).

The HIV-1 *env* gene codes for gp160 which is cleaved into two major envelope glycoproteins, gp120 and gp41. Soluble gp120 can induce apoptosis in a wide variety of cells including lymphocytes, cardiomyocytes and neurons [15,16]. HIV-1 gp120 may be directly neurotoxic at high concentrations [17]. Gp120-induced apoptosis has been demonstrated in studies in cortical cell cultures, in rat hippocampal slices and by intracerebral injections *in vivo* [18]. Gp120 binds neuron cell membrane co-receptors (CCR3, CCR5 and CXCR4) and elicits apoptosis, apparently *via* G-protein-coupled pathways [19,20]. Soluble gp120 also increases glial cell release of arachidonate, which impairs neuron and astrocyte reuptake of glutamate [21], leading to prolonged activation of NMDA receptor with consequent disruption of cellular Ca^{2+} homeostasis [22]. This process involves generation of superoxide and peroxide species, with resultant oxidative stress, and leads to neuron cell death after mitochondrial permeabilization, cytochrome c release and activation of caspases and endonucleases [2].

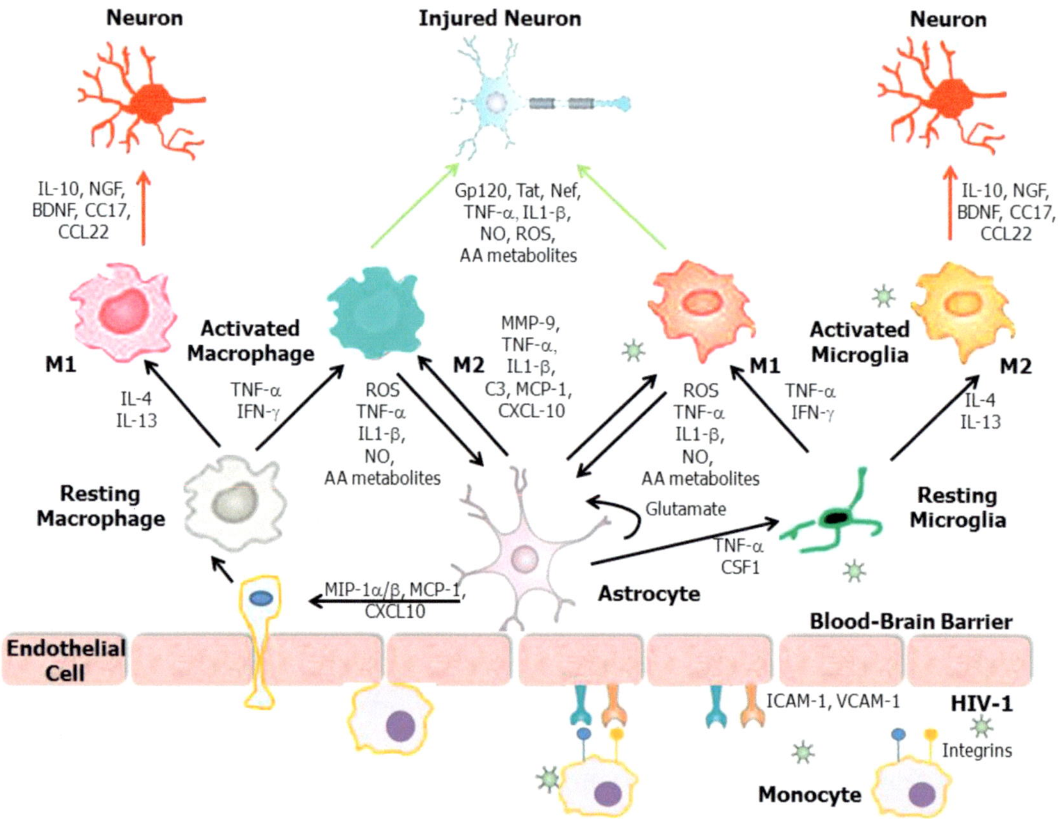

Fig. (1). Pathogenesis of HIV-1 in the brain. Activated monocytes are attracted to the brain by chemokines and pass the blood-brain barrier. HIV-1 infects microglia and macrophages, releasing HIV-1 proteins, most likely neurotoxins, gp120 and Tat among others. These proteins can induce apoptosis through a cell death cascade as well as trigger production of pro-inflammatory cytokines and chemokines. Astrocytes and resident microglia are activated during the CNS infection, resulting in the spreading of infection to neighboring cells with concomitant neuroinflammation. Activated microglia polarize to either an M1 or M2 phenotype, leading to a neurotoxic or neurotrophic microglial phenotype (modeled after Figure **1** in Reference [175] and [176]).

The trans-membrane protein gp41 is elevated in the brains of patients with HAD [23,24]. *In vitro*, gp41 induces a cascade of events that is toxic to primary neuronal cultures through NO-dependent mechanism, depletion of glutathione and disruption of mitochondrial function [23,24].

The HIV-1 *trans*-acting protein Tat, an essential protein for viral replication, is a key mediator of neurotoxicity. Brain areas that are particularly susceptible to Tat toxicity include the CA3 region and the dentate gyrus of the hippocampus and the striatum. Tat is internalized by neurons primarily through lipoprotein related protein receptor (LRP) and by activation of N-methyl-D-aspartate (NMDA) receptor [25,26]. It also interacts with several cell membrane receptors, including integrins, Vascular Endothelium Growth Factor (VEGF) receptor in endothelial cells and possibly CXCR4 [27].

Tat can directly depolarize neuron membranes, independently of Na^+ flux [28] and may potentiate glutamate- and NMDA-triggered calcium fluxes and neurotoxicity [28]. It promotes excitotoxic neuron apoptosis [29,30] by activating endoplasmic reticulum pathways to release intracellular calcium ($[Ca^{2+}]i$) [31]. Consequent dysregulation of calcium homeostasis [19,29,32] leads to mitochondrial calcium uptake, caspase activation and, finally, neuronal death. Tat also increases levels of lipid peroxidation [33] by generating the reactive oxygen species (ROS) superoxide (O_2^-) and hydrogen peroxide (H_2O_2). It activates inducible nitric oxide synthase (iNOS) to produce nitric oxide (NO), which binds superoxide anion to form the highly reactive peroxynitrite (ONOO) [34].

Tat neurotoxicity has been reported in cultured cells, but fewer studies have demonstrated its neurotoxic properties *in vivo* [35-40]. Despite evidence that Tat has been detected in the striatum of patients with HIV encephalitis [41,42], it is difficult to know the exact levels of Tat generated. Although mRNA for Tat was detected by RT-PCR in brain extracts from half [42] or more [41] of patients with HIV encephalitis, protein levels could not be measured by ELISA [42]. The lesions of HAND reflect chronic injury caused by ongoing production of Tat, as well as other substances, by HIV-1-infected cells.

Other HIV-1 proteins (Vpr, Nef, Rev) are also involved in HAND neuropathogenesis. HIV-1 viral protein r (Vpr) is thought to be important for effective viral replication in the early stages of the infection. Vpr is present as a soluble protein in the blood serum and the CSF of patients infected with HIV-1 [43-45] and accumulates within these compartments to increasing concentrations as disease progresses toward the later stages of disease. As an extracellular protein, HIV-1 Vpr has been shown to negatively affect the survival of brain-resident cells, especially neurons and astrocytes, which are the cell types most sensitive to local insult; they become dysfunctional and are gradually lost as patients infected with HIV-1 advance towards AIDS [46]. Some studies have shown that Vpr can directly induce neuronal apoptosis [47,48], and that Vpr can deregulate calcium secretion in neural cells [49].

The non-structural protein Nef is required for the proper budding of virions from HIV-infected cells. *In vitro*, Nef can be lethal for astrocytes and neurons and can increase the expression of matrix metalloproteinases (MMPs) [50]. Abundant Nef expression has been shown in astrocytes of HIV-1-infected patients with neuronal damage [11,51].

The HIV-1 phosphoprotein Rev is involved in the nuclear export of unspliced viral mRNAs. Extracellular Rev has neurotoxic properties as demonstrated in rodents by intracerebroventricular injection of a synthetic peptide spanning the basic region of Rev causing neuronal death [52].

ANIMAL MODELS OF HAND

There are no perfect models for HAND. Several animal systems have been used to study the pathogenesis of HIV-1-induced neurological disease. Many of them are based on other lentiviruses (*i.e.*, simian immunodeficiency virus (SIV) infection of macaques, feline immunodeficiency virus (FIV) infection of cats, Visna-Maedi virus infection in sheep) [53-55]. However, only small percentages of animals develop neurological manifestations in these models and the costs for using these species may be high. Transgenic expression of gp120 in mice has been studied [56], but the gp120 in that model is mainly expressed in astrocytes, whereas in humans HIV-1 mostly infects microglial cells. Other models based on introduction of HIV-infected macrophages into the brains of SCID mice have been proposed, but they suffer from the fact of human macrophages delivered into a murine brain [57]. HIV-1-infected NOD/scid-IL-2Rγ(c)(null) humanized mice can, at least in part, recapitulate lentiviral neuropathobiology. This model of neuroAIDS reflects the virological, immunological, and early disease-associated neuropathological components of human disease [58]. Some models of ongoing exposure to Tat have been developed. For example, GFAP-driven, doxycycline-inducible Tat transgenic mice have been useful for mechanistic studies of Tat contribution to HAND. However, the reported data concerning neuronal TUNEL positivity are still debated [59].

We [40,60,61] and others [36,62] have used model systems in which recombinant gp120, or Tat, proteins are directly injected into the striatum. The neurotoxicity of such recombinant proteins is highly reproducible and can be used as an interesting tool for testing novel therapeutic interventions. Administration of recombinant proteins is useful in understanding the effects of HIV-1 gene products, and so their individual contribution to the pathogenesis of HAND. However, HIV-1 infection of the brain is a chronic process, and its study would benefit from a model system allowing longer term exposure to HIV-1 gene product. Moreover, there are important differences between the situation in the striatum of patients with AIDS and models where Tat, for example, is directly injected into the CP. In these models, Tat is localized initially in extracellular space following intra-CP injection, then it is internalized in neurons and in some microglial cells, while the sites of production are focal in patients with HAND (*i.e.*, microglial cells and infected macrophages). Direct injection of Tat results in acute injury, while production of Tat is more protracted in the brain of patients with HAND.

This is in part the reason why we developed experimental models of chronic HIV-1 neurotoxicity based on recombinant SV40 (rSV40) vector-modified expression of gp120 [63] or Tat [40] in the brain.

RSV40 VECTORS DELIVER LONG-TERM TRANSGENE EXPRESSION

We previously demonstrated that SV40-derived vectors deliver long-term transgene expression to brain neurons and microglia, when administered by several different routes. rSV40s were employed in the current study because they transduce a wide range of cell types from humans and other mammals and deliver genes to cells efficiently, including neurons, whether they are resting or dividing, to achieve long-term transgene expression *in vitro* and *in vivo* [64-67]. However, they transduce astrocytes and skeletal muscle fibers poorly [64]. Several studies demonstrated that rSV40 transduction of several organs has proven long-lived [59,60,64-67,69]. Moreover, they do not elicit detectable immune response on the part of normal animals and so can be used to deliver multiple transgenes over time and in sequence [68]. For example, rSV40s do not trigger the formation of antibodies compared to other viral vectors [64]. They integrate and are not susceptible to transgene silencing [64]. Large T antigen, proto-oncogen derived from SV40, was deleted from the rSV40s we generated and used: rSV40s were not susceptible to induce tumors and tumors were never observed in animals injected with the rSV40s we used [64,66]. rSV40s transduce > 95% of cultured human NT2-derived neurons, primary human neurons [69,70] and microglia [71] without detectable toxicity.

rSV40s have some advantages compared to other vector systems. Adenovirus-mediated gene transfer to the brain is limited by innate immunity and acquired immune responses against the virus, and against foreign transgenes as well, that limit the duration of transient gene expression. Development of gutted vectors, manipulation of host immune responses and use of less immunogenic transgenes may help to circumvent these limitations, but success to date has been limited. Gene transfer to rodent and primate CNS *in vivo* has been demonstrated with lentiviral vectors derived from HIV and other lentiviruses, delivering both marker and potentially therapeutic genes to neurons [reviewed in 59,60,62]. Vectors derived from adeno-associated viruses (AAV) may deliver long term transgene expression in the brain, with little, if any, inflammatory response after intracerebral injection. Cell tropism and transduction efficiency of AAVs can be modified by using different AAV serotypes. However, transgene size is limited to under 4 kb [reviewed in 59,60,62]. In the case of the transduction of the caudate-putamen by rSV40s, the estimated number of cells that expressed the rSV40-delivered transgene was similar to figures obtained using AAV2/5, perhaps the best rAAV for transducing the striatum so far [60]. Moreover, the number of transgene-positive cells was stable throughout the 6 month study period after injection, while transgene expression reportedly declines over time with adenovirus and rAAV vectors [60].

OXIDATIVE STRESS IN HAND

Under physiologic conditions, reactive oxygen species (ROS), which include superoxide (O_2^-), hydrogen peroxide (H_2O_2) and hydroxyl radical (OH-), are generated at low levels and play important roles in signaling and metabolic pathways [72]. ROS levels are controlled by antioxidants such as superoxide dismutases (SOD), glutathione peroxidase (GPx1), glutathione and catalase. The tripeptide glutathione (γ-L-glutamyl-L-cysteinylglycine, GSH) is the key low molecular thiol antioxidant involved in the defense of brain cells against oxidative stress. Oxidative stress arises due to the disturbances of the balance in pro-oxidant/antioxidant homeostasis that further causes the generation of ROS which are potentially toxic for neurons.

Abnormalities in oxidative metabolism have been reported in many nervous system diseases. These include neurodegenerative diseases (Parkinson's disease, Alzheimer's disease, Huntington's disease, amyotrophic lateral sclerosis and cerebellar degeneration) [73-77], vascular diseases (ischemia-reperfusion) [78] or toxic reactions (chronic alcoholism) [79], as well as aging [80].

Oxidative stress plays a role in the development of HAND as well [81,82]. Fig. (**2**) shows the role of oxidative stress in HAND. Oxidative stress in HIV-1 dementia has been documented by analyses of brain tissue, including increased levels of lipid peroxidation product [*i.e.*, by immunodetection of 4-hydroxynonenal (HNE) or measurement of malondialdehyde (MDA) levels] and the presence of oxidized proteins [*i.e.*, dinitrophenol (DNP)]. Serum levels of GSH and GPx1 are decreased in HIV-1 patients while MDA levels are increased [83]. A characteristic of patients infected with HIV-1 in late stage disease is diffuse intracellular oxidation in the form of decreased availability of GSH, the main cellular antioxidant and redox buffer, and augmented lipid oxidation, which triggers a cascade of downstream signaling events.

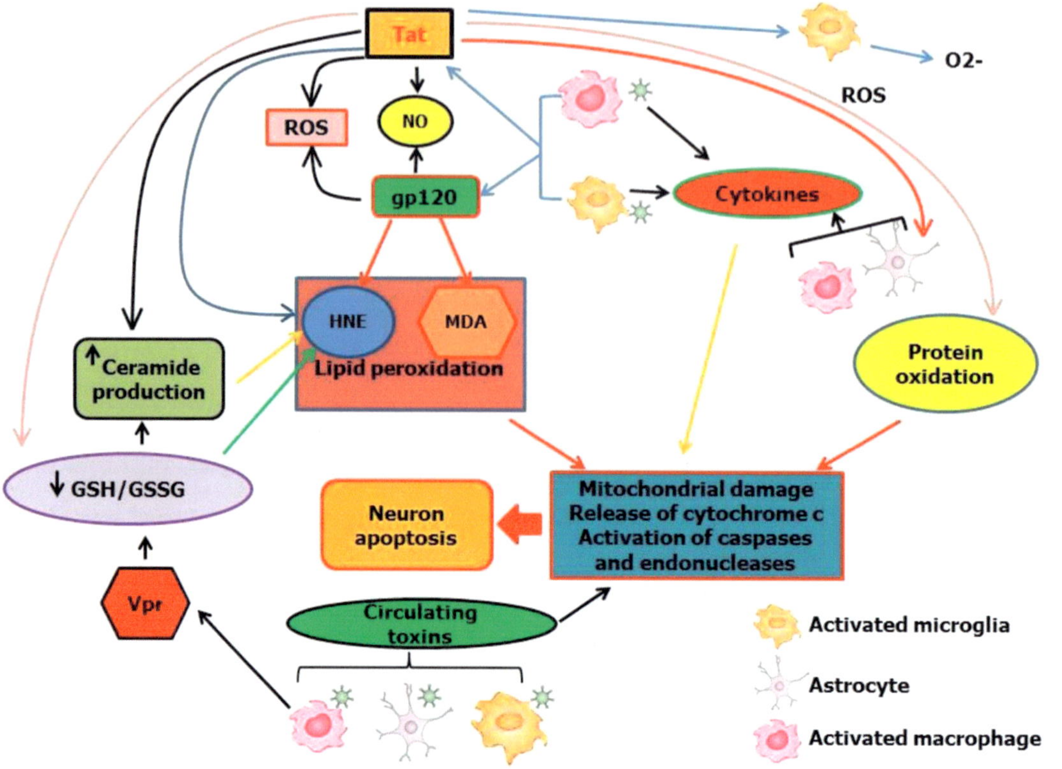

Fig. (2). Role of oxidative stress in HAND. Once in the brain, HIV-1 infects microglia and macrophages, releasing HIV-1 proteins, most likely neurotoxins, gp120, and Tat among others. Gp120 and Tat induce formation of ROS as well as peroxynitrite from NO. Gp120 and Tat cause lipid peroxidation with increase of 4-hydroxynonenal (HNE) and malondialdehyde (MDA). Tat and gp120 induce directly formation of ceramide and sphingomyelin. γ-L-glutamyl-L-cysteinylglycine (GSH) is the key low molecular thiol antioxidant involved in the defense of brain cells against ROS and thus oxidative stress. Tat and Vpr can decrease GSH, thus increasing the formation of ceramide and HNE. Tat can trigger protein oxidation by protein carbonyl formation. Tat can also induce the formation of superoxide by microglia. Lipid and protein oxidation are two elements leading to apoptosis by different ways. Cytokines released from activated microglia/macrophages upon HIV-1 infection can amplify apoptosis.

Membrane-associated oxidative stress correlates with HIV-1 dementia pathogenesis and cognitive impairment [1]. HNE-positive neurons have been demonstrated in the brains of patients with HIV-1 encephalitis [33,82,84]. In the case of HIV-1 infection, Tat and gp120 can elicit such oxidative stress [1,85] which can induce apoptosis in cultured neurons [86]. It can also damage neurons and cause cognitive dysfunction *in vivo* [87]. Tat and gp120 induce ceramide production in cultured neurons by triggering sphingomyelinase activity *via* a mechanism that involves induction of oxidative stress by CXCR4 activation [1,88]. Oxidative stress can play a role in HAND in other ways as well. Circulating toxins in the CSF, derived from HIV-1-infected cells, may damage mitochondria, leading to release of cytochrome c and then to a cascade of events leading to apoptosis [81,82]. HIV-1 gp120 and Tat can cause free radical production, possibly as part of the signal-transduction pathways they activate [1,85].

It is still unclear whether oxidative stress is the primary initiating event associated with neurodegeneration. However, a growing body of evidence implicates it as being involved in at least the propagation of cellular injury that leads to neuron death [89]. Earlier reports support the hypothesis that oxidative modifications of macromolecular cell components (lipids, proteins and nucleic acids) may be an early step in the mechanism of Tat and gp120 neurotoxicity [37,38].

ANTIOXIDANT THERAPEUTIC APPROACHES IN HAND

Rationale and Therapeutic Options

As HIV-1 infection of the brain lasts the lifetime of affected individuals, and as eradication of CNS HIV-1 is currently not possible, control of the damage caused by the virus may represent a useful approach to treatment. This could entail limiting oxidative stress-related neurotoxicity.

Experimental Data

Antioxidant therapeutic options targeting oxidative stress can be artificially divided as targeting upstream and downstream pathways. Fig. (**3**) illustrates different antioxidant therapeutic strategies against oxidative stress in the brain.

Upstream Antioxidant Therapy

Upstream preventive treatment is based on prevention of free radical generation, regulation of neuronal protein interaction with redox metals (*i.e.*, Fe) and maintaining normal cellular metabolism. Our daily diet contains several natural antioxidants (lipoic acid, vitamins E and C, β-carotene). Antioxidant therapy involving endogenous enzymes and some anti-inflammatory drugs constitute upstream therapy in ROS generation and can prevent downstream neurodegeneration. Oxyradicals have a very short life and thus can be inactivated by antioxidants before they can inflict damage to proteins, lipids or nucleic acids. Two mechanisms can be described: inactivation of oxyradicals by dietary antioxidant like vitamin E, vitamin C, and replacement of esterified membrane phospholipids with polyunsaturated fatty acids by dietary supplementation with essential fatty acids [89].

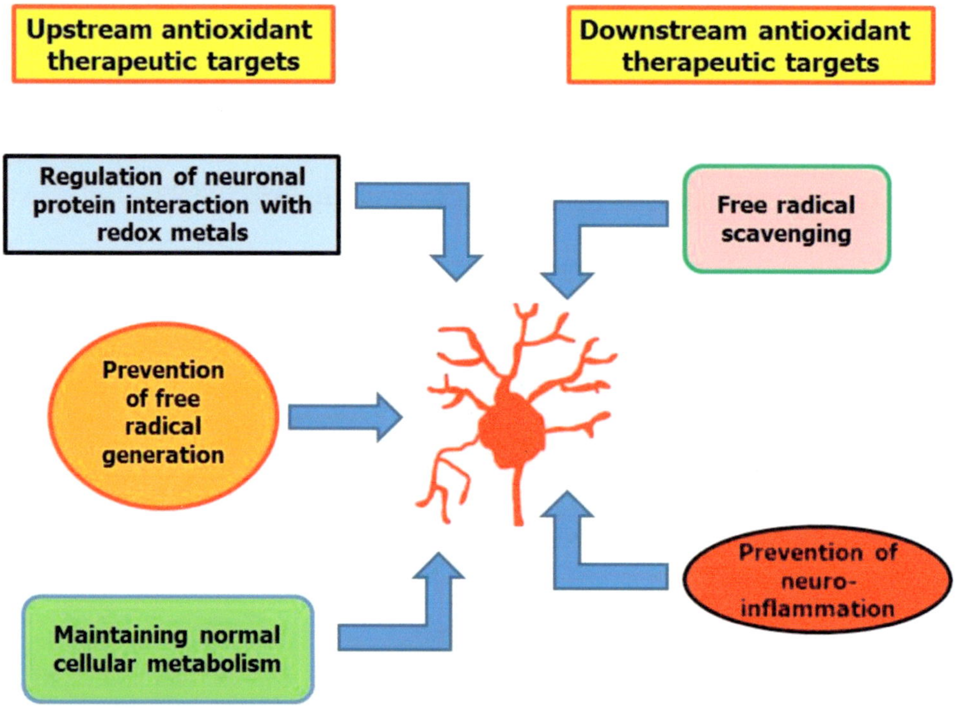

Fig. (3). Different antioxidant therapeutic strategies against oxidative stress leading to neuronal degeneration (modeled after Fig. **4** in ref. [89]).

Some components have been studied in models of HAND or can be useful in this context. Vitamin E can block the neurotoxicity induced by CSF of patients with HIV dementia [82]. Flavonoids are a group of compounds made by plants that have antioxidant and neuroprotective properties. This class of molecules has weak estrogen-receptor-binding properties and thus, do not have the side effects of estradiol. It has been described that diosgenin, a plant-derived estrogen present in yam and fenugreek can prevent neurotoxicity by HIV-1 proteins and by CSF from patients with HIV dementia [82]. Other interesting molecules include resveratrol, found in grape skins, red wine, and peanuts, as well as genistein and quercetin, found in soybeans. Polyphenols are a group of compounds with antioxidant properties. Other polyphenols like curcumin can induce stress response-protective genes, such as heme oxygenase 1 (HO-1), and can protect against heavy-metal insult to the brain and 6-hydroxydopamine (6-OHDA) in a model of Parkinson's disease, probably through reduction of lipid peroxidation and inhibition of iNOS, NF-kappaB and cyclooxygenase-2 [83]. Selenium is a key molecule in GPx1 metabolism. Some HIV-infected patients have low levels of selenium. Because selenium supplementation increases GPx1 activity, it might be beneficial in these patients [89]. N-acetyl-L-cysteine (NAC) is a nutritional supplement precursor in the formation of the antioxidant glutathione in the body and its sulfhydryl group confers antioxidant effects and is able to reduce free radicals. NAC injected i.p. into rodents increases glutathione levels in the brain and protects the CNS against the damaging effects of hydroxyl radicals and lipid peroxidation product acrolein [90]. However, NAC itself does not cross the BBB easily. In addition, bioavailability of NAC is very low because its carboxylic group loses its proton at physiological pH, making the compound negatively charged and consequently less permeable [83]. N-acetylcysteine amide (NACA), a modified form of NAC, where the carboxyl group has been replaced by an amide group, has been found to be more effective in neurotoxic cases because of its ability to permeate cell membranes and the blood-brain barrier (BBB). Treatment of animals injected intravenously with gp120, Tat and methamphetamine METH by NACA significantly rescued the animals from oxidative stress. Further, NACA-treated animals had significantly less BBB permeability as compared to the group treated with gp120+Tat+METH alone, indicating that NACA can protect the BBB from oxidative stress-induced damage in gp120, Tat and METH exposed animals [91].

Downstream Antioxidant Therapy

The therapeutic coverage of post oxidative stress events can be done by downstream antioxidant therapy. Non steroidal anti-inflammatory drugs (NSAIDS) limit the infiltration of macrophages and can reduce the inflammatory cascade induced by oxidative stress. CPI-1189, a nitrone related compound, is believed to regulate the pro-inflammatory cytokine cascade of genes in primary glial cells [89]. Minocycline is a tetracycline-derived compound that demonstrated neuroprotective profile in several models of neurodegeneration. The molecule has significant anti-inflammatory actions and can easily cross the BBB. *In vitro* data show that minocycline protected mixed neuronal cultures in an oxidative stress assay and has effective antioxidant properties with radical-scavenging potency similar to that of vitamin E [92]. Furthermore, minocycline treatment suppressed viral load in the brain, decreased the expression of CNS inflammatory markers and reduced the severity of encephalitis in a SIV model of HIV dementia [93]. A chemical moiety that resembles vitamin E in its chemical structure is the female sex hormone estrogen (estradiol) that contains a phenolic free radical scavenging site and acts as an antioxidant. It is beneficial in neurodegeneration and oxidative stress [89]. Estrogen replacement may result in improvement of cognitive function in several neurodegenerative disorders and conversely estrogen deficiency has been considered as a risk factor in some of them. Estradiol can protect against the neurotoxic effects of HIV-1 proteins in human neuronal cultures, probably by protecting the neuronal mitochondria in a receptor-independent manner [82]. However, estradiol has well known side effects in women (potential risk of developing breast or uterine cancer), and cannot be used in men or children because of feminizing effects [83]. It has been shown that several novel antioxidants (ebselen, diosgenin) can protect *in vitro* against neurotoxicity induced by CSF from patients with HIV dementia [82].

It is likely that neuroprotective therapies should benefit from multiple and combination approaches targeting different aspects and pathways of the oxidative-stress insult. For example, coupling a potent antioxidant with a compound that modifies downstream signaling pathways (*i.e.*, minocycline) could provide a synergistic neuroprotective effect, at lower doses (and thus with less toxicity) that each molecule could achieve alone. The combination of HAART with an antioxidant compound and a molecule involved in downstream antioxidant therapy could be a promising avenue in the treatment of HAND [83]. However, it should be reminded that one of the challenges in designing antioxidants to protect the CNS against ROS is the crossing of the BBB.

Clinical Trials

A few antioxidants have been tried in small prospective controlled studies in HAND. However, the findings have all been relatively disappointing so far. Selegiline (L-deprenyl), which mechanism of action is speculative, albeit it might decrease the production of ROS and serve as an anti-apoptotic factor, was used in 2 double-blind controlled studies in the pre-HAART era. The first trial involving patients with minor cognitive and motor dysfunction (MCMD) showed improvement in verbal learning and trends for improvement in recall [94,95]. The second study was a smaller study in patients with MCMD and HIV dementia and showed significant improvement in delayed recall. However, other tests were not improved. A slight improvement was noted in patients treated with OPC-14117, a lipophilic compound structurally similar to vitamin E that acts as an antioxidant by scavenging superoxide radicals [96]. CPI-1189, a lipophilic antioxidant that scavenges superoxide anion radicals and block the neurotoxicity of gp120 and TNF-alpha [97], showed no effect on neurocognition in patients with MCMD and HIV dementia [98].

Gene Delivery of Antioxidant Enzymes in HAND

Introduction

In order to deliver potent antioxidant compounds to the brain, we used gene transfer of antioxidant enzymes. Gene transfer of antioxidant enzymes has been studied in numerous models of neurological disorders by using diverse viral vectors [99-101]. We used rSV40 vectors to deliver SV(SOD1) or SV(GPx1) carrying the antioxidant enzymes Cu/Zn superoxide dismutase (SOD1) or glutathione peroxidase (GPx1) respectively, into the rat caudate putamen (CP). The safety of SV(SOD1) and SV(GPx1) delivered intra-CP has been demonstrated in rats and in Rhesus macaques monkeys, and resulting transgene expression is very durable [102]. Patterns of transgene expression are featured on Fig. (**4**). Transgene expression of antioxidant enzymes can also be achieved through intravenous injection [103].

Mitochondria are a major site of production of superoxide in normal cells and probably contribute to increased oxidative stress in numerous diseases.

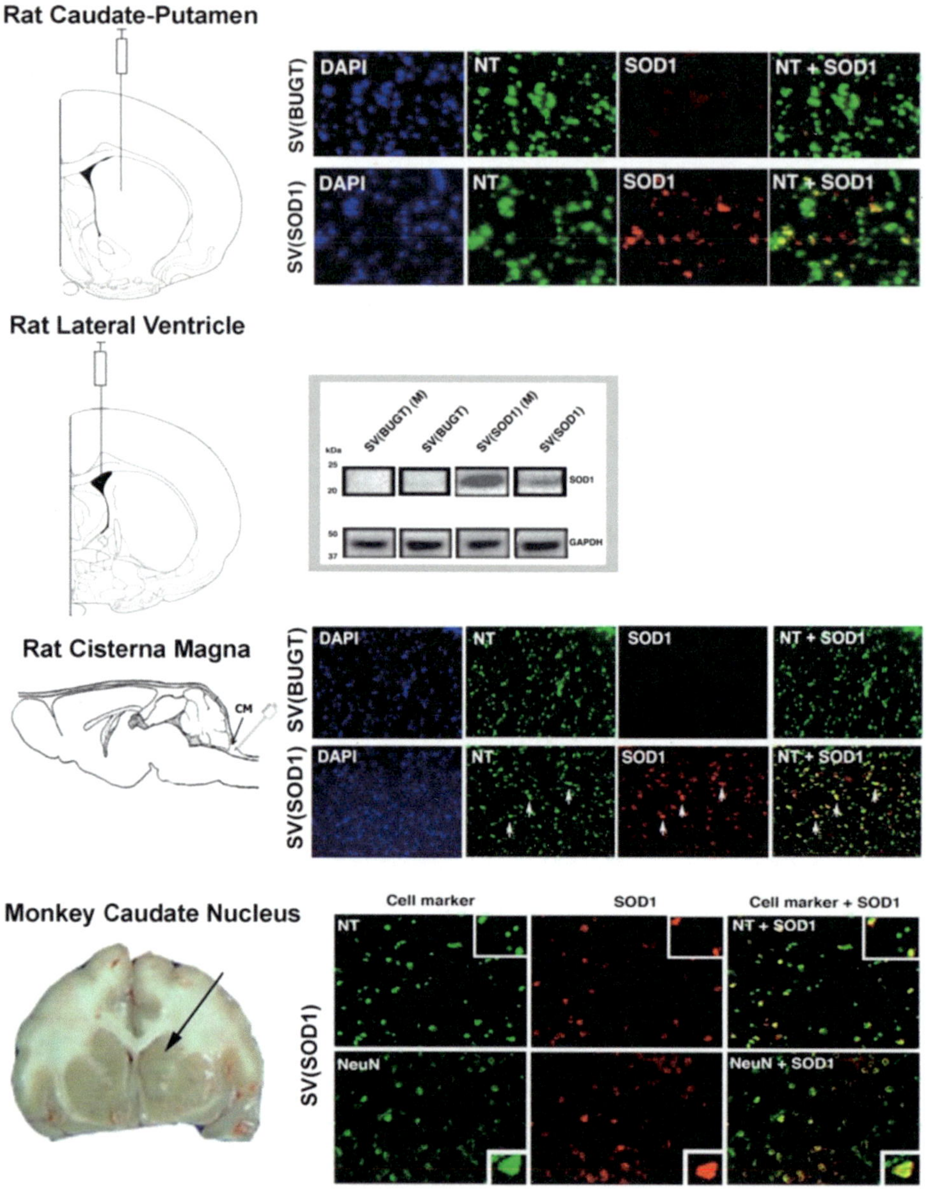

Fig. (4). SV40-mediated expression of superoxide dismutase (SOD1) in the brain of Rats and Macaques in different experimental procedures. SV(SOD1) was injected in the Caudate-Putamen, in the Lateral Ventricle or in the Cisterna Magna of Rats (with or without prior intraperitoneal injection of mannitol (M) for these 2 injections), as well as in the Caudate Nucleus of Monkeys. Transgene expression (SOD1) was assessed by immunocytochemistry or by Western blotting. SV(BUGT) is a control vector carrying an irrelevant transgene, Bilirubin-UDP-Glucuronosyl-Transferase. Nuclei were stained by 4',6-diamidino-2-phenylindole (DAPI). Neurotrace (NT) and NeuN are neuronal markers.

Overexpression of mitochondrial Mn^{2+}-superoxide dismutase results in moderate reductions in infarction in temporary ischemia. Glutathione, the major water-soluble antioxidant, is localized in both the cytosol and the mitochondria. Mice overexpressing the cytosolic enzyme $Cu^{2+}Zn^{2+}$-superoxide dismutase develop smaller infarcts than wild-type ones, with a decrease in multiple events associated with mitochondrially mediated apoptosis, including the release of cytochrome c [104]. It is thus possible that cytosolic overexpression of antioxidant enzymes delivered by SV40-derived vectors can mitigate the apoptotic events linked to mitochondria.

Gene Delivery of Antioxidant Enzymes Mitigates Oxidative Stress in Animal Models of HAND

We studied acute exposure to Tat by injecting recombinant Tat protein into the CP. Acute Tat exposure induced lipid peroxidation assessed by measuring MDA levels. Prior administration of recombinant SV40 vectors carrying antioxidant enzymes SOD1 or GPx1 protected from Tat-induced oxidative injury: MDA levels were lower in the animals given the vectors [40].

We also used a model of more chronic exposure to gp120, based on recombinant SV40 (rSV40) vector-modified expression of gp120. Prior administration of recombinant SV40 vectors carrying antioxidant enzymes, SOD1 or GPx1, was similarly protective against SV(gp120)-induced oxidative injury assessed by MDA levels and immunostaining for HNE [63]) a marker of oxidative stress [105].

However, a more direct proof of the protective effect of gene delivery of SOD1 and GPx1 was needed to be established. In the following paragraphs, we will examine this effect on gp120-induced neurotoxicity first, then on Tat-related neuronal loss.

Protection Against gp120-Elicited Apoptosis and Neuronal Loss by SV40-Mediated Gene Delivery of Antioxidant Enzymes

We first established that gp120-induced apoptosis of striatal neurons is mitigated by SV(SOD1) and SV(GPx1).

Intracerebral injection of SV(SOD1) or SV(GPx1) into the rat caudate putamen (CP), induces long-lasting transgene expression and significantly protects neurons from apoptosis and neuronal loss caused by subsequent inoculation of recombinant HIV-1 envelope glycoprotein, gp120 at the same location [60,61,106,107] (Fig. **5A**, **B**, **D**, **E**). Vector administration into the lateral ventricle (LV) [106] or cisterna magna (CM) [108], particularly if preceded by intraperitoneal mannitol, protects from intra-CP gp120-induced neurotoxicity comparably to intra-CP vector administration.

In a more chronic setting, antioxidant enzymes gene delivery mitigates SV(gp120)-induced apoptosis of striatal neurons SV(SOD1) and SV(GPx1) were administered into the CP one month before the injection of SV(gp120) in the same structure. Gene delivery of antioxidant enzymes protected against apoptosis in this animal model of protracted exposure to gp120 [63].

Finally, we also examined the role of ROS in the loss of dopaminergic neurons (DNs) from the substantia nigra (SN) in HAND. The frequency of Parkinson-like symptomatology [109-111], and DN loss, in HAND is often attributed to nonspecific DN fragility to oxidative stress. Cultured DN were more sensitive to ROS than non-dopaminergic neurons (RN): DN underwent apoptosis at far lower H_2O_2 concentrations than RN. Gene delivery of GPx1, which detoxifies H_2O_2, largely protected both neuron types. HIV-1 envelope, gp120, which elicits oxidative stress in neurons, caused apoptosis more readily in DN than in RN. However, unlike apoptosis caused by H_2O_2, gp120-induced DN apoptosis was specific: DNs were specifically more sensitive than RN to receptor-mediated [Ca(2+)](i) fluxes triggered by gp120. Gp120-induced Ca(2+) signaling in both neuron types was inhibited by GPx1 or SOD1, implicating superoxide and peroxide in ligand (gp120)-induced signaling upstream of Ca(2+) release from intracellular stores. *In vivo*, rats given 10 ng of gp120 stereotaxically showed rapid DN loss within the SN, while loss of RN in the SN and CP was slower and required > or =100 ng of gp120. Furthermore, gp120 injected into the CP was transported axonally retrograde to the SN, causing delayed DN loss there. This, too, was prevented by SOD1 or GPx1. DNs are therefore specifically hypersensitive to gp120-induced apoptosis, signaling for which involves ROS

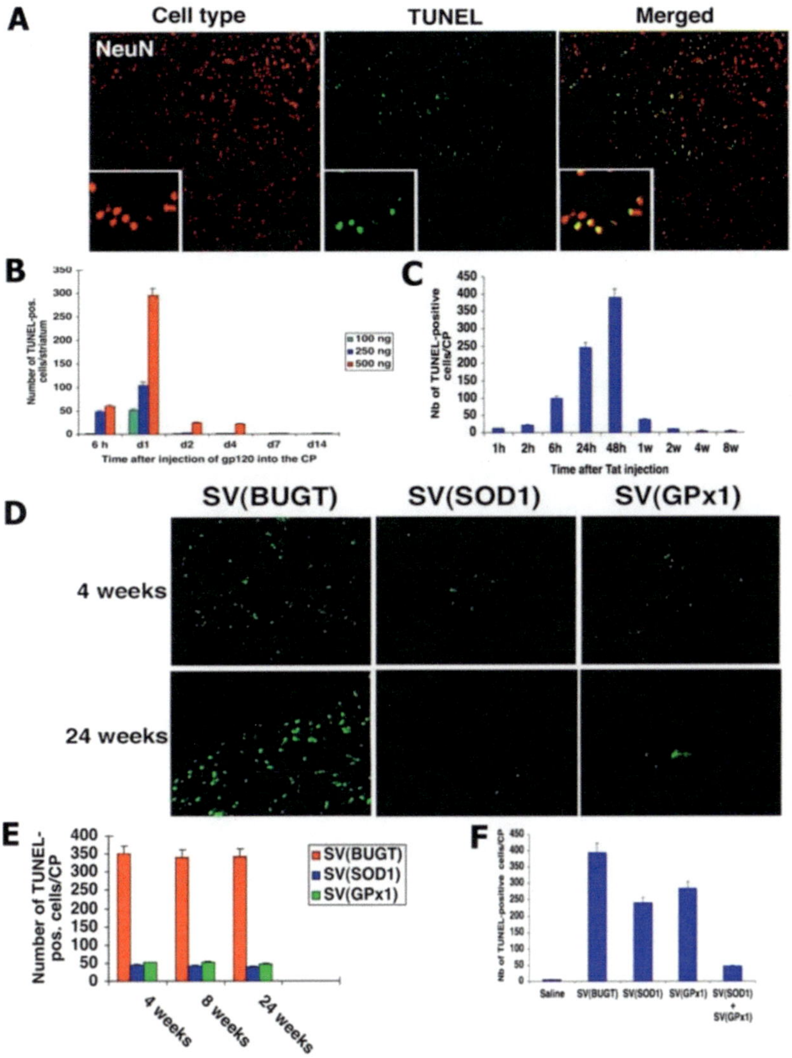

Fig. (5). SV40 mediated-overexpression of SOD1 and GPx1 protects against gp120- and Tat-induced apoptosis. **A**. Two days after injection of 10 ng Tat into the caudate-putamen (CP) of Rat, apoptototic cells (positive for TUNEL) were mainly neuronal cells, immunostained for neuN. Similar results were observed with gp120 (not shown). Apoptosis peaked one and two days after injection of gp120 (**B**) and Tat (**C**) respectively. **D**. Four and 24 weeks after injection of SV(SOD1) and SV(GPx1) into the CP, brains were injected with 500 ng 120 and assessed for TUNEL one day later. Significantly less TUNEL-positive (apoptotic) cells were observed in the CPs injected with SV(SOD1) or SV(GPx1) compared to the one administered with the control vector SV(BUGT). **E**. Reduction in the number of gp120-induced apoptotic cells after prior injection of SV(SOD1) and SV(GPx1). **F**. Prior administration of SV(SOD1), SV(GPx1) and combination of the two, reduced the number of TUNEL-positive cells observed after injection of Tat.

intermediates. These findings may help explain why DN loss and Parkinson's-like dysfunction predominate in HAND [109-111] and may apply to other neurodegenerative diseases involving the SN [112].

Gene Delivery of Antioxidant Enzymes Inhibits HIV-1 gp120-Induced Expression of Caspases

Caspases are implicated in neuronal death in neurodegenerative and other CNS diseases. The caspases family of proteases is conserved from nematodes through mammals. They are central to apoptotic death and are expressed as inactive zymogens that become cleaved during apoptosis [113]. Initiator caspases (among them caspases 8 and 9) autoactivate and self-process upon recruitment to adaptor proteins. Then, they proceed to cleave and thereby activate the executioner/effector caspases (among them caspases 3 and 6). Activated executioner/effector caspases proceed to process key structural and nuclear proteins and thereby cause the disassembly and death of the cell [114]. Two major caspases pathways have been described: the intrinsic pathway is initiated by cytochrome c release from the mitochondrion while the extrinsic pathway is initiated by the binding of ligands to plasma-membrane death receptors [104].

Intrinsic apoptosis pathway is required for fetal and postnatal brain development, but is downregulated through the suppression of the expression of one of its key mediator, caspase-3 [114]. During stroke and neurodegenerative diseases, some caspases are upregulated in the brain [113]. Cerebral ischemia triggers both the intrinsic and extrinsic pathways of apoptosis [72,104]. Mounting evidence suggests the involvement of caspases in the disease process associated with neurodegenerative diseases such as Alzheimer's disease (AD) [115] and amyotrophic lateral sclerosis (ALS) [114].

The involvement of caspases in HIV-1 neurotoxicity has been documented *in vitro* and *in vivo*. Higher levels of caspase-3 and caspase-6 have been shown in the brains of patients with HAD [12,116-118]. Both HIV-1 neurotoxins gp120 and Tat significantly increase caspase-3 activation in striatal neurons *in vitro*. However, gp120 acts in large part through the activation of caspase(s), while Tat-induced neurotoxicity is also accompanied by activating an alternative pathway involving endonuclease G [119]. Tat can induce both caspases 3/7 and 9 in hippocampal cell cultures [120]. Increased expression of caspase-3 has been shown in neurons following exposure to Tat [19,29,119,121] and to gp120 [122-125]. In HIV-1 transgenic mice, Tat induction increased the percentage of neurons expressing caspase-3 [59]. Caspase-3-positive cells were also observed in a model of protracted exposure to gp120, SV(gp120) [63].

However, so far, no study was focused on the expression of different caspases following gp120 injection. We studied the effect of gp120 on different caspases (3, 6, 8, 9) expression. Caspases production increased in the rat CP 6h after gp120 injection into the same structure. The expression of caspases peaked by 24h. Caspases colocalized mainly with neurons. There was a relationship with the concentration of gp120 injected. Both initiator (caspases 8 and 9) and effector/executioner (caspases 3 and 6) were increased after gp120 injection. We showed that about 70% of caspase-8- and 9-positive cells were TUNEL-positive while about 60% of caspase-3- and 6-positive cells were TUNEL-positive one day after intra-CP injection of gp120 [126]. These results suggest that not all caspases-positive cells undergo apoptosis, at least as assessed by the methods used here and/or at the time points we considered. It is also possible that apoptosis will occur in the remaining caspases-positive cells at later time points. Gp120-induced caspase-3 activity may also be causing nonlethal neuron injury. As previously noted [59], if cell death in response to caspase-3 depends on total enzyme activity within a cell, the caspase-3 activity detected may be below the threshold required to initiate neuron death. This is difficult to determine based on immunocytochemistry. It has also been shown that activated caspase-3 rapidly degrades itself [127].

As previously described, a link between oxidative stress and activation of some caspases seems highly probable. Prior gene delivery of the antioxidant enzymes SOD1 or GPx1 into the CP before injecting gp120 there reduced levels of gp120-induced caspases, recapitulating the effect of antioxidant enzymes on gp120-induced apoptosis observed by TUNEL. Thus, HIV-1 gp120 increased caspases expression in the CP. Prior antioxidant enzyme treatment mitigated production of these caspases, probably by reducing ROS levels. However, additional studies are needed to determine the relative contribution of the various caspases to neuronal demise in HAND.

Gp120-Mediated Abnormalities of the Blood-Brain Barrier are Mitigated by SV(SOD1) and SV(GPx1)

Reduction of MMPs Levels

Reactive oxygen species are important in the pathogenesis of HIV-induced CNS injury [105] and can be induced in brain endothelial cells by HIV-1 gp120 and Tat [128-130]. Although damage to the BBB has been documented in patients with HIV-related encephalopathy [131-133], the exact mechanism by which this injury occurs is still debated [26,134-143]. We used animal models of HAND to characterize abnormalities of the BBB in this context. Exposure to gp120, whether acute (by direct intra-CP injection) or chronic (using SV(gp120), an experimental model of ongoing production of gp120) disrupted the BBB, and led to leakage of vascular contents into the area of gp120 exposure. Gp120 was directly toxic to brain endothelial cells and gp120-mediated BBB abnormalities were related to lesions of brain microvessels [144,145]. Abnormalities of the BBB may reflect the activity of proteolytic enzymes, particularly matrix metalloproteinases (MMPs). MMPs are a family of neutral proteases that are grouped according to their protein structures. MMP-2 and MMP-9 are considered gelatinases [145], and are enzymatically activated by the cleavage of precursor propeptides. These target laminin, a major BBB component, and attack the tight junctions between endothelial cells and BBB basal laminae. MMP-2 and MMP-9 were upregulated following intra-CP gp120-injection. Gp120 greatly diminished total CP content of laminin and tight junction proteins. Reactive oxygen species have been reported to activate MMPs. Injecting gp120 into the CP induced lipid peroxidation, assessed by increased MDA levels. One product of gp120-triggered lipid peroxidation, HNE, was immunolocalized to vascular endothelial cells. Moreover, gene transfer of antioxidant enzymes using recombinant SV(SOD1) and SV(GPx1) protected against gp120-induced BBB abnormalities, including MMP-9 production [144,145]. BBB injury has also been linked to NMDA, which upregulates the proform of MMP-9 and increases MMP-9 gelatinase activity [146]. Using the NMDA receptor (NMDAR-1) inhibitor, memantine, we observed partial protection from gp120-induced BBB injury [144].

MMPs are upregulated in different neurological diseases and models of CNS injury [147-153]. Various factors, such as ROS, NO, and proteases such as plasmin and stromelysin-1, are involved in MMP activation and upregulation in CNS injury [154-156]. MMPs have been reported in the cerebrospinal fluid of HIV-1 infected patients [157,158] as well as in models of HIV-1 encephalopathy [159-162]. In rapidly progressing simian immunodeficiency virus-infected monkeys, MMP-9 levels correlate with motor and cognitive deficits [163]. Moreover, cerebrospinal fluid levels of the urokinase-type plasminogen activator receptor, which plays an important role in degradation of extracellular matrix, and hence BBB injury, are elevated in patients with HIV dementia [164].

Restoring the Balance Between MMPs and TIMPs

Relatively little is known about the roles of ROS and oxidative stress in the balance between MMPs and their endogenous tissue inhibitors (TIMPs). More than 20 MMPs and four TIMPs act together to control tightly temporally restricted, focal proteolysis of extracellular matrix (ECM) [165]. Once activated, MMPs are subject to inhibition by specific TIMPs that bind MMPs non-covalently [164]. Tissue destruction by MMPs is regulated by TIMPs and TIMPs prevent excessive MMP-related degradation of extracellular matrix components. The balance between MMPs and TIMPs is linked to ECM remodeling and imbalance between TIMPs and MMPs can lead to excessive degradation of matrix components as in rheumatoid arthritis. Tumor metastasis and angiogenesis may also reflect such imbalances. In the myocardium, ROS activate MMPs, decrease TIMPs levels and collagen synthesis [166].

A relationship between oxidative damage, MMP production and BBB disruption has been found in some lesions of the striatum [156]. We reported above that prior gene transfer of antioxidant enzymes mitigates gp120-induced MMP-9 production and BBB leakiness [143]. We studied the effect of gp120 on TIMP1- and TIMP-2 production. TIMP-1 and TIMP-2 levels increased 6h after gp120 injection into rat CP. TIMP-1 and TIMP-2 colocalized mainly with neurons (92 and 95% respectively). By 24h, expression of these protease inhibitors diverged, as TIMP-1 levels remained high but TIMP-2 subsided. Gene delivery of the antioxidant enzymes SOD1 or GPx1 into the CP before injecting gp120 there reduced levels of gp120-induced TIMP-1 and TIMP-2, recapitulating the effect of antioxidant enzymes on gp120-induced MMP-2 and MMP-9 [166]. A significant correlation was observed between MMP/TIMP upregulation and BBB leakiness. Thus, HIV-1 gp120 upregulated TIMP-1 and TIMP-2 in the CP. Prior antioxidant enzyme treatment mitigated production of these TIMPs, probably by reducing MMP expression. This might be explained by reduced ROS generation, either as effectors of damage or as signaling intermediates, or both, by antioxidant gene transfer with subsequent decrease in MMP expression. Moreover, there was a significant correlation between gp120-related BBB disturbances and MMP/TIMP upregulation. Following prior antioxidant gene delivery, a relationship was also seen between the reduction in Evans Blue (EB) extravasation and MMP-9/TIMP-1 decreased production [167].

Thus, MMPs and their inhibitors, TIMPs, are upregulated in response to oxidative stress produced in a rat model of HIV encephalopathy. In this setting, increased TIMPs may counterbalance the increase in MMPs. The centrality of ROS to this process is demonstrated by the fact that prior gene delivery of antioxidant enzymes mitigates production of TIMPs, possibly by reducing MMP expression. These results suggest that gp120-related oxidative stress induces MMP upregulation, potentially which triggers TIMP production.

SV40-Mediated Gene Delivery of Antioxidant Enzymes Reduces gp120-Induced Neuroinflammation

If neuron loss [36,61,62,107] and astrogliosis [36] have been described in animals receiving gp120 directly into their brains, a temporal relationship between neuronal degeneration, astrocytic reaction, proinflammatory cytokine production and microglial proliferation remained to be established. Rat CPs were challenged with 100-500 ng HIV-1BaL gp120, with or without prior rSV40-delivered SOD1 or GPx1. CD11b-positive microglia were increased 1 day post-challenge; Iba-1- and ED1-positive cells peaked at 7 days and 14 days respectively. Astrocyte infiltration was maximal at 7-14 days. MIP-1alpha was produced immediately, mainly by neurons. ED1- and GFAP-positive cells correlated with neuron loss and gp120 dose. We also tested the effect of more chronic gp120 exposure on neuroinflammation using an experimental model of continuing gp120 exposure.

SV(gp120), a recombinant SV40-derived gene transfer vector was inoculated into the rat CP, leading to chronic expression of gp120, ongoing apoptosis in microglia and neurons, and oxidative stress. Increase in microglia and astrocytes was seen following intra-CP SV(gp120) injection, suggesting that continuing gp120 production increased neuroinflammation. SV(SOD1) or SV(GPx1) significantly reduced MIP-1alpha and limited neuroinflammation following gp120 administration into the CP, as well as microglia and astrocytes proliferation after injection of SV(gp120) in the striatum. Thus, gp120-induced CNS injury, neuron loss and inflammation may be mitigated by antioxidant gene delivery [168].

Free radical production may be accompanied by elevated expression of MIP-1 alpha contributing to microglial recruitment and delayed neuronal death in several models of CNS injury [155,169-172]. The radical scavengers, like vitamin E analogs, may inhibit free radicals and MIP-1 alpha production, and recruitment of microglia in the injured area [172]. In models of ischemia/reperfusion injury, transgenic mice that overexpressed antioxidant enzymes, such as SOD-1 and GPx1 showed less upregulation of MIP-1 alpha and MCP-1 and less neuron loss and inflammation [173,174]. Our findings extend the principle of antioxidant protection from neuroinflammation to HIV-related injury, and suggest that rSV40 antioxidant gene delivery may be therapeutically applicable in the case of ongoing injury and neuroinflammation such as HAND.

HIV-1 envelope gp120 induces neuroinflammation when injected in the rat CP. Gp120-induced neuroinflammation correlates with neuron loss. An increase in expression of MIP-1alpha may play a role in this phenomenon, as well as ROS, as evidenced by the protective effects of rSV40-delivered antioxidant enzymes. The participation of other chemokines/cytokines in gp120-induced lesions *in vivo* remains to be established. The modulation of the interaction between these chemokines/cytokines and their ligands needs to be investigated.

Neuroprotection Against Tat-Induced Brain Injury by SV(SOD1) and SV(GPx1)

Tat activates multiple signaling pathways, in one of which superoxide acts as an intermediate, while the other utilizes peroxide [85]. Tat elicits lipid peroxidation (induced by generation of ROS), one of the elements leading to cell death. In culture, SV(SOD1) and SV(GPx1) not only increase levels of antioxidant enzymes and decrease lipid peroxidation but also have an effect on Tat-induced cytosol calcium fluxes [85]. Neuroprotection from apoptosis caused by Tat requires detoxification of both O_2^- and H_2O_2 *via* SOD1 and GPx1. Combining SV(SOD1) and SV(GPx1) provides such protection.

We studied acute exposure by injecting recombinant Tat protein into the CP. Ongoing Tat expression, which more closely mimics HIV-1 infection of the brain, was studied by delivering Tat-expression over time using an SV40-derived gene delivery vector, SV(Tat). Both acute and chronic Tat exposure induced lipid peroxidation and neuronal apoptosis. Prior administration of recombinant SV40 vectors carrying antioxidant enzymes SOD1 or GPx1 protected from Tat-induced oxidative injury and apoptosis (Fig. **5C**, **F**). Thus, injection of recombinant HIV-1 Tat and the expression vector, SV(Tat), into the rat CP cause respectively acute or ongoing apoptosis and oxidative stress in neurons and may represent useful animal models for studying the pathogenesis and, potentially, treatment of HIV-1 Tat-related damage [40].

CONCLUSIONS

HIV-1-associated neurocognitive disorder (HAND) is an increasingly common, progressive disease characterized by progressively deteriorating CNS function. HIV-1 gene products, particularly gp120 and Tat, elicit ROS that lead to oxidant injury, cause neuron apoptosis, as well as subsequent consequences (*e.g.* neuroinflammation, abnormalities of the BBB). Understanding of, and developing therapies for, HAND requires accessible models of the disease. We have devised experimental approaches to studying the acute and chronic effects of gp120 and Tat on the CNS. Even though HIV-1 gp120 and Tat cannot be solely responsible for the pathogenesis of HAND, the animal models used in the present study are able to recapitulate many aspects of HAND. These approaches to gp120 and Tat administration may therefore represent useful animal models for studying the pathogenesis and treatment of HIV-1 gp120- and Tat-related damage. Gene delivery of antioxidant enzymes by recombinant SV40-derived vectors protects against gp120 and Tat-induced oxidative stress and neuronal apoptosis, opening new avenues for potential therapeutics of HAND.

ACKNOWLEDGEMENTS

This work was supported by NIH grants MH70287, MH69122 and AH48244 to DS.

CONFLICT OF INTEREST

The authors state that there is no conflict of interest.

REFERENCES

[1] Mattson MP, Haughey NJ, Nath A. Cell death in HIV dementia. Cell Death Diff 2005; 12: 893-904.
[2] Major EO, Rausch D, Marra C, Clifford D. HIV-associated dementia. Science 2000; 288: 440-42.
[3] McArthur JC, Hoover DR, Bacellar H, *et al.* Dementia in AIDS patients: incidence and risk factors. Multicenter AIDS Cohort Study. Neurology 1993; 43: 2245-52.
[4] Koutsilieri, E; Sopper, S; Scheller, C; *et al.* Parkinsonism in HIV dementia. J Neural Transm 2002; 109: 767-75.
[5] Antinori A, Arendt G, Becker JT, *et al.* Updated research nosology for HIV-associated neurocognitive disorders. Neurology 2007; 69: 1789-99.
[6] Woods SP, Moore DJ, Weber E, Grant I. Cognitive neuropsychology of HIV-associated neurocognitive disorders. Neuropsychol Rev 2009; 19: 152-168.
[7] McArthur JC, Brew BJ, Nath A. Neurological complications of HIV infection. Lancet Neurol 2005; 4: 543-55.
[8] Nath A, Sacktor N. Influence of highly active antiretroviral therapy on persistence of HIV in the central nervous system. Curr Opin Neurol 2006; 19: 358-61.
[9] Ances BM, Ellis RJ. Dementia and neurocognitive disorders due to HIV-1 infection. Semin Neurol 2007; 27: 86-92.
[10] Rumbaugh JA, Nath A. Developments in HIV neuropathogenesis. Curr Pharm Des 2006; 12: 1023-44.
[11] Gonzalez-Scarano F, Martin-Garcia J. The neuropathogenesis of AIDS. Nat Rev Immunol 2005; 5: 69-81.
[12] Kaul M, Garden GA, Lipton SA. Pathways to neuronal injury and apoptosis in HIV-associated dementia. Nature 2001; 410: 988-94.
[13] van de Bovenkamp M, Nottet HS, Pereira CF. Interactions of human immunodeficiency virus-1 proteins with neurons: possible role in the development of human immunodeficiency virus-1 associated dementia. Eur J Clin Invest 2002; 32: 619-27.
[14] King, JE; Eugenin, EA; Buckner, CM, Berman JW. HIV Tat and neurotoxicity. Microbes Infect 2006; 8: 1347-57.

[15] Garden GA, Guo W, Jayadev S, *et al.* HIV associated neurodegeneration requires p53 in neurons and microglia. FASEB J 2004; 18: 1141-43.

[16] Xu, Y; Kulkosky, J; Acheampong, E, Nunnari G, Sullivan J, Pomerantz RJ. HIV-1-mediated apoptosis of neuronal cells: proximal molecular mechanisms of HIV-1-induced encephalopathy. Proc Natl Acad Sci US*A* 2004; 101: 7070-75.

[17] Meucci O, Fatatis A, Simen AA, Bushell TJ, Gray PW, Miller RJ. Chemokines regulate hippocampal neuronal signaling and gp120 neurotoxicity. Proc Natl Acad Sci USA 1998; 95: 14500-505.

[18] Regulier EG, Reiss K, Khalili K, *et al.* T-cell and neuronal apoptosis in HIV infection: implications for therapeutic intervention. Int Rev Immunol 2004; 23: 25-59.

[19] Kruman II, Nath A, Mattson MP. HIV-1 protein Tat induces apoptosis of hippocampal neurons by a mechanism involving caspase activation, calcium overload, and oxidative stress. Exp Neurol 1998; 154: 276-88.

[20] Kaul M, Lipton SA. Chemokines and activated macrophages in HIV gp120-induced neuronal apoptosis. Proc Natl Acad Sci USA 1999; 96: 8212-16.

[21] Lipton SA, Choi YB, Pan ZH, *et al.* A redox-based mechanism for the neuroprotective and neurodestructive effects of nitric oxide and related nitrosocompounds. Nature 1993; 364: 626-32.

[22] Dreyer EB, Kaiser PK, Offermann JT, Lipton SA. HIV-1 coat protein neurotoxicity prevented by calcium channel antagonists. Science 1990; 248: 364-67.

[23] Adamson DC, Wildemann B, Sasaki MD; *et al.* Immunologic NO synthase elevation in severe AIDS dementia and induction by HIV-1 gp41. Science 1996; 274: 1917-20.

[24] Adamson DC, Kopnisky KL, Dawson TM, Dawson VL. Mechanisms and structural determinants of HIV-1 coat protein, gp41-induced neurotoxicity. J Neurosci 1999; 19: 64-71.

[25] Eugenin EA, D'Aversa TG, Lopez L, Calderon TM, Berman JW. MCP-1 (CCL2) protects human neurons and astrocytes from NMDA or HIV-tat-induced apoptosis. J Neurochem 2003; 85: 1299-311.

[26] Eugenin EA, King JE, Nath A, *et al.* HIV-tat induces formation of an LRP-PSD-95-NMDAR-nNOS complex that promotes apoptosis in neurons and astrocytes. Proc Natl Acad Sci USA 2007; 104: 3438-43.

[27] Ghezzi S, Noolan DM, Aluigi MG, *et al.* Inhibition of CXCR-3-dependent HIV-1 infection by extracellular HIV-1 Tat. Biochem Biophys Res Commun 2000; 270: 992-96.

[28] Magnuson DS, Knudsen BE, Geiger JD, Brownstone RM, Nath A. Human immunodeficiency virus type 1 tat activates non-N-methyl-o-aspartate excitatory amino receptors and causes neurotoxicity. Ann Neurol 1995; 37: 373-80.

[29] Bonavia R, Bajetto A, Barbero S, Albini A, Noonan DM, Schettini G. HIV-1 Tat causes apoptosis death and calcium homeostasis alterations in rat neurons. Biochem Biophys Res Commun 2001; 288: 301-8.

[30] Haughey NJ, Nath A, Mattson MP. HIV-1 tat through phosphorylation of NMDA receptors potentiates glutamate excitotoxicity. J Neurochem 2001; 78: 457-67.

[31] Norman JP, Perry SW, Reynolds HM, *et al.* HIV-1 Tat activates neuronal ryanodine receptors with rapid induction of the unfolded protein response and mitochondrial hyperpolarization. PLoS ONE 2008; 3: e3731.

[32] Nath A, Haughey NJ, Jones M, Anderson C, Bell JE, Geiger JD. Synergistic neurotoxicity by human immunodeficiency virus proteins tat and gp120: protection by memantine. Ann Neurol 2000; 47: 186-94.

[33] Haughey NJ, Cutler RG, Tamara A, *et al.* Perturbation of sphingolipid metabolism and ceramide production in HIV-dementia. Ann Neurol 2004; 5: 257-67.

[34] Bonfoco E, Krainc D, Ankarcrona M, Nicotera P, Lipton SA. Apoptosis and necrosis: two distinct events induced, respectively, by mild and intense insults with N-methyl-D-aspartate or nitric oxide/superoxide in cortical cell cultures. Proc Natl Acad Sci USA 1995; 92: 7162-66.

[35] Jones M, Olafson K, Del Bigio MR, Peeling J, Nath A. Intraventricular injection of human immunodeficiency virus type 1 (HIV-1) tat protein causes inflammation, gliosis, apoptosis, and ventricular enlargment. J Neuropathol Exp Neurol 1998; 57: 563-70.

[36] Bansal AK, Mactutus CF, Nath A, Maragos W, Hauser KF, Booze RM. Neurotoxicity of HIV-1 proteins gp120 and Tat in the rat striatum. Brain Res 2000; 879: 42-49.

[37] Aksenov MY, Hasselrot U, Bansal AK, *et al.* Oxidative damage induced by the injection of HIV-1 Tat protein in the rat striatum. Neurosci Lett 2001; 305: 5-8.

[38] Aksenov MY, Hasselrot U, Wu G, *et al.* Temporal relationship between HIV-1 Tat-induced neuronal degeneration, OX-42 immunoreactivity, reactive astrocytosis, and protein oxidation in the rat striatum. Brain Res 2003; 987: 1-9.

[39] Theodore S, Cass WA, Maragos WF. Methamphetamine and human immunodeficiency virus protein Tat synergize to destroy dopaminergic terminals in the rat striatum. Neuroscience 2006; 137: 925-35.

[40] Agrawal L, Louboutin JP, Reyes BAS, VanBockstaele EJ, Strayer DS. HIV-1 Tat neurotoxicity: a model of acute and chronic exposure, and neuroprotection by gene delivery of antioxidant enzymes. Neurobiol Dis 2012; 45: 657-70.

[41] Wiley CA, Baldwin M, Achim CL. Expression of HIV regulatory and structural mRNA in the central nervous system. AIDS 1996; 10: 843-47.

[42] Hudson L, Liu J, Nath A, *et al.* Detection of the human immunodeficiency virus regulatory protein tat in CNS tissues. J Neurovirol 2000; 6: 144-55.

[43] Hoshino S, Sun B, Konishi M, *et al.* Vpr in plasma of HIV type 1-positive patients is correlated with the HIV type 1 RNA titers. AIDS Res Hum Retroviruses 2007; 23: 391-97.

[44] Levy DN, Refaeli Y, MacGregor RR, Weiner DB. Serum Vpr regulates productive infection and latency of human immunodeficiency virus type 1. Proc Natl Acad Sci U S A 1994; 91, 10873-77.

[45] Levy DN, Refaeli Y, Weiner DB. Extracellular Vpr protein increases cellular permissiveness to human immunodeficiency virus replication and reactivates virus from latency. J Virol 1995; 69: 1243-52.

[46] Ferrucci R, Nonnemacher MR, Cohen EA, Wiqdahl B. Extracellular human immunodeficiency 1 virus type 1 viral protein R causes reductions in astrocytic ATP and glutathione levels compromising the antioxidant reservoir. Virus Res 2012; 167: 358-69.

[47] Patel CA, Mukhtar M, Pomerantz RJ. HIV-1 Vpr induces apoptosis in human neuronal cells. J Virol 2000; 74: 9717-26.

[48] Sabbah EN, Roques BP. Critical implication of the (70-96) domain of human immunodeficiency virus type 1 Vpr protein in apoptosis of primary rat cortical and striatal neurons. J Neurovirol 2005; 11: 489-502.

[49] Rom I, Deshmane SL, Mukerjee R, Khalili K, Amini S, Sawaya BE. HIV-1 Vpr deregulates calcium secretion in neural cells. Brain Res 2009; 1275: 81-86.
[50] Trillo-Pazos G, McFarlane-Abdulla E, Campbell IC, Pilkington GJ, Everall IP. Recombinant nef HIV-IIIB protein is toxic to human neurons in culture. Brain Res 2000; 864: 315-26.
[51] Saito Y, Sharer LR, Epstein LG, *et al*. Overexpression of nef as a marker for restricted HIV-1 infection of astrocytes in postmortem pediatric central nervous tissues. Neurology 1994; 44: 474-81.
[52] Mabrouk K, Van Rietschoten J, Vives, E, Darbon H, Rochat H, Sabatier JM. Lethal neurotoxicity in mice of the basic domains of HIV and SIV Rev proteins. Study of these regions by circular dichroism. FEBS Lett 1991; 289: 13-17.
[53] Hurtrel M, Ganiere JP, Guelfi JF, *et al*. Comparison of early and late feline immunodeficiency virus encephalopathies. AIDS 1992: 6: 399-406.
[54] Thormar H. Maedi-Visna virus and its relationship to human deficiency virus. AIDS Rev 2005; 7: 233-45.
[55] Lackner AA, Veazey RS. Current concepts in AIDS pathogenesis: Insights from the SIV/macaque model. Annu Rev Med. 2007; 58: 461-76.
[56] Toggas SM, Masliah E, Rockenstein EM, Rall GF, Abraham CR, Mucke L. Central nervous system damage produced by expression of the HIV-1 coat protein gp120 in transgenic mice. Nature 1994; 367: 188-93.
[57] Avgeropoulos N, Kelley B, Middaugh L, *et al*. SCID mice with HIV encephalitis develop behavioral abnormalities. J Acquir Immune Defic Syndr 1998; 18: 13-20.
[58] Gorantla S, Makarov E, Finke-Dwyer J, *et al*. HIV-1 infection of humanized mice and viral neuropathogenesis by Gorantla *et al*., Am J Pathol, 2010; 177: 2938-49
[59] Bruce-Keller AJ, Turchan-Cholewo J, Smart EJ, *et al*. Morphine causes rapid increases in glial activation and neuronal injury in the striatum of inducible HIV-1 Tat transgenic mice. Glia 2008; 56: 1414-27.
[60] Agrawal L, Louboutin JP, Reyes BAS, Van Bockstaele E, Strayer DS. Antioxidant enzyme gene delivery to protect from HIV-1 gp120-induced neuronal apoptosis. Gene Ther 2006; 13: 1645-56.
[61] Louboutin JP, Agrawal L, Reyes BAS, Van Bockstaele EJ, Strayer DS. Protecting neurons from HIV-1 gp120-induced oxidant stress using both localized intracerebral and generalized intraventricular administration of antioxidant enzymes delivered by SV40-derived vectors. Gene Ther 2007; 14: 1650-61.
[62] Nosheny RL, Bachis A, Acquas E, Mocchetti I. Human immunodeficiency virus type 1 glycoprotein gp120 reduces the levels of brain-derived neurotrophic factor *in vivo*: potential implication for neuronal cell death. Eur J Neurosci 2004; 20: 2857-64.
[63] Louboutin JP, Agrawal L, Reyes BAS, Van Bockstaele EJ, Strayer DS. A rat model of human immunodeficiency virus 1 encephalopathy using envelope glycoprotein gp120 expression delivered by SV40 vectors. J Neuropathol Exp Neurol 2009; 68: 456-73.
[64] Strayer DS. Gene therapy using SV40-derived vectors: what does the future hold? J Cell Physiol 1999; 181: 375-84.
[65] Strayer DS, Kondo R, Milano J, Duan LX. Use of SV40-based vectors to transduce foreign genes to normal human peripheral blood mononuclear cells. Gene Ther 1997; 4: 219-25.

[66] Strayer DS, Lamothe M, Wei D, Milano J, Kondo R. Generation of recombinant SV40 vectors for gene transfer. SV40 protocols. In: Raptis L, ed. *Methods in Molecular biology.* Humana Press, Totowa, NJ, 2001; vol. 165, pp. 103-117.

[67] Sauter BV, Parashar B, Chowdhury NR, *et al.* A replication-deficient rSV40 mediates liver-directed gene transfer and a long-term amelioration of jaundice in gunn rats. Gastroenterology 2000; 119: 1348-57.

[68] McKee HJ, Strayer DS. Immune responses against SIV envelope glycoprotein, using recombinant SV40 as a vaccine delivery vector. Vaccine 2002; 20: 3613-25.

[69] Cordelier P, Calarota SA, Pomerantz RJ, Xiaoshan J, Strayer DS. Inhibition of HIV-1 in the central nervous system by IFN-alpha2 delivered by an SV40 vector. J Interferon Cytokine Res 2003; 23: 477-88.

[70] Cordelier P, Van Bockstaele E, Calarota SA, Strayer DS. Inhibiting AIDS in the central nervous system: gene delivery to protect neurons from HIV. Mol Ther 2003; 7: 801-10.

[71] Cordelier P, Strayer DS. Using gene delivery to protect HIV-susceptible CNS cells: inhibiting HIV replication in microglia. Virus Res 2006; 118: 87-97.

[72] Broughton BRS, Reutens DC, Sobey CG. Apoptotic mechanisms after cerebral ischemia. Stroke 2009; 40: e331-e339.

[73] Dexter DT, Carter CJ, Wells FR, *et al.* Basal lipid peroxidation in substantia nigra is increased in Parkinson's disease. J Neurochem 1987; 52: 381-89.

[74] Rosen DR, Siddique T, Patterson D; *et al.* Mutations in Cu/Zn superoxide dismutase are associated with familial amyotrophic lateral sclerosis. Nature 1993; 362: 59-62.

[75] Beal MF. Aging, energy, and oxidative stress in neurodegenerative diseases. Ann Neurol 1995; 38: 357-66.

[76] Smith MA, Perry G. Free radical damage, iron, and Alzheimer's disease. J Neurol Sci 1995; 134: 92-94.

[77] Smith MA, Sayre LM, Monnier VM, Perry G. Radical ageing in Alzheimer's disease. Trends Neurosci 1995; 18: 172-76.

[78] Cao W, Carney JM, Duchon A, Floyd RA, Chevion M. Oxygen free radicals involvement in ischemia and reperfusion of the brain injury to brain. Neurosci Lett 1998; 88: 233-38.

[79] Montoliu C, Valles S, Renau-Piqueras J, Guerri C. Ethanol-induced oxygen radical formation and lipid peroxidation in rat brain: effect of chronic alcohol consumption. J Neurochem 1994; 63: 1855-62.

[80] Smith CD, Carney JM, Starke-Reed PE, *et al.* Excess brain protein oxidation and enzyme dysfunction in normal aging and in Alzheimer's disease. Proc Natl Acad Sci USA 1991; 88: 10540-43.

[81] Mollace V, Nottet HS, Clayette P, *et al.* Oxidative stress and neuroAIDS: triggers, modulators and novel antioxidants. Trends Neurosci 2001; 24: 411-16.

[82] Turchan J, Pocernich CB, Gairola C, *et al.* Oxidative stress in HIV demented patients and protection *ex vivo* with novel antioxidants. Neurology 2003; 60: 307-14.

[83] Steiner J, Haughey N, Li W, *et al.* Oxidative stress and therapeutic approaches in HIV dementia. Antioxid Redox Sign 2006; 8: 2089-100.

[84] Cutler RG, Haughey NJ, Tammara A, *et al.* Dysregulation of sphingolipids and sterol metabolism by ApoE4 in HIV dementia. Neurology 2004; 63: 626-30.

[85] Agrawal L, Louboutin JP, Strayer DS. Preventing HIV-1 Tat-induced neuronal apoptosis using antioxidant enzymes: mechanistic and therapeutic implications. Virology 2007; 363: 462-72.

[86] Kruman I, Bruce-Keller AJ, Bredesen D, Waq G, Mattson MP. Evidence that 4-hydroxynonenal mediates oxidative stress-induced neuronal apoptosis. J Neurosci 1997; 17: 5089-100.
[87] Bruce-Keller AJ, Li YJ, Lovell MA, *et al.* 4-Hydroxynonenal, a product of lipid peroxidation, damages cholinergic neurons and impairs visuospatial memory in rats. J Neuropathol Exp Neurol 1998; 57: 257-67.
[88] Bruce-Keller AJ, Barger SW, Moss NI, Pham JT, Keller JN, Nath A. Proinflammatory and pro-oxidant properties of Tat in a microglial cell line: attenuation by 17β-estradiol. J Neurochem 2001; 78: 1315-24.
[89] Uttara B, Singh AV, Zamboni P, Mahajan RT. Oxidative stress and neurodegenerative diseases: a review of upstream and downstream antioxidant therapeutic options. Curr Neuropharmacol 2009; 7: 65-74.
[90] Pocernich CB, La Fontaine M, Butterfield DA. *In vivo* glutathione elevation protects against hydroxyl free radical-induced protein oxidation in rat brain. Neurochem Int. 2000; 36: 185-91.
[91] Banerjee A, Zhanq X, Manda KR, Banks WA, Ercal N. HIV proteins (gp120 and Tat) and methamphetamine in oxidative stress-induced damage in the brain: potential role of the thiol antioxidant N-acetylcysteine amide. Free Rad Biol Med 2010; 48: 1388-98.
[92] Kraus RL, Pasieczny R, Lariosa-Willingham K, Turner MS, Jiang A, Trauger JW. Antioxidant properties of minocycline: neuroprotection in an oxidative stress assay and direct radical-scavenging activity. J Neurochem 2005; 94: 819-27.
[93] Zink MC, Uhrlaub J, DeWitt J, *et al.* Neuroprotective anti-human immunodeficiency virus activity of minocycline. JAMA 2005; 293: 2003-11.
[94] Consortium D. A randomized, double-blind, placebo-controlled trial of deprenyl and thioctic acid in human immunodeficiency virus-associated cognitive impairment: Dana Consortium on the therapy of HIV dementia and related cognitive disorders. Neurology 1998; 50: 645-51.
[95] Sacktor N, Schifitto G, McDermott MP, Marder K, McArthur JC, Kieburtz K. Transdermal seleginine in HIV-associated cognitive impairment: pilot, placebo-controlled study. Neurology 2000; 54: 233-35.
[96] Consortium D. Safety and tolerability of the antioxidant OPC-14117 in HIV-associated cognitive impairment: the Dana Consortium on the therapy of HIV dementia and related cognitive disorders. Neurology 1997; 49: 142-46.
[97] Pulliam L, Irwin I, Kusdra L, Rempel H, Flitter WD, Garland WA. CPI-1189 attenuates effects of suspected neurotoxins associated with AIDS dementia: a possible role for ERK activation. Brain Res 2001; 893: 95-103.
[98] Clifford DB, McArthur JC, Schifitto G, *et al.* A randomized clinical trial of CPI-1189 for HIV-associated cognitive-motor impairment. Neurology 2002; 59: 1568-73.
[99] Watanabe Y, Chu Y, Andresen JJ, Nakane H, Faraci FM, Heistad DD. Gene transfer of extracellular superoxide dismutase reduces cerebral vasospasm after subarachnoid hemorrhage. Stroke 2003; 34: 434-40.
[100] Hoehn B, Yenari MA, Sapolsky RM, Steinberg GK, *et al.* Glutathione peroxidase oveexpression inhibits cytochrome, e C release and proapoptotic mediators to protect neurons from experimental stroke. Stroke 2003; 34: 2489-94.

[101] Ridet JL, Bensadoun JC, Deglon N, Aebischer P, Zurn AD. Lentivirus-mediated expression of glutathione peroxidase: neuroprotection in murine models of Parkinson's disease. Neurobiol Dis 2006; 21: 29-34.
[102] Louboutin JP, Marusich E, Fisher-Perkins J, Dufour JP, Bunnell BA, Strayer DS. Gene transfer to the Rhesus monkey brain using SV40-derived vectors is durable and safe. Gene Ther 2011; 18: 682-91.
[103] Louboutin JP, Chekmasova AA, Marusich E, Chowdhury JR, Strayer DS. Efficient CNS gene delivery by intravenous injection. Nature Meth 2010; 7: 905-07.
[104] Sims NR, Muyderman H. Mitochondria, oxidative metabolism and cell death in stroke. Biochim Biophys Acta 2010; 1802: 80-91.
[105] Sacktor N, Haughey N, Cutler R, *et al.* Novel markers of oxidative stress in actively progressive HIV dementia. J Neuroimmunol 2004; 157: 176-84.
[106] Louboutin JP, Reyes BAS, Agrawal L, Van Bockstaele EJ, Strayer DS. Strategies for CNS-directed gene delivery: *in vivo* gene transfer to the brain using SV40-derived vectors. Gene Ther 2007; 14: 939-49.
[107] Louboutin JP, Agrawal L, Reyes BAS, Van Bockstaele EJ, Strayer DS. HIV-1 gp120 neurotoxicity proximally and at a distance from the point of exposure: Protection by rSV40 delivery of antioxidant enzyme. Neurobiol Dis 2009; 34: 462-76.
[108] Louboutin JP, Reyes BAS, Agrawal L, Van Bockstaele EJ, Strayer DS. Intracisternal rSV40 administration provides effective pan-CNS transgene expression. Gene Ther 2012; 19: 114-18.
[109] Mirsattari SM, Power C, Nath, A. Parkinsonism with HIV infection. Mov Disord 1998; 13: 684-89.
[110] Ramachandran G, Glickman L, Levenson J, Rao C. Incidence of extrapyramidal syndromes in AIDS patients and a comparison group of medically ill patients. J Neuropsychiatry Clin Neurosci 1997; 9: 579-83.
[111] Sardar AM, Czudek C, Reynolds GP. Dopamine deficits in the brain: the neurochemical basis of parkinsonism symptoms in AIDS. Neuroreport 1996; 7: 9-12.
[112] Agrawal L, Louboutin JP, Marusich, E, Reyes BAS, Van Bockstaele, EJ, Strayer DS. Dopaminergic neurotoxicity of HIV-1 gp120: reactive oxygen species as signaling intermediates. Brain Res 2010; 1306: 116-30.
[113] Ribe EM, Serrano-Saiz E, Akpan N, Troy CM. Mechanisms of neuronal death in disease: defining the models and the players. Biochem. J 2008; 415: 165-82.
[114] Madden SD, Cotter TG. Cell death in brain development and degeneration: control of caspase expression may be key! Mol Neurobiol 2008; 37: 1-6.
[115] Rohn TT. The role of caspases in Alzheimer's disease: potential novel therapeutic opportunities. Apoptosis 2010; 15: 1403-09.
[116] Petito CK, Roberts B. Evidence of apoptotic cell death in HIV encephalitis. Am J Pathol. 1995; 146: 1121-30.
[117] James HJ, Sharer LR, Zhang Q, *et al.* Expression of caspase-3 in brains from paediatric patients with HIV-1 encephalitis. Neuropathol Appl Neurobiol 1999; 25: 380-86.
[118] Noorbakhsh F, Ramachandran R, Barsby N, *et al.* MicroRNA profiling reveals new aspects of HIV neurodegeneration: caspase-6 regulates astrocyte survival. FASEB J 2010; 24: 1799-812.

[119] Singh IN, Goody RJ, Dean C, *et al.* Apoptotic cell death of striatal neurons induced by human immunodeficiency virus-1 Tat and gp120: Differential involvement of caspase-3 and endonuclease G. J Neurovirol 2004; 10: 141-51.

[120] Aksenov MY, Aksenova MV, Mactutus CF, Booze RM. Attenuated neurotoxicity of the transactivation-defective HIV-Tat protein in hippocampal cell cultures. Exp Neurol 2009; 219: 586-90.

[121] Kruman II, Mattson MP. Pivotal role of mitochondrial calcium uptake in neural cell apoptosis and necrosis. J Neurochem 1999; 72: 529-40.

[122] Nosheny RL, Bachis A, Aden SA, De Bernardi MA, Mocchetti I. Intrastriatal administration of human immunodeficiency virus-1 glycoprotein 120 reduces glial cell-line derived neurotrophic factor levels and causes apoptosis in the substantia nigra. J Neurobiol 2006; 66: 1311-21.

[123] Nosheny RL, Ahmed F, Yakoviev A, *et al.* Brain-derived neurotrophic factor prevents the nigrostriatal degeneration induced by human immunodeficiency virus-1 glycoprotein 120 *in vivo*. Eur J Neurosci 2007; 25: 2275-84.

[124] Bachis A, Aden SA, Nosheny RL, Andrews PM, Mocchetti I. Axonal transport of human immunodeficiency virus type 1 envelope protein glycoprotein 120 is found in association with neuronal apoptosis. J Neurosci 2006; 26: 6771-80.

[125] Ahmed F, McArthur L, De Bernardi M, Mocchetti I. Retrograde and anterograde transport of HIV protein gp120 in the nervous system. Brain Behav Immun 2009; 23: 355-64.

[126] Louboutin JP, Reyes BAS, Agrawal L, Van Bockstaele EJ, Strayer DS. Gene delivery of antioxidant enzymes inhibits HIV-1 gp120-induced expression of caspases. Neuroscience 2012; 214: 68-77.

[127] Cribbs DH, Poon WW, Rissman RA, Blurton-Jones M. Caspase-mediated degeneration in Alzheimer's disease. Am J Pathol 2004; 165: 353-55.

[128] Ullrich CK, Groopman JE, Ganju RK. HIV-1 gp120- and gp160-induced apoptosis in cultured endothelial cells is mediated by caspases. Blood 2000; 96: 1436-42.

[129] Price TO, Ercal, N, Nakaoke R, Banks WA. HIV-1 viral proteins gp120 and Tat induce oxidative stress in brain endothelial cells. Brain Res 2005; 1045: 57-63.

[130] Price TO, Uras F, Banks WA, Ercal N. A novel antioxidant N-acetylcysteine amide prevents gp120- and Tat-induced oxidative stress in brain endothelial cells. Exp Neurol 2006; 201: 193-202.

[131] Petito CK, Cash KS. Blood-brain barrier abnormalities in the acquired immunodeficiency syndrome: immunohistochemical localization of serum proteins in postmortem brain. Ann Neurol 1992; 32: 658-66.

[132] Power C, Kong PA, Crawford TO, *et al.* Cerebral white matter changes in acquired immunodeficiency syndrome dementia: alterations of the blood-brain barrier. Ann Neurol 1993; 34: 339-50.

[133] Avison MJ, Nath A, Greene-Avison R, Schmitt FA, Greenberg RN, Berger JR, *et al.* Neuroimaging correlates of HIV-associated BBB compromise. J Neuroimmunol 2004; 157: 140-46.

[134] Toneatto S, Finco O, van der Putten H, Abrignani S, Annunziata P. Evidence of blood-brain barrier alteration and activation in HIV-1 gp120 transgenic mice. AIDS 1999; 13: 2343-48.

[135] Huang MB, Hunter M, Bond VC. Effect of extracellular human immunodeficiency virus type 1 glycoprotein 120 on primary human vascular endothelium cell cultures. AIDS Res Hum Retroviruses 1999; 15: 1265-77.

[136] Dallasta LM, Pisarov LA, Esplen JE, *et al.* Blood-brain barrier tight junction disruption in human immunodeficiency virus-1 encephalitis. Am J Pathol 1999; 155: 1915-27.

[137] Banks WA, Ibrahimi F, Farr SA, Flood JF, Morley JE. Effects of wheatgerm agglutinin and aging on the regional brain uptake of HIV-1 gp120. Life Sci. 1999; 65: 81-89.

[138] Banks WA, Freed EO, Wolf KM, Robinson SM, Franko M, Kumar VB. Transport of human immunodeficiency virus type 1 pseudoviruses across the blood-brain barrier: role of envelope proteins and adsorptive endocytosis. J Virol 2001; 75: 4681-91.

[139] Banks WA, Robinson SM, Nath A. Permeability of the blood-brain barrier to HIV-1 Tat. Exp Neurol 2005; 193: 218-27.

[140] Cioni C, Annunziata P. Circulating gp120 alters the blood-brain barrier permeability in HIV-1 gp120 transgenic mice. Neurosci Lett 2002; 330: 299-301.

[141] Annunziata P. Blood-brain barrier changes during invasion of the central nervous system by HIV-1. Old and new insights into the mechanism. J Neurol 2003; 250: 901-06.

[142] Kanmogne GD, Primeaux C, Grammas P. HIV-1 gp120 proteins alter tight junction protein expression and brain endothelial cell permeability: implications for the pathogenesis of HIV-associated dementia. J Neuropath Exp Neurol 2005; 64: 498-505.

[143] Kanmogne GD, Schall K, Leibhart J, Knipe B, Gendelman HE, Persidsky Y. HIV-1 gp120 compromises blood-brain barrier integrity and enhance monocyte migration across blood-brain barrier: implication for viral neuropathogenesis. J Cereb Blood Flow Meta 2007; 27: 123-34.

[144] Louboutin JP, Agrawal L, Reyes, BAS, Van Bockstaele EJ, Strayer DS, *et al.* HIV-1 gp120-induced injury to the blood-brain barrier: role of metalloproteinases 2 and 9 and relationship to oxidative stress. J Neuropathol Exp Neurol 2010; 69: 801-16.

[145] Louboutin JP, Reyes, BAS Agrawal L, Van Bockstaele EJ, Strayer DS. Blood-brain barrier abnormalities caused by exposure to HIV-1 gp120- Protection by gene delivery of antioxidant enzymes. Neurobiol Dis 2010; 38: 313-25.

[146] Manabe S, Gu Z, Lipton SA. Activation of matrix metalloproteinase-9 *via* neuronal nitric oxide synthase contributes to NMDA-induced retinal ganglion cell death. Invest Ophtalmol Vis Sci 2005; 46: 4747-53.

[147] Rosenberg GA. Matrix metalloproteinases in neuroinflammation. Glia 2002; 39: 279-91.

[148] Gu Z, Kaul M, Yan B, *et al.* S-nitrosylation of matrix metalloproteinases: signaling pathway to neuronal cell death. Science 2002; 297: 1186-90.

[149] Yong VW, Power C, Forsyth P, Edwards DR. Metalloproteinases in biology and pathology of the central nervous system. Nat Rev Neurosci 2001; 2: 502-11.

[150] Lo EH, Wang X, Cuzner MI. Extracellular proteolysis in brain injury and inflammation: role for plasminogen activators and matrix metalloproteinases. J Neurosci Res 2002; 69: 1-9.

[151] Gursoy-Ozdemir Y, Qiu J, Matsuoka N, *et al.* Cortical spreading depression activates and upregulates MMP-9. J Clin Invest 2004; 113: 1447-55.

[152] Zozulya AL, Reinke E, Baiu DC, Karman J, Sandor M, Fabry Z. Dendritic cell transmigration through brain microvessel endothelium is regulated by MIP-1α chemokine and matrix metalloproteinases. J Immunol 2007; 178: 520-29.

[153] Haorah J, Schall K, Ramirez S, Persidsky Y. Activation of protein kinases and matrix metalloproteinases causes blood-brain barrier injury: novel mechanisms for neurodegeneration associated with alcohol abuse. Glia 2008; 56: 78-88.

[154] Asahi M, Asahi K, Jung J-C, del Zoppo GJ, Fini ME, Lo EH. Role for matrix metalloproteinase 9 after focal cerebral ischemia: effects of gene knockout and enzyme inhibition with BB-94. J Cereb Blood Flow Metab 2000; 20: 1681-89.

[155] Gasche Y, Copin J-C, Sugawara T, Fujimura M, Chan PH. Matrix metalloproteinases inhibition prevents oxidative stress-associated blood-brain barrier disruption after transient focal cerebral ischemia. J Cereb Blood Flow Metab 2001; 21: 1393-400.

[156] Kim GW, Gasche Y, Grzeschik S, Copin JC, Maier CM, Chan PH. Neurodegeneration in striatum induced by the mitochondrial toxin 3-nitropropionic acid: role of matrix metalloproteinase-9 in early blood-brain barrier disruption? J Neurosci 2003; 23: 8733-42.

[157] Sporer B, Paul R, Koedel U, *et al.* Presence of matrix metalloproteinase-9 activity in the cerebrospinal fluid of human immunodeficiency virus-infected patients. J Infect Dis 1998; 178: 854-57.

[158] Liuzzi GM, Mastroianni CM, Santacroce MP, *et al.* Increased activity of matrix metalloproteinases in the cerebrospinal fluid of patients with HIV-associated neurological diseases. J Neurovirol 2000; 6: 156-63.

[159] Marshall DCL, Wyss-Coray TW, Abraham CR. Induction of matrix metalloproteinase-2 in human immunodeficiency virus-1 glycoprotein 120 transgenic mouse brains. Neurosci Lett 1998; 254: 97-100.

[160] Toschi E, Barillari G, Sgadari C, *et al.* Activation of matrix-metalloproteinase-2 and membrane-type-1-matrix-metalloproteinase in endothelial cells and induction of vascular permeability *in vivo* by human immunodeficiency virus-1 Tat protein and basic Fibroblast Growth Factor. Mol Biol Cell 2001; 12: 2934-46.

[161] Conant K, St Hillaire C, Anderson C, Galey D, Wang J, Nath A. Human immunodeficiency virus type 1 Tat and methamphetamine affect the release and activation of matrix-degrading proteinases. J Neurovirol 2004; 10: 21-28.

[162] Russo R, Siviglia E, Gliozzi M, *et al.* Evidence implicating matrix metalloproteinases in the mechanism underlying accumulation of IL-1β and neuronal apoptosis in the neocortex of HIV/gp120-exposed rats. Int Rev Neurobiol 2007; 82: 407-21.

[163] Berman NE, Marcario JK, Yong C, *et al.* Microglial activation and neurological symptoms in the SIV model of neuroAIDS: association with MHC-II and MMP-9 expression with behavioral deficits and evoked potential changes. Neurobiol Dis 1999; 6: 486-98.

[164] Cinque P, Nebuloni M, Santovito ML, *et al.* The urokinase receptor is overexpressed in the AIDS dementia complex and other neurological manifestations. Ann Neurol 2004; 55: 687-94.

[165] Dzwonek J, Rylski M, Kaczmarek L. Matrix metalloproteinases and their endogenous inhibitors in neuronal physiology of the adult brain. FEBS Lett 2004; 567: 129-35.

[166] Siwik DA, Colucci WS. Regulation of matrix metalloproteinases by cytokines and reactive oxygen/nitrogen species in the myocardium. Heart Fail Rev 2004; 9: 43-51.

[167] Louboutin JP, Reyes BAS, Agrawal L, Van Bockstaele EJ, Strayer DS. HIV-1 gp120 upregulates matrix metalloproteinases and their inhibitors in a rat model of HIV encephalopathy. Eur. J. Neurosci. 2011; 34: 2015-23.

[168] Louboutin JP, Reyes BAS, Agrawal L, Van Bockstaele EJ, Strayer DS. HIV-1 gp120-induced neuroinflammation: relationship to neuron loss and protection by rSV40-delivered antioxidant enzymes. Exp Neurol 2010; 221: 231-45.
[169] Chan PH, Schmidley JW, Fishman RA, Longar SM. Brain injury, edema, and vascular permeability changes induced by oxygen-derived free radicals. Neurology 1984; 34: 315-20.
[170] Chan PH, Yang GY, Carlson E, Epstein CJ. Cold-induced brain edema and infarction are reduced in transgenic mice overexpressing CuZn-superoxide dismutase. Ann Neurol 1991; 29: 482-86.
[171] Aoki T, Sumii T, Mori T, Wang X, Lo EH. Blood-brain barrier disruption and matrix metalloproteinase-9 expression during reperfusion injury: mechanical *versus* embolic focal ischemia in spontaneously hypertensive rats. Stroke 2002; 33: 2711-17.
[172] Wang HK, Park UJ, Kim SY, *et al.* Free radical production in CA1 neurons induces MIP-1alpha expression, microglial recruitment, and delayed neuronal death after transient forebrain ischemia. J Neurosci 2008; 28, 1721-27.
[173] Ishibashi N, Prokopenko O, Weisbrot-Lefkowitz M, Reuhl KR, Mirochnitchenko O. Glutathione peroxidase inhibits cell death and glial activation following experimental stroke. Brain Res Mol Brain Res 2002; 109: 34-44.
[174] Nishi T, Maier CM, Hayashi T, Saito A, Chan PH. Superoxide dismutase 1 overexpression reduces MCP-1 and MIP-1 alpha expression after transient focal cerebral ischemia. J Cereb Blood Flow Metab 2005; 25: 1312-24.
[175] Kraft-Terry SD, Buch SJ, Fox HS, Gendelman HE. A coat of different colors: neuroimmune cross talk in human immunodeficiency virus infection. Neuron 2009; 64: 133-45.
[176] Saijo K and Glass CK. Microglial cell origin and phenotypes in health and disease. Nature Rev. Immunol. 2011; 11: 775-87.

Frontiers in CNS Drug Discovery, 2013, *2*, 118-145

CHAPTER 5

Transient Receptor Potential Ion Channels as Promising Therapeutic Targets: An Overview

Merab G. Tsagareli*

Pain Research Group, Department of Neurophysiology, Ivane Beritashvili Center for Experimental Biomedicine, Tbilisi, Georgia

Abstract: Transient receptor potential (TRP) ion channels have been extensively investigated over the past few years and they are being ardently pursued as targets for drug discovery. Several factors make TRP ion channels appealing as drug targets. First, they are the largest group of noxious stimulus detectors in pain receptors (nociceptors). Second, although pain is currently the most advanced TRP channel-related field, an increasing number of gene deletion researches in animals and genetic association studies in humans have demonstrated that the pathophysiological roles of TRP channels extend well beyond the sensory nervous system (vision, olfaction, taste, mechano- and thermosensation, and osmoregulation). Many studies implicate them in other body systems, including pulmonary, cardiovascular, renal, and bladder systems.

Many TRP channels are expressed by the central nervous system; some are expressed at the spinal cord level (for example TRPA1, TRPM8 and TRPV1 channels), whereas others are expressed at high levels in the cerebrum (*e.g.*, TRPC3 in cerebellar Purkinje cells, and TRPC5 in the hippocampus and amygdala). TRPM2 and TRPM7 are expressed in brain neurons and microglia and are implicated in various pathologies related to oxidative stress, including the focal ischemia model of stroke. Therefore, TRPM7 antagonists may have a role in the treatment of stroke. The TRPM2 gene is also a candidate risk factor gene for bipolar disorder.

Recent findings in the field of pain have established a subset of TRP channels that are activated by temperature (the so-called thermoTRP ion channels) and are capable of initiating sensory nerve impulses following the detection of thermal, as well as mechanical and chemical irritant stimuli. At least, a family of six thermoTRP channels (TRPA1, TRPM8, TRPV1, TRPV2, TRPV3, and TRPV4) exhibits sensitivity to increases or decreases in temperature as well as to chemical substances that elicit similar hot or cold sensations. Such irritants include menthol from mint, cinnamaldehyde, gingerol, capsaicin from chili peppers, mustard oil, camphor, eugenol from cloves, and others.

***Address correspondence to Merab G. Tsagareli:** Beritashvili Exp Biomed Center, 14 Gotua Street, 0160 Tbilisi, Georgia; Tel: 995-32-237-1149; Fax: 995-32-237-3410;
E-mails: tsagareli@biphysiol.ge, merab.tsagareli@caucasus.net

Atta-ur-Rahman & M. Iqbal Choudhary (Eds.)

This review focuses on recent developments in the TRP ion channel-related area and highlights evidence supporting TRP channels as promising targets for new analgesic drugs at the periphery and central levels and opportunities for therapeutic intervention.

Keywords: Allodynia, cold pain, heat pain, sensory neurons, signal transduction, nociception.

INTRODUCTION

Transient receptor potential (TRP) cation channels, a large family of receptor channel proteins, are one of the most extensively studied in neuroscience. They initially attracted researchers in the field of pain as key molecules in nociception (sense of pain), but later they became known as more general transducer molecules for various physical stresses [1]. At the end of 1960s, the seminal findings in abnormal electro-retinograms from a mutant fruit-fly *Drosophila melanogaster* led to an explosion of interest in photo-transduction [2,3]. Some of *Drosophila* mutants had defects in the photoreceptor cells while others had been interpreted as lacking some important neural events following light reception [4]. Later, Minke and Montell, independently of each other, provided the direct evidence that *Drosophila* TRP comprises a subunit of Ca^{2+} permeable channel [5,6]. These works represented the most rigorous demonstration that a member of the TRP superfamily functioned as a cation channel in a native system [7,8].

The TRP channels were not on the main stream of pain study, however, until 1997, when Caterina and coworkers, in the Julius lab, cloned a vanilloid receptor and found that its structure was closely related to TRP channels [9]. Sensitivity to capsaicin, the hot natural ingredient of capsicum peppers, was believed to be one of the key features of nociceptors (pain receptors), and the protein responsible had been long sought. The vanilloid receptor found in this study was activated not only by capsaicin but also by noxious heat, which made it a perfect fit with nociceptor-related protein [10]. Since then, a tremendous amount of pain-related investigations has been dedicated to the vanilloid receptor and other TRP channels.

PHYLOGENIC ASPECTS OF TRP CHANNELS

Combined molecular and physiological analyses of nociceptive transduction have revealed important mechanisms in a few species. The TRP channels have demonstrated their importance for nociceptive transduction in both vertebrates and invertebrates [11]. The repertoires of temperature sensitive (thermoTRP) homologous have changed through vertebrate evolution. Since thermoTRPs are involved in thermosensation as well as other kinds of sensory detection variability of repertoires may be associated with adaptation of the organisms to their respective habitat environments [12].

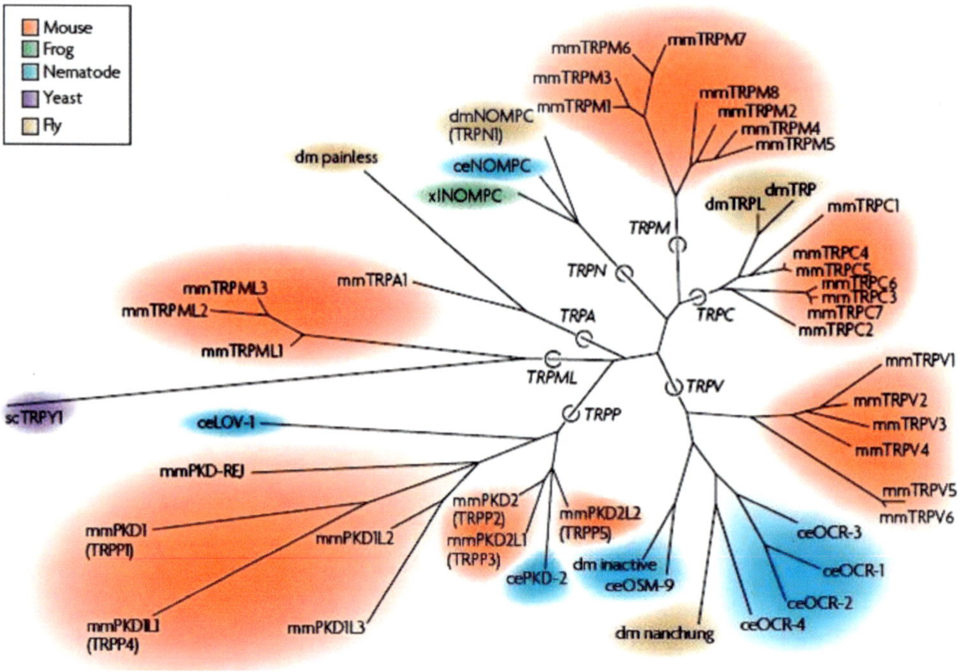

Fig. (1). Phylogeny of representative TRP channels. A phylogenic tree was generated in ClustalX by aligning the transmembrane domains of all 33 transient receptor potential (TRP) channels from mouse and some from other species. The seven main branches are denoted by circles at the branch roots. The letters and numbers following TRP denote TRP subfamily and member, respectively. Different species are indicated by colours and by prefixes. ce, *Caenorhabditis elegans*; dm, *Drosophila melanogaster*; mm, *Mus musculus*; sc, *Saccharomyces cerevisiae*; xl, *Xenopus laevis*. (Reproduced from [13]).

There are 33 TRP channel genes in mammals (nearly 60 in zebrafish, 30 in sea squirts, 24 in nematodes, 16 in fruit flies and 1 in yeast). They are subdivided into seven subfamilies on the basis of sequence similarity [13] (Fig. **1**). Distinct members of the thermoTRP families are present in the invertebrates *C. elegans* and *Drosophila* as illustrated in Fig. (**2**). At least some of the invertebrate TRP channels appear to be playing a role in thermosensation as well [14].

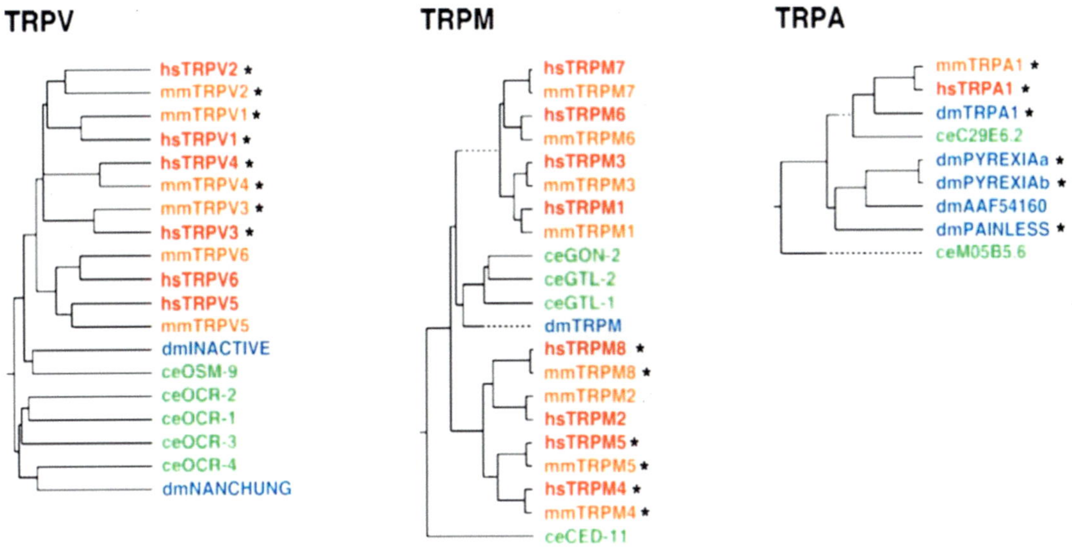

Fig. (2). Phylogenies are shown for three families of TRP cation channels: TRPV, TRPM, and TRPA. *H. sapiens*, *M. musculus*, *D. melanogaster*, and *C. elegans* members of these families are color coded. Channels implicated in thermosensation are labeled with an asterisk. (Reproduced from [14]).

STRUCTURAL CHARACTERISTICS OF TRP CHANNELS

The TRP channel superfamily is mostly classified into six related subfamilies: TRP cation channel subfamily A (ankyrin, TRPA), TRP cation channel subfamily C (canonical, C), TRP cation channel subfamily M (melastatin, M), TRP cation channel subfamily V (vanilloid, TRPV), TRP cation channel polycystin subfamily (TRPP), and TRP cation channel mucolipin subfamily (TRPML). The TRPML and TRPP subfamilies were named after the human diseases that are associated with mucolipidosis and polycystic kidney disease, respectively. The founding member of the TRPM subfamily, TRPM1, was identified *via* comparative analysis of genes that distinguish benign nevi from malignant melanoma. The TRPA subfamily has only one known member (TRPA1) and its name refers to the usually high number of ankyrin repeats at the amino terminus of the channel protein (Fig. **3**). Mammalian TRP channels those are most similar to the product of the *Drosophila* TRP gene, are referred to as TRPC proteins [15,16]. The TRPV subfamily, as we mentioned above, was identified following expression cloning of TRPV1, which is the receptor for the prototypical chemical irritant vanilloid, capsaicin.

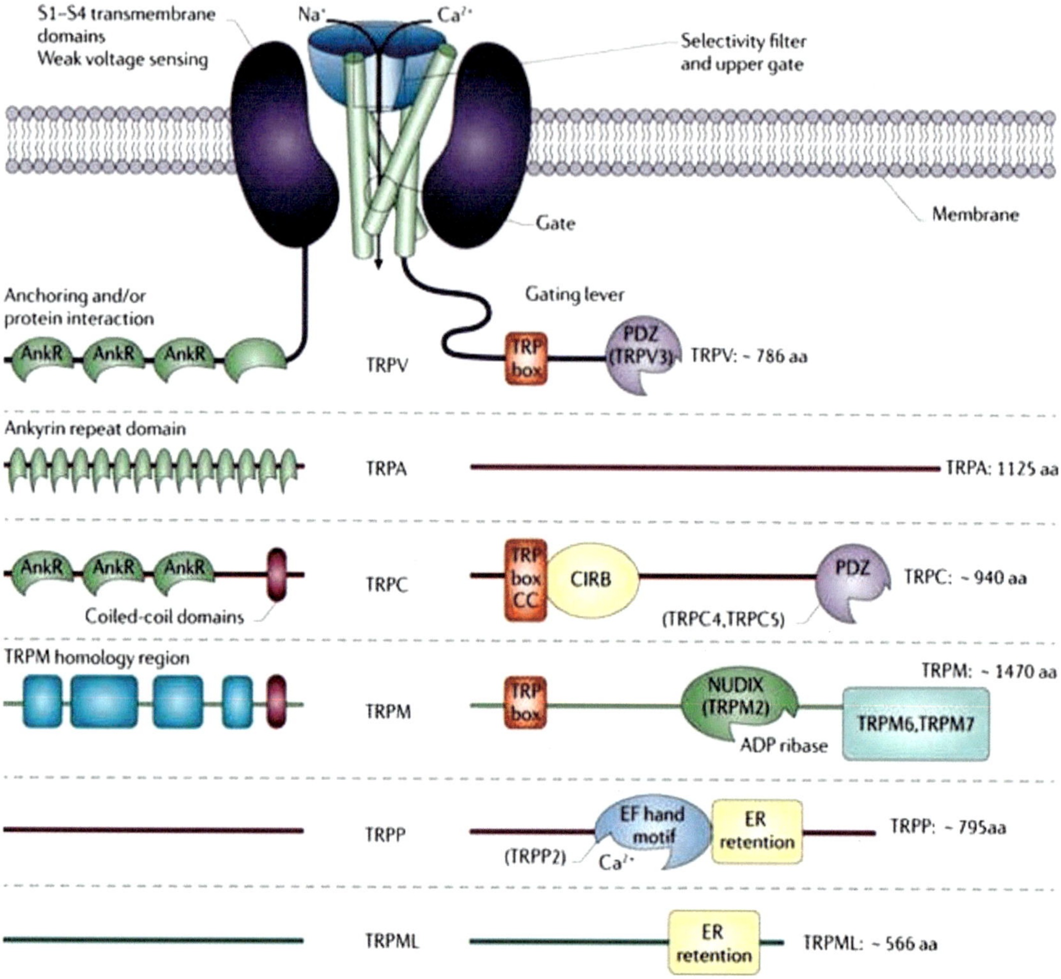

Fig. (3). The six transient receptor potential (TRP) cation families contain very different motifs in their amino and carboxyl termini. The TRPV, TRPA and TRPC families have amino terminal ankyrin repeat (AnkR) domains that are not present in other TRP channel subfamilies. The TRP box, which is found in the TRPV, TRPM and TRPC families, is thought to be involved in gating. TRP cation channel TRPP and TRPML proteins both have endoplasmic reticulum (ER) retention domains that may be due to their functional localization on intracellular organelles. aa, amino acids; CIRB, calmodulin/inositol-1,4,5-trisphosphate ($Ins(1,4,5)P_3$) receptor binding domain; NUDIX, nucleoside diphosphate-linked moiety X; PDZ, acronym for postsynaptic density protein 95 (PSD95), Drosophila disc large tumour suppressor (DLGA) and zonula occludens protein 1 (ZO1). (Reproduced from [15]).

Most members of the TRP channel superfamily share a low level of structural similarity, but some channels –such as TRPC3 and TRPC7, as well as TRPV5 and TRPV6 – are highly homologous to each other. Most of the channels are predicted to have six transmembrane domains and large intracellular amino and carboxyl termini (Fig. **3**). Many TRP channels form functional channels as homo-tetramers, although hetero-multi-merization is not uncommon [15,16]. The latter phenomenon may have important implications in drug discovery as it is crucial for understanding the endogenous subunit composition of the ion channels so that TRP can be appropriately targeted with a pharmacological agent [15].

TRP CHANNELS AS THERAPEUTIC AND ANALGESIC TARGETS

Consistent with their diverse structure, TRP channels also serve diverse functions. Although most members of the TRP channel superfamily are cation channels with limited selectivity for calcium, both calcium-selective, such as TRPV5 and TRPV6, and sodium-selective, such as TRPM4 and TRPM5, members of the TRP channel subfamilies exist [15,16]. In addition, some TRP channels transport non-canonical cations such as iron (TRPML1) or magnesium (TRPV6) [15]. Temperature also exerts profound effects on several TRP channels (Fig. **4**). Although, TRPV1 and TRPM8 channels have been clearly demonstrated to serve as sensors for changes in environmental temperature, many other TRP channels have thermal coefficients such that a change in temperature of 10°C has profound effects on channel activity. These include TRPV2, TRPV3, TRPV4, TRPM2, TRPM4, TRPM5 and TRPA1 [1,15,17].

Data from animal models and human genetics (and probably in the near future clinical trials) will serve as the final arbiters of utility of TRP channel modulators as therapeutics in channel dysfunction (known as TRP channelopathy). Current evidence indicates that channelopathies contribute to the development and/or progression of the symptoms of many diseases. Among them are inherited pain syndrome and neuropathic pain, itch, multiple kidney disease, skeletal disorders, overactive bladder, asthma, and anxiety disorders. Therefore, TRP ion channels could be therapeutic targets that are amenable to blockade by small molecules [15,18,19].

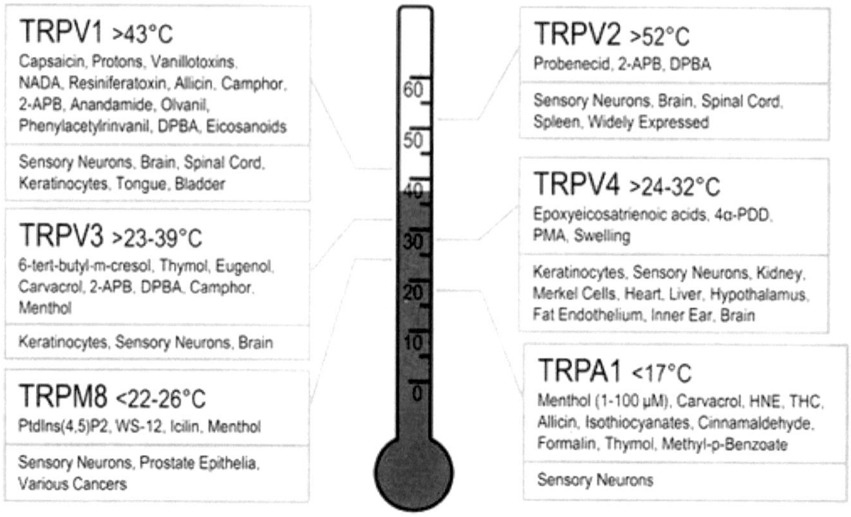

Fig. (4). Temperature thresholds, chemical agonists, and tissue distribution of six temperature-sensitive TRP channels. NADA, N-arachidonoyl-dopamine; 2-APB, 2-aminoethoxydiphenyl borate; DPBA, diphenylboronic anhydride; 4α-PDD, 4α-phorbol 12,13-didecanoate; PMA, phorbol 12-myristate 13-acetate; PtdIns (4,5)P2, phosphatidylinositol 4,5-bisphosphate; HNE, 4-hydroxynonenal; THC, tetrahydrocannabinol. (Reproduced from [1]).

TRP Channels in Physiological Nociception

The role of TRP channels is best understood in pain physiology and pharmacology. We feel a wide range of temperatures spanning from cold to heat. Within this range, temperatures over about 43°C and below about 15°C evoke not only a thermal sensation, but also a feeling of pain. The neurons that allow us to sense temperatures are located in the dorsal root ganglia (DRG) and within cranial nerve ganglia such as the trigeminal ganglion (TG) (Fig. **5**).

It has been hypothesized that cutaneous nociceptor endings detect temperature, chemicals, mechanical and other physical stimuli by means of TRP ion channels responsive to these stimuli [17].

HEAT RECEPTORS

TRPV1

Exposure to capsaicin evokes a painful burning sensation through the vanilloid TRPV1 receptor, that is also activated by noxious thermal stimuli above 43°C or

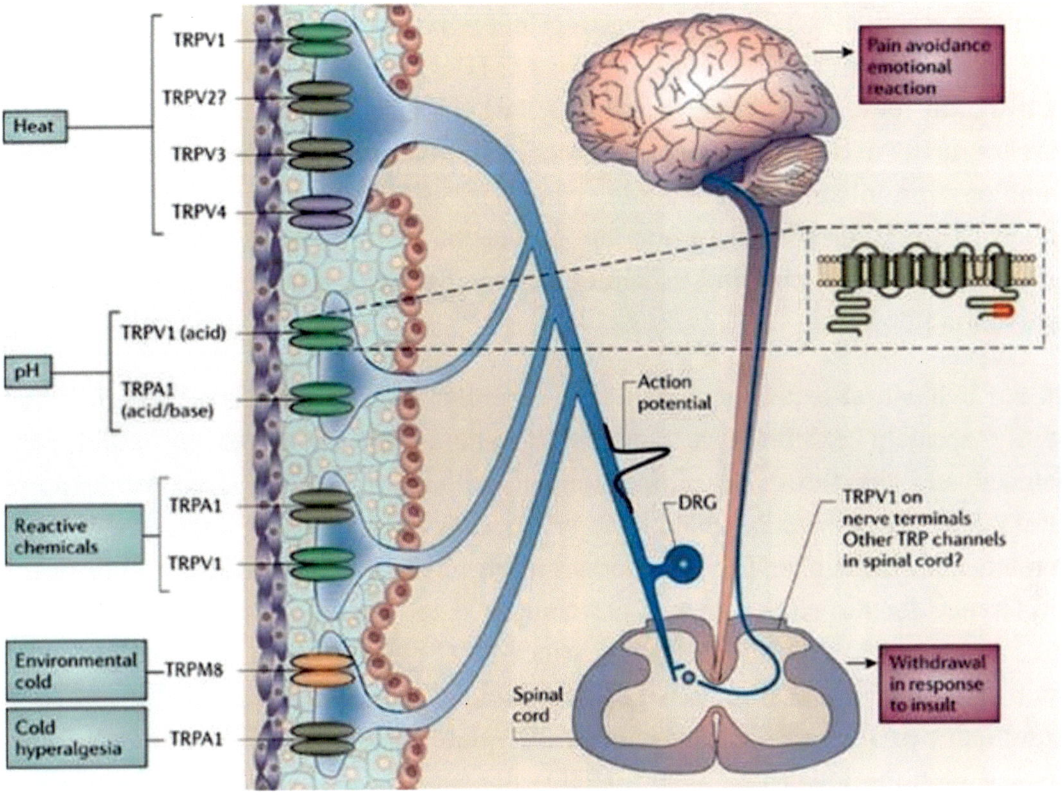

Fig. (5). Sensory neurons express multiple transient receptor potential (TRP) channels. TRP cation channel subfamily V, member 1 (TRPV1), TRPV3 and TRPV4 all respond to warming temperatures. Noxious heat activates TRPV2, but the physiological relevance of this is unclear. Acids are robust activators of TRPV1 and bases have emerged as activators of TRP cation channel subfamily A, member 1 (TRPA1). TRPA1 is a key chemoreceptor that responds to scores of reactive chemicals. At higher concentrations, some of these chemicals also activate TRPV1. TRP cation channel subfamily M, member 8 (TRPM8) serves as the key receptor for environmental cold, although TRPA1 also has a role in cold hyperalgesia. Activation of any of these TRP cation channels can trigger action potentials in the sensory neuron. Some of these channels, such as TRPV1, are also expressed in the spinal cord, where they seem to have an important role in the central nervous system as well. DRG, dorsal root ganglion. (Reproduced from [15]).

by an acidic environment of pH 5.4 [10,17]. In addition to its sensitivity to various pain-inducing stimuli such as capsaicin, heat, and protons, the TRPV1 ion channel has many features that a receptor related to nociception is supposed to have, such as its preferential distribution in the central nervous system (CNS) within small to medium-sized DRG and TG neurons, which are believed to serve as nociceptive nerve cells [20]. Phosphatidylinositol 4,5-bisphosphate (PIP_2) bound to the C-terminus inactivates TRPV1, suggesting that conditions which remove or degrade PIP_2, such as activation of phospholipase C (PLC) during inflammation, can also activate or potentiate TRPV1 [1]. TRPV1 is also expressed by an alkaline environment and by various chemical stimulants including resinferatoxin, vanillotoxins, olvanil, anandamide, camphor, allicin, eicosanoids, eugenol and others [21,22]. But the most important aspects of TRPV1 is that it can integrate all of these noxious stimuli and inflammatory mediators to modulate its threshold of activation [23-26].

In our behavioral experiments we have recently found that the hind paw injected with capsaicin exhibited a concentration-dependent decrease in withdrawal latency and the threshold of mechanical withdrawal reflex. Two temperature preference tests have revealed that when exposed to 30° *vs* 15°C plates, rats treated with the higher (0.3%) concentration of capsaicin exhibited a significant preference for the colder 15°C plate compared to vehicle-treated rats ($P<0.001$), *i.e.*, they significantly avoided the warmer 30°C plate (Fig. **6**). Another group of rats treated with the highest (0.4%) capsaicin exhibited an opposite effect, a significant preference for the warmer 30° plate ($P<0.001$). Two groups of rats treated with the lower (0.1% and 0.2%) concentrations of capsaicin exhibited no significant preference for the warmer or colder plates, though the lowest (0.1%) concentration treated rats had a strong trend to preference for the colder 15°C plate compared to vehicle-treated rats (Fig. **6**).

Our data provide an additional comprehensive view of the effects of intraplantar injections of capsaicin on thermal and mechanical sensitivity. They showed a dose-dependent heat hyperalgesia and mechanical allodynia lasting >2 hours; also different concentrations of capsaicin exhibited different effects in thermal preference test [27].

Thus, the TRPV1 ion channel has been a promising target in the field of pain research. Understanding how TRPV1 transduces various noxious chemical irritants and mechanical stimuli into an electrical signal in the peripheral endings of nociceptive neurons could lead to better understanding of the nature of pain sensation, and blocking the activation TRPV1 could be a very effective analgesic strategy [1,15]. Nowadays, as the desensitization of sensory nociceptive neurons to capsaicin has analgesic potential, the cloning of the vanilloid receptor TRPV1, has spurred considerable efforts in the pharmaceutical community to find TRPV1 antagonists. In particular, several TRPV1 antagonists (ABT-102, AMG-517, AZD-1386, GRC-6211 and others) have already advanced to clinical trials [15].

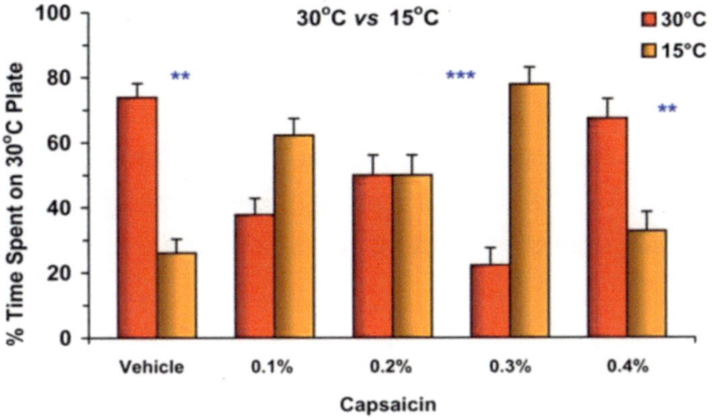

Fig. (6). Biphasic effects of capsaicin on thermal preference. Graph plots % time rat stood on 30°C *vs* 15°C plate. At higher (0.3%) capsaicin concentration rats spent significantly more time on the 15°C plate (yellow bar) compared to the 30°C plate (red bar) (P<0.001), indicating cold hyposensitivity. However, at the highest (0.4%) capsaicin concentration rats spent significantly more time on the 30°C plate (red bar) compared to the 15°C plate (yellow bar) (P<0.01), indicating cold hypersensitivity. At the lower (0.1%, and 0.2%) concentrations, there was no significant difference between the warm (30°C, red bars) and cold (15°C, yellow bars) plates.

TRPV2, TRPV3 and TRPV4

TRPV2 is widely expressed in sensory neuronal cells (mostly fast Aδ fibers and a small portion of slow C fibers) and non-neuronal cells. It is activated by temperature above 52°C and has a higher threshold than that of TRPV1. However, its role in nociception has been debated because it is not sensitive to capsaicin or protons, and nociceptors lacking both TRPV1 and TRPV2 channels showed normal heat responses in *ex vivo* recordings, suggesting that mechanisms other than TRPV1 and TRPV2 might be more important in the intact physiological environment [1,28-31]. Just recently, the neuroanatomical distribution of TRPV2 in the adult male rat brain has been reported, focusing on the hypothalamus, hindbrain and forebrain regions. Based on their immunostaining results, the authors concluded that TRPV2 may play an important role in several CNS networks that regulate body fluid homeostasis, autonomic function, and metabolism [32].

Two other TRPV members, TRPV3 and TRPV4, can be activated at warm temperatures, which can hardly be perceived as nociceptive. TRPV3 is activated at 32-39°C and shows an increased response to higher temperature or repetitive stimuli. It shares 40-50% homology with TRPV1 and has certain common features such as activation and sensitization by camphor and 2-APB. Other agonists of TRPV3 include carvacrol, eugenol and thymol. TRPV4 has an even lower threshold of 27-34°C and has a variety of chemical ligands, such as phorbol esters, low pH, citrate, endocannabinoids, arachidonic acid metabolites, and nitric oxide [1,33-35].

Both TRPV3 and TRPV4 are expressed most extensively in skin keratinocytes, indicating that keratinocytes may signal to sensory neurons, instead of thermal stimuli acting directly on neurons. Furthermore, TRPV3-deleted mice lack camphor-induced activation of keratinocytes and exhibit strong deficits in response to innocuous and noxious heat. Thus, TRPV3 expressed in skin keratinocytes may have an important role in mammalian thermosensation [36].

COLD RECEPTORS

An early psychophysical study in humans reported that temperatures of around and below 15°C are perceived as pain [37], but unlike the discrete temperature threshold of hot nociception, the transition from cool to painfully cold is less well defined [38]. However, almost all nociceptive neurons are sensitive to cold, although some are activated at temperature as low as 0°C, which might be due to a nonspecific response following tissue damage from freezing [38].

TRPM8

The search for the cold receptor began with menthol, the chemical derived from the plants of the mint family. The cooling sensation of menthol was established as early 1951 by the classic work of Hensel & Zotterman [39]. Later, two independent research groups cloned and characterized a cold- and menthol-sensitive TRP channel, TRPM8 [40-43], which had been found in the prostate without a known function [1]. TRPM8 is mostly expressed in small DRG and TG neurons. It is activated by temperature below 25°C and by various chemicals including menthol, eucalyptol, and icilin [44-47].

We have recently used behavioral methods to investigate the effects of topical menthol on thermal (hot and cold) pain and innocuous cold and mechanical sensitivity in rats [48]. Menthol dose-dependently increased the latency for noxious heat-evoked withdrawal of the treated hindpaw with a weak mirror-image effect, indicating antinociception (Fig. **7**).

Menthol at the highest concentration (40%) reduced mechanical withdrawal thresholds, with no effect at lower concentrations (Fig. **8**).

It was interesting that menthol had a biphasic effect on cold avoidance (thermal preference test). At high concentrations (10% and 40%) menthol reduced avoidance of colder temperatures (15°C and 20°C) compared to 30°C, while at lower concentrations (0.01–1%) menthol enhanced cold avoidance (Fig. **9**).

In a−5°C cold plate test, 40% menthol significantly increased the nocifensive response latency (cold hypoalgesia) while lower concentrations were not different from vehicle controls (Fig. **10**).

The behavioral effects of topical menthol application seen in our study are consistent with effects on TRPM8 channels. An important role for TRPM8 becomes apparent when this channel is missing. TRPM8 null mice exhibit a deficit in cold avoidance and in general, deficient response behaviors to moderately cool temperatures [43,44].

These results, thus, are generally consistent with neuro-physiological and human psychophysical data and support TRPM8 as a potential peripheral target of pain modulation.

TRPA1

The role of TRPA1 channel in thermal and mechanical transduction is also controversial. TRPA1 was found to be cold sensitive, being activated at temperatures

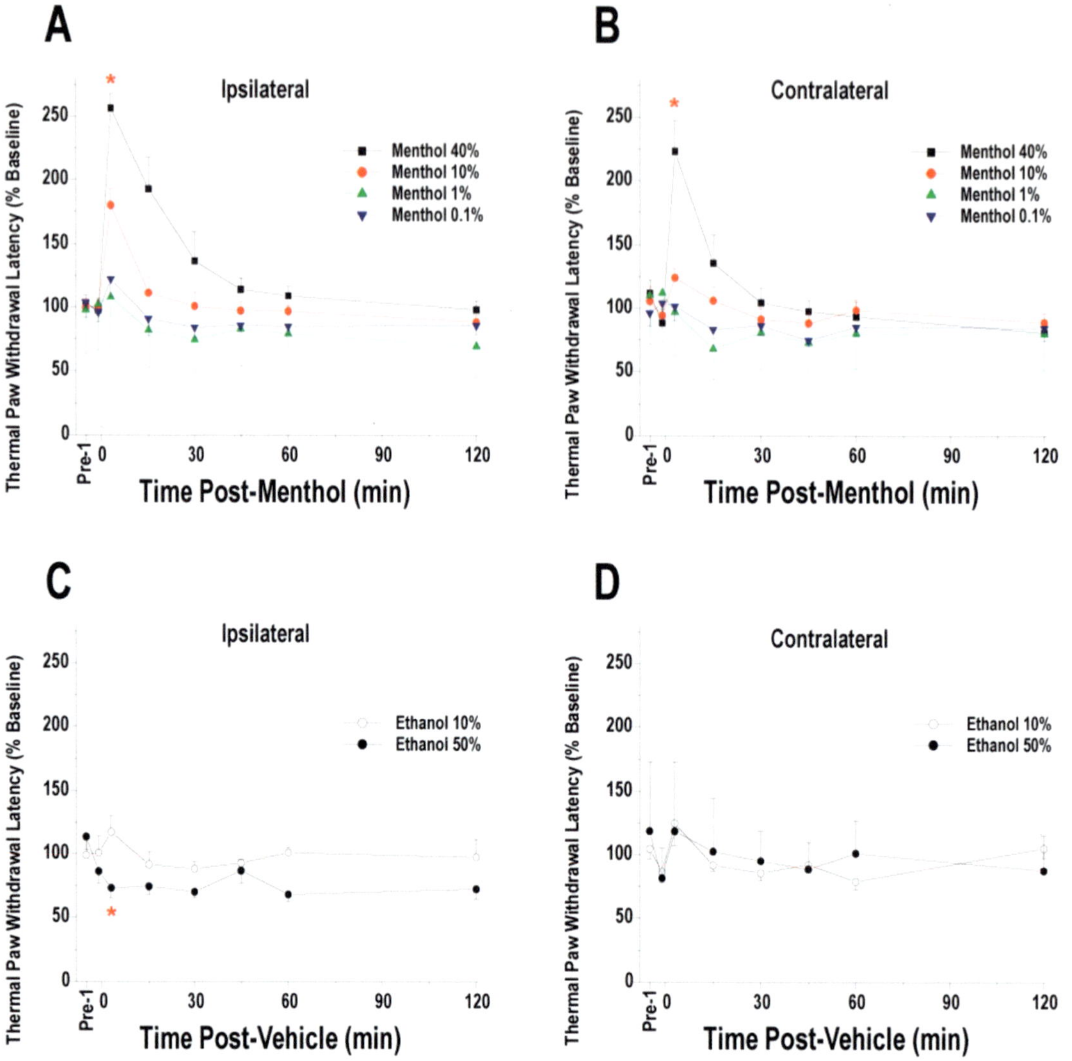

Fig. (7). Concentration-dependent antinociceptive effect of menthol on thermal hindpaw withdrawal latency (Hargreave's test). (**A**): Ipsilateral hindpaw. The hindpaw receiving topical menthol exhibited a concentration-dependent increase in withdrawal latency (analgesia). Groups of rats tested at concentrations of 40%, 10% and 1% menthol were significantly different from vehicles. The 40%, menthol was different from all other concentrations (*$p < 0.01$, repeated-measures ANOVA), while 10% menthol was not different from 1% menthol ($p = 0.07$). Error bars: SEM; n = 8/group. (**B**) Contralateral hindpaw. There was a weak mirror-image effect. The 40% menthol group was significantly different from all other concentrations (*$p < 0.01$), which were not different from vehicle. (**C**) Vehicle controls: ipsilateral hindpaw. There was a significant difference between groups (*$p < 0.01$). (**D**) Vehicle controls: contralateral hindpaw. There was no significant difference between ethanol concentrations, both of which were ineffective. (Adapted from [48]).

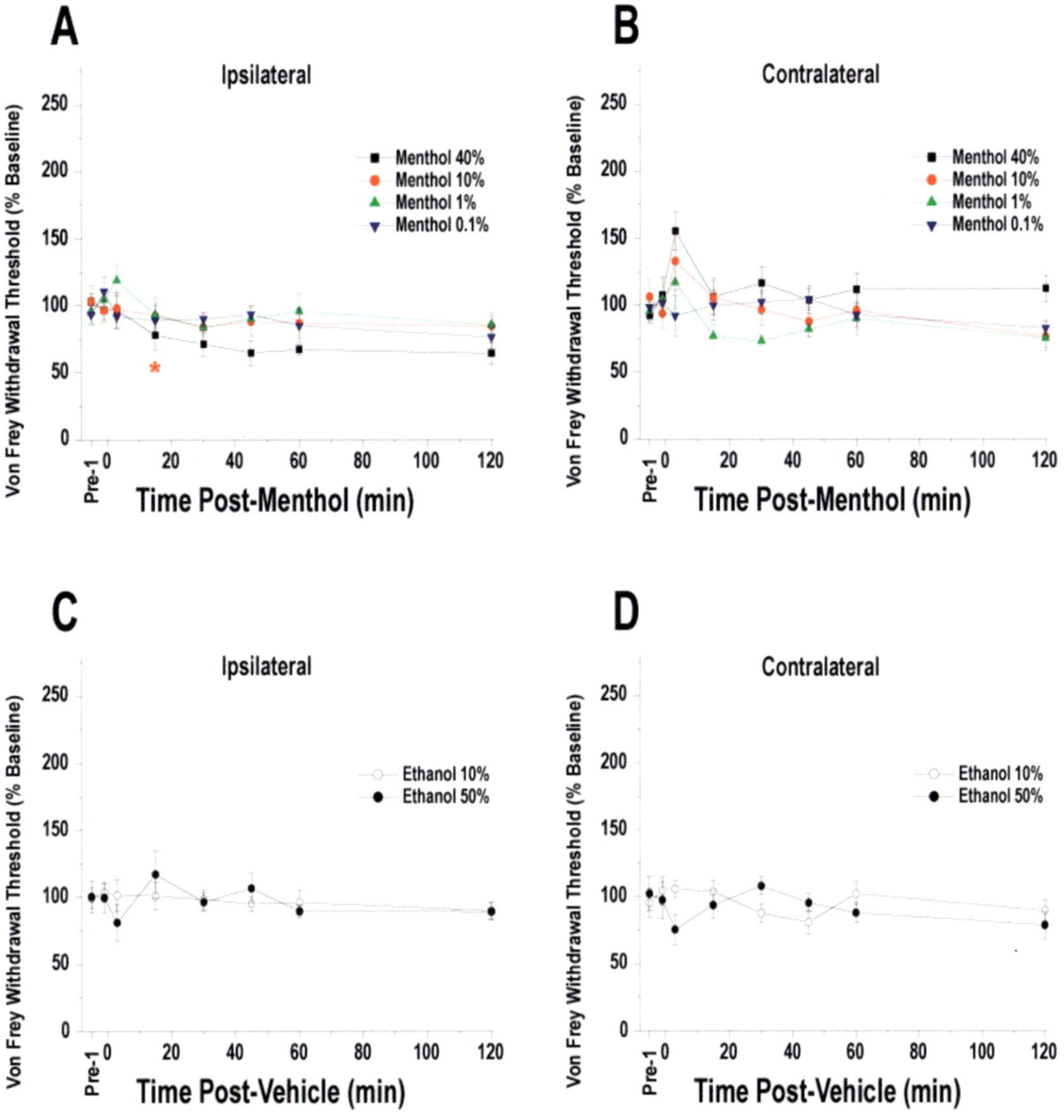

Fig. (8). Mechanical paw withdrawal latencies (von Frey's test) and the lack of concentration-dependent effect of menthol. (**A**): ipsilateral hindpaw. The 0.1–10% menthol groups were not significantly different from vehicle (10% ethanol). Only the 40% menthol group was significantly different from all other groups (*$p < 0.05$, repeated-measures ANOVA) indicating allodynia. (**B**) Contralateral hindpaw. None of the menthol concentration groups were significantly different from the vehicles. (**C**) Vehicle controls: ipsilateral hindpaw. There was no significant difference between 10% + 1% Tween-80 and 50% ethanol + 5% Tween-80 vehicle groups. (**D**) Vehicle controls: contralateral hindpaw. No significant difference between ethanol concentrations. n = 8/group. (Adapted from [48]).

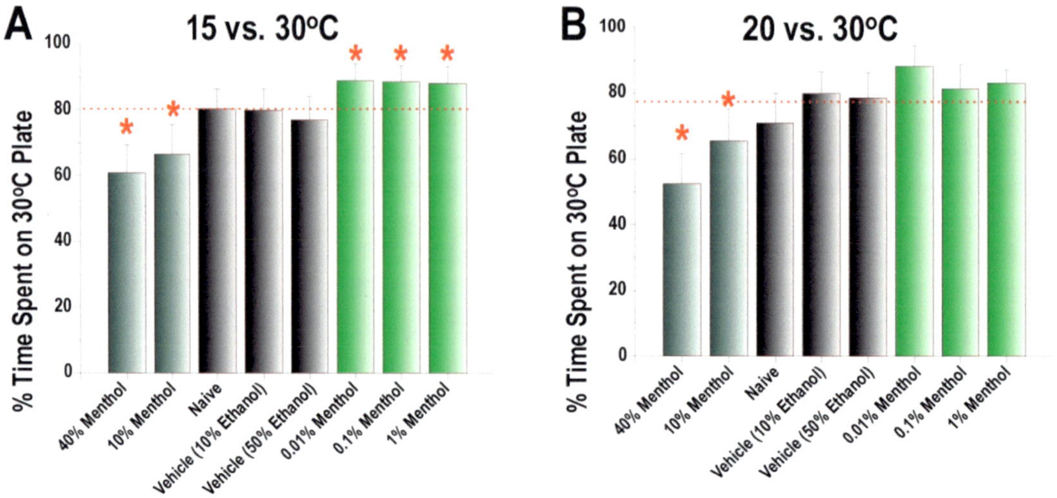

Fig. (9). Biphasic effects of menthol on thermal preference. (**A**) Graph plots % time rat stood on 30°C *vs* 15°C plate. Horizontal dashed line indicates that naive and vehicle treated rats avoided the colder plate ~80% of the time as a reference. At high (40%, 10%; dark green bars) menthol concentrations rats spent significantly less time on the 30°C plate compared to vehicle controls (dark gray bars) ($p < 0.05$), indicating cold hyposensitivity. At lower concentrations (0.01–1%; light green bars), rats spent significantly more time on the 30°C plate ($p < 0.05$), indicating cold hypersensitivity. *Significantly different *vs* vehicle ($p < 0.05$, n = 16/ group). (**B**) as in (**A**) for 20°C *vs* 30°C preference test. Note significant cold hyposensitivity with 40% menthol and significant hypersensitivity at the lowest menthol concentration of 0.01%. *Significantly different *vs* vehicle ($p < 0.05$, n = 16/group). (Adapted from [48]).

below 17°C, which is lower than the temperature threshold of TRPM8 [17]. As most of the expression of TRPA1 overlaps with that of TRPV1, it seemed reasonable to link TRPA1 to cold nociception (Fig. **11**).

Several chemical irritants can activate TRPA1 channel, among them is icilin, a synthetic compound that induces intense cold sensation when applied to human mucous membrane [50]. Other pungent cysteine-reactive chemicals, such as isothiocyanates (from horseradish and mustard), cinnamaldehyde (cinnamon), and allicin (garlic), activate TRPA1 through covalent modification of cysteine, regardless of their overall structures [51].

We have recently investigated behavioral responses to see whether cinnamaldehyde affects sensitivity to thermal and mechanical stimuli in rats [52]. Unilateral intraplantar injection of cinnamaldehyde (5–20%) induced a significant, concentration-dependent reduction in latency for ipsilateral paw withdrawal from a noxious heat stimulus, peaking by 30 min with partial recovery at 120 min (Fig. **12A**, **B**).

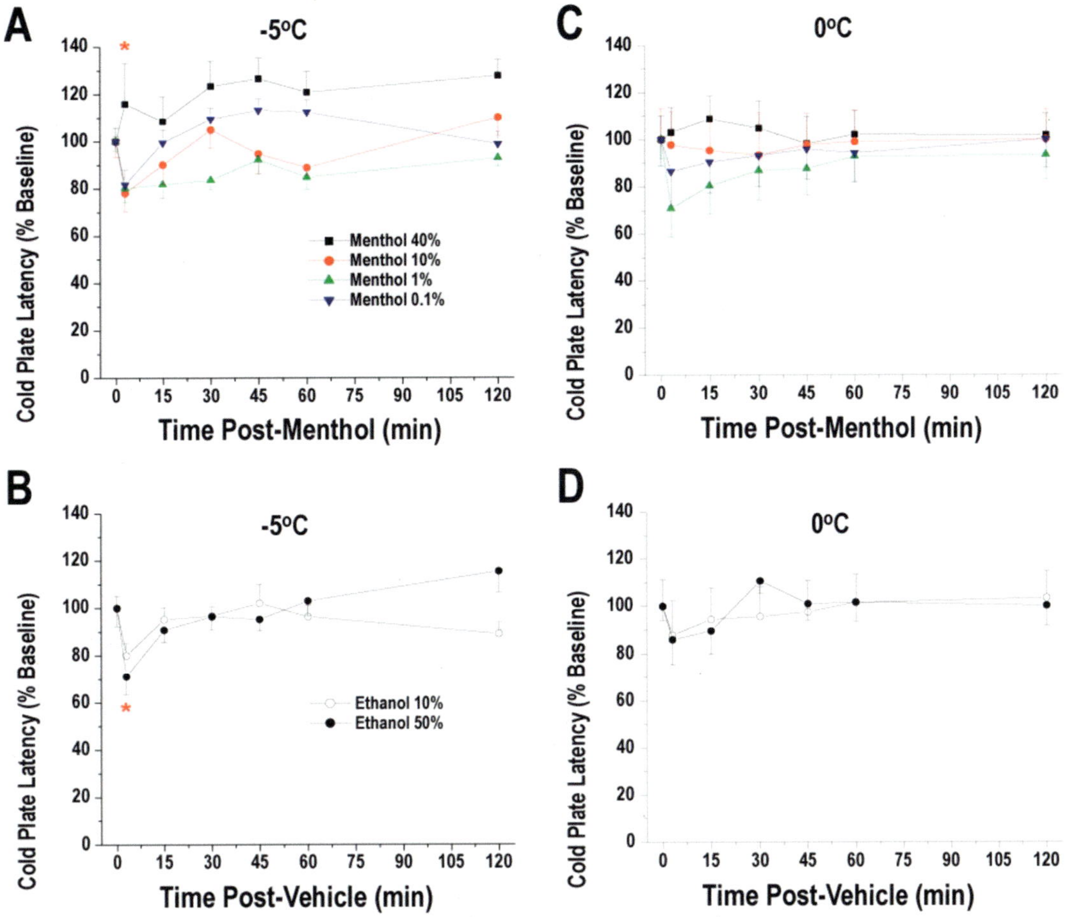

Fig. (10). Antinociceptive effect of 40% menthol in −5C cold plate test. (**A**) Cold plate −5°C: menthol. Graph plots change in cold plate latency (% of pre-menthol baseline) *vs* time after topical menthol application at indicated concentrations. Rats were tested 3min after menthol or vehicle, and again at 15-min intervals out to 60 min and once more at 120 min. The 40% menthol group was significantly different from all other concentrations (*p < 0.001, repeated-measures ANOVA) which did not differ from each other or vehicle. This indicates a cold antinociceptive effect of 40% menthol. Error bars: SEM, n=8/group. (**B**) Cold plate −5°C: vehicle. There was a significant difference between 10% and 50% ethanol (*p < 0.001, ANOVA). The ~20% reduction in cold plate latency seen at 3 min post-10% ethanol was comparable to the latency reductions in the 0.1–10% menthol groups at the same 3-min time point (**A**). (**C**) Cold plate 0°C: menthol. There was no significant difference among menthol concentration groups. (D) Cold plate 0°C: vehicle. There was no significant difference between ethanol concentrations. (Adapted from [48]).

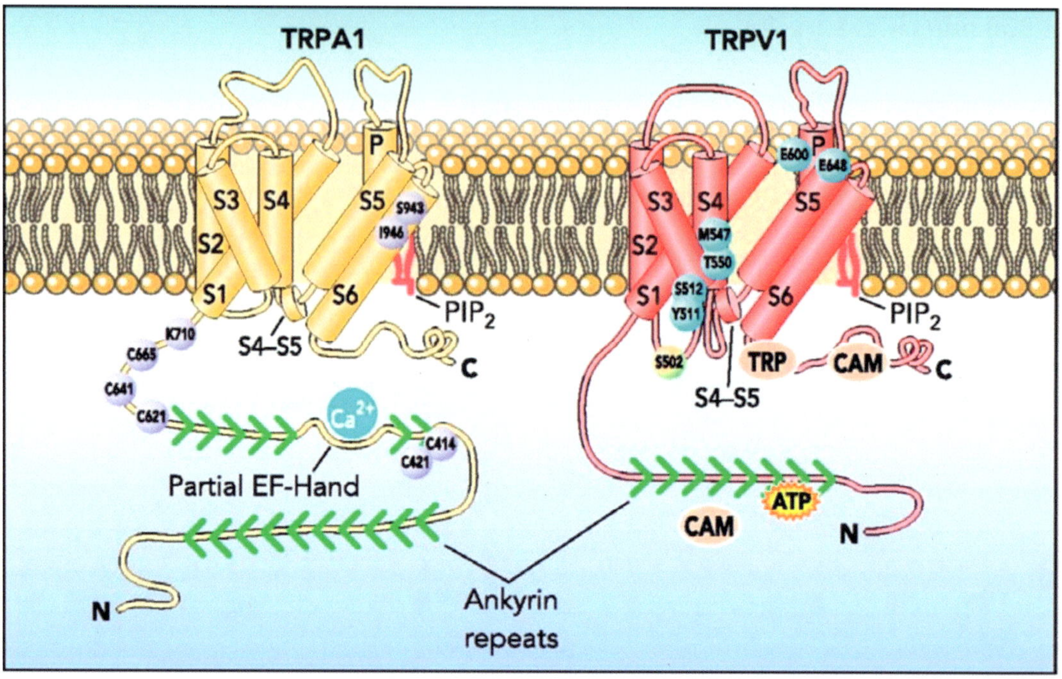

Fig. (11). Structures of TRPA1 (*left*) and TRPV1 (*right*) monomers, modeled after the X-ray crystal structure of the potassium channel (Kv1.2). The intracellular NH_2-terminal segment of TRPA1 has ~15 ankyrin repeats, containing several cysteine and lysine residues (gray) crucial for activation by reactive agonists, as well as a partial EF-hand domain implicated in calcium-dependent gating. Sites in transmembrane domain S6 are essential for gating by antagonists and agonists. TRPV1 is gated by vanilloids and endogenous inflammatory fatty acid metabolites binding to sites close to the intracellular face of the membrane. Protons interact with sites at the extracellular end of S5 and within the channel pore loop. NH_2- and COOH-termini have interaction sites for calmodulin (CaM) and ATP. Positively charged domains within the COOH termini of TRPA1 and TRPV1 may serve as interaction sites for phosphatidyl-inositol-4,5-bisphosphate (PIP_2), the substrate of phospholipase C, exerting an inhibitory effect on channel function. (Reproduced from [49]).

The highest dose of cinnamaldehyde also significantly reduced the contralateral paw withdrawal latency. Cinnamaldehyde significantly reduced mechanical withdrawal thresholds of the injected paw that peaked sooner (3 min) and was more profound (44.4% of baseline), with no effect contralaterally (Fig. **12C**, **D**). Cinnamaldehyde did not increase cold avoidance in the thermal preference test when compared to control (Fig. **13**).

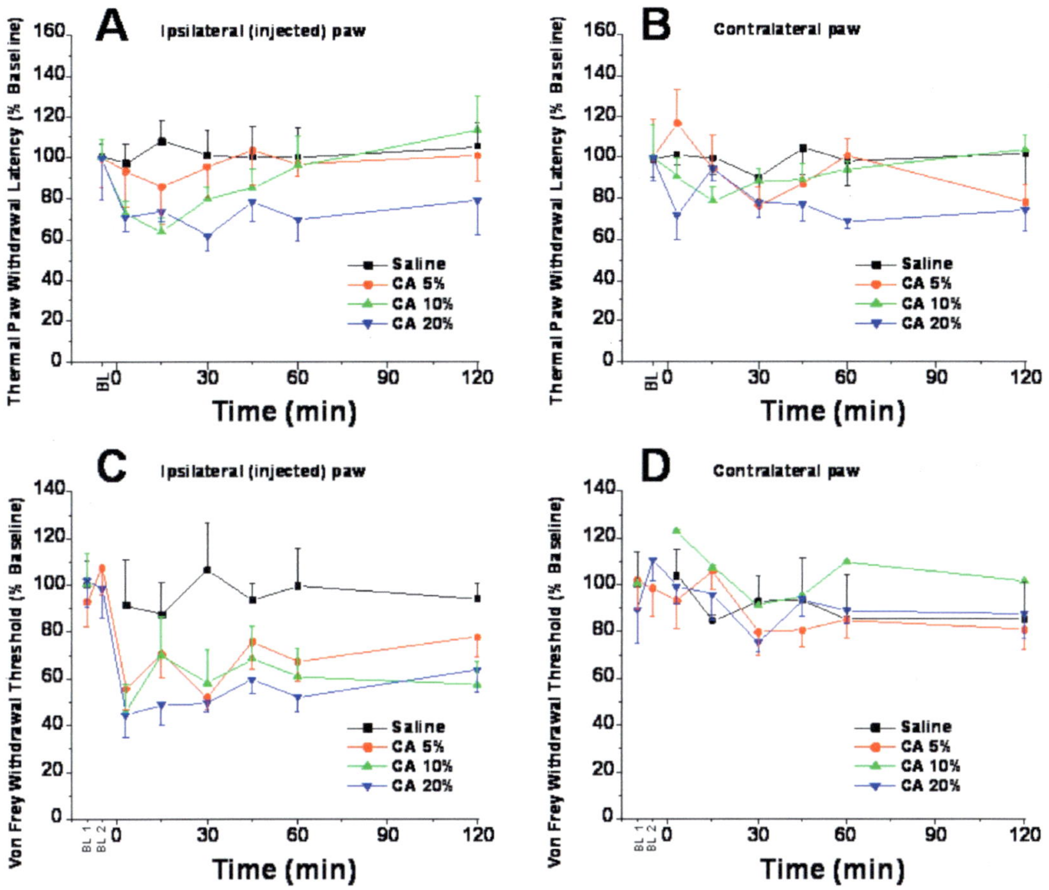

Fig. (12). (**A**): Normalized mean thermal paw withdrawal latency *vs* time following ipsilateral intraplantar injection of vehicle (control) or cinnamaldehyde (CA) at each indicated concentration. There was a significant effect of CA concentration with the 20% CA group significantly different from vehicle and 5% CA groups (LSD; $p < 0.05$ for both). BL: pre-injection baseline. Error bars: SEM (n = 8/group). (**B**): As in (**A**) for paw contralateral to CA injection. There was a significant effect of CA concentration with the 20% group significantly different from vehicle and 5% groups (LSD; $p < 0.05$ for both). (**C**): As in (**A**) for von Frey mechanically-evoked withdrawal of the injected paw. There was a significant effect of CA concentration with 5%, 10% and 20% CA all different from vehicle but not from each other. (**D**): As in (**C**) for contralateral paw. There was no significant effect of CA concentration. ($P>0.05$). (Adapted from [52]).

However in other experiments with allylisothiocyanate, (AITC) chemical compound of mustard oil, we have found that in the 30° *vs* 15°C plates, rats treated with the higher (10% and 15%) concentrations of AITC exhibited a significant preference for the colder 15°C plate compared to vehicle- and 5% concentration treated rats (Fig. **14**), *i.e.*, they significantly avoided the warmer

30ºC plate [27]. The data are consistent with roles for TRPA1 in thermal (hot and cold) hyperalgesia and mechanical allodynia.

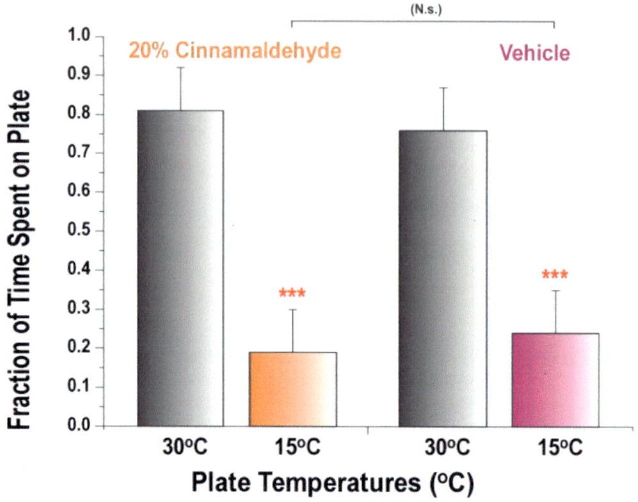

Fig. (13). Cinnamaldehyde does not affect cold sensitivity. In the 30°C *vs* 15°C temperature preference test, both CA- and vehicle-treated rats significantly avoided the colder plate. There was no significant difference between treatments, although there was a very weak trend towards greater cold avoidance by CA-treated rats. (*** P <0.001; n = 8/group). (Adapted from [52]).

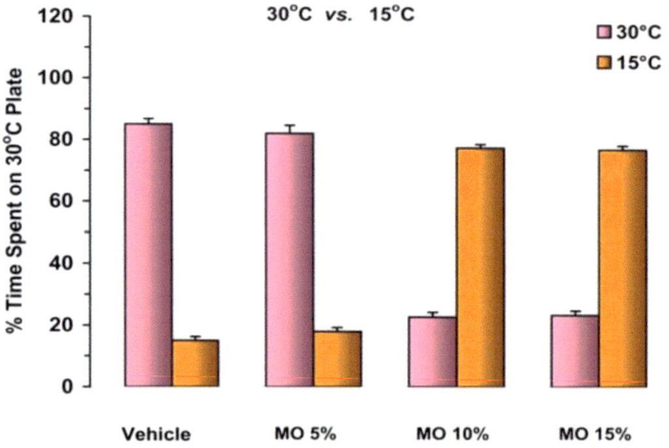

Fig. (14). Biphasic effects of mustard oil (MO) on thermal preference. Graph plots % time rat stood on 30°C *vs* 15°C plate. At high (10% and 15%) AITC concentrations rats spent significantly more time on the 15°C plate (yellow bars) compared to the 30°C plate (purple bars) (P<0.05, and P<0.01, respectively), indicating cold hyposensitivity. At the lower (5%, and vehicle) concentration, rats spent significantly more time on the 30°C plate (p<0.001), indicating cold hypersensitivity. (Adapted from [27]).

Concerning the mechanical sensitivity of TRPA1 channels, Pertovaara and colleagues have recently shown that TRPA1 channels in the skin contribute to sustained as well noxious mechanical stimulus-evoked post-operative pain whereas the spinal TRPA1 channels contribute predominantly to innocuous mechanical stimulus evoked postoperative pain [53]. Furthermore, the spinal TRPA1 is responsible for central pain hypersensitivity in various patho-physiological conditions, such as inflammatory and neuropathic pain [54-57]. However, our abovementioned behavioral data with cinnamaldehyde support a role for TRPA1 in cold detection [52]. These results are consistent with the possibility that TRPA1 agonists can enhance cold-evoked gating of TRPA1 channel to increase cold sensitivity [58,59].

Very interesting data were reported by Carstens' group. They investigated the extracellular spike responses of neurons in the trigeminal subnucleus caudalis (Vc) to intraoral cooling and agonists of TRPM8 and TRPA1 receptor channels. They found that all neuronal units responded to noxious heat and ~90% responded to menthol. Noxious cold evoked responses were significantly enhanced after menthol in a concentration-dependent manner. Most menthol-responsive units also responded to the TRPA1 agonists, cinnamaldehyde and mustard oil, and the TRPV1 agonist capsaicin. The authors concluded that neuronal units in superficial Vc receive convergent input from primary afferents that express TRPM8, TRPA1, and/or TRPV1 channels, either directly or indirectly *via* inter-subnuclear pathways, and that the convergent nature of these units suggests a general role in signaling noxious stimuli [60]. Furthermore, this group of researchers has indicated that the mutual cross-desensitization between cinnamaldehyde (TRPA1 agonist) and menthol (TRPM8 agonist) and differential modulation of cold- *vs* heat-evoked responses, suggests a direct inhibition of TRPM8 and TRPA1 expressed in peripheral nerve endings by cinnamaldehyde and menthol, respectively, rather than a central site of interaction [61]. Their recent findings support the argument that the perceived reductions in oral sensitivity and cross-interactions between menthol and cinnamaldehyde can be largely accounted for by the properties of trigeminal sensory neurons innervating the tongue [62].

TRP CHANNELS IN THE BRAIN

Many TRP ion channels are expressed by brain tissue; some of them are expressed in higher brain centers (for example, TRPC3 and TRPC5), whereas others are expressed in lower brain centers (for example, TRPV1) [15]. The function of these channels remains to be fully elucidated, but there is evidence that several TRP channels may contribute to neuronal excitability and neurotransmitter-mediated signaling in the brain [1,15].

TRPV Subfamily

Members of vanilloid TRP subfamily are found in various brain areas. Interestingly, TRPV1 is highly expressed in central terminals of primary sensory neurons and some brain structures such as hippocampal pyramidal neurons CA1 and CA3 areas, the dentate gyrus, the thalamic and hypothalamic nuclei, the locus coeruleus, periaqueductal grey, cerebellum, central amygdala and caudate putamen [63,64]. However, recent research – that relies on a powerful combination of reporter mice, *in situ* hybridization, whole cell voltage-clamp recordings and calcium imaging – suggests that TRPV1 receptor channel expression is restricted to very few regions of the brain, most notably in a contiguous band of cells within and adjacent to the caudal hypothalamus [15,65]. Consequently, additional research will need to be carried out to explain the differences that have been noted in the behavioral responses between wild-type and TRPV1 null mice [15].

TRPV1 knockout mice adapt more easily than their wild-type littermates to aversive light, and they explore the open arm of the elevated maze more freely; these results are indicative of a reduced unconditioned fear response in TRPV1-deficient mice. Moreover, the latter type of mice exhibits less freezing than wild-type mice in auditory fear conditioning assays [15,66]. These findings imply that TRPV1 antagonists have therapeutic potential as novel anxiolytic drugs. Further behavioral studies that directly compare selective TRPV1 antagonists with differential CNS penetrances are needed to elucidate the role of TRPV1 receptor channel in the brain [15].

Although less intensively studied, TRPV2, TRPV3, and TRPV4 are also found in the CNS [10]. TRPV2 is found co-expressed with TRPV1 in layers IV, V, and VI of the cerebral cortex [67]. TRPV3 expressed in the cortex, thalamus, striatum, hippocampal pyramidal neurons, and cerebellum [68]. TRPV4 is found in the optic chiasm, cerebellum, basal ganglia, and hippocampal pyramidal neurons [69]. However, there is still controversy concerning the functions and roles of TRPV2, TRPV3, and TRPV4 receptor channels in the brain.

TRPC Subfamily

TRPC3 is the most abundant TRP channel of the TRPC subfamily in cerebellar Purkinje cells. Like TRPC6 and TRPC7, TRPC3 channel is activated by diacylglycerol, and G-protein-coupled receptors (GPCRs) are likely to be crucial regulators of channel activity *in vivo* [15,16]. In addition, receptor tyrosine kinases activate TRPC3 *in vitro* and brain-derived neurotrophic factor (BDNF)-mediated survival of cerebellar granular cells depends on functional TRPC3 expression [15,70].

TRPC3 null mice show considerably attenuated inward currents in response to activation of metabotropic glutamate receptor 1 (mGluR1), which is a GPCR that is thought to be upstream of TRPC3 channels in the cerebellum [15,71,72]. TRPC3 deficient mice also display impairments in walking behavior, although – as predicted – the TRPC3-knockout phenotype is less severe than the ataxia observed in mGluR1 null animals [15,71,73]. Overall, these data indicate that TRPC3 channels have important role in synaptic transmission to cerebellar Purkinje cells and in the survival of these cells. Identification of selective pharmacological agents will be useful for determining whether TRPC3 channels have a broader role in cerebellar dysfunction like ataxia [15].

High levels of TRPC5 ion channel are expressed in the hippocampus and amygdala. The TRPC5 knockout mice show less innate fear behavior than their wild-type littermates in an open-field test, an elevated plus maze test and a nose bumping assay. In addition, their conditioned fear memory is unaffected in a single fear conditioning paradigm [15,74]. These behavioral data are consistent with electrophysiological findings of these authors in which brain slices from TRPC5 null mice showed normal membrane excitability and synaptic responses to activation of mGluRs and cholecystokinin (CCK) receptors [15,74]. These results provide a potential link between TRPC5 and the CCK signaling pathway, the activation of which induces anxiety in rodents and humans. This suggests that TRPC5 antagonists might be useful as anxiolytic agents [15].

TRPM Subfamily

In the brain, TRPM2 is expressed by neurons and microglia. Consistent with the concept that TRPM2 functions as a redox sensor, TRPM2 null mice are protected against various pathologies related to oxidative stress, including the focal ischemia model of stroke [15,75]. The TRPM2 channel is also a candidate risk factor gene for bipolar disorder [15,76]. Knockdown of TRPM7 reduces cell death that is caused by oxygen- and/ or glucose deprivation in isolated neuronal cultures, which implies that TRPM7 antagonists may have a role in the treatment of stroke [15,77].

TRP CHANNELS IN HUMAN DISEASES

Mutations in at least six of the 30 members of the TRP channel superfamily are associated with genetic diseases in humans [15,16,18]. The diversity of pathologies caused by TRP channel dysfunction highlights the range of roles TRP channels have in normal physiology and underscores the importance of cation (sodium, calcium) signaling in the peripheral and CNS. Some of the rare mutations may also point to a more general role for TRP channels in these genetic pathologies. In a situation in which a gain-of function mutation underlies the pathology of a TRP channelopathy, the potential utility of an antagonist is evident. However, TRP channels agonists could also have therapeutic benefits in situations in which one gene allele is intact or the gene mutation reduces the probability of the channel being open but leaves TRP channels functioning intact [15]. In addition to the therapeutic areas of genetic diseases, TRP channels have been implicated in various other diseases, such as cancer, cardiovascular, pulmonary, metabolic and other disorders [15].

CONCLUSIONS

The recent expansion of investigation into TRP ion channels has resulted in the identification some of potential drug targets and has elucidated roles for TRP channels in diverse therapeutic areas including pain, pulmonary function, oncology, neurology, visceral organs and genetic diseases [15]. Interest is mounting as a result of emerging data from animal models, human genetic disorders and, in some cases, compounds entering clinical trials. At this early stage, with very limited clinical data available regarding the effects of some antagonists (blockers) to several channels, it is deceptively easy to speculate on the therapeutic potential of TRP channel modifiers [15,18]. Specifically, the new methodology could be used to identify amino acid residues in certain TRP ion channel proteins and G-protein-coupled receptors that are involved in interactions with small molecules that affect their function. Therefore, it provides a framework for high-throughput approaches for future studies on the structural and functional relationships of cellular proteins. Through emerging technologies and concerted efforts across industry and academia, there is reason to believe novel TRP drugs are on the horizon [78,79]. In the meantime, better understanding of the role of TRP ion channels in the CNS will help clinical researchers to predict and screen for possible side effects [1].

ACKNOWLEDGEMENT

None declared.

CONFLICT OF INTEREST

The author states that there is no conflict of interest.

REFERENCES

[1] Chung G, Jung SJ, Oh SB. The transient receptor potential (TRP) family in pain and temperature sensation. In: Beaulieu P, Lussier D, Porreca F, Dickenson AH, Eds. Pharmacology of Pain, Seattle: IASP Press 2010; pp. 327-46.

[2] Cosens DJ, Manning A. Abnormal electroretinogram from a *Drosophila* mutant', Nature 1969; 22: 285-7.

[3] Pak WL, Grossfield J, White NV. Nonphototactic mutants in a study of vision of *Drosopkila'*. Nature 1969; 333: 351-4.

[4] Heisenberg M. Separation of receptor and lamina potentials in the electroretinogram of normal and mutant *Drosophila*. J Exp Biology 1971; 55: 85-100.

[5] Minke B, Selinger Z. Inositol lipid pathway in fly photoreceptors: excitation, calcium mobilization and retinal degeneration. In: Osborne NA, Chader GJ, Eds. Progress in Retinal Research. Oxford: Pergamon Press 1991; pp. 99-124.

[6] Montell C, Rubin GM. Molecular characterization of the *Drosophila* trp locus: a putative integral membrane protein required for phototransduction. Neuron 1989; 2: 1313-23.
[7] Minke B. The history of the Drosophila TRP channel: the birth of a new channel superfamily. J Neurogenetics 2010; 24: 216-33.
[8] Montell C. The history of TRP channels, a commentary and reflection. Pflügers Archive 2011; 461: 499-506.
[9] Caterina MJ, Schumacher MA, Tominaga M, *et al.* The capsaicin receptor: a heat-activated ion channel in the pain pathway. Nature 1997; 389: 816-24.
[10] Caterina MJ. Transient receptor potential ion channels as participants in thermosensation and thermoregulation. American J Physiology: Regul Integr Comp Physiol 2007; 292: R64-R76.
[11] Walters ET. Evolutionary aspects of pain. In: Basbaum AI, Bushnell MC, Eds. Science of Pain, San Diego: Elsevier 2009; pp. 175-84.
[12] Saito S, Shingai R. Evolution of thermoTRP ion channel homologs in vertebrates. Physiol Genomics 2006, 27: 219-30.
[13] Christensen AP, Corey DP. TRP channels in mechano-sensation: direct or indirect activation? Nature Review Neuroscience 2007; 8: 510-21.
[14] Dhaka A, Veena Viswanath V, Patapoutian A. TRP ion channels and temperature sensation. Annual Review Neuroscience 2006; 29: 135-61.
[15] Moran MM, McAlexander MA, Bíró T, Szalassi A. Transient receptor potential channels as therapeutic targets. Nature Review Drug Discovery 2011; 10: 601-20.
[16] Wu LJ, Sweet TB, Clapham DE. Current progress in the mammalian TRP ion channel family. Pharmacology Review 2010; 62: 381-404.
[17] Tominaga M. Thermal sensation (cold and heat) through thermosensitive TRP channel activation. In: Basbaum AI, Bushnell MC, Eds. Science of Pain. San Diego: Elsevier 2009; pp. 127-32.
[18] Nilius B, Owsianik G. Transient receptor potential channelopathies. Pflügers Archive 2010; 460: 437-50.
[19] Patapoutian A, Tate S, Woolf CJ. Transient receptor potential channel: targeting pain at the source. Nature Review Drug Discovery 2009; 8: 55-68.
[20] Carstens E, Klein A, Tsagareli MG, *et al.* Effects of thermo-sensitive transient receptor potential (TRP) channel agonists on the neural coding of touch, temperature and pain sensation, In: Proc. 9th "Gagra Talks", Intern. Conference on Fundamental Problems of Neuroscience. Tbilisi, 2010; pp. 267-80.
[21] Chung M-K, Güler AD, Caterina MJ. TRPV1 shows dynamic ionic selectivity during agonist stimulation. Nature Neuroscience 2008; 11: 555-64.
[22] Willis WD. The role of TRPV1 receptors in pain evoked by noxious thermal and chemical stimuli. Exp Brain Research 2009; 196: 5-11.
[23] Cortright DN, Krause JE, Broom DC. TRP channels and pain. Biochim Biophys Acta 2007; 1772: 978-88.
[24] Dhaka A, Uzzell V, Dubin AE, *et al.* TRPV1 is activated by both acidic and basic pH. J Neuroscience 2007; 29, 159-58.
[25] Levine JD, Alexandri-Haber N. TRP channels: targets for the relief of pain. Biochim Biophys Acta 2007; 1772: 989-1003.
[26] Tominaga M, Caterina MJ, Malberg AB, *et al.* The cloned capsaicin receptor integrates multiple pain producing stimuli. Neuron 1998; 21: 531-43.

[27] Tsagareli MG, Nozadze IR, Carstens MI, Tsiklauri NJ, Carstens EE. Behavioral and electrophysiological study of thermal and mechanical pain modulation by TRP channel agonists. Neurophysiology 2013; 45 (in press).

[28] Lewinter RD, Skinner K, Julius D, Basbaum AI. Umminoreactive TRPV-2, a capsaicin receptor homolog, in the spinal cord of the rat. J Comparative Neurology 2004; 470: 400-8.

[29] Stokes AJ, Wakano C, Del Carmen KA, Koblan-Huberson M, Turner H. Formation of physiological complex betweenTRPV2 and TGA protein promotes cell surface expression of TRPV2. J Cell Biochem 2005; 94: 669-83.

[30] Wainwright A, Rutter AR, Seabrook GR, Relly K, Oliver KR. Discrete expression of TRPV2 within the hypothalamo-neurohypophysial system: implications for regulatory activity within the hypothalamic-pituitary-adrenal axis. J Comparative Neurology 2004; 474: 24-42.

[31] Woodbury CJ, Zwink M, Wang S, *et al.* Nociceptors lacking TRPV1 and TRPV2 have normal heat responses. J Neuroscience 2004; 24: 6410-15.

[32] Nedungadi TP, Dutta M, Bathina CS, Caterina MJ, Cunningham JT. Expression and distribution of TRPV2 in rat brain. Exp Neurology 2012; 237: 223-37.

[33] Vriens O, Appendino G, Nilius B. Pharmacology of vanilloid transient receptor potential cation channels. Molecular Pharmacology 2009; 75:1262-79.

[34] Xu H, Delling M, Jun JC, Clapham DE. Oregano, thyme and clove-derived flavors and skin sensitizers activate specific TRP channels. Nature Neuroscience 2006; 9: 628-35.

[35] Vogt-Eisele AK, Weber K, Sherkheli MA, *et al.* Monoterpenoid agonists of TRPV3. British J Pharmacology 2007; 151: 530-40.

[36] Moqrich A, Hwang SW, Early TJ, *et al.* Impaired thermosensation in mice lacking TRPV3, a heat and camphor sensor in the skin. Science 2005; 307: 1468-72.

[37] Morin C, Bushnell MC. Temporal and qualitative properties of cold pain and heat pain: a psychophysical study. Pain 1998; 74: 67-73.

[38] Foulkes T, Wood JN. Mechanisms of cold pain. Channels (Austin) 2007; 1: 154-60.

[39] Hensel H, Zotterman Y. The effects of menthol on the chemoreceptors. Acta Physiol Scand 1951; 24: 27-34.

[40] McKemy DD, Neuhausser WM, Julius D. Identification of a cold receptor reveals a general role for TRP channels in thermosensation. Nature 2002; 416: 52-8.

[41] McKemy DD. How cold is it? TRPM8 and TRPA1 in the molecular logic of cold sensation. Molecular Pain 2005; 1, 16.

[42] Peier A, Moqrich A, Hergarden AC, *et al.* A TRP channel that senses cold stimuli and menthol. Cell 2002; 108: 105-15.

[43] Dhaka A, Murray AN, Mathur J, Earley TE, Petrus MJ, Patapoutian A. TRPM8 is required for cold sensation in mice. Neuron 2007; 54: 371-8.

[44] Bautista DM, Siemens J, Joshua M, *et al.* The menthol receptor TRPM8 is the principal detector of environmental cold. Nature 2007; 448, 204-9.

[45] Belmonte C, Brock JA, Viana F. Converting cold into pain. Experimental Brain Research 2009; 196: 13-30.

[46] Gerhold KA, Bautista DM. Molecular and cellular mechanisms of trigeminal chemosensation. In: Annals NY Academy Sciences 2009; 1170, pp. 184-189

[47] McCoy DD, Knowlton WM, McKemy DD. Scraping through the ice: uncovering the role of TRPM8 in cold transduction. American J Physiology: Regul Integr Comp Physiology 2011; 300: R1278-R1287.

[48] Klein AH, Sawyer CM, Iodi Carstens M, Tsagareli MG, Tsiklauri N, Carstens E. Topical application of L-menthol induces heat analgesia, mechanical allodynia, and a biphasic effect on cold sensitivity in rats. Behavioural Brain Research 2010; 212:179-86.

[49] Bessac BF, Jordt S-E. Breathtaking TRP channels: TRPA1 and TRPV1 in airway chemosensation and reflex control. Physiology 2008; 23: 360-70.

[50] Rawls SM, Gomez T, Ding Z, Raffa RB. Differential behavioral effect of the TRPM8/TRPA1 channel agonist icilin (AG-3-5). Eur. J Pharmacology 2007; 575: 103-4.

[51] Macpherson LJ, Dubin AE, Evans MJ, *et al.* Noxious compounds activate TRPA1 ion channels through covalent modification of cysteines. Nature 2007; 445: 541-5.

[52] Tsagareli MG, Tsiklauri N, Zanotto KL, *et al.* Behavioral evidence of thermal hyperalgesia and mechanical allodynia induced by intradermal cinnamaldehyde in rats. Neuroscience Letters 2010; 473: 233-6.

[53] Wei H, Karimaa M, Korjamo T, *et al.* Transient receptor potential ankyrin 1 ion channel contributes to guarding pain and mechanical hypersensitivity in a rat model of postoperative pain. Anesthesiology 2012; 117: 137-48.

[54] Pertovaara A, Koivisto A. TRPA1 ion channel in the spinal dorsal horn as a therapeutic target in central pain hypersensitivity and cutaneous neurogenic inflammation. European J Pharmacology 2011; 666: 1-4.

[55] Wei H, Koivisto A, Saarnilehto M, *et al.* Spinal transient receptor potential ankyrin 1 channel contributes to central pain hypersensitivity in various pathophysiological conditions in the rat. Pain 2011; 152: 582-91.

[56] Eid S, Crown E, Moore E, *et al.* HC-030031, a TRPA1 selective antagonist, attenuates inflammatory- and neuropathy-induced mechanical hypersensitivity. Molecular Pain, 2008, 4: 48-57.

[57] Kerstein P, del Camino D, Moran M, *et al.* Pharmacological blockade of TRPA1 inhibits mechanical firing in nociceptors. Molecular Pain 2009; 5: 19-31.

[58] Karashima Y, Talavera K, Everaerts W, *et al.* TRPA1 acts as a cold sensor *in vitro* and *in vivo*. Proc Natl Acad Sciences 2009; 106: 1273-8.

[59] Story GM, Peier AM, Reeve AJ, *et al.* ANKTM1, a TRP-like channel expressed in nociceptive neurons, is activated by cold temperatures. Cell 2003; 112: 819-29.

[60] Zanotto KL, Merrill AW, Iodi Carstens M, Carstens E. Neurons in superficial trigeminal subnucleus caudalis responsive to oral cooling, menthol, and other irritant stimuli. J Neurophysiology 2007; 97: 966-78.

[61] Zanotto KL, Iodi Carstens M, Carstens E. Cross-desensitization of responses of rat trigeminal subnucleus caudalis neurons to cinnamonaldehyde and menthol. Neuroscience Letters 2008; 430: 29-33.

[62] Klein AH, Iodi Carstens M, Zanotto KL, *et al.* Self- and cross-desensitization of oral irritation by menthol and cinnamaldehyde (CA) *via* peripheral interactions at trigeminal sensory neurons. Chemical Senses 2011; 36: 199-208.

[63] Alter BJ, Gereau RW. Hotheaded: TRPV1 as mediator of hippocampal synaptic plasticity. Neuron 2008; 57: 629-31.

[64] Starowicz K, Cristino L, Di Marzo V. TRPV1 receptors in the central nervous system: potential for previously unforeseen therapeutic applications. Current Pharmaceutical Design 2008; 14: 42-54.

[65] Cavanaugh DJ, Chesler AT, Jackson AC, *et al.* 'Trpv1 reporter mice reveal highly restricted brain distribution and functional expression in arteriolar smooth muscle. J Neuroscience 2011; 31: 5067-77.

[66] Marsch R, Foeller E, Rammes G, *et al.* Reduced anxiety, conditioned fear, and hippocampal long-term potentiation in transient receptor potential vanilloid type 1 receptor-deficient mice. J Neuroscience 2007; 27: 832-9.

[67] Venkatachalam K, Montell C. TRP channels. Annual Review Biochemistry 2007; 76: 387-417.

[68] Smith GD, Gunthorpe MJ, Kelsell RE, *et al.* TRPV3 is a temperature-sensitive vanilloid receptor-like protein. Nature 2002; 418: 186-90.

[69] Nilius B, Vriens J, Prenen J, Droogmans G, Voets T. 'TRPV4 calcium entry channel: a paradigm for gating diversity. American J Physiology, Cell Physiology 2004; 286: C195-C205.

[70] Jia Y, Zhuo J, Tai Y, Wang Y. TRPC channels promote cerebellar granule neuron survival. Nature Neuroscience 2007; 10: 557-67.

[71] Hartmann J, Konnerth A. Mechanisms of metabotropic glutamate receptor-mediated synaptic signaling in cerebellar Purkinje cells, Acta Physiologica (Oxford) 2008 (Cited by [15]).

[72] Hartmann J, Dragicevic E, Adelsberger H, *et al.* TRPC3 channels are required for synaptic transmission and motor coordination. Neuron 2008; 59: 392-8.

[73] Hartmann J, Henning HA, Konnerth A. mGluR1/ TRPC3-mediated synaptic transmission and calcium signaling in mammalian central neurons. Cold Spring Harbor Perspectives in Biology 2011; 3(4). doi: 10.1101/ cshperspect.a006726

[74] Riccio A, Li Y, Moon J, *et al.* Essential role for TRPC5 in amygdala function and fear-related behavior. Cell 2009; 137: 761-72.

[75] Miller BA, Zhang W. TRP channels as mediators of oxidative stress. Advances Exp Medicine and Biology 2011; 704: 531-44.

[76] Xu C, Pottle JE, Taylor JT, *et al.* TRPM2 variants and bipolar disorder risk: confirmation in a family-based association study. Bipolar Disorders 2011; 11: 1-10.

[77] Asrar S, Aarts M. TRPM7, the cytoskeleton and neuronal death. Channels (Austin) 2012; 7: 6-16.

[78] Chen J, Reilly RM, Kym PR, Joshi S. *In vitro* and *in vivo* assays for the discovery of analgesic drugs targeting TRP channels. In: Zhu MX, Ed. TRP Channels, Boca Raton, FL: CRC Press 2011, chapter 18.

[79] Hu H, Bandell M, Grandl J, Petrus M. High-throughput approaches to studying mechanisms of TRP channel activation. In: Zhu MX, Ed., TRP Channels, Boca Raton, FL: CRC Press 2011, chapter 12.

 Frontiers in CNS Drug Discovery, 2013, 2, 146-210

CHAPTER 6

Antipsychotic Polypharmacy in Schizophrenia, from Empirical Associations to Combined Selective Treatments

Alessandro De Risio[*,1] **and Davide Carlino**[2]

[1]NSH Health Trust No. 10 "Veneto Orientale", Unit of Psychiatry of Portogruaro, Via Forlanini, 2, 30026 Portogruaro, Venezia, Italia; [2]Department of Morphological, Technological and Clinical Science, Clinic of Psychiatry, University of Trieste, Via De Ralli, 5 34128 Trieste, Italia

Abstract: Treatment with antipsychotics, APs has been a cornerstone of schizophrenia and other severe mental disorders for more than fifty years. Antipsychotics have been used in monotherapy or in a combination of two, or more drugs. Empirical polypharmacy, common after First Generation Antipsychotics, FGAs introduction, in 1960s, was replaced by monotherapy and the principle of "*Minimally effective APs drug strategies*" later on, at the end of the 20th Century. Despite current guidelines recommendations, promoting monotherapy with the newly introduced Second Generation Antipsychotics, SGAs, the practice of combining two antipsychotic drugs is routinely utilized. The aim of this review is to address the boundaries of the polypharmacy with APs, from epidemiological features to its clinical significance. At first APs prescription patterns in Italy and other countries were outlined. Then, a comparison between the theoretical rationale of monotheraphy and the pharmacokinetic and pharmachodynamic properties of the combined selective associations of two APs was performed, to assess if this practice might help in the care of treatment-resistant forms of schizophrenia. Finally, a PubMed literature search from 1957 to February 2013 led to the extraction of 118 papers regarding APs combined treatment, with data from larger RCTs to single case reports described in detail to provide reasons for rationale use of polypharmacy in routine practice. Although RCTs led to inconclusive results, case series revisions outlined the feasibility of combining APs with a complementary pharmacodynamic profile. The need for adequately targeted, clinically effective, low-cost APs combinations improving functional autonomy of schizophrenic persons is warranted.

Keywords: Antipsychotics, combinations, metabolism, monotherapy, polypharmacy, schizophrenia, efficacy.

Address correspondence to Alessandro De Risio: Health Trust No. 10 "Veneto Orientale", Unit of Psychiatry of Portogruaro, *Via* Forlanini, 2 30026 Portogruaro, Venezia, Italia. Phone: 39-0421-761311-30; Fax: 39-0421-761342; E-mails: Alessandro.DeRisio@ulss10.veneto.it; alessandro.derisio@gmail.com

Atta-ur-Rahman & M. Iqbal Choudhary (Eds.)

INTRODUCTION

Schizophrenia is a long-lasting protracted disease with an unpredictable course, whose main symptoms are auditory hallucinations, hearing thoughts spoken aloud, thought withdrawal, insertion or broadcasting, actions experienced as preformed or influenced by external agents, ideas of reference, delusion of persecutions, flattening of affect and lack of insight. Excess of dopamine activity in brain mesolimbic system is still the most plausible hypothesis of the origin of the disease, as well as other conjectures, such as hypofunction of glutamate systems at NMDA glutamate receptor or hyperfunction of 5-HT_2 receptors. Blockade of mesolimbic D_2 receptors is the way used by antipsychotic drug to enact their clinical activity [1, 66].

It is common knowledge that there has been a discordance between the theory and routine practice in the pharmacological treatment of schizophrenia since its early developments. At least three main factors might influence the correct prescription and use of antipsychotic drugs on the persons affected by this disease. The first is the appropriateness of the diagnosis. When the current operationalized diagnostic criteria had not yet been developed, a psychiatric diagnosis showed so much variation between the operators that multiple diagnoses were performed on the same patient [1]. The second feature is represented by the pharmacokinetic and pharmacodynamic characteristics of antipsychotic drugs. For most antipsychotics, interindividual variation in pharmacokinetics accounts for a more than 20-fold discrepancy in medication's steady state concentration at the same dosage, as patients show different absorption, distribution, metabolism and excretion. To overcome this problem, it is necessary to achieve dose titration by using an adequate Therapeutic Drug Monitoring to quantify drug concentration in blood plasma or serum [2]. The third issue is, then, the attitude of the psychiatrists on the prescription of their drugs. A wide discrepancy has been noted between the scarce theoretical evidence on APs combinations and their increasing empirical use in routine practice [3]. This last aspect is particularly interesting, for its dual implication in the activity of the prescribing physicians and on the attitude of the patients who are bound to be treated with APs. Although the majority of current guidelines on schizophrenia promote monotherapy - the prescription of only one antipsychotic drug [4-9] in the real world it often happens that a psychiatrist may prescribe two or more APs on the same patients. Antipsychotic combination treatment, also termed as polypharmacy, is a not explicitly forbidden practice that may have pros and cons. Treatment-resistant schizophrenia patients might take advantage from being treated with two or more drugs acting on different pharmacodynamic targets, while the pharmaceutical expenditure for multiple antipsychotic prescription will obviously increase [10-11]. This might be a great disadvantage, especially when the health systems face a severe economic downturn. Furthermore, warnings have been raised on the possible impact of APs polypharmacy on patients' physical health, with the increased risk of diabetes, cardiovascular diseases and premature death [12-14].

In this review, the extent of polypharmacy with APS will be first described, by outlining how the prescription patterns of these drugs may vary within the health systems of the main industrialized countries. Then, a short history of antipsychotic combination treatment will be illustrated, with particular regard to the empirical widespread polypharmacy of 1960s, that later on became replaced - at least theoretically - by the *"Minimally effective"* monotherapy principle. Afterwards, a comparison between monotherapy and polypharmacy will be attempted by outlining pharmacokinetic and pharmacodynamic reasons supporting the first and the latter prescription modality. In the end, an overview of the combined selective associations of APs supported by controlled studies will be presented, to show which of them might become favourable in the care of treatment-resistant forms of schizophrenia.

ALL THE MAIN HEALTH SYSTEMS OF INDUSTRIALIZED COUNTRIES HAVE TO DEAL WITH ANTIPSYCHOTIC POLYPHARMACY

Apart from the reasons to justify this controversial habit, that will be explained further on, it is important to say that polypharmacy is often practiced in the care of complex illnesses, such as diabetes, epilepsy, cardiovascular diseases, rheumatic disorders, HIV and other multifactorial chronic-degenerative disorders [10]. APs polypharmacy for schizophrenia had developed from empirical observations to become a routine clinical practice, despite a host of controlled researches promoting sequential treatments with single drugs [6-14]. This practice is neither confined to a single country or to a group of countries with a similar cultural or economical profile, nor is a preferred style of care in some nations as compared to others, *i.e.,* western Europe *vs* North America. As a matter of fact, APs polypharmacy is a widespread phenomenon involving all the health systems, not only in the western world, but also in the emerging industrialized countries. To describe the extension of the occurrence, a short overview of use of polypharmacy with APs in the health systems of a group of countries representative of the principal macro-regions of the world will be presented.

The pioneristic study of Tibaldi *et al.* [15] was the first research that in Italy addressed on a rational basis of the prescription patterns of APs. This study outlined how APs polypharmacy was more frequent in general hospital psychiatric wards than in community outpatient services. Although the average mean daily drug dose was low, younger age, higher education, being diagnosed as suffering of schizophrenia and having a longer duration of the illness emerged as predictors of being treated with a higher dosage of APs. The reason to explain multiple prescription patterns was, according to the Authors, a combination of difficulties in achieving scientifically-based data on APs and inadequate undergraduate or postgraduate training for the psychiatrists, associated to the influence of advertising and sale promotion strategies of pharmaceutical companies. The retrospective study of Mauri *et al.* [16], that was set in a general hospital psychiatric ward, evidenced how the polypharmacy of two or more APs was frequent on discharge, with an increase in mean drug daily dosage from 1989 to 2002 and the prevalence of a combination of an FGA plus an SGA. APs prescription patterns in Italy were also investigated in Non-Hospital Residential Facilities, NHRFs. Two other studies displayed how multiple APs prescriptions are only loosely associated to diagnosis and tended to escalate over time during the stay of psychotic patients in NHRF settings [17-18].

Analysis of APs prescription patterns in other western Europe countries displayed how SGAs prescriptions increased over time and became predominant from 1990s onwards, with adjunctive FGAs for sedative purposes becoming predominant in France, Germany, Spain and Greece, without being influenced by ethnical or racial prejudice when drugs were administered to immigrants [19-27].

The analysis of APs prescription patterns in northern European countries had provided interesting results. Two Norwegian studies [28-29] found that at least one third of schizophrenia patients admitted to hospital were mainly treated with a combination of two SGAs or SGA plus FGA. The associations of an FGA plus another FGA or of more than two APs were uncommon. Among the significant predictors of polypharmacy were the number of hospital admissions, the severity of disease, the comorbidities with mental retardation and personality disorder, plus a previous hospital admission within 12 months.

Polypharmacy with FGAs had become the rule, rather than the exception in eastern Europe countries, with the reported purpose to contrast the main symptoms and iatrogenic side effects of single APs [30-32].

The habit of co-prescribing more than one APs in persons with schizophrenia is common in extra-European countries as well. In South Africa, the study of Koen *et al.* [33] evidenced how in Xhosa persons with schizophrenia, polypharmacy was customary for at least one third of the participants. The most common APs combination was haloperidol and a long-acting preparation. Even one fifth of persons being administered with clozapine had a concurrent prescription of a FGA. The Indian study of Ramadas *et al.* [34], conducted in the Thrissur district of the state of Kerala, whose economy and health systems are akin to the developed countries, evidenced a proportion of schizophrenia patients on polypharmacy with APs comparable to other studies. The average mean dose of combined prescription, however, exceeded the recommended doses, raising questions on the sustainability of the risk of adverse effects.

In Australia and New Zealand co-administration of more than one antipsychotic drug is a less utilized option than in other countries. Regional guidelines for the treatment of schizophrenia strongly discourage improper use of antipsychotic drugs and emphasize their careful administration in first episode cases, close integration of drug therapy with psychosocial treatments and clinical audit to prevent questionable practice [35]. As a consequence, the proportion of persons with schizophrenia on polypharmacy or treated with higher doses is lower than in other western countries [36-39].

Research on APs prescription patterns is relatively recent in Asia. Although use of SGAs steadily increased over time from 1990s onwards in People's Republic of China, antipsychotics polypharmacy with oral and depot FGAs involved a relevant proportion of prescriptions, higher than in western Europe, in at least nine Asian countries. A greater severity in schizophrenia symptomatology, especially positive and negative symptoms, as well as higher drug dosage and younger age characterized the patients administered with more than one AP [40-41].

The trend in polypharmacy with APs observed in United States from the introduction of SGAs onwards evidenced an uneven distribution. Some studies showed an increase in multiple APs prescription during hospital stay rather than at discharge, while others outlined the evolution from the standard combination of two FGAs in 1990s, to the association of an FGA plus a SGA, and later to the polypharmacy with two SGAs, that became current after 2000 [10, 42]. According to insurance registries, the overall proportion of people treated with AP polypharmacy in United States increased four times, from 3.3% in 1999 to 13.7% in 2005, with the percentage of schizophrenia sufferers administered with two or more APs raising from 32% in 1998 to 41% in 2000. In single studies, the prevalence of combined treatments ranged from 10% to 50% [43-46]. Persistent APs polypharmacy associated to excessive dosing was reported in a Canadian outpatient study in more than one third of a sample of schizophrenia spectrum disorder as well [47].

Multisite studies comparing APs prescription patterns underscored how polypharmacy was associated to the difficulty in treating the patient, the length of the illness and lack of family support. The concurrent prescription of FGAs plus SGAs was predictive of higher daily drug dosage [48-49]. Females tended to receive lower doses of co-prescribed APs than males in at least one multicentre study [50]. The proportion of polypharmacy was reduced when low-potency FGAs were ruled out in another multisite survey, denoting a derivative use of these drugs as hypnotics [51]. An overview of the studies reporting data on APs prescription patterns and polypharmcy in people affected by schizophrenia is shown in Table **1**.

Table 1. Outline of Studies Reporting APs Prescription Patterns in the Health Systems of Industrialized Countries

Country	Study	No. of Participants	Setting	Mean Daily Drug Dose	Polypharmacy (%)	Comments
Italy	Tibaldi *et al.*, 1997 [15]	437	Cross-sectional, PWGH; CMHC	mg/CPZ/day <500	Inpatients: 45 Outpatients: 28	Predictors of higher APs daily drug dose were younger age, higher education, a diagnosis of schizophrenia
	Mauri *et al.*, 2005 [16]	1,696	Retrospective, PWGH	2002 >1999 >1989	20.63 (1989); 31.24 (1999); 23.09 (2002)	The combination FGA plus SGA increased from 4.04% in 1999 to 13.06% in 2002
	Tomasi *et al.*, 2006 [17]	2,692	Cross-sectional, NHRF	NA	83	No association to APs prescriptions and users diagnosis
	Ghio *et al.*, 2011 [18]	362	Cross-sectional, NHRF	mg/CPZ/day, all pts: admission: 465.6±513.5; census day: 503.2±586.2 mg/CPZ/day, stay 1-3 yrs: admission, 491.9 ±503; census day, 620.2±593.8; mg/CPZ/day, stay 4-5 yrs:admission, 521.1 ±659.3; census day, 622.8±497.9; mg/CPZ/day, stay>6yrs: admission, 401.7±381.4; census day, 581.9±502.9	Overall: admission, 50.8; census day, 57.2; stay 1-3 yrs: admission, 52.0; census day, 56.9; stay 4-5 yrs: admission, 40.9; census day, 50.0; stay>6 yrs: admission, 56.8; census day, 66.4	The study reported a trend in the increase of polypharmacy and daily drug dosage correlated to the length of stay in NHRF. A plausible reason for this trend may be the intent to avoid monotherapy at high doses. Concerns over the increased costs of APs polypharmacy
France	Bret *et al.*, 2007 [20]	527	Cross-sectional, PH	Mean (SD) daily dosage, mg: CLZ: 386 (169); RIS: 6.8 (3.2); AMI: 877 (424); OLZ: 15.9 (5.9)	60.8	FGAs (levomepromazine, cyamemazine) most frequently associated to SGAs to provide treatment for anxiety and to induce sedation
	Bret *et al.*, 2009 [21]	2,192	Naturalistic, PH	NR	49.3	A sedative FGA nearly always associated to a SGA, annulling the expected benefit of the latter on cognition and neurological side effects
Germany	Weinbrenner *et al.*, 2009 [22]	3,121	Retrospective, PH	NA	20.7	Surprisingly high proportion of SGAs as compared to other studies; no gender differences; combinations most frequently composed of FGAs plus SGAs

(Table 1) contd…..

Country	Study	No. of Participants	Setting	Mean Daily Drug Dose	Polypharmacy (%)	Comments
Spain	Lerma-Carrillo *et al.*, 2008 [24]	209	Retrospective, PH	NA	Mean of 1.61 APs at discharge	Amisulpride most frequently used as adjuvant AP
	Molina *et al.*, 2009 [25]	52	Retrospective, PH	-	17.5	Amisulpride most frequently associated to a SGA or a depot FGA
Greece	Douzenis *et al.*, 2011 [26]	153	Cross-sectional, PH	NR	Greek participants: 3.80 APs (SD=1.59) Non-Greek participants: 3.95 APs (SD=1.22)	APs prescription not influenced by ethnicity
	Kontis *et al.*, 2010 [27]	53	Cross-sectional, PH	mg/Eq/CPZ/day >1000	NR	No difference between polypharmacy and monotherapy in cognitive impairment
Norway	Bolstad *et al.*, 2011 [28]	329	Cross-sectional, PH	mg/Eq/CPZ/day: **SGAs**: OLA:288; RIS:244; QUE: 698; ARI: 189; ZIP: 137; AMI: 616; CLZ: 391; SER: 342 **FGAs**: PER: 111; CTX: 233; ZUC: 80; LEV: 120; CPZ: 120; FLU: 50	2 APs: 30.7; 3 or more APs: 3.2%	Predictors of polypharmacy were: two or more previous hospital admissions, low psychosocial functioning, higher negative symptoms
	Kroker *et al.*, 2009 [29]	486	Cross-sectional, PWGH	mg/Eq/CPZ/day: 450	35.6 (2 or more FGAs: 6.5; 2 or more SGAs: 9.4; FGA + SGA: 19.8)	Predictors of polypharmacy were: younger age, admission to hospital in the previous 12 months, comorbidity with personality disorders and mental retardation
Eastern Europe (*Albania, Croatia, Macedonia, Serbia, Romania*)	Jordanova *et al.*, 2011 [30]	1,304	Retrospective, PH	NA	93.2 (2 APs: 23.2; 3 APs: 42.1; 4 or more APs: 22.1)	FGAs prescribed to 63% of persons with psychosis; more evidence-based practices in psychiatric care required for countries participating to the survey
Serbia	Divac *et al.*, 2007 [31]	198	Retrospective, PH	NA	67.7	Polypharmacy rate higher than in western Europe; persons on monotherapy with a higher number of hospital admission than polypharmacy

(Table 1) contd…..

Country	Study	No. of Participants	Setting	Mean Daily Drug Dose	Polypharmacy (%)	Comments
Bosnia-Herze-govina	Loga-Zec and Loga, 2011 [32]	216	Cross-sectional, PH	NA	All participants taking 2 or more APs	Polypharmacy approach considered customary and inevitable; adjunctive treatment set to cover adverse effects of the main AP
South Africa	Koen *et al.*, 2008 [33]	510	Retrospective, PH	mg/Eq/CPZ/day: 233.2	28.6	Use of Clozapine lower than in United States and other industrialized countries; need to adequate current psychiatric care to international guidelines
India	Ramadas *et al.*, 2010 [34]	29	Retrospective, PWGH	NR	31	Risk of prescribing higher than recommended doses with 2 or more APs; risk of EPS, TD, hyperprolactinaemia and QT prolongation in polypharmacy users
Australia and New Zealand	Humberstone *et al.*, 2004 [36]	3,178	Retrospective, CMHC	mg/Eq/CPZ/day: 360 (polypharmacy: 601; monotherapy: 312)	8.4	Reported variation in prescribed dose of APs among the different catchment areas of the survey
	Wheeler *et al.*, 2006 [37]	2,300	Retrospective, CMHC	-	14.3	Polypharmcy associated to higher doses of APs; reported change towards prescription patterns recommended by guidelines over time
	Wheeler *et al.*, 2009 [38]	794	Prospective, CMHC, clinical audit	mg/Eq/CPZ/day: 699	10.6	Prescription patterns of users with polypharmacy followed for 10 months and reviewed by two independent raters: in 46.9% of cases "lacked justification". At the end of clinical audit poly-pharmacy dropped to 3.5%
Asia and China	Xiang *et al.*, 2011 [41]	6,761	Retrospective, PH	NA	46.8 (2001); 38.3 (2004); 43.4 (2009)	Clinical and socio-cultural factors play a role in determining APs polypharmacy in the 9 Asian states and territories participating to the survey
United States	Centorrino *et al.*, 2002 [42]	698	Retrospective, PH	mg/Eq/CPZ/day:371	43	Total dose at discharge increased of 46% from 1993 to 1998 due to polypharmacy; need for further studies to assess costs and benefits of polypharmacy

(Table 1) contd…..

Country	Study	No. of Participants	Setting	Mean Daily Drug Dose	Polypharmacy (%)	Comments
	Gilmer *et al.*, 2007 [43]	15,962	Retrospective, Administrativ e Database	NR	3.3 (1999); 13.7 (2004)	Increase in polypharmacy led to a 27% increase of pharmaceutical costs, with a 274% increment of SGAs co-prescription costs
	Ganguly *et al.*, 2004 [46]	31,435	Retrospective, Administrativ e Database	NR	40 (long-term APs polypharmacy prevalence: 23)	Statistically significant difference with current treatment guidelines rejecting polypharmacy; SGAs polypharmcy significantly associated with QUE and CPZ
	Eisen *et al.*, 2008 [44]	6,666	Retrospective, Administrativ e Database	NR	7.90	The survey investigates polypharmacy with SGAs, reporting adjunctive co-prescription of anticholinergic medication reflecting higher APs dosage
	Megna *et al.*, 2007 [45]	117	Retrospective, PH	NA	22.2	Polypharmacy with SGAs is a frequent practice despite scientific support of guidelines
Canada	Procyshyn *et al.*, 2010 [47]	435	Retrospective, Administrativ e Database	PDD/DDD ratio >1.5 denoting excessive daily drug dose	25.7	Mean PDD/DDD ratio significantly higher for users with APs polypharmacy than monotherapy, denoting APs polypharmacy is associated to excessive dosing
Multisite studies	Barbui *et al.*, 2006a [48] (*UK, Italy, The Netherlands, Germany*)	390	Cross-sectional, CMHC	PDD/DDD >1.5 at baseline and T1 (12 months)	<15	Participants on polypharmacy showed higher psychopathology and were less frequently treated with SGAs
	Barbui *et al.*, 2006b [49] (*UK, Italy, The Netherlands, Germany*)	375	Prospective, CMHC	PDD/DDD >1.5 at baseline and T1 (12 months)	13	Persistent polypharmacy predicted by baseline administration of FGAs + SGAs
	Kiivet *et al.*, 1995 [50] (*Spain, Sweden, Estonia*)	300	Retrospective, PH	Mg/Eq/CPZ/day: 505 (Spain); 515 (Estonia); 399 (Sweden)	76 (Spain) 59 (Sweden) 56 (Estonia)	Low-potency FGAs often used in low doses as sedative; combined AP treatment used to quench side effects

(Table 1) contd.....

Country	Study	No. of Participants	Setting	Mean Daily Drug Dose	Polypharmacy (%)	Comments
	Broekema *et al*., 2007 [51] (*Belgium, Denmark, France, Germany, The Netherlands, Scotland*)	2,725	Cross-sectional, hospital database	Total median dose not calculated	42.1 (24.4 excluding low-potency APs)	APs polypharmacy partially explained by use of low-potency APs as sedative drugs
	Mundt *et al*., 2011 [23] (*Germany, Uzbekistan*)	1,767	Cross-sectional, PH	NA	44 (Germany); 67 (Uzbekistan)	Polypharmacy with CLZ + HAL more common in Uzbekistan; combination of OLZ, CLZ, QUE, RIS, HAL more used in Germany

Abbreviations: **PWGH** = Psychiatric Ward in General Hospital; **CMHC** = Community Mental Health Centre; **PH** = Psychiatric Hospital (outside Italy); **NHRF** = Non Hospital Residential Facility; **mg/Eq/CPZ/day** = milligrams Equivalents of Chlorpromazine per day; **AP** = Antipsychotic Drug; **FGA** = First Generation Antipsychotic; **SGA** = Second Generation Antipsychotic; **EPS** = Extrapiramidal Effects; **TD** = Tardive Dyskinesia; **OLZ** = Olanzapine;**RIS** = Risperidone; **QUE** = Quetiapine; **SER** = Sertindole; **CLZ** = Clozapine; **ZIP** = Ziprasidone; **ARI** = Aripiprazole; **AMI** = Amisulpride; **HAL** = Haloperidol; **PER** = Perphenazine; **CTX** = Clorprothixene; **ZUC** = Zuclopenthixole; **LEV** = Levomepromazine; **CPZ** = Chlorpromazine; **FLU** = Flupenthixole; **PDD** = Prescribed Daily Dose; **DDD** = Defined Daily Dose; **NA** = not available; **NR** = not reported.

THE THEORETICAL CONCEPT OF MONOTHERAPY FACES WITH EMPIRICAL POLYPHARMACY OF APS IN THE TREATMENT OF SCHIZOPHRENIA

Almost a decade after the discovery of FGAs, in 1960s, the utilization of combined APs in the treatment of schizophrenia became widely accepted and recommended [52-57]. It was believed that a combination of two FGAs, a high potency drug associated with a low potency antipsychotic could decrease the side effects of both drugs and, on the other hand, display an adjunctive antipsychotic efficacy. Studies on combinations of a low potency plus a high potency AP, however, were unsystematic and were also lacking the necessary characteristics to assess clinical effectiveness required in today's research practice [52]. Use of combination of antipsychotics became so common that, in 1970s, in United States the prescription of up to six APs had become a routine practice. The most frequent reason put forward to justify combinations of APs was the ineffectiveness of the first used drugs, leading to the necessity to add another one to a failing chemotherapy regimen. As no reasonable difference in terms of clinical effectiveness had been demonstrated by clinical research, older FGAs were mainly chosen for their side effects profile [58]. Polypharmcy in persons with schizophrenia became therefore an "universal" practice, with high-potency neuroleptics being administered at 3.5-fold rate higher than low-potency ones, up to a dosage of 1,200 mg equivalents of chlorpromazine per day, with scarce evidence in favour of a real clinical improvement [52, 57-59].

In 1980s, the increased awareness of the occurrence of adverse side effects and of the risks of tardive dyskinesia and malignant neuroleptic syndrome, induced clinician to discard the practice of combining three or more APs in favour of the principle of the "*Minimally effective APs drug strategies*" of a single drug. For legal reasons, in fact, a reduction of daily APs dosage was warranted. It was recognized that equal or lower than 300 mg equivalents of chlorpromazine per day were as effective as "maxipharmacy", with decreased clinical risks [52, 61]. However, studies on schizophrenic subjects treated with two combined APs displayed how it was difficult to prevent relapses after suspending one of the two drugs [62-63].

During the 1990s, the National Institute of Mental Health, after a close revision of the issues of the literature, established the Schizophrenia Patients Outcomes Research Team, PORT [64-65] to assess effective pharmacological and psychosocial treatment for schizophrenia. At pharmacological level, two were the leading mainframes of PORT: (*i*) each APs was no better than any other in terms of clinical effectiveness, while a minimal effective dose ranging from 300 to 1,000 mg equivalents of chlorpromazine per day; (*ii*) clozapine was the antipsychotic drug of choice in case of lack of response *i.e.,* the persistence of symptoms after two 6-weeks trials of up to 1,000 mg equivalents of chlorpromazine per day to two trials with two different classes of APs. If the treatments with APs are sequential, this means they should be carried out with a single drug. For this reason, NICE Guidelines reaffirmed how APs should not be prescribed concurrently, except for short periods to cover the switch to another drug [4-5]. The principle of monotherapy has been also put forward by American Psychiatric Association guidelines, and by PORT guidelines last update, that explicitly discourages concurrent APs treatment [8-9]. Texas Medication Algorithm Project considers APs polypharmacy only after the failure of four consecutive trials of monotherapy, comprehensive of clozapine [7]. In Austria, Finland, Norway and Singapore local guidelines explicitly forbid APs combinations, that are instead allowed in Denmark and South Africa [6, 212]. Other regional guidelines have overlooked to provide suggestions on polypharmacy [212].

To explain why APs polypharmacy continues to be so common and widespread in the current clinical practice of persons with schizophrenia, some hypotheses have been proposed by field trials [28-29, 51], including inadequate treatment response with a single AP, hesitancy in discontinuing medication in persons with enduring psychotic symptoms, too low doses of single APs. An interesting reason to justify polypharmacy may be the so-called "cross-titration trap", a switch from an AP to another one that never ends, as the clinicians become aware that the patient responds better when the two drugs are co-prescribed and desist from the tapering of the first AP [10]. Low-potency FGAs, such as phenothiazines, as well as some SGAs, like quetiapine are most often prescribed in low doses as hypnotics, and this practice contributes to increase APs polypharmacy [50-51].

There are at least three main ways to combine the different APs: (*i*) two or more drugs of the same class; (*ii*) two drugs in different classes at full dose; (*iii*) adjunctive and augmentation, *i.e.,* a low dose of one AP combined with a standard dose of another [66]. To further understand why clinicians decide to enact this practice, it might be appropriate to explain the pros and cons of APs polypharmacy. Some of the advantages and disadvantages of APs polypharmacy are described in Table **2**.

Table 2. The Pros and Cons of APs Polypharmacy

Advantages of APs Combinations	**Disadvantages of APs Combinations**
Helpful in contrasting side effects of a single AP	Excessive sedation
Low doses to reduce insomnia and/or anxiety	Masking of single APs adverse effects
Helpful in treating violence in high-risk patients	Increasing costs of prescribing two or more drugs
Useful in treating severe recurrences of the disease	Improper alternative to adequate psychiatric services (NHRFs, inpatient crisis units) or effective non-pharmacological treatments (integrated psychosocial interventions with Cognitive Behaviour Therapy for psychoses, CBTp or Behavioural Family Treatments, BFT)
Useful in treating clozapine-resistant patients	Too often empirically enacted[§]

[§]"because he's a big chap"[66].

As up to two thirds of persons with resistant schizophrenia are partial or poor responders to clozapine treatment, to overcome clozapine resistance is the main clinical reason that nowadays justifies co-prescription of APs [4, 7, 67-68]. Clozapine intolerance, with the second AP as augmentation of a low clozapine dose, is another motivation to combine antipsychotic drugs [66]. From this view, an adequate and sustainable polypharmacy should only be enacted when confronting with a person resistant to clozapine, with an absolute necessity to contrast severely disabling psychotic symptoms. There are, however, a few open and controlled trials of combinations of different APs than clozapine, with contrasting results [4, 10]. To better understand the rationale sustaining these combinations, a brief overview of the main aspects of some pharmacokinetic and pharmacodynamic properties of APs is required.

THE MAIN PHARMACOKINETIC AND PHARMACODYNAMIC ASPECTS IN APS POLYPHARMACY

It is known that drugs may interact through pharmacokinetic and pharmacodynamic mechanisms. The concurrent administration of two or more drugs may lead to their impaired action, with a therapeutic failure and/or the occurrence of side effects. This has been observed in APs polypharmacy as well [3].

Pharmacokinetic interactions may first occur during absorption by altering the available proportion of the drugs. Other interactions may take place during distribution. In this context, current research highlighted the importance of the drug efflux transporter P-glycoprotein, P-gp, a protein belonging to ATP-cassette binding transporter protein family encoded by the multidrug resistance gene (MDR1; ABCB1) [2]. This protein acts as a drug efflux pump, greatly altering substrate absorption, distribution and excretion [69]. Polymorphism in genes encoding for P-gp, influencing activity of this protein in the intestinal mucosa and blood-brain barrier, accounted for variations in plasma levels of 9-hydroxyrisperidone and quetiapine in patients with schizophrenia [2, 70-71]. Among SGAs amisulpride, aripiprazole, olanzapine, perospirone, risperidone and paliperidone are substrates for P-gp in therapeutic concentrations, while clozapine and quetiapine are not substrates for P-gp [72]. On the other hand, loxapine is not a substrate of P-gp *in vitro* [69]. SNRI antidepressants, such as venlafaxine, are substrates of P-gp as well [2].

In APs polypharmacy, however, the most important pharmacokinetic interactions take place during hepatic metabolism, *i.e.,* the process of biotransformation from an active compound to an inactive metabolite that can be eliminated through excretion. The majority of APs is metabolized through Cytocrome P450, CYP enzymatic system. Although CYP 450 isoenzyme are principally located in the liver, their activity has been detected in other tissues, such as brain or small intestine mucosa [2, 66]. More than 200 CYP 450 isoenzymes catalyze phase-I reactions, allowing the introduction in the compound of a polar functional group, that permits a phase-II conjugation reaction with highly polar molecules such as glucuronic or sulphuric acid [2]. CYP 450 isoenzymes are characterized by genetic polymorphism, that is there are in the population subgroups, or phenotypes of different metabolic capacities according to the genetic features of their CYP enzymes. Functional alleles are deficient in Poor metabolizers, PM, while Intermediate metabolizers, IM might either carry an active and an inactive allele, or have two reduced activity alleles. Two active alleles are present in Extensive metabolizers, EM, whereas an intensification of functional alleles is the feature of ultra-rapid metabolizers, UM [2]. PM are exposed to the risk of reaching higher concentration of the drugs, with adverse or toxic reactions, while UM might not show the requested therapeutic effects due to reduced plasma concentrations [2, 73]. Enzymatic inhibition and induction are the two main conditions influencing drug metabolism. Enzymatic inhibition, due to a competition for binding to a specific CYT P450 enzymatic site, induce a reduction in the enzyme activity, leading to a fast increase in the hematic concentration of a drug, that is displaced from the enzyme for its lower receptor affinity. A slower process is, instead, enzymatic induction, for the involvement of genetic transcription mechanisms, with an increase in the enzymatic protein synthesis eventually determining a reduction of drug plasma concentrations. Metabolic interactions on CYP 450 isoenzymes are usually observed in studying co-administration of APs with antidepressants, mood stabilizers, cigarette smoking and particular aliments [66]. For CNS drugs, the most relevant CYP 450 isoenzymes are CYP 1A2, CYP 2B6, CYP 2C9, CYP 2C19 and CYP 3A4/5 [2].

In general, APs are mainly metabolized by CYP 1A2, CYP 2D6, CYP 2C19 and CYP 3A4, except amisulpride, that has a linear kinetic, being excreted with urine without a remarkable metabolization. Clinically relevant inhibitory properties are shown only by some APs, such as perazine, that inhibits CYP 1A2, or melperone, a strong inhibitor of CYP 2D6 [2, 183, 231, 232]. The association between clozapine and aripiprazole or ziprasidone has complementary basis, for the two drugs become metabolized by different CYP isoenzymes than clozapine [73, 160-161]. As isoenzymes such as CYP 3A4 and P-gp are co-expressed in the enterocytes, liver, kidneys, blood-brain barrier and neurons, it is conceivable that they act synergistically in limiting absorption, metabolism and bioavailability [225]. Co-occurrence of CYP 3A4 and P-gp in endothelial cells and neurons may represent a cytoprotective mechanism [228]. An overview of the principal CYP 450 isoenzymes involved in APs polypharmacy, with the different drugs mainly acting as substrates, inhibitors and inducers, their relationship with APs combinations and the clinical consequences, is presented in Table **3**.

Pharmacodynamic interactions usually take place between drugs with overlapping therapeutic or adverse effects or among drugs acting on the same physiological system [66]. When combining two or more APs, the risk of adverse effects rises proportionally to the number of combined drugs. For this reasons, APs combinations should be used only as a last resort, when monotherapies have failed, or have proved inadequate, carefully monitoring the outcomes with the commitment to discontinue them once no clinical improvement is seen [7, 66]. Drugs with a similar mechanism of action should not be combined [10].

Among the motivations that put forward the choice of APs polypharmacy, there are several pharmacodynamic issues. First of all, APs combinations may be prescribed to obtain multiple receptor agonism, then to exert agonism preferentially on specific, targeted receptors and finally to intensify block of dopamine D_2 receptor. A further pharmacodynamic rationale is the choice of drugs with a favourable metabolic burden profile to avoid hyperglycemia, weight gain and the other common side effects of SGAs [10, 77]. Multireceptorial agonism is usually chosen to minimize disturbing side effects, such as daytime sedation or to control anxiety and insomnia. With older FGAs, it was a customary

Table 3. The Principal CYP 450 Isoenzymes, their Involvement in the Metabolism of APs and the Relation to APs Polypharmacy

Isoenzyme	% of Cyto-chrome Activity	Genetic Polymorphysm	Substrate(s)	Inhibitor(s)	Inducer(s)	Relation to APs Poly-pharmacy	Clinical Conse-quences
CYP 2D6	5	7% of Caucasians, 4.5% of Hispanics, 1.9% of African Americans and 1% of Asians are poor metabolizers, PMs; ultrarapid metabolizers, UMs (10-29%) are common in North Africa and Middle East	**Antidepressants**: amitriptyline, clomipramine, fluoxetine, fluvoxamine, imipramine, maprotiline, mianserine, paroxetine, trimipramine, venlafaxine; **Opiates**: codeine, dextrometorphane, idrocodone, methadone tramadole; **FGAs**:***chlorpromazine, flupenthixol, fluphenazine, levomepromazine, perphenazine, thioridazine, zuclopenthixol*** **SGAs**: ***aripiprazole***[†]**,** ***iloperidone, risperidone, sertindole***	**Antidepressants**: bupropione, duloxetine, fluoxetine, moclobemide, paroxetine; **SGAs:** ***melperone***[(i)]***;*** **Others**: amiodarone, chinidine, cimetidin, metoclpramide, metoprolol, pergolide, propafenone, propanlol, ritonavir	-	Concurrent aripiprazole administration should not cause significant metabolic interactions in patients taking clozapine; Augmentation with melperone increase levels of a second AP in CYP 2D6 UM patients [183]	Absence of pharmaco-kinetic interactions might favour SGA clozapine-aripiprazole combination; Melperone augmentation as a possible pharmacological strategy in CYP 2D6 UM patients not responding to APa metabolized by this isoenzyme [183]
CYP 2B6	1-10	Functionally deficient allele CYP 2B6*6 occurs in 15-60% of various populations, inactive allele CYP 2B6*18 occurs predominantly in Africans (4-12%) [224]	**Antidepressants:** bupropione sertraline; **Opiates**: methadone; **Others**: cyclophosfamide, efavirenz, selegiline	Clopidogrel, itraconazol, moclobemide	Bromocriptine, rifampicine	Relation to APs polypharmacy yet to be established	Unrelated to clinical consequences of APs polypharmacy
CYP 3A4	30	This isoenzyme metabolizes at least 50% of all marketed drugs and accounts for 50-60% of the total liver P450 [66]. Until recently little	**Antidepressants**: trazodone; **Benzodiazepines**: alprazolam, brotizolam, midazolam; **Opiates**: buprenorphine, levomethadon	**Antidepressants**: fluvoxamine; **Antifungines**: ketoconazole, itraconazole, fluconazole; **Others**: amiodarone, bromocriptin,	Carbamazepine, cigarette smoking, dexamethason, efavirenz, oxybutynin, Phenobarbital, phenytoin, primidon,	Concurrent ziprasidone administration should not cause significant metabolic interactions in patients taking clozapine	Absence of pharmacokinetic interactions might favour SGA clozapine-ziprasidone combination

(Table 3) contd…..

Isoenzyme	% of Cyto-chrome Activity	Genetic Polymorphysm	Substrate(s)	Inhibitor(s)	Inducer(s)	Relation to APs Poly-pharmacy	Clinical Conse-quences
		genetic polymorphism was identified. However, Single Nucleotide Polymorphism, SNPs have been identified in Africans (54%) and Caucasians (5%) [225]	**FGAs**: ***bromperidol haloperidol, pimozide***; **SGAs**: ***aripiprazole***†, ***quetiapine****, ***risperidone***+, ***sertindole, ziprasidone***#, ***zotepine;*** **Others**: buspirone, bromocriptine, buspirone, dihydroergocriptine, zaleplone, zolpidem, zopiclone	cimetidine, claritromycin, erythromycin, grapefruit juice, indinavir, isoniazid, mifepriston, nelfinavir, ritonavir, saquinavir, troleandomycin, verapamil, voriconazol;	rifabutin, ritonavir, St. John's wort		
CYP 1A2	10-15	12-13% of African Americans, Asians and Caucasians are PMs [66]	**Antidepressants**: agomelatine, duloxetine, fluvoxamine, imipramine; **FGAs**: ***chlorpromazine, thioridazine***; **SGAs**: ***asenapine***±, ***clozapine***‡, ***olanzapine***§; **Others**: caffeine, rasagiline, ropirinole	**Antidepressants**: fluvoxamine, sertraline; **FGAs**: ***perazine***; **Others**: cimetidine, ciprofloxacin, enoxacin, grapefruit juice, isoniazid, norfloxacine, propafenone	Omeprazole, charcoal-broiled food, cigarette smoking	No pharmacokinetic reason to combine olanzapine with clozapine, FGAs, SGAs. Relevant increase in clozapine serum levels after co-administration with CYP 1A2 inhibitor perazine [231, 232]	Combinations of olanzapine plus FGAs/SGAs might not be clinically useful§ Unwanted side effects due to increase in clozapine serum levels after add-on with perazine [231, 232]
CYP 2C9	18	Significant polymorphism (10%) identified in Europeans, while SNPs were monomorphic in African and Asian populations [226]	**Antidepressants**: doxepin, fluoxetine **Others**: zolpidem	**Antidepressants**: fluvoxamine **Others**: amiodarone, fluconazole, miconazol, saquinavir, valproate, voriconazl	Dexamethason, Phenobarbital, phenytoin, primidon, rifampicin, warfarin	Unrelated to APs polypharmacy	Unrelated to clinical consequences of APs polypharmacy
CYP 2C19	4	3-5% of Caucasians + 8-23% of Asians show a lack of this isoenzyme	**Antidepressants**: citalopram, clomipramine, dothiepin/dosulepin, doxepin, escitalopram, fluoxetine, imipramine,	**Antidepressants**: fluoxetine, fluvoxamine, moclobemide; **Others**: esomeprazole, felbamate, fluconazole,	Ginkgo Biloba, St. John's wort, Phenobarbital, phenytoin, primidon, rifampicin	Unrelated to APs polypharmacy	Unrelated to clinical consequences of APs polypharmacy

(Table 3) contd.....

Isoenzyme	% of Cytochrome Activity	Genetic Polymorphysm	Substrate(s)	Inhibitor(s)	Inducer(s)	Relation to APs Polypharmacy	Clinical Consequences
			moclobemide, sertraline, trimipramine **Benzodiazepines**: diazepam; **FGAs**: ***perazine***; **SGAs**: ***clozapine***; **Opiates**: methadone; **Others**: propanolole, omeprazole, lansoprazole, progesterone	isoniazid, miconazol, omeprazole			
CYP 2 E1	9	CYP 2E1*7 allele more frequent (33.9%) in Chinese Han, Japanese and Asians than in Germans (3.7%) [227]	Acetaminophene, acetone, benzene, choloform, fatty acids, ethanol, isoniazid, styrene	Disulfiram	Ethanol, isoniazid, acetaldehyde, benzene	CYP 2E1 polymorphism associated to schizophrenia but not related to risperidone response [226]. No information about association with APs polypharmacy	Relation to clinical consequences of APs polypharmacy yet to be established

†aripiprazole has a dual metabolic pathway through CYP 2D6 and CYP 3A4. Antidepressants might increase aripiprazole concentrations by inhibiting CYP 2D6, while CYP 3A4 inducers like carbamazepine might reduce aripiprazole levels down to 70% [72-73]; ‡clozapine and olanzapine have a common metabolic pathway through CYP 1A2, with this isoenzyme showing a major role for clozapine, due to the presence of a direct secondary glucurnation pathway leading to olanzapine excretion as a soluble metabolite. Antidepressants might, however, increase the levels of olanzapine from 54 to 77%. As cigarette smoking increases clearance of high-potency FGAs and several SGAs by inducing cytochromes 1A2 and 3A4, abrupt smoking cessation might increase levels of clozapine up to toxic range with unpredictable consequences [72-73]; *quetiapine is metabolized to an inactive compound *via* 3A4 isoenzyme, with 3A4 inhibitors increasing quetiapine level up to 3-fold [73]; +clinical evidence reporting no increase in clozapine levels after co-administration of risperidone contrasts with the theoretical possibility to optimize clozapine dosage by adding another AP aimed at increasing clozapine level through effects on Cytochrome P450 metabolism [10, 135]; #ziprasidone is only partially (33%) metabolized by 3A4 isoenzyme, with its major metabolizing pathway through aldehyde oxidase system, that is neither saturable, nor inhibitable [74]; § olanzapine show a common metabolizing pathway with most FGAs and clozapine. A retrospective chart review of the olanzapine-haloperidol combination [75] and a randomized controlled trial of olanzapine-sulpiride association [76] failed in showing pharmacokinetic data supporting clinical improvement of psychotic symptoms; ±asenapine has an alternative metabolizing pathway trough glucuronosyl transferase [2]; (i) melperone can inhibit metabolism of other commonly prescribed CNS drugs that are substrates of CYP 2D6 isoenzyme, such as venlafaxine, whose serum levels can increase up to 52% after co-prescription with this AP [233]. Increase in plasma levels of a SSRI or a SNRI might induce a Serotonin syndrome, whose symptoms may include mental status change (agitation, hallucinations, coma), autonomic instability (tachycardia, labile blood pressure, hyperthermia), neuromuscular aberrations (hyperreflexia, incoordination) and/or gastrointestinal symptoms (nausea, vomiting, diarrhea). On the other hand, SSRIs and SNRIs can independently increase serotonin levels when coprescribed with triptans, 5-HT agonists [234]. Contrariwise, aripiprazole may exert an activity against serotonin syndrome with its high affinity to postsynaptic 5HT2A and 5HT1A receptors, that would be protected against a surplus of serotonin, especially if aripiprazole is co-administered with a CYP 2D6 inhibiting SSRI [235].

practice to prescribe high-potency D_2-blocking drugs during the day associated to small doses of low-potency phenothiazines at bedtime to spread side effects and to take advantage of sedation induced by their histaminergic and antimuscarinic activity [50]. In this context, doubts have been raised whether hypnotic use of low-potency phenothiazines should be considered a form of APs polypharmacy [28-29]. Older phenothiazines as hypnotics have been replaced by olanzapine and quetiapine, two SGAs with comparable antimuscarinic and histaminergic properties [78]. As optimal antipsychotic action is generally achieved with a 60-80% level of D_2 receptor occupancy, with a balanced activity on cortical 5-HT_2 and mesolimbic D_2 receptors, it might be a reasonable therapeutic strategy to combine clozapine and quetiapine, two APs usually reaching a degree of D_2 occupancy around 70%, with more potent SGAs, such as risperidone [10, 66]. The last pharmacodynamic useful strategy is to combine APs to preferentially act on specific receptors with alleged therapeutic advantages. This is the rationale of the combinations between clozapine and other SGAs, such as sulpiride, with a targeted D_2/D_3 antagonism, ziprasidone, with a favourable agonistic activity on 5-HT_{1A} serotoninergic receptors and, most of all, aripiprazole, a D_2 partial agonist SGA also active on 5-HT_{1A} receptors. The associations involving 5-HT_{1A} serotonin receptors, in fact, might improve anxiety, negative depressive symptoms and especially cognitive dysfunctions [79-83]. The complementary nature of the associations between clozapine and ziprasidone or aripiprazole also allow the reduction of metabolic adverse effects, such as hyperglycemia, dyslipidemia and weight gain [84].

This outline has demonstrated that pharmacokinetic and pharmacodynamic complementary properties may be an essential feature when there is the need to combine these drugs. Although guidelines do not show conclusive evidence on the effectiveness and the feasibility of APs combinations [4-9], a host of researches has attempted to demonstrate that APs polypharmacy might be useful, at least in treatment resistant schizophrenia. An overview of controlled evidence in support of combined AP treatment might provide further elements to correctly enact this practice.

THE RESEARCH ON APS POLYPHARMACY: DO EVIDENCE SUPPORT CLINICAL EFFECTIVENESS?

Although a host of studies on APs polypharmacy has outlined how this practice is extensive, still there is not enough evidence to support its clinical use, despite a small number of adequately conducted randomized controlled trials whose results have attempted to shed light on the effectiveness of combinations of antipsychotic drugs. The extent of APs polypharmacy has been described in reviews and investigated by meta-analyses that have evaluated the randomized trials published on this topic. Reviews on APs polypharmacy have investigated combinations of SGAs plus FGAs [85, 88], SGA polypharmacy [10, 84, 86-88, 211], combinations of clozapine plus FGAs/SGAs [85-89] and the impact of systematic, practice-based interventions to reduce the prevalence of combining APs [212]. In all the review papers were given details on randomized controlled trials, as well as on open studies, case series studies and case reports. Combined antipsychotic treatment has been also evaluated by several critical reviews and meta analyses [90-94]. The critical reviews have evidenced how augmentation with risperidone or sulpiride, as well as a longer duration of the trial favoured the activity of clozapine [90-91]. The need for augmentation trials of adequate length, longer than 6 weeks in patients partially responding to clozapine has been outlined in the meta-analysis of Paton *et al.* [92]. Three other meta-analyses involved the evaluation not only of studies conducted in the Western hemisphere, but of Chinese trials also, with contrasting results [68, 93]. Correll *et al.* [93] evidenced a regional effect in Chinese studies, in which clozapine and the second APs were started together, and antipsychotic co-treatment resulted superior to monotherapy, in contrast with Western trials, where the other AP is added to treatment-resistant persons already taking clozapine. These interesting results were contradicted by Barbui *et al.* [68] and Honer *et al.* [89], who displayed that the methodology of Chinese polypharmacy trials was poorer than Western ones, with "sequential" or absent randomization, no evidence of placebo controls and very limited use of blinding. The evidence supporting the effectiveness of adjunctive AP treatment in clozapine resistance is - consequently - poor, with modest or absent clinical benefit [68, 89, 92]. Even the duration of the trials, that apparently influenced the results of earlier researches, had no impact on the clinical effectiveness of APs combinations, according to the meta-analysis of Taylor *et al.* [94], fostering the necessity to develop longer and larger controlled studies on APs polypharmacy in the future. The characteristics of the main review and meta-analytic papers on APs polypharmacy are reported in Table **4**.

Table 4. Outline of the Main Reviews and Meta-Analyses on Antipsychotic Polypharmacy Published from 2002 Onwards

Type of Study	Reference	No. of Reports	No. of Double Blind RCTs	No. of Open Studies	No. of Case Series	No. of Case Reports	Comments
Reviews[a]	Freudenreich and Goff, 2002	12	2	6	1	-	Empirical support to augment clozapine with a D_2-blocker drug like RIS. Use of APs polypharmacy unsupported by evidence
	Lerner *et al.*, 2004	19	1	2	8	19	CLZ combined to RIS (*n*=69), SUL (*n*=35), OLZ (*n*=3), QUE (*n*=65), ZIP (*n*=11); other associations were OLZ+SUL (*n*=7), OLZ+QUE (*n*=1), RIS+OLZ (*n*=9), RIS+QUE (*n*=1). Combinations of SGAs clinically effective and well tolerated, but more double-blind RCTs needed
	Patrick *et al.*, 2005	52	4	13	-	35	Only 1 open label trial and 2 case reports used effective criteria for evaluation of drug combination and used standardized instruments to assess outcome; in 3 out of 4DBRCT (75%) and in 9 out of 13(69%) open label trials APs polypharmacy improved symptoms. APs polypharmacy not supported by EBM practice but feasible for clinical use
	Zink, 2005	14	1	2	2	9	Outline of the combination of OLZ plus HAL (*n*=40), FLU (*n*=1), PIM (*n*=1), CLZ (*n*=3), RIS (*n*=6), SUL (*n*=23), AMI (*n*=8), ARI (*n*=1). In the only DB RCT (OLZ + SUL) there was improvement of mood, but not of psychotic symptoms. In another prospective trial (OLZ + SUL), psychopathology improved
	Chan and Sweeting, 2007	21	-	4	5	12	Limited literature highlighting some SGAs combinations (OLZ + AMI; QUE + RIS), with emphasis on isolated case reports supporting worsening of psychosis after ARI add-on. Improvement observed with APS with pharmacodynamic complementary receptor profile.
	Englisch and Zink, 2008	11	-	4	1	6	Outline of the combination of OLZ plus ARI (*n*=94). Combination CLZ + ARI shows a favourable profile for the absence of metabolic side effects and the reduction of heavy clozapine-associated adverse effects. Standardized instruments evidence improvement of clozapine-induced obsessive symptoms in 1 case reports and quality of life in one open study.

(Table 4) contd…..

Type of Study	Reference	No. of Reports	No. of Double Blind RCTs	No. of Open Studies	No. of Case Series	No. of Case Reports	Comments
	Pandurangi and Dalkilic, 2008	75	6[§]	4	24	41	A comprehensive review addressing the need of regulating APs polypharmacy through evidence-based prescribing algorithms. Extensive coverage of cases (*n*=678). Evidence of psychopathology improvement when adding a strong D_2-blocker drug like RIs to CLZ from RCTs. Evidence of significant weight loss from the CLZ + QUE combination. Exacerbation of psychotic symptoms in some combinations with ARI.
	Honer *et al.*, 2009	7[#]	-	-	-	-	4 DB, placebo-controlled RCTs were on the CLZ + RIS combination: in 3 of them there was no statsistically improvement in psychopathology in RIS arm compared to placebo arm, while one favoured RIS. In 2 RCTs (CLZ + AMI and CLZ + ARI) there was no difference with the placebo arm. In one RCT (CLZ + SUL) SUL was slightly better that placebo.
"Critical" reviews[b]	Kontaxakis *et al.*, 2005	11	3	8	-	-	This review also explored the add-on of other than APs drugs (lithium, lamotrigine, d-cycloserine, *etc.*) to clozapine. CLZ augmentation with SUL had a favourable outcome, as well as augmentation with other psychoactive drugs
	Kontaxakis *et al.*, 2006	15	2	3	8	-	A comprehensive review covering pharmacological, clinical and methodological issues in APs polypharmacy, in persons with schizophrenia or schizoaffective disorder (*n*=86), administered with CLZ + RIS combination. A lower dose of RIS and a longer duration of trials are associated to better outcomes.
	Barnes and Paton, 2011	15	9[†]	4	-	2	This comprehensive, critical review addresses not only studies on pharmacological and clinical aspects of APs polypharmacy, but also interventions to reduce use of combined APs, focusing on questionable practices such as "p.r.n./as required" medication, effectiveness of clinical audits and the role of non medical psychiatric staff in changing APs prescribing practices
Meta-analyses[c]							
	Paton *et al.*, 2007	12	4	8	-	-	The analysis revealed 4 adequate RCTs, whose participants (n=166) were taking CLZ and augmented with another AP. Two RCTs with a duration of more than 10 weeks showed higher odds ratios, as well as 8 open studies. RCT on APs polypharmacy should be longer than those for AP monotherapy.

(Table 4) contd…..

Type of Study	Reference	No. of Reports	No. of Double Blind RCTs	No. of Open Studies	No. of Case Series	No. of Case Reports	Comments
	Correll *et al.*, 2009	19	16*	2*	-	-	Superiority of AP co-treatment with 2 APs started at the same time in trials lasting more than 10 weeks. Regional effect of Chinese studies using costart of CLZ + FGA/SGA suggested that CLZ + FGA combination was superior to SGA or FGA monotherapy. However, due to a rater bias, combination treatments were not more effective than CLZ monotherapy
	Barbui *et al.*, 2009	21	6	15	-	-	6 RCTs conducted in the Western hemisphere were adequately conducted and showed minimal effects of CLZ + APs combination on outcome measures, with the reverse was true for 15 Chinese studies, lacking double blindness and use of placebo. Meta-analysis conducted on an adequate sample of patients (n=624), with single studies however showing a limited number of participants. Adding a second AP to clozapine has modest to absent benefit
	Taylor and Smith, 2009	10	10	-	-	-	Meta-analysis conducted on an adequate sample size (*n*=522). CLZ + AP combinations were superior to placebo only in mean effect size for psychopathology rating scales score. Duration of the study was not associated to outcome, with marginal therapeutic benefit of CLZ + APs in trials whose duration was up to 16 weeks.

§5 DB + 1SB study; #all studies are double blind, placebo-controlled trials; *one SB study [205] + 1 study with "unclear" binding [99]; a[84-88]; [10]; [89]; b[90-91]; [212]; c[68]; [92-94]; †one SB study [205] + 8 DB studies.

To further provide useful details, a description of single studies on APs combinations will be enacted, with the purpose of shedding light on a controversial, somewhat desultory clinical practice that is however so common to have been considered a continue, deliberately performed treatment choice [95].

METHODOLOGY

From a PubMed search on the literature and on the bibliographies of earlier appearing reviews and meta-analyses, 162 reports on APs polypharmacy were obtained. The literature search was conducted from June, 1957 to February, 2013. Keywords used for the search, together with logical operators "AND"; "IN", were: antipsychotics, combinations, metabolism, monotherapies, polypharmacy, schizophrenia, efficacy.

To be included in this chapter, each study was required to meet the criteria of being divided according to the possible combination category: (*i*) Clozapine plus FGA; (*ii*) Clozapine plus SGA, (*iii*) FGA plus FGA; (*iv*) SGA plus SGA; (*v*) FGA plus SGA; (*vi*) Multiple APs. Full revision of all 162 papers lead to drawing out the following data [10, 84, 87]: type of report and trial design (randomized double blind study, open study, case series, case report, *etc.*), change in psychopathology, doses (if available), duration of treatment, outcome and relevant observations. The revision led to the selection of 118 papers of interest for this chapter. In particular, there were reviewed 16 double blind RCTs [79, 96-98, 109, 129, 139-142, 157, 159, 162, 173, 175, 208], 17 open, case series studies [100-101, 118-119, 122-123, 128, 129, 134, 135, 143, 149, 178, 186, 201, 202, 206, 231], 20 open, randomized studies [76, 102-108, 125, 126, 130, 133, 137, 138, 160, 165, 176, 203, 209], 6 open, non randomized studies [115, 151, 153, 156, 166, 200], one open, case-control study [124], 7 retrospective case series reports [144-145, 155, 161, 168, 195, 204], one retrospective non randomized study [158] and 46 open case reports [110-114, 116, 117, 120, 121, 127, 131, 132, 136, 146-148, 150, 152, 154, 163, 164, 167, 169-171, 177, 179-194, 196-199, 232]. A case report [207] was retrospectively assessed. The literature search also allowed to obtain one triple blind [172] and two single blind RCTs [174, 205]. A detailed overview of the reports involving APs combinations is presented in Table **5**.

Table 5. Outline of Antipsychotics Combined Treatment Involving Two or More Drugs

Combination	Reference	*N*	Country	Design	Dose[§]	Psycho-pathology	Duration of Treatment (Weeks)	Out-come	Comment
CLZ + FGA									
CLZ + CPZ	Zhang and Xu, 1989 [96]	57	China	DB	CLZ: 256 mg/d; CPZ: 355 mg/d	NA	8	Improve-ment	CPZ administered as costart, not in add-on, regional bias
CLZ + CPZ	Potter *et al.*, 1989 [97]	57	China	DB	CLZ, R: 50-400 mg/d; CPZ, R:100-400 mg/d	Positive and depressive symptoms improved in combi-nation arm	8	Improve-ment	CPZ administered as costart, not in add-on, regional bias

(Table 5) contd…..

Combination	Reference	*N*	Country	Design	Dose[§]	Psycho-pathology	Duration of Treatment (Weeks)	Out-come	Comment
CLZ + SUL	Wang *et al.*, 1994 [98]	105	China	DB	CLZ: 52.7 mg/d; SUL: 738.5 mg/d	NA	8 (follow-up at wk 12, 52 and 156)	Improve-ment	SUL administered as costart, not in add-on, regional bias
CLZ + SUL	Liu *et al.*, 1996 [99]	63	China	Open R[#]	CLZ>400 mg/d; SUL: 1127 mg/d	>20% BPRS or more reduction	12	Improve-ment	Poor methodologic quality
CLZ + LOX	Mowerman and Siris, 1996 [100]	7	United States	Open, CS	CLZ: NA; LOX: NA	BPRS reduction	18 to 50 wks	Improve-ment	No effects of LOX to CLZ serum levels in 4 cases
CLZ + SUL	Shiloh *et al.*, 1997a [79]	28	Israel	DB	CLZ: 403 mg/d; SUL, R: 100-600 mg/d	CLZ + SUL arm: 42.4% BPRS and 50.4% SAPS reduction	10	Improve-ment	First RCT outlining the effectiveness of APs with pharmacodynamic compementarity
CLZ + SUL	Shiloh *et al.*, 1997b [101]	6	Israel	Open, CS	CLZ:, SUL: 600 mg/d	Reduction in positive and negative symptoms	10	Partial improve-ment	Amelioration of positive and negative symptoms in 4/6 patients
CLZ + CPZ	Cha *et al.*, 1999 [102]	200	China	Open R	CLZ: NA; CPZ: NA	BPRS used to assess psycho-pathology	6	Improve-ment	Poor methodologic quality
CLZ + SUL	Si and Yuan, 1999 [103]	100	China	Open R	CLZ<400 mg/d; SUL: 1390 mg/d	>20% BPRS or more reduction	12	Improve-ment	Poor methodologic quality
CLZ + SUL	Zhu *et al.*, 1999 [104]	59	China	Open R	CLZ<400 mg/d; SUL: 100 mg/d	BPRS reduction	12	Improve-ment	Poor methodologic quality
CLZ + SUL	Xao, 1999 [105]	42	China	Open R	CLZ<400 mg/d; SUL: 800 mg/d	BPRS reduction	6	Improve-ment	Poor methodologic quality
CLZ+ PIP	Jia *et al.*,2000 [106]	50	China	Open R	CLZ>400 mg/d; PIP:100 mg/d	BPRS used to assess psycho-pathology	12	Improve-ment	Poor methodologic quality
CLZ + PIP	Zhu and Deng, 2002 [107]	84	China	Open R	CLZ>400 mg/d; PIP:100 mg/d	BPRS used to assess psycho-pathology	24	Improve-ment	Poor methodologic quality

(Table 5) contd…..

Combination	Reference	*N*	Country	Design	Dose§	Psycho-pathology	Duration of Treatment (Weeks)	Out-come	Comment
CLZ + SUL	Zou *et al.*, 2003 [108]	61	China	Open R	CLZ: NR; SUL:1200 mg/d	>20% BPRS or more reduction	12	Improve-ment	Poor methodologic quality
CLZ + PIM	Friedman *et al.*, 2011 [109]	53	United States	DB	CLZ: 378 ng/ml; PIM: 6.48 mg/d	Lower PANSS positive, negative and total score	12	No improve-ment	CLZ dose should be optimized before any add-on treatment
CLZ + PER	Schaller *et al.*, 2009 [231]	1	Germany	Open, CR	CLZ: NA PER: NA	NA	NA	No improve-ment	Elevation of serum CLZ levels up to 400% after add-on with PER
CLZ + PER	Fischer *et al.*, 2013 [232]	4	Germany	Open, CS	CLZ: 75-350 mg/d (140/101 - 1,542/656 ng/ml); PER: 150-350 mg/d (219-273 ng/ml)	Increase of agitation, fear, irritability after co-administrat ion with PER in patients suffering for catatonic schizo-phrenia	7	No improve-ment	Sialorrhea, confusion, fatigue due to increased clozapine levels after add-on with PER
CLZ + SGA									
CLZ + RIS	Koreen *et al.*, 1995 [110]	1	United States	Open, CR	CLZ: 675 mg/d; RIS: 2 mg/d	NA	NA	Improve-ment	Reported mild oculogyric crisis
CLZ + RIS	Tyson *et al.*, 1995 [111]	1	United States	Open, CR	CLZ: 300 mg/d; RIS: 2 mg/d	NA	2	Improve-ment	Increase in CLZ plasma level after add-on with RIS probably due to CYP2D6 interaction
CLZ + RIS	McCarthy and Terkelsen, 1995 [112]	2	United States	Open, CR	CLZ: NA; RIS: NA	NA	NA	Improve-ment	Amelioration of psychopatholog y reported in both cases
CLZ + RIS	Chong *et al.*, 1996 [113]	1	Singapor e	Open, CR	CLZ: 200 mg/d; RIS: 6 mg/d	NA	16	No improve-ment	Agitation and compulsive behaviours

(Table 5) contd.....

Combination	Reference	*N*	Country	Design	Dose§	Psycho-pathology	Duration of Treatment (Weeks)	Out-come	Comment
CLZ + RIS	Godleski and Sernyak, 1996 [114]	1	United States	Open, CR	CLZ: 900 mg/d; RIS, R: 4-6 mg/d	NA	6	No improve-ment	Agranulocytosis after 6 wks of combined RIS+CLZ, both drugs stopped
CLZ + RIS	Henderson and Goff, 1996 [115]	12	United States	Open, NR	CLZ: NA; RIS: NA	>20% BPRS or more reduction	4	Improve-ment	Reported side effects of akathisia and hypersalivation
CLZ + RIS	Chong *et al.*, 1997 [116]	1	Singapor e	Open, CR	CLZ: NA; RIS: NA	NA	NA	No improve-ment	Atrial ectopics
CLZ + RIS	Patel *et al.*, 1997 [117]	1	United States	Open, CR	CLZ: 275 mg/d; RIS: 6 mg/d	NA	12	Improve-ment	Better functional outcome, weight gain
CLZ + RIS	Manto-nakis *et al.*, 1998 [118]	4	Greece	Open, CS	CLZ: NA; RIS: NA	NA	NA	Partial improve-ment	2/4 patients on RIS-CLZ combination showed improvement, 1 person developed tremor
CLZ + RIS	Zervas *et al.*, 1998 [119]	12	Greece	Open, CS	CLZ: NA; RIS: NA	NA	NA	Partial improve-ment	6/12 patients on RIS-CLZ combination improved
CLZ + RIS	Morera *et al.*, 1999 [120]	2	Spain	Open, CR	CLZ: NA; RIS: NA	NA	NA	Improve-ment	Reported clinical efficacy of combination
CLZ + RIS	Adesanya and Pantelis, 2000 [121]	2	Australia	Open, CR	CLZ: NA; RIS: NA	NA	NA	Improve-ment	Reported clinical efficacy of combination
CLZ + RIS	Raskin *et al.*, 2000 [122]	3	Israel	Open, CS	CLZ: NA; RIS: NA	PANSS improve-ment	NA	Improve-ment	No signs of adverse effects
CLZ + RIS	de Groot *et al.*, 2001 [123]	12	The Netherla nds	Open, CS	CLZ: NA; RIS: NA	NA	NA	No improve-ment	One patient developed orthostatic hypotension
CLZ + RIS	Henderson *et al.*, 2001 [124]	20	United States	Open, CC	CLZ: NA; RIS: NA	NA	NA	No improve-ment	Mild increment of serum prolactin levels in co-treatment arm

(Table 5) contd…..

Combination	Reference	*N*	Country	Design	Dose[§]	Psycho-pathology	Duration of Treatment (Weeks)	Out-come	Comment
CLZ + RIS	Liu and Li, 2001 [125]	64	China	Open R	CLZ<400 mg/d; RIS:4.5 mg/d	BPRS reduction	10	No improve-ment	Poor methodologic quality
CLZ + RIS	Ni *et al.*, 2001 [126]	215	China	Open R	CLZ<400 mg/d; RIS:3 mg/d	>30% PANSS reduction	8	Improve-ment	Poor methodologic quality
CLZ + RIS	Raju *et al.*, 2001 [127]	2	India	Open, CR	CLZ: R: 600-800 mg/d; RIS, R:2-10 mg/d	PANSS improve-ment	NA	Improve-ment	Combination more effective than monotherapy
CLZ + RIS	Taylor *et al.*, 2001 [128]	13	United States	Open, CS	CLZ: NA; RIS: NA	PANSS improve-ment	NA	Improve-ment	One person with increased compulsive behavior
CLZ + RIS	Xie and Ni, 2001 [129]	40	China	DB	CLZ: 141 mg/d; RIS, R: 4-6 mg/d	NA	8	No improve-ment	RIS administered as costart, not in add-on, regional bias
CLZ + RIS	Xin *et al.*, 2001 [130]	64	China	Open R	CLZ<400 mg/d; RIS:4 mg/d	BPRS reduction	12	Improve-ment	Poor methodologic quality
CLZ + RIS	Beauchemin *et al.*, 2002 [131]	1	Canada	Open, CR	CLZ: 750 mg/d; RIS: 4 mg/d	NA	1	Worse-ning	Neuroleptic malignant syndrome
CLZ + RIS	Kontaxakis *et al.*, 2002 [132]	1	Greece	Open, CR	CLZ: 100 mg/d; RIS: 16 mg/d	NA	1	Worse-ning	NMS developed after add-on of CLZ to RIS
CLZ + RIS	Peng *et al.*, 2002 [133]	66	China	Open R	CLZ<400 mg/d; RIS:6 mg/d	>20% BPRS or more reduction	8	Improve-ment	Poor methodologic quality
CLZ + RIS	Procyshyn *et al.*, 2002 [134]	8	Canada	Open, CS	CLZ: NA; RIS: NA	NA	NA	No improve-ment	Co-administration of RIS and CLZ reduces smoking
CLZ + RIS	Raaska *et al.*, 2002 [135]	18	Finland	Open, CS	CLZ: 451±207 mg/d; RIS: 2.9±0.9 mg/d	NA	NA	No improve-ment	No activity of RIS on serum CLZ levels
CLZ + RIS	Senechal *et al.*, 2002 [136]	1	Canada	Open, CR	CLZ: 100 mg/d; RIS: 2 mg/d	NA	1	Worse-ning	Neutropenia, patient had been already taking HAL

(Table 5) contd.....

Combination	Reference	*N*	Country	Design	Dose[§]	Psycho-pathology	Duration of Treatment (Weeks)	Out-come	Comment
CLZ + RIS	Wu, 2002 [137]	67	China	Open R	CLZ<400 mg/d; RIS:4 mg/d	PANSS reduction	12	No improve-ment	Poor methodologic quality
CLZ + RIS	Yue *et al.*, 2004 [138]	46	China	Open R	CLZ<400 mg/d; RIS:2.1 mg/d	PANSS reduction	96	No improve-ment	Poor methodologic quality
CLZ + RIS	Anil Yagcioglu *et al.*, 2005 [139]	30	Turkey	DB	CLZ: 515.6 mg/d; RIS:3 mg/d	Significant PANSS positive subscale reduction	6	Improve-ment	Increase of sedation, prolactin levels and cognitive performance in combination arm
CLZ + RIS	Josiassen *et al.*, 2005 [140]	40	United States	DB	CLZ: 529mg/d; RIS. 4.4 mg/d	>20% reduction in BPRS; significant reduction in BPRS positive subscale	12	Improve-ment	CLZ dose higher in combination arm
CLZ + RIS	Honer *et al.*, 2006 [141]	68	Multisite *	DB	CLZ: 494 mg/d; RIS: 3 mg/d	No significant reduction in psycho-pathology	8	No improve-ment	Increase in fasting glucose in combination arm
CLZ + RIS	Freund-enreich *et al.*, 2007 [142]	24	United States	DB	CLZ: 456 mg/d; RIS: 4 mg/d	Significant PANSS thought subscale reduction	6	Improve-ment	Routine RIS add-on to CLZ unsupported by study outcomes
CLZ + AMI	Agelink *et al.*, 2004 [143]	7	United States	Open, CS	CLZ: 293 mg/d; AMI: 543 mg/d	Significant BPRS and SAPS reduction	36	Improve-ment	Concomitant medication with lithium in 2 patients and lorazepam in 3 patients
CLZ+ AMI	Zink *et al.*, 2004a [144]	15	Germany	Retr, CS	CLZ: 375 mg/d; AMI: 527 mg/d	Amelio-ration of positive and negative symptoms	NA	Improve-ment	Reduction of CLZ side effects by augmenting AMI
CLZ + AMI	Kämpf *et al.*, 2005 [145]	14	Germany	Retr, CS	CLZ: NA; AMI: NA	Reduction of mean CGI-I score	20	Improve-ment	Reversible CLZ-induced leucopenia in 1 patient, 1/15 patient did not improve

(Table 5) contd…..

Combination	Reference	*N*	Country	Design	Dose§	Psycho-pathology	Duration of Treatment (Weeks)	Out-come	Comment
CLZ + ARI	Lim *et al.*, 2004 [146]	3	United States	Open, CR	CLZ: 150 mg/d; ARI: 30mg/d	BPRS reduction	2	Improve-ment	Persistent positive symptoms despite augmentation and BPRS reduction, no side effects
CLZ + ARI	Ashton, 2005 [147]	2	United States	Open, CR	CLZ: 600 mg/d; ARI: 52.5 mg/d	Psycho-pathology reduction	52	Improve-ment	Consistent weight loss (20 kg) in one case, marked psychosocial improvement in both cases
CLZ + ARI	Ziegenbein *et al.*, 2005 [148]	2	Germany	Open, CR	CLZ: 762.5 mg/d; ARI: 15 mg/d	Psycho-pathology reduction	22	Improve-ment	Weight loss, reduction of hypersalivation and sedation
CLZ + ARI	Abu-Tair *et al.*, 2006 [149]	5	Israel	Open, CS	CLZ: 570 mg/d; ARI: 26 mg/d	PANSS reduction	31	Improve-ment	Amelioration of psycho-pathology
CLZ + ARI	Clarke *et al.*, 2006 [150]	3	United States	Open, CR	CLZ: 466.6 mg/d; ARI: 30 mg/d	Reduction of negative symptoms	22.6	Improve-ment	Amelioration of psycho-pathology in 3 patients and of body hygiene in one case
CLZ + ARI	Henderson *et al.*, 2006 [151]	10	United States	Open, NR	CLZ: 455±83 mg/d; ARI: 18±6 mg/d	PANSS Stable	6	Improve-ment	Amelioration of metabolic parameters (Cholesterol, triglycerides, insulin), improvement in QoL, increase of anxiety in 3/10 patients
CLZ + ARI	Rocha and Hara, 2006 [152]	3	Brazil	Open, CR	CLZ: 300 mg/d; ARI: 15 mg/d	Reduction of negative symptoms and obsessive-compul-sive symptoms in one case	52	Improve-ment	In one case <diabetes and weight loss (30 kg); in one case < weight (3.5 kg); psycho-pathology improvement

(Table 5) contd…..

Combination	Reference	*N*	Country	Design	Dose§	Psycho-pathology	Duration of Treatment (Weeks)	Out-come	Comment
CLZ + ARI	Ziegenbein *et al.*, 2006 [153]	11	Germany	Open, NR	CLZ: 736.4±93.1 mg/d; ARI:26.4±6.4 mg/d	Significant reduction of BPRS, total score, with >20% BPRS positive symptoms reduction	12	Improve-ment	No alteration of QTc improvement; one patient with headache, vomiting, nausea, insomnia and agitation
CLZ + ARI	Zink *et al.*, 2006 [154]	1	Germany	Open, CR	CLZ: 500 mg/d; ARI: 30 mg/d	PANSS and YBOCS reduction	24	Improve-ment	Reduction of CLZ-induced obsessive-compulsive symptoms
CLZ+ ARI	Karun-akaran *et al.*, 2007 [155]	26	United Kingdo m	Retr, CS	CLZ:393.8 mg/d; ARI: 19.8 mg/d	Improve-ment of hallu-cinations, delusions, and CGI-S	33.88	Improve-ment	Amelioration of metabolic parameters and weight loss, slight HDL increase, two dropouts due to TD and NMS
CLZ + ARI	Mitsonis *et al.*, 2007 [156]	28	Greece	Open, NR	CLZ: 438 mg/d; ARI: 15 mg/d	Significant PANSS reduction	16	Improve-ment	Significant improvement in QLS
CLZ + ARI	Chang *et al.*, 2008 [157]	62	South Corea	DB	CLZ>400 mg/d; ARI, R: 5-30 mg/d	BPRS negative symptoms and SANS improve-ment	8	Improve-ment	Prolactin and triglycerides level lower in ARI arm
CLZ + ARI	Benedetti *et al.*, 2010 [158]	7	Italy	Retr, NR	CLZ: 292.9±220.7 mg/d; ARI: 6.8±3.7 mg/d	BPRS total score, "thought disorder" and "anergia" subscales improved	24	Improve-ment	Add-on of ARI may improve dopamine projections firing by removing inhibitory control
CLZ + ARI	Fleisch-hacker *et al.*, 2010 [159]	207	Multisite †	DB	CLZ: 363 mg/d; ARI: 11.1 mg/d	No significant differences in PANSS total score; CGI and IAQ scores favoured ARI arm	16 (placebo controlled) + 12 (open label)	Partial improve-ment	Significant cholesterol and weight loss in ARI arm

(Table 5) contd…..

Combination	Reference	*N*	Country	Design	Dose§	Psycho-pathology	Duration of Treatment (Weeks)	Out-come	Comment
CLZ + ARI	Barbui *et al.*, 2011 [160]	106	Italy	Open, R	CLZ + ARI and CLZ + HAL arm: standard doses according to clinical necessities	No improvement in BPRS in CLZ +ARI arm *vs* CLZ + HAL arm; statistically significant decrease of LUNSERS in CLZ + ARI arm	12	No improve-ment	No clinical benefits of add-on with ARI on CLZ-treated schizophrenic patients; advantages in the perception of less side effects with ARI
CLZ + ARI	De Risio *et al.*, 2011 [161]	16	Italy	Retr, CS	CLZ: 275.56±100.61 mg/d; ARI: 11.7±6.75 mg/d	Significant reduction of BPRS total and positive, negative, dis-organized, elevated affect and negative affect subscales	6	Improve-ment	Metabolic parameters improved after 6 wks, BPRS and HoNOS n. 11, autonomy in everyday life scores predictive of global functioning at PSP scale
CLZ + ARI	Musca-tello *et al.*, 2011 [162]	31	Italy	DB	CLZ>400 mg/d; ARI: 15 mg/d	BPRS total score and SAPS "thought disorders" subscale reduction	24	Improve-ment	No significant difference between CLZ and control group for cognitive symptoms
CLZ + ZIP	Kaye, 2003 [163]	11	United States	Open, CR	CLZ:>400 mg/d; ZIP: 160 mg/d	No improv-ement of psycho-pathology	NA	Improve-ment	Amelioration of motivation and initiative, reduction of weight loss and CLZ dosage after ZIP add-on
CLZ + ZIP	Zink *et al.*, 2004b [164]	1	Germany	Open, CR	CLZ: NA; ZIP: NA	Reduction of positive and negative symptoms	NA	Improve-ment	Cotreatment better than monotherapy with both drugs
CLZ + ZIP	Zink *et al.*, 2009 [165]	12	Germany	Open, R	CLZ: NA; ZIP: NA	Reduction of positive and negative symptoms	6	Improve-ment	Improvement in psychosocial functioning, small elongation of QTc, reduced EPS

(Table 5) contd…..

Combination	Reference	*N*	Country	Design	Dose[§]	Psycho-pathology	Duration of Treatment (Weeks)	Out-come	Comment
CLZ + ZIP	Ziegen-bein *et al.*, 2005 [166]	9	Germany	Open, NR	CLZ: NA; ZIP: NA	Reduction in mean BPRS score in 7/9 patients	24	Improve-ment	No increment in side effects
CLZ + ZIP	Ziegenbei n and Calliess, 2006 [167]	2	Germany	Open, CR	CLZ: 675 mg/d; ZIP: 80 mg/d	>20% reduction of BPRS scale	24	Improve-ment	Add-on of ZIP allowed reduction of CLZ dosage after 24 wks.; CLZ adverse effects subsided
CLZ + QUE	Reinstein *et al.*, 1999 [168]	65	United States	Retr, CS	CLZ: 200-800 mg/d; QUE: 100-400 mg/d	No changes in psycho-pathology	40	Improve-ment	Significant weight loss (mean: 4.2 kg), amelioration of CLZ-induced diabetes mellitus in 13/65 patients
CLZ + QUE	Diaz and Hogan, 2001 [169]	1	United States	Open, CR	CLZ: 400 mg/d; QUE: 250 mg/d	Clinical deterio-ratiom	5	Worse-ning	Granulocytopen ia
CLZ + OLZ	Gupta *et al.*, 1998 [170]	2	United States	Open, CR	CLZ: 800 mg/d; OLZ: 15 mg/d	35 % BPRS reduction	72	Improve-ment	Reported hypersalivation in one patient
CLZ + OLZ	Rhoads, 2000 [171]	1	United States	Open, CR	CLZ: 100 mg/d; OLZ: 10 mg/d	Improve-ment of positive symptoms	72	Improve-ment	Amelioration of psychopatholog y
FGA + FGA									
CPZ + RES	Barrett *et al.*, 1957 [172]	30	United States	TB	CPZ: 230 mg/day; RES: 2.3 mg/day	Reduction in psycho-pathology	12	Improve-ment	Superiority of cotreatment *vs* monotherapies
CPZ + TRI	Talbot, 1964 [173]	77	United States	DB	CPZ; 150 mg/d (2m); 300 mg/d (4m); TRI: 10 mg/d (2m); 20 mg/d (4m)	Reduction in psycho-pathology	32	Improve-ment	Combination treatment as costart, no diagnostic instrument, baseline group features not compared
CPZ + FLU	Chien and Cole, 1973 [174]	46	United States	SB	CPZ: 350 mg/d; FLU: 26 mg/d	Reduction in psycho-pathology	4	Improve-ment	No diagnostic instrument

(Table 5) contd…..

Combination	Reference	*N*	Country	Design	Dose§	Psycho-pathology	Duration of Treatment (Weeks)	Out-come	Comment
PIM + THI	Nishi-kawa, 1985 [175]	106	Japan	DB	PIM: 4.1 mg/d; THI: 50.5 mg/d	Reduction in psychopath ology	52	Improve-ment	Poorly defined outcome criteria of relapse/adverse effects
HAL + LEV	Higashima *et al.*, 2004 [176]	19	Japan	Open, R	HAL: 5.4 mg/d; LEV: 54 mg/d	Reduction in psycho-pathology	8	Improve-ment	Drug-free participants at enrollment, efficacy data reported for 2 wks only
FGA + SGA									
PIM + OLZ	Takhar, 1999 [177]	1	Canada	Open, CR	OLZ: 20 mg/d; PIM: 3 mg/d	40% BPRS improve-ment	104	Improve-ment	No weight gain, good psychosocial outcome
SUL + OLZ	Raskin *et al.*, 2000 [178]	6	Israel	Open, CS	OLZ: 27 mg/d; SUL: 377 mg/d	33% PANSS and 37% BPRS improve-ment	10	Improve-ment	No remarkable side effects noticed
HAL + OLZ	Mujica and Weiden, 2001[179]	1	United States	Open, CR	OLZ: 10 mg/d; HAL: 23 mg/d	Psychopat hology not assessed	<1	Worse-ning	Combination induced NMS
HAL + OLZ	Abdullah *et al.*, 2003 [180]	1	United States	Open, CR	OLZ: 20 mg/d; HAL: 10 mg/d	Psychopat hology not assessed	1	Worse-ning	Neutropenia
FLU + OLZ	Tofler and Ahmed, 2003 [181]	1	United States	Open, CR	OLZ: 30 mg/d; FLU: 20 mg/d	Psychopat hology not assessed	<1	Worse-ning	Combination induced NMS
SUL + OLZ	Kotler *et al.*, 2004 [76]	17	Israel	Open, R	OLZ: 22.2 mg/d; SUL: 600 mg/d	No changes in PANSS and HAM-A; HAM-D improved	10	Improve-ment	No changes in SAS, BAS; surprisingly low weight gain
HAL + ARI	Grover *et al.*, 2006 [182]	1	India/United Kingdom	Open, CR	HAL: 30 mg/d; ARI: 20 mg/d	Increase of psychotic symptoms (CGI> 2pts.)	8	Worse-ning	A hypodopaminergic milieu may increase ARI dopamine-agonist activity

(Table 5) contd…..

Combination	Reference	*N*	Country	Design	Dose[§]	Psycho-pathology	Duration of Treatment (Weeks)	Out-come	Comment
HAL + MEL	Gahr *et al.*, 2012 [183]	1	Germany	Open, CR	HAL: 30 mg/d; MEL: 100 mg/d	Pheno-typing test with dextrome-thorphan revealed CYP 2D6 UM status after failure in treatment with AMI, 1200 mg/d	2	Improve-ment	Increase in HAL serum levels, probably induced by MEL CYP 2D6 inhibition
SGA + SGA									
OLZ + RIS	John *et al.*, 1998 [184]	1	United States	Open, CR	OLZ: 10 mg/d; RIS: 3 mg/d	Improve-ment of aggressive behavior and psycho-motor agitation	1	Improve-ment	Add-on of RIS after injection of HAL decanoas, 100 mg i.m. Agitation induced by "D_2-supersensitivity" psychosis
RIS + ARI	Gaston *et al.*, 2008 [185]	1	United Kingdom	Open, CR	RIS: 6 mg/d; ARI: 20 mg/d	Improved psycho-pathology, urinary inconti-nence, type II diabetes mellitus occurred after previous treatment with olanzapine, 25 mg/d	12	Improve-ment	Combination reduced psychotic symptoms, but added intolerable side effects, improvement in diabetes
OLZ + RIS	Lerner *et al.*, 2000 [186]	5	Israel	Open, CS	OLZ, R: 10-15 mg/d; RIS, R: 1-5 mg/d	25-38% BPRS improvement	NA	Improve-ment	Combination proved effective in selected patients
RIS + QUE	Chue *et al.*, 2001 [187]	1	Canada	Open, CR	RIS: 8 mg/d; QUE: 800 mg/d	Improved psychopathology	NA	Improve-ment	Good psychosocial outcome, sexual dysfunction with RIS 8 mg/d
OLZ + RIS	Seger and Lamberti, 2001 [188]	1	United States	Open, CR	OLZ: 7.5 mg/d; RIS: 6 mg/d	Improved psychopathology	12	Improve-ment	Priapism

(Table 5) contd…..

Combination	Reference	*N*	Country	Design	Dose[§]	Psycho-pathology	Duration of Treatment (Weeks)	Out-come	Comment
OLZ + QUE	Hedges and Jeppson, 2002 [189]	1	United States	Open, CR	OLZ: 15 mg/d; QUE: 100 mg/d	No evaluation of psychopath ology	NA	Worse-ning	The abrupt onset of seizures raises caution issues on SGAs
QUE + AMI	Jones, 2002 [190]	1	United States	Open, CR	AMI: 100 mg/d; QUE: NA	Stable psychopath ology, worsening on AMI suspension	NA	Worse-ning	Patient improved when combination was resumed
RIS + QUE	Bozikas *et al.*, 2003 [191]	1	Greece	Open, CR	RIS: 12 mg/d; QUE: 500 mg/d	63% BPRS reduction	6	Improve-ment	Antiaggression activity of QUE probably due to its pro-serotoninergic properties
RIS + QUE	Nelson *et al.*, 2003 [192]	1	United States	Open, CR	RIS: NA; QUE: NA	Improved psychopath ology	10	Improve-ment	Combination reduced tardive dyskinesia symptoms
QUE + AMI	O'Shea *et al.*, 2003 [193]	1	New Zealand	Open, CR	QUE: 150 mg/d; AMI: 200 mg/d	Psychopat hology not reported	1	Worse-ning	Trigemny ventricular ectopic beats developed afted add-on of QUE to AMI. After AMI stopping and QUE reduction, ventricular ectopic beats continued for 5 days more, with QTc prolongation (465 ms). Spontaneous stop of ectopic beats and QTc normalization on 6th day
QUE + ZIP	Minov, 2004 [194]	1	Germany	Open, CR	QUE: NA; ZIP: NA	Psychopat hology not reported	NA	Worse-ning	Developing of severe cardiac arrhythmia with extrasystole and QTc prologation after add-on of ZIP

(Table 5) contd…..

Combination	Reference	*N*	Country	Design	Dose§	Psycho-pathology	Duration of Treatment (Weeks)	Out-come	Comment
OLZ + AMI	Zink *et al.*, 2004b [195]	7	Germany	Retr, CS	OLZ: 21.4 mg/d; AMI: 485.7 mg/d	Improve-ment of positive and negative symptoms	NA	Improve-ment	OLZ dose <21% and AMI <26% compared to monotherapy; 29% GAF increment; 61% CGI reduction; weight gain: 6.2%
OLZ + ARI	Duggal, 2004 [196]	1	United States	Open, CR	OLZ: 20 mg/d; ARI: 15 mg/d	59% PANSS reduction;	2	Improve-ment	Clinical efficacy probably due to ARI activity on D2 autoreceptors contrasting negative symptoms
QUE + ARI	Reeves and Mack, 2004 [197]	1	United States	Open, CR	QUE: 800 mg/d; ARI: 15-30 mg/d	Worsening of grandiosity and halluci-nations	1	Worse-ning	QUE may have induced a hypodopaminergic environment on which ARI acted as a dopamine agonist, exacerbating psychosis
OLZ + ARI	DeQuardo, 2005 [198]	1	United States	Open, CR	OLZ: 60 mg/d; ARI: 10 mg/d	Worsening of halluci-nations and paranoid symptoms	NA	Worse-ning	Highlighting of risks associated to polypharmacy
OLZ +QUE	Dunkley and Reveley, 2005 [199]	1	United Kingdom	Open, CR	OLZ: 30 mg/d; QUE: 750 mg/d	Improve-ment of psychopathology, except of auditory halluci-nations	NA	Improve-ment	Patient affected by a prolactin-secreting pituitary microadenoma, combination effective and respectful of the basic disease
OLZ + RIS	Suzuki *et al.*, 2008 [200]	17	Japan	Open, NR	OLZ: 12.9-14.5 mg/d; RIS: 3.14-5.5 mg/d	>30% BPRS reduction in 7/17 patients	8	Partial improve-ment	9/17 participants showed a premature drop-out; GAF improvement in responders; significant increase in weight, prolactin and cholesterol

(Table 5) contd…..

Combination	Reference	*N*	Country	Design	Dose§	Psycho-pathology	Duration of Treatment (Weeks)	Out-come	Comment
Multiple APs									
RIS + Drugs affecting CYP 3A4	Bork *et al.*, 1999 [201]	2	United States	Open, CS	RIS: NA; Other drugs: NA	NA	NA		Part of a larger CS (*n*=33; 13 RIS + 20 CC for CYP2D6 genotype) of RIS patients investigated for CYP2D6 and 3A interactions, no change in RIS plasma levels. CYP2D6 poor metabolizers (2/13 in CS and 3/20 in the CC arm) did not tolerate RIS. Drugs affecting CYP3A4 induced a 2-fold decrease or increase in RIS levels.
RIS + CLZ, OLZ, CLZ-OLZ, HAL	Margolese *et al.*, 2000 [202]	10	Canada	Open, CS	RIS: NA; Other drugs: NA	For 6/10 patients (CLZ: *n*=1; OLZ: *n*=2; CLZ + OLZ: *n*=2; HAL: *n*=1): add-on of RIS: no improvement; add-on of QUE: partial improvement (very much: *n*=1; much improved: *n*=2; minimal: *n*=3); For 4/10 patients, previously added with	NA	No improve-ment	Patients continued to show psychotic symptoms after add-ons (mean CGI-S: 5.17)

(Table 5) contd…..

Combination	Reference	*N*	Country	Design	Dose§	Psycho-pathology	Duration of Treatment (Weeks)	Out-come	Comment
						RIS (OLZ: *n*=2; CLZ + OLZ: *n*=2): add-on of OLZ: partial improve-ment (much improved: *n*=2; minimal: *n*=2)			
QUE + HAL, RIS, THI	Potkin *et al.*, 2002 [203]	36	United States	Open, R	QUE: 600 mg/d; HAL: 7.5 mg/d; RIS: 3 mg/d; THI: 200 mg/d	Stable psycho-pathology	1		Clearance of QUE increased by THI; HAL and RIS had no pharmacokinetic effects on QUE; 25% of partici-pants reported sedation or increased sleep duration
HAL + OLZ + antidepres-sant, mood stabilizers, anxiolytics	Mc Cue *et al.*, 2003 [204]	38	United States	Retr, CS	OLZ: NR; HAL: NR	Psycho-pathology not reported	NA	No improve-ment	Reported CS was part of a larger survey (*n*=435) on change in prescription patterns and adverse drug reactions in psychotic patients
CLZ + AMI; CLZ + QUE	Genç *et al.*, 2007 [205]	50	Turkey	SB	NA	Improve-ment in BPRS, SAPS, SANS	8	Improve-ment	Participants already on CLZ randomized to CLZ + AMI or CLZ + QUE; psycho-pathology and side effects improved better with CLZ + AMI combination
ARI +SGAs	Ramaswamy *et al.*, 2004 [206]	4	United States	Open, CS	ARI (7.5-30 mg/D) + RIS (3mg/d)/OLZ (15-20 mg/d)/ QUE (100 mg/ d)/ ZIP (160 mg/d)	Increase of psychotic symptoms	NA	Worse-ning	A hypo-dopaminergic milieu may increase ARI dopamine-agonist activity

(Table 5) contd…..

Combination	Reference	*N*	Country	Design	Dose§	Psycho-pathology	Duration of Treatment (Weeks)	Out-come	Comment
AMI + SGAs	Lerner *et al.*, 2005 [207]	15	Israel	Retr, CR	AMI (693.3±279.6 mg/d) + CLZ (490 mg/d)/OLZ (15 mg/d)/RIS (6mg/d)/ZIP (160 mg/d)	Marked improve-ment (7/15); mild improve-ment (5/15), no improve-ment (3/15)	25.4 (before AMI add-on)	Improve-ment	80% of participants reported improvement in mental states; two patients (RIS + AMI) had, respectively, mild tremor and constipation
ARI + RIS; ARI + QUE	Kane *et al.*, 2009 [208]	323	United States	DB	ARI (2-15 mg/d) + RIS (4-8 mg/d)/QUE (400-800 mg/d)	No statistically significant PANSS reduction	16	No improve-ment	In RIS arm, reported statistically significant reduction of serum prolactin, add-on of ARI resulted safe and well-tolerated
CLZ + ZIP; CLZ + RIS	Kuwilsky *et al.*, 2010 [209]	24	Germany	Open, R	NA	Improvem ent in SANS, PANSS and HAM-D	26 and 52 wks	Improve-ment	Sample study reduced by dropouts after 26 wks (ZIP:4/24; RIS: 2/24) and after 52 wks (ZIP:no drop; RIS:5/24); slight increase of akathisia in CLZ + ZIP arm; improvement in CLZ- associated side effects

§for randomized and double blind studies doses are referred to the APs combination arm. Doses are expressed in mg Eq CPz/day, mg/day, ng/ml or DDD according to the single study; #the blindness of this study has been difficult to ascertain [93] *Canada, Germany, China and UK; †55 centres in 10 European countries and South Africa.

Abbreviations: Drugs, **AMI**=Amisulpride; **ARI**=Aripiprazole; **CLZ**=Clozapine; **CPZ**=Chlorpromazine; **FLU**=Fluphenazine; **HAL**=Haloperidol; **LEV**=Levomepromazine; **LOX**=Loxapine; **MEL**=Melperone; **OLZ**=Olanzapine; **PER**=Perazine; **PIM**=Pimozide; **QUE**=Quetiapine; **THI**=Thioridazine; **TRI**=Trifluoperazine; **RIS**=Risperidone; **ZIP**=Ziprasidone; Studies: **DB**=Double blind; **Open, CC**=Open, Case Control study; **Open, CS**=Open, Case Series study; **Open, CR**=Open, Case Report; **Open, NR**=Open, Non Randomized study; **Open, R**=Open, Randomized study; **Retr, CS**=Retrospective, Case Series study; **Retr, CR**=Retrospective, Case Report; Scales: **BPRS**=Brief Psychiatric Rating Scale; **CGI**=Clinical global Impression Scale; **GAF**=Global Assessment of Function scale; **HAM-D**=Hamilton Rating for Depression Scale; **HoNOS**=Health of the Nations Outcome Scale; **LUNSERS**=Liverpool University Neuroleptic Side Effect Rating Scale; **PANSS**=Positive and Negative Symptoms Scale; **PSP**=Personal and Social Performance Scale; **SANS**=Scale for the Assessment of Negative Symptoms; **SAPS**=Scale for the Assessment of Positive Symptoms; **YBOCS**=Yale-Brown Obsessive Compulsive Scale; Other abbreviations: **QoL**=Quality of Life; **NMS**=Neuroleptic Malignant Syndrome; **NA**=Not Available.

RESULTS

Clozapine Plus FGAs Combinations

Five double blind RCTs [79, 96-98, 109], three open, case series studies [100-101, 232], eight open, randomized studies [99, 102-108] and one case report [232] on persons taking a clozapine-FGAs combination were reviewed, for a total of 17 reports. Three Chinese double-blind trials [96-98] have outlined the effectiveness of the combination of clozapine with, respectively, chlorpromazine and sulpiride. An Israeli trial [79] evidenced how clozapine-sulpiride combination had a favourable outcome on schizophrenia symptoms, by acting on the complementary pharmacodynamic interaction between serotonin and D_2 activity [4]. Eight Chinese open, case series studies [99, 102-108] also outlined that clozapine-sulpiride, clozapine-chlorpromazine or, respectively, clozapine-pipothiazine combinations were all effective in reducing psychopathology. An American open trial [100] showed that clozapine-loxapine had no pharmacokinetic effects on clozapine serum levels, while a double-blind RCT, conducted in the United States [109] on clozapine-pimozide association, did not support the efficacy of this combination, but outlined how optimal baseline plasma concentration of clozapine should be ruled out before starting a RCT on clozapine-APs associations. A German case report highlighted that co-administration with perazine inhibited CYP 1A2 isoenzyme metabolizing clozapine, strongly increasing its serum levels [231]. Perazine-induced increase in clozapine serum levels caused loss of therapeutic efficacy and unwanted side effects in a German open case series [232].

Clozapine Plus SGAs Combinations

Data extracted from meta-analyses [68, 92-94] and reviews [10, 84-91] on clozapine plus SGAs combinations allowed to obtain eight double blind RCTs [139-142, 157, 159, 162]; nine open, case series studies [118-119, 122-123, 128, 134-135, 143, 149]; nine open, randomized studies [125-126, 130, 133, 137-138, 160, 165, 176]; five open, non randomized studies [115, 151, 153, 156, 166]; one open, case-control study [124]; five retrospective, case series studies [144-145, 155, 161, 168]; one retrospective, non randomized study [158] and 25 open case reports [110-114, 116-

117, 120-121, 127, 131-132, 136, 146-148, 150, 152, 154, 163-164, 167, 169-171]. Thirty-three reports concerned the clozapine-risperidone association [110-142], 17 described persons taking a clozapine-aripiprazole combination [146-162], 5 papers were about the clozapine-ziprasidone combination [163-167], in 2 reports clozapine had been associated to quetiapine [168-169], while in two more papers clozapine had been combined to olanzapine [170-171]. Although augmentation with risperidone was methodologically well-conducted in 4 double blind, placebo-controlled studies [139-142], improvement in psychopathology was not statistically significant in three of them after the add-on with the second SGA, while in only one report risperidone had a favourable impact on symptoms [89, 140]. Several case reports outlined how the combinations of clozapine and aripiprazole was effective in reducing hyperglycemia, hypertriglyceridemia, weight gain [151-155], while a retrospective, non randomized study [158] and a small double blind study [162] demonstrated the amelioration of thought disorganization positive symptoms. Two case series studies explicitly denoted an improvement in quality of life [156] and functional autonomy [161]. Larger double blind [157, 159] and randomized controlled studies [160] had, however, evidenced that add-on of aripiprazole to clozapine had modest benefits, confirming the results of the meta-analyses [68, 94]. Adjunctive ziprasidone to clozapine improved psychopathology, sexual dysfunction and allowed clozapine dose reduction in selected cases [163-164, 167] and in two open studies [165-166], while a retrospective case series outlined a statistically significant weight loss in persons administered with a combination of clozapine and quetiapine [168]. One patient showed granulocytopenia, however, when taking the same combination [169]. Mixed adverse effects and improvement of psychopathology are described in the two case reports of clozapine combined to olanzapine [170-171].

FGAs Plus FGAs Combinations

Combined FGA treatment was investigated in only 5 methodologically well-conducted studies [172-176], one of which, realized in the United States, even showed a triple blind design, associating chlorpromazine to reserpine in the combination arm [172]. In another American double blind study [173] it was, instead, investigated the association of chlorpromazine to trifluoperazine, while a third, single blind report from United States [174] concerned a chlorpromazine-fluphenazine combination. A Japanese double blind study [175] investigated the association of pimozide to thioridazine, while another open, Japanese report [176] described the use of haloperidol combined to levomepromazine. Although outdated, these studies reported an amelioration of psychopathology and outcomes. At least one meta-analysis [93] had utilized data from these studies to support the superiority of cotreatment with respect to monotherapies.

FGAs Plus SGAs Combinations

One open, Israeli randomized study [76], one open, Israeli case series [178] and 6 case reports [177, 179-183] evaluated the combination of olanzapine with various FGAs. In the Israeli reports, the combination of olanzapine with sulpiride displayed improvement in psychotic and depressive symptoms, reduced weight gain and few adverse effects. Combining olanzapine to haloperidol [179] or to fluphenazine [181] induced neuroleptic malignant syndrome, while in another report, the association of haloperidol to olanzapine provoked reversible neutropenia [180]. An increase in psychotic symptoms was evidenced in a case report on the add-on of aripiprazole to haloperidol [182], in which an haloperidol-generated hypodopaminergic milieu might have increased aripiprazole dopamine-agonist activity. Augmentation of haloperidol with melperone, a potent CYP 2D6 inibitor [2, 183] was considered a possible pharmacological strategy in a CYP 2D6 ultrarapid metabolizer with resistant psychotic symptoms.

SGAs Plus SGAs Combinations

Seventeen reports of combined, coupled, SGAs [184-200] were obtained by the search, with one open, case series of olanzapine plus risperidone combination [186], another retrospective case series on a olanzapine plus amisulpride association [195] and fourteen more case reports [184-185, 187-194, 196-200]. The association of amisulpride to olanzapine proved effective, with improvement in positive and negative symptoms, increased psychosocial functioning and reduced weight gain [195]. Amelioration of psychopathology was also noticed in the risperidone plus olanzapine case series [184, 186, 188, 200], evidencing how SGAs with complementary pharmacodynamic properties may have favourable effects on psychotic symptoms in selected cases. Olanzapine plus risperidone association provoked, however, increase in body weight, cholesterol and serum prolactin despite a better psychosocial functioning in at least one third of a Japanese open, non randomized study sample [200]. Add-on of risperidone to a schizophrenic patient treated with aripiprazole induced intolerable urinary incontinence despite control of psychotic symptoms [185], while a combination of quetiapine and olanzapine induced seizures in a person with schizophrenia [189]. Ziprasidone combined to quetiapine induced a severe arrhythmia with elongation of electrocardiographic QT/QTc complex in another German case report [194]. Aripiprazole combined to quetiapine caused worsening of grandiosity and hallucinations in one person [197], by probably acting as a dopamine agonist in a hypodopaminergic environment. An increase in paranoid symptoms was also observed in a person taking an association of olanzapine and aripiprazole in the United States [198], denoting how SGA combinations may highlight the risks associated to polypharmacy. The association of olanzapine and quetiapine triggered, instead, the improvement of psychotic symptoms in a United Kingdom case report [199], as well as the olanzapine plus aripiprazole combination in the United States [196]. Pro-serotoninergic quetiapine activity might have caused reduction of psychomotor agitation when added to risperidone in a Greek patient [191], while in another case, the same combination reduced tardive dyskinesia in the United States [192]. Add-on of amisulpride to quetiapine normalized psychopathologic symptoms in another American case report [190], in which psychotic features worsened when the second SGA was briefly suspended. Sexual dysfunctions and, respectively, priapism were noticed in two case reports in which risperidone was added to quetiapine [187] and olanzapine to risperidone [188].

Multiple APs Combinations

Nine reports described the activity of multiple APs combinations [201-209]. A Turkish single blind randomized study [205] had randomized add-on with amisulpride and add-on with quetiapine to 50 schizophrenic resistant patients already taking clozapine. A statistically significant improvement was noticed in both groups. The clozapine plus amisulpride combination displayed better control of psychopathology, while in the clozapine-quetiapine arm the amelioration of psychopathology was smaller. In an open, randomized study conducted in Germany, Kuwilsky *et al.* [209] outlined how the add-on of ziprasidone (n=12) and risperidone (n=12) to patients on clozapine achieved a comparable reduction of psychotic and depressive symptoms, both alleviating clozapine-induced side effects. Another pharmacokinetic open randomized study [203] in which haloperidol, risperidone or thioridazine were added to quetiapine displayed that, although haloperidol or risperidone showed no effects on quetiapine clearance, thioridazine significantly increased oral quetiapine clearance, with at least one quarter of the participants reporting sedation or increment in sleep duration. In a study comparing the add-on of risperidone to CYP 3A4 affecting drugs [201], a 2-fold decrease or increase in risperidone levels was induced in the participants according to the nature of the CYP 3A4 influencing drug. CYP2 D6 poor metabolizers were impaired in tolerating this SGA. A Canadian open case series study [202] explored the subsequent add-on of risperidone and quetiapine in participants already taking clozapine, olanzapine or a combination of clozapine plus olanzapine, highlighting multiple, different outcomes, while psychopathology did not globally improve. No amelioration of psychopathology was also reported in a retrospective case series [204] investigating the association of haloperidol and olanzapine in 38 patients that were part of a larger survey (n=435) about changes in prescription patterns of multiple drugs acting on Central Nervous System, including antidepressants, mood stabilizers and anxiolytics. In an open, case series study [206] aripiprazole was added on to participants already taking risperidone, olanzapine, quetiapine or ziprasidone. The results reported no improvement in psychopathology. Such a condition may be triggered by aripiprazole dopamine-agonist activity, that is more likely to take place in the hypodopaminergic milieu created by some multireceptor SGAs. Add-on of aripiprazole, although well-tolerated, did not seem to improve psychopathology and social outcomes in patients already taking risperidone or quetiapine at stable doses in a large randomized American placebo-controlled double blind trial [208]. Finally, amisulpride was associated to patients administered with clozapine, olanzapine, risperidone or ziprasidone [207]. Global improvement of psychopathology was reported, with participants taking risperidone plus amisulpride combination reporting, respectively, mild tremor and constipation.

DISCUSSION

After reviewing this series of reports on APs polypharmacy, it appears that the different ways in which these drugs may be combined may reflect prescribers' different intentions according to the perceived dissimilarities in pharmacokinetic properties, pharmacodynamic use and in the expected clinical results.

The non-clozapine APs associations were mainly described in open studies and case reports, with the exception of the five RCTs on FGAs [172-176], whose results supported the clinical effectiveness of the combined older drugs. A reason put forward to justify these findings relies on the relatively longer (>10 weeks) duration of the trials, but more research is needed to prove that a protracted combined treatment with two FGAs is more effective than monotherapy [93]. In three out of the five combined FGAs studies [173, 175-176], the second AP was a low-potency phenothiazine administered in relatively small doses, supporting the practice of prescribing multireceptor-acting FGAs as hypnotic drugs [50]. In some studies on APs prescription patterns [28-29] the rate of polypharmacy dropped of more than ten points when low-potency FGAs prescriptions of less than 100 mg equivalents of chlorpromazine were ruled out, raising questions on how bedtime use of the older phenothiazines should really be considered as an example of polypharmacy. The open, non randomized studies on combined FGAs [102-108] used few diagnostic instruments and unconventional outcome criteria, with questions arising about their reported effectiveness on resistant schizophrenia. Some researches have, in fact, postulated that the good outcome results of these trials were skewed by regional biases [68]. In Chinese trials, in fact, two different FGAs are often prescribed as costart and not in add-on, with unclear randomization procedures [77, 94]. A small effect size favouring antipsychotic combinations in reducing rehospitalization of chronic schizophrenic or schizoaffective patients has been, however, noticed in a current trial mainly reporting the effectiveness of monotherapy with long-acting perphenazine [210]. In the examination of open studies or case reports involving SGAs plus FGAs, or SGAs plus SGAs combinations, the benzamides, that is sulpiride, a FGA and amisulpride, a SGA, have shown remarkable pharmacodynamic properties when associated to other APs. Sulpiride has proved to improve psychopathology and reduce remarkable side effects, such as weight gain, when combined to olanzapine [76, 178], while amisulpride managed in reducing psychopathology and increasing psychosocial outcomes in association with olanzapine [195]. Another issue put forward by studies about non-clozapine APs combination is that add-on of aripiprazole may worsen psychotic symptoms, probably due to its dopamine-agonist properties in the hypodopaminergic environment generated by transient D_2 receptor occupancy of multireceptor-acting SGAs, such as olanzapine [196] or quetiapine [197]. A large, placebo-controlled randomized double blind American study [208] seem, however, to contradict case report results, evidencing that add-on with aripiprazole was associated to reduction of some adverse effects of other SGAs, such as serum prolactin decrease, without influencing psychopathology. A careful approach in balancing the benefits and the risks of prescribing non-clozapine APs combinations is therefore warranted [211].

Combinations of APs plus clozapine have instead obtained more interest, due to their perceived importance in the treatment of persons with resistant schizophrenia [5, 7, 10-11, 66, 72]. The advantages of complementary pharmacokinetic and pharmacodynamic properties of some FGAs, such as sulpiride and some SGAs, mainly amisulpride, quetiapine, ziprasidone and, most of all, aripiprazole have determined the good results of small open and non randomized studies combining these APs to clozapine [101, 143, 151, 153, 168]. Although unsystematic observations have seemed to favour especially the clozapine plus aripiprazole combination [147-150, 153-155], a pioneristic small, but well-conducted double blind RCT proved the effectiveness of the add-on of sulpiride to clozapine [79], while another double blind study outlined the positive results of augmentation with risperidone [140], and a single blind study evidenced the good augmenting properties of amisulpride [205]. The larger trials have disregarded the effectiveness of aripiprazole plus clozapine combination, indicating how the adjunct of aripiprazole gave no better reduction in global psychopathology than haloperidol [160] or placebo [159]. Resistant schizophrenia patients added on with aripiprazole reported, however, an improvement in negative symptoms in a South Korean double blind study [157]. Two small randomized Italian studies have also displayed a statistically significant improvement of psychotic symptoms in resistant schizophrenic patients taking clozapine and adjuncted with aripiprazole [158, 162], while an amelioration of cholesterol, tryglicerides and glicemia hs been observed in an open study [151] and in a retrospective case series [155] with this combination. What is more, another open study [156] highlighted an improvement in quality of life for residual schizophrenic patients taking a clozapine plus aripiprazole combination. A statistically significant reduction of metabolic indices, associated to an improvement in functional autonomy in persons with schizophrenia administered with adjunct aripiprazole to clozapine has finally been observed in another retrospective case series report [161]. Such a result, albeit contrasting with trials investigating the effectiveness of this combination in real-world [160], is in accordance with randomized studies proving the tolerability of add-on of aripiprazole to other SGAs [208].

A sensible reason to put forward the clinical use of combining amisulpride, aripiprazole, sulpiride or ziprasidone to clozapine is their pharmacokinetic and pharmacodynamic complementary nature [79, 161, 164-165]. Amisulpride is pharmacodynamically acting by binding to D_2 and D_3 dopamine receptors, with the former distributed throughout the whole brain and the latter concentrated in limbic and cortical areas involved in the pathogenesis of schizophrenia, and its metabolism does not involve hepatic cytochromes, being cleared by renal excretion. For these reasons, when combined to clozapine, amisulpride may allow a reduction of clozapine dose up to 13% and may also counteract clozapine's muscarinic side effects, such as hypersalivation [213]. Aripiprazole-clozapine combination is supported by the favourable complementary pharmacodynamic receptor profile, that strengthens aripiprazole's partial agonist activity, tackling anxiety, negative depressive symptoms and cognitive dysfunctions [161]. Ziprasidone exhibits a D_2 plus serotonin 5-HT_2 antagonist activity, associated to a 5-HT_{1A} receptor agonism and infrequent QTc elongation [167], that renders effective the combination with clozapine, allowing to reduce clozapine dose and its unfavourable side effects.

Sales promotion initiative of pharmaceutical companies, postgraduate inadequate training or the management of disturbed behaviour of inpatients, with "as required", or prn, *pro re nata* prescriptions, have been proposed as the real cause of APs polypharmacy [15, 212]. The comorbidity with mental retardation and personality disorders, two conditions often associated to psychomotor agitation, physical assaults and disturbed behaviour, were in fact recognized as predictors of combined APs polypharmacy [28-29]. As inward nurse staff tend to request or favour prescriptions of FGAs, such as haloperidol or chlorpromazine to deal with hallucinations, delusions, thought disorders and behavioural disturbance, a host of research emphasized the role of clinical audits in changing prescribing practices, such as prn medications, with the involvement of senior nursing staff in finding alternative decisions of care [35, 39, 212]. In countries where clinical audits on APs polypharmacy were routinely enacted, the rate of multiple APs prescriptions lowered and co-administration of these drugs tended to be regarded as unjustified [37-38]. A relevant issue in coprescription of two or more APs is the use of long-acting prescriptions plus an oral drug to control physically aggressive forensic patients [66]. Therapeutic drug monitoring may also be of help in assessing adherence to prescribed medications to reduce the risk of aggressive or violent behavior in these patients [2, 66, 214].

Despite more than fifty years of use, in the prescription of APs there are still some peculiar aspects that render medication a complex, individualized process tailored for specific clinical necessities. This condition dramatically impacts with the need to standardize the treatment put forward by clinical guidelines. A most relevant feature, in this context, is the skepticism of psychiatrists, that tend to relay on clinical experience instead of guidelines when prescribing antipsychotic drugs [215]. Nevertheless, some guidelines recognized that combining APs is necessary in selected conditions. NICE guidelines [4-5] allow APs combinations for the short period covering a switch, while TMAP algorithms [7] permit APs polypharmacy after 4 consecutive failings of monotherapies, including clozapine. Barnes and Paton [212] evidenced, however, that some regional guidelines development groups deliberately overlooked APs coprescription issues [216-217]. Clozapine augmentation in treatment resistant schizophrenia had been explicitly permitted in at least one current British guideline [218]. From this condition, it is possible to state that some guidelines have begun to take into account the clinicians' experience. Essock *et al.*'s trial on patients taking two APs randomized to switching from APs polypharmacy to monotherapy or staying on polypharmacy [219] evidenced that after six months at least 69% of participants assigned to monotherapy by discontinuing one AP were still taking the same drug. In the remaining one third of participants returning to an APs combination, discontinuation of monotherapy was subjectively attributed to change in symptoms and side effects, despite the absence of significant differences in psychopathology among the two groups. In line with Essock *et al.*'s conclusions, efforts in healthcare policy should be made to build up guidelines that endorse the switch from APs combinations to monotherapy and consent patients to return to their original polypharmacy if monotherapy reveals inadequate.

Besides, considering simple pharmacological concepts, such as pharmacokinetic and/or pharmacodynamic complementary nature, might help to rationalize the prescription of two or more antipsychotics, avoiding high dose excessive sedation and severe adverse effects. In this context, therapeutic drug monitoring may be a valuable tool in augmentation strategies with drugs showing complex pharmacokinetic interactions due to metabolism *via* CYP 450 isoenzymes altering plasma concentrations [2, 88]. To exemplify this issue, add-on of melperone, a potent inhibitor of CYP 2D6 isoenzyme, proved a possible pharmacological strategy in the treatment of a CYP 2D6 ultrarapid metabolizer patient with schizophrenia [183]. CYP 2D6 and 2C19 are, in fact, the most relevant isoenzymes in antipsychotics and other CNS drugs metabolism [183, 229]. In other situations, such as clozapine augmentation with perazine, which inhibits CYP 1A2, therapeutic drug monitoring may be of help in controlling unwanted side effects induced by increase in serum clozapine levels [231, 232]. However, pharmacokinetic optimization of APs has been questioned by some authors [10] and therapeutic drug monitoring may be unavailable for extensively utilized drugs like antipsychotics, as it happens in Italy [2, 230]. A thorough consideration of the complementary profile in D_2 and non- D_2 receptor affinity or binding profiles, half-life, cytocrome P450 metabolization, side effects and costs is needed in any case to find out a targeted, personalized APs combination [220]. The "start low and go slow" prescription approach may be a useful reminder to contrast metabolic interactions [66].

Ideally, the treatment of schizophrenia should include different agents that match the different expression of the illness [221]; as dopaminergic antagonism is still the leading pharmacodynamic mechanism with proven antipsychotic efficacy [222], effective combinations should take into account a pharmacodynamic effect aimed at increasing frontal dopaminergic transmission and reverting the reduction in mesocortical dopaminergic transmission [223]. In this context, the careful administration of selected associations of antipsychotic drugs may prove an useful tool for obtaining clinical benefits and improving quality of life of the patients [161, 165].

ACKNOWLEDGMENT

None declared.

CONFLICT OF INTEREST

The authors state that there is no conflict of interest.

REFERENCES

[1] Kendell RE, Cooper JE, Gourlay AJ, *et al.* Diagnostic criteria of American and British psychiatrists. Arch Gen Psychiatry 1971; 25: 123-30.

[2] Hiemke C, Baumann P, Bergemann N, *et al.* AGNP Consensus Guidelines for Therapeutic Drug Monitoring in Psychiatry: Update 2011. Pharmacopsychiatry 2011; 44: 195-235.

[3] Miller A, Craig CS. Combination antipsychotics, pros, cons and questions. Schizophr. Bull. 2002; 28: 105-109.

[4] National Institute for Clinical Excellence. Schizophrenia. Full national clinical guideline on core interventions in primary and secondary care. London: Gaskell, pp.1-252. 2003.

[5] National Institute for Clinical Excellence. Schizophrenia. Core interventions in the treatment and management of schizophrenia in adults in primary and secondary care. National Institute for Clinical Excellence 2009 [cited 2011 Nov 26] Available from: www.nccmh.org.uk

[6] Gaebel W, Weissman S, Sartorius N, *et al.* Schizophrenia practice guidelines: international survey and comparison. Br J Psychiatry 2005; 187: 248-255.

[7] Moore TA, Buchanan RW, Buckley PF, *et al.* The Texas Medication Algorithm Project antipsychotic algorithm for schizophrenia: 2006 update. J Clin Psychiatry 2007; 68: 1751-62.

[8] Buchanan RW, Kreyenbuhl, J, Kelly DL, *et al.* The 2009 Schizophrenia PORT Psychopharmacological Treatment Recommendations and Summary Statements. Schizophr Bull 2010; 36: 71-93.

[9] Lehman AF, Lieberman JA, Dixon LB, *et al.* Practice guideline for the treatment of patients with schizophrenia, second edition. Am J Psychiatry 2004; 161: 1-56.

[10] Pandurangi AK, Dalkilic A. Polypharmacy with Second-Generation Antipsychotics: A Review of Evidence. J Psychiatr Pract 2008; 14: 345-67.

[11] Patel JK, Pinals DA, Breier A. Schizophrenia and other Psychotic Disorders. In: Tasman A, Kay J, Lieberman JA, First MB, Maj M, Eds. Psychiatry, Third Edition. England: Wiley-Blackwell 2009.

[12] Correll CU, Frederickson AM, Kane JM, *et al.* Does Antipsychotic Polypharmacy Increase the Risk for Metabolic Syndrome? Schizophr Res 2007; 89: 91-100.

[13] Citrome L, Jaffe A, Levine J, *et al.* Relationship between antipsychotic medication and new cases of diabetes among psychiatric inpatients. Psychiatr Serv 2004; 55: 1006-13.

[14] Joukamaa M, Heliovaara M, Knekt P, *et al.* Schizophrenia, neuroleptic medication and mortality. Br J Psychiatry 2006; 188: 122-27.

[15] Tibaldi G, Munizza C, Bollini P, *et al.* Utilization of neuroleptic drugs in Italian mental health services: a survey in Piedmont. Psychiatr Serv 1997; 48: 213-7.

[16] Mauri MC, Regispani F, Beraldo S, *et al.* Patterns of clinical use of antipsychotics in hospitalized psychiatric patients. Prog Neuropsychopharmacol Biol Psychiatry 2005; 29: 957-63.

[17] Tomasi R, de Girolamo G, Santone G, *et al.* The prescription of psychotropic drugs in psychiatric residential facilities: a national survey in Italy. Acta Psychiatr Scand. 2006; 113: 212-23.

[18] Ghio L, Natta W, Gotelli S, *et al.* Antipsychotic utilisation and polypharmacy in Italian residential facilities: a survey. Epidemiol Psychiatr Sci 2011; 20: 171-9.

[19] Bret P, Bonnet F, Bret MC, *et al.* Use of atypical antipsychotics in Charles Perrens psychiatric hospital (Bordeaux) analysis of prescribing practices for Amisulpride, Clozapine, Olanzapine and Risperidone. Encephale 2002; 28: 329-42.

[20] Bret MC, Bret P, Pariente A, *et al.* The use of atypical antipsychotics in French psychiatric hospitals. Pharm World Sci 2007; 29: 551-6.

[21] Bret P, Bret MC, Queuille E. Prescribing patterns of antipsychotics in 13 French psychiatric hospitals. Encephale 2009; 35: 129-38.

[22] Weinbrenner S, Assion HJ, Stargardt T, *et al.* Drug prescription patterns in schizophrenia outpatients: analysis of data from a German health insurance fund. Pharmacopsychiatry. 2009; 42: 66-71.

[23] Mundt AP, Aichberger MC, Fakhriddinov S, *et al.* Prescription patterns of patients diagnosed with schizophrenia in mental hospitals in Tashkent/Uzbekistan and in four German cities. Pharmacoepidemiol Drug Saf. 2011 Jul 1. doi: 10.1002/pds.2166.

[24] Lerma-Carrillo I, de Pablo Brühlmann S, del Pozo ML, *et al.* Antipsychotic polypharmacy in patients with schizophrenia in a brief hospitalization unit. Clin Neuropharmacol 2008; 31: 319-32.

[25] Molina JD, Lerma-Carrillo I, Leonor M, *et al.* Combined treatment with amisulpride in patients with schizophrenia discharged from a short-term hospitalization unit: a 1-year retrospective study. Clin Neuropharmacol 2009; 32: 10-5.

[26] Douzenis A, Apostoulopolos A, Seretis D, *et al.* The effect of ethnicity on prescribing practice and treatment outcome in inpatients suffering from schizophrenia in Greece. BMC Psychiatry 2011; 11: 66.

[27] Kontis D, Theochari E, Kleisas S, *et al.* Doubtful association of antipsychotic polypharmacy and high dosage with cognition in chronic schizophrenia. Prog Neuropsychopharmacol Biol Psychiatry 2010; 34: 1333-41.

[28] Bolstad A, Andreassen OA, Røssberg JI, *et al.* Previous hospital admissions and disease severity predict the use of antipsychotic combination treatment in patients with schizophrenia. BMC Psychiatry 2011, 11: 126.

[29] Kroker RA, Johnsen E, Ruud T, *et al.* Treatment of schizophrenia with antipsychotics in Norwegian emergency wards, a cross-sectional national study. BMC Psychiatry 2009, **9**: 24 doi: 10.1186/1471-244X-9-24.

[30] Jordanova V, Maric NP, Alikaj V, *et al.* Prescribing practices in psychiatric hospitals in Eastern Europe. Eur Psychiatry 2011; 26: 414-8.

[31] Divac N, Jasović-Gasić M, Samardzić R, *et al.* Antipsychotic polypharmacy at the University Psychiatric Hospital in Serbia. Pharmacoepidemiol Drug Saf 2007; 16: 1250-1.

[32] Loga-Zec S, Loga S. Polypharmacy in the treatment of schizophrenic patients in three University Centers in the Federation of Bosnia and Herzegovina (F/BH). Psychiatr Danub 2011; 23: 60-3.

[33] Koen L, Magni P, Niehaus DJH, *et al.* Antipsychotic prescription patterns in Xhosa patients with schizophrenia or schizoaffective disorder. Afr J Psychiatry 2008; 11: 287-90.

[34] Ramadas S, Kuttichira P, Sumesh TP, *et al.* A study of an antipsychotic prescription pattern of patients with schizophrenia in a developing country. Indian J Psychol Med 2010; 32: 13-16.

[35] Royal Australian and New Zealand College of Psychiatrists clinical practice guidelines for the treatment of schizophrenia and related disorders. Royal Australian and New Zealand College of Psychiatrists Clinical Practice Guidelines Team for the Treatment of Schizophrenia and Related Disorders. Aust N Z J Psychiatry 2005; 39: 1-30.

[36] Humberstone V, Wheeler A, Lambert T. An audit of outpatient antipsychotic usage in the three health sectors of Auckland, New Zealand. Aust N Z J Psychiatry 2004; 38: 240-5.

[37] Wheeler A, Humberstone V, Robinson G. Trends in antipsychotic prescribing in schizophrenia in Auckland. Australas Psychiatry 2006; 14: 169-74.

[38] Wheeler A. Explicit *versus* implicit review to explore combination antipsychotic prescribing. J Eval Clin Pract 2009; 15: 685-91.

[39] Yamin S, Vaddadi K. Are we using excessive neuroleptics? An argument for systematic neuroleptic dose reduction in stable patients with schizophrenia with specific reference to clozapine. Int Rev Psychiatry 2010; 22: 138-47.

[40] An FR, Xiang YT, Wang CY, *et al.* Change of psychotropic drug prescription for schizophrenia in a psychiatric institution in Beijing, China between 1999 and 2008. Int J Clin Pharmacol Ther 2010; 48: 270-4.

[41] Xiang YT, Wang CY, Si TM, *et al.* Antipsychotic Polypharmacy in Inpatients with Schizophrenia in Asia (2001-2009). Pharmacopsychiatry. 2011 Oct 11. [Epub ahead of print].

[42] Centorrino F, Eakin M, Won-Myong B, *et al.* Inpatient Antipsychotic Drug Use in 1998, 1993, and 1989. Am J Psychiatry 2002; 159: 1932-35.

[43] Gilmer TP, Dolder CR, Folsom DP, *et al.* Antipsychotic polypharmacy trends among Medicaid beneficiaries with schizophrenia in San Diego County, 1999-2004. Psychiatr Serv 2007; 58: 1007-10.

[44] Eisen C, Shaner R, Unützer J, *et al.* Datapoints: second generation antipsychotic medication combinations for schizophrenia. Psychiatr Serv 2008; 59: 235.

[45] Megna JL, Kunwar AR, Mahlotra K, *et al.* A study of polypharmacy with second generation antipsychotics in patients with severe and persistent mental illness. J Psychiatr Pract 2007; 13: 129-37.

[46] Ganguly R, Kotzan JA, Miller LS, *et al.* Prevalence, trends, and factors associated with antipsychotic polypharmacy among Medicaid-eligible schizophrenia patients, 1998-2000. J Clin Psychiatry 2004; 65: 1377-88.

[47] Procyshyn RM, Honer WG, Wu TK, *et al.* Persistent antipsychotic polypharmacy and excessive dosing in the community psychiatric treatment setting: a review of medication profiles in 435 Canadian outpatients. J Clin Psychiatry 2010; 71: 566-73.
[48] Barbui C, Nosè M, Mazzi MA, *et al.* Determinants of first- and second-generation antipsychotic drug use in clinically unstable patients with schizophrenia treated in four European countries. Int Clin Psychopharmacol 2006a; 21: 73-9.
[49] Barbui C, Nosè M, Mazzi MA, *et al.* Persistence with polypharmacy and excessive dosing in patients with schizophrenia treated in four European countries. Int Clin Psychopharmacol 2006b; 21: 355-62.
[50] Kiivet RA, Llerena A, Dahl ML, *et al.* Patterns of drug treatment of schizophrenic patients in Estonia, Spain and Sweden. Br J Clin Pharmacol 1995; 40: 467-76.
[51] Broekema WJ, de Groot IW, van Harten PN. Simultaneous prescribing of atypical antipsychotics, conventional antipsychotics and anticholinergics—a European study. Pharm World Sci 2007; 29: 126-30.
[52] Borison RL, Pathiranja A, Haverstock S, *et al.* Classical and New Antipsychotic Drugs in the Treatment of Schizophrenia. In: Shriqui CL, Nasrallah HA, Eds. Contemporary Issues in the Treatment of Schizophrenia. Washington, D.C. and London, England: American Psychiatric Press, Inc. 1996.
[53] Casey JLF, Hollister LE, Klett CJ, *et al.* Combined drug therapy of chronic schizophrenics. Am J Psychiatry 1961; 7: 997-1003.
[54] Terrel MS. Response to trifluoperazine and chlorpromazine, singly and in combinations, in chronic "back-ward" patients. Dis Nerv Syst 1962; 23: 41-8.
[55] Swanson DW, Smith JA, Perez H. A fixed combination of chlorpromazine and trifluoperazine in psychotic patients. Dys Nerv Sys 1967; 28: 756.
[56] Jones B, Lehman HE, Saxena BM, *et al.* Treatment of chronic schizophrenic patients with haloperidol and chlorpromazine. Curr Ther Res 1968; 10: 276-78.
[57] Sheppard C, Beyel V, Fracchia J, *et al.* Polypharmacy in psychiatry: a multi-state comparison of psychotropic drug combinations. Dis Nerv Syst. 1974; 35: 183-9.
[58] Davis JM, Garver DL. Neuroleptics: clinical use in psychiatry. In: Iversen L, Iversen S, Snyder S, Eds. Handbook of Psychopharmacology. New York: Plenum Press 1978.
[59] Wilson WH, Ban TA, Guy W. Pharmacotherapy of chronic hospitalized schizophrenics: prescription practices. Neuropsychobiology. 1985; 14: 75-82.
[60] Baldessarrini RJ, Katz B, Cotton P. Dissimilar dosing with high-potency and low-potency neuroleptics. Am J Psychiatry 1984; 141: 748-52.
[61] Baldessarrini RJ, Kando JC, Centorrino F. Hospital use of antipsychotic agents in 1989 and 1993: stable dosing with decreased length-of-stay. Am J Psychiatry 1995; 152: 1038-44.
[62] Godleski LS, Kerler K, Barber JW, *et al.* Multiple *versus* single antipsychotic drug treatment in chronic psychosis. J Nerv Dis 1989; 177: 689-89.
[63] Soni SD, Sampath G, Shah A, *et al.* Rationalising neuroleptic polypharmacy in chronic schizophrenics: effects of changing to a single depot preparation. Acta Psychiatr Scand 1992; 85: 354-59.
[64] Lehman AF, Steinwachs DM, PORT Project Investigators. At Issue: Translating Research Into Practice: The Schizophrenia Patient Outcomes Research Team (PORT) Treatment Recommendations. Schizophr Bull 1998; 24: 1-10

[65] Lehman AF, Steinwachs DM, PORT Project Investigators. Patterns of Usual Care for Schizophrenia: Initial Results From the Schizophrenia Patient Outcomes Research Team (PORT) Client Survey. Schizophr Bull 1998; 24: 11 -20.

[66] Bazire S. Psychotropic drug directory, 2005. The professionals' pocket handbook & aide memoire. Salisbury, UK: Fivepin Limited; 2005.

[67] Chakos M, Lieberman J, Hoffman E, *et al.* Effectiveness of secondgeneration antipsychotics in patients with treatment-resistant schizophrenia: a review and meta-analysis of randomized trials. Am J Psychiatry 2001; 158: 518-26.

[68] Barbui C, Signoretti A, Mulè S, *et al.* Does the addition of a second antipsychotic drug improve clozapine treatment? Schizophr Bull 2009; 35: 458-68.

[69] Reed A, Huie K, Perloff ES, *et al.* Loxapine P-glycoprotein Interactions *In vitro*. Drug Metabol Lett 2012; 6: 26-32.

[70] Gunes A, Spina E, Dahl ML, *et al.* ABCB1 polymorphisms influence steady-state plasma levels of 9-hydroxyrisperidone and risperidone active moiety. Ther Drug Monit. 2008; 30: 628-633.

[71] Nikisch G, Baumann P, Oneda B, *et al.* Cytochrome P450 and ABCB1 genetics: association with quetiapine and norquetiapine plasma and cerebrospinal fluid concentrations and with clinical response in patients suffering from schizophrenia. A pilot study. J Psychopharmacol. 2011; 25: 896-907.

[72] Moons T, de Roo M, Claes S, *et al.* Relationship between P-glycoprotein and second-generation antipsychotics. Pharmacogenomics. 2011; 12: 1193-1211.

[73] Spina E, de Leon J. Metabolic drug interactions with newer antipsychotics: a comparative review. Basic Clin Pharmacol Toxicol 2007; 100: 4-22.

[74] Meyer J. Drug-drug interactions with antipsychotics. CNS Spectr 2007; 12: 12 (Suppl 21) 6-9.

[75] McCue RE, Waheed R, Urcuyo L. Polypharmacy in patients with schizophrenia. J Clin Psychiatry 2003; 64: 984-9.

[76] Kotler M, Strous RD, Reznik I, *et al.* Sulpiride augmentation of olanzapine in the management of treatment-resistant chronic schizophrenia: evidence for improvement of mood symptomatology. Int Clin Psychopharmacol 2004; 19: 23-6.

[77] Correll CU, Frederickson AM, Kane JM, *et al.* Does Antipsychotic Polypharmacy Increase the Risk for Metabolic Syndrome? Schizophr Res. 2007 J; 89: 91-100.

[78] Kane JM, Correll CU. Past and Present Progress in the Pharmacologic Treatment of Schizophrenia. J Clin Psychiatry. 2010; 71(9): 1115-1124.

[79] Shiloh R, Zemishlany Z, Aizenberg D, *et al.* Sulpiride augmentation in people with schizophrenia partially responsive to clozapine. A double-blind, placebo-controlled study. Br J Psychiatry 1997; 171: 569-73.

[80] King D, Zigmond MJ, Finlay JM. Effects of dopamine depletion in the medial prefrontal cortex on the stress-induced increase in extracellular dopamine in the nucleus accumbens core and shell. Neuroscience 1997; 77: 141-53.

[81] Tidey JW, Miczek KA. Social defeat stress selectively alters mesocorticolimbic dopamine release: an *in vivo* microdialysis study. Brain Res 1996; 721: 140-9

[82] Moretti L. Real life experiences: a doctor's account. Giorn Ital Psicopat 2009; 15: 310-13.

[83] Stip E, Tourjman V. Aripiprazole in schizophrenia and schizoaffective disorder: A review. Clin Ther 2010; 32: Suppl 1: S3-20.

[84] Englisch S, Zink, M. Combined antipsychotic treatment involving clozapine and aripiprazole. Progr Neuro-Psychopharmacol Biol Psychiatry 2008; 32: 1386-92.
[85] Freudenreich O, Goff DC. Antipsychotic combination therapy in schizophrenia: a review of efficacy and risk of current combinations. Acta Psychiatr Scand 2002; 106: 323-30.
[86] Lerner L, Libov I, Kotler M, *et al.* combination of “atypical” antipsychotic medication in the management of treatment-resistant schizophrenia and schizoaffective disorder. Prog Neuropsychopharmacol Biol Psychiatry 2004; 28: 89-98.
[87] Patrick V, Levin E, Schleifer S. Antipsychotic polypharmacy: is there evidence for its use? J Psychiatr Pract 2005; 11: 248-57.
[88] Zink M. Augmentation of olanzapine in treatment-resistant schizophrenia. J Psychiatry Neurosci 2005; 30(6): 409-15.
[89] Honer WG, Procyshyn RM, Chen EYH, *et al.* A translational research approach to poor treatment response in patients with schizophrenia: clozapine-antipsychotic polypharmacy. J Psychiatry Neurosci 2009; 34(6): 433-42.
[90] Kontaxakis VP, Ferentinos PP, Havaki-Kontaxaki BJ, *et al.* Randomized controlled augmentation trials in clozapine-resistant schizophrenic patients: a critical review. Eur Psychiatry 2005; 20: 409-15.
[91] Kontaxakis VP, Ferentinos PP, Havaki-Kontaxaki BJ, *et al.* Risperidone augmentation of clozapine: a critical review. Eur Arch Psychiatry Clin Neurosci 2006; 256: 350-5.
[92] Paton C, Whittington C, Barnes TR. Augmentation with a second antipsychotic in patients with schizophrenia who partially respond to clozapine: a meta-analysis. J Clin Psychopharmacol 2007; 27: 198-204.
[93] Correll CU, Rummel-Kluge C, Corves C, *et al.* Antipsychotic combinations *vs* monotherapy in schizophrenia: a meta-analysis of randomized controlled trials. Schizophr Bull 2009; 35: 443-57.
[94] Taylor DM, Smith L. Augmentation of clozapine with a second antipsychotic — a meta-analysis of randomized, placebo-controlled studies. Acta Psychiatr Scand 2009; 119: 419-25.
[95] Faries D, Ascher-Svanum H, Zhu B, *et al.* Antipsychotic monotherapy and polypharmacy in the naturalistic treatment of schizophrenia with atypical antipsychotics. BMC Psychiatry 2005; 5: 26
[96] Zhang L, Xu Y. A comparison study on treatment effect of clozapine, chlorpromazine and the combination of clozapine and chlorpromazine in schizophrenia. Chin J Nerv Ment Dis. 1989; 5(5): 306-308.
[97] Potter WZ, Ko GN, Zhang LD, *et al.* Clozapine in China: a review and preview of US/PRC collaboration. Psychopharmacology. 1989; 99: 87-91.
[98] Wang CH, Qin TF, Lin YL, *et al.* A clinical effect and following-up study about sulpiride and clozapine for 105cases of the schizophrenia type. J Xinxiang Med Coll. 1994; 11(2): 148-51.
[99] Liu Q, Li X, Zhang Y. A control study of clozapine in combination with sulpiride in alleviating the negative symptoms of schizophrenia. Chin J Psychiatry. 1996; 29: 87-90.
[100] Mowerman S, Siris SG. Adjunctive loxapine in a clozapine-resistant cohort of schizophrenic patients. Ann Clin Psychiatry. 1996 Dec; 8(4): 193-7.
[101] Shiloh R. Sulpride adjunction to clozapine in treatment resistant schizophrenic patients: A preliminary case series study. Eur Psychiatry 1997; 12: 152-5.

[102] Cha C, Hui G, Quing G. Evaluation of therapeutic effect with chlorpromazine and clozapine for treatment of schizophrenia. Xinxiang Med Stud. 1999; 16: 311-16.

[103] Si S, Yuan C. A comparative trial of the effects of sulpiride combined with clozapine in the treatment of schizophrenia. Shandong Arch Psychiatry. 1999; 12: 17-20.

[104] Zhu Y, Zhang S, Zhang D. A controlled trial comparing chlorimipramine and sulpiride as adjunct to clozapine in the treatment of negative symptoms of schizophrenia. J Clin Psychol Med. 1999; 9: 204-5.

[105] Xao H. A double-blind comparative study of the effects of sulpiride combined with clozapine in the treatment of schizophrenia. Sichuan Ment Health. 1999; 12: 250-251.

[106] Jia Z, Zhang Z, Jin S. A controlled trial for comparing clozapine combined with pipothiazine palmitate to clozapine alone in the treatment of negative symptoms in schizophrenic patients. Herald Med. 2000; 19: 142-43.

[107] Zhu H, Deng D. A study of clozapine combined with or without pipotiazine palmitate in refractory schizophrenia. J Clin Psychol Med. 2002; 12: 15-17.

[108] Zou G, Huang Y, Zou S, *et al.* A comparative trial of the beneficial effects of sulpiride combined with clozapine in the treatment of refractory schizophrenia. J Yichun Univ. 2003; 25: 94-96.

[109] Friedman JI, Lindenmayer JP, Alcantara F, *et al.* Pimozide Augmentation of Clozapine In Patients With Schizophrenia And Schizoaffective Disorder Unresponsive To Clozapine Monotherapy. Neuropsychopharmacology. 2011 May ; 36(6): 1289-95.

[110] Koreen AR, Lieberman JA, Kronig M, *et al.* Cross-tapering clozapine and risperidone. Am J Psychiatry 1995; 152: 1690.

[111] Tyson SC, Devane CL, Risch SC. Pharmacokinetic interaction between risperidone and clozapine. Am J Psychiatry 1995; 152: 1401-2.

[112] McCarthy RH, Terkelsen KG. Risperidone augmentation of clozapine. Pharmacopsychiatry 1995; 28: 61-3.

[113] Chong SA, Tan CH, Lee HS. Hoarding and clozapine-risperidone combination. Can J Psychiatry 1996; 41: 315-6.

[114] Godleski LS, Sernyak MJ. Agranulocytosis after addition ofrisperidone to clozapine treatment. Am J Psychiatry 1996; 153: 735-6.

[115] Henderson DC, Goff DC. Risperidone as an adjunct to clozapine therapy in chronic schizophrenics. J Clin Psychiatry 1996; 57: 395-7.

[116] Chong SA, Tan CH, Lee HS. Worsening of psychosis with clozapine and selective serotonin reuptake inhibitor combination: Two case reports. J Clin Psychopharmacol 1997; 17: 68-9.

[117] Patel JK, Salzman C, Green AI, *et al.* Chronic schizophrenia: Response to clozapine, risperidone, and paroxetine. Am J Psychiatry 1997; 154: 543-6.

[118] Mantonakis I, Kattan K, Zervas IM. Risperidone augmentation of clozapine and olanzapine for refractory schizophrenia. Eur Neuropsychopharmacol 1998; 8: 233.

[119] Zervas IM, Kattan K, Mantonakis I. Risperidone-clozapine combination for refractory schizophrenia. Eur Neuropsychopharmacol 1998; 8: S37.

[120] Morera AL, Barreiro P, Cano-Munoz JL. Risperidone and clozapine combination for the treatment of refractory schizophrenia. Acta Psychiatr Scand 1999; 99: 305-6.

[121] Adesanya A, Pantelis C. Adjunctive risperidone treatment in patients with 'clozapine resistant schizophrenia'. Aust N Z J Psychiatry 2000; 34: 533-4.

[122] Raskin S, Katz G, Zislin Z, *et al.* Clozapine and risperidone: Combination/augmentation treatment of refractory schizophrenia: A preliminary observation. Acta Psychiatr Scand 2000; 101: 334-6.
[123] de Groot IW, Heck AH, van Harten PN. Addition of risperidone to clozapine therapy in chronically psychotic inpatients. J Clin Psychiatry 2001; 62: 129-30.
[124] Henderson DC, Goff DC, Connolly CE, *et al.* Risperidone added to clozapine: Impact on serum prolactin levels. J Clin Psychiatry 2001; 62: 605-8.
[125] Liu Q, Li X. A comparative study on the efficacy of combining risperidone and clozapine in the treatment of schizophrenia. Shandong Arch Psychiatry. 2001; 14: 28-30.
[126] Ni J, Jang L, Hong X. Therapeutic effects of clozapine, risperidone and their combination in the treatment of schizophrenia. Health Psychol J. 2001; 3: 181-82.
[127] Raju GVL, Kumar R, Khanna S. Clozapine-risperidone combination in treatment-resistant schizophrenia. Aust N Z J Psychiatry 2001; 35: 543.
[128] Taylor CG, Flynn SW, Altman S, *et al.* An open trial of risperidone augmentation of partial response to clozapine. Schizophr Res 2001; 48: 155-8.
[129] Xie C, Ni XL. The compared study of treating schizophrenia with risperidone combining clozapine. J Prev Med Inform. 2001; 17(4): 245.
[130] Xin X, Du B, Zeng Z. A controlled clinical study of risperidone and low dose of clozapine in treating schizophrenia. Herald Med. 2001; 20: 501-2.
[131] Beauchemin MA, Millaud F, Nguyen KA. A case of neuroleptic malignant syndrome with clozapine and risperidone. Can J Psychiatry 2002; 47: 886.
[132] Kontaxakis VP, Havaki-Kontaxaki BJ, Stamouli SS, *et al.* Toxic interaction between risperidone and clozapine: A case report. Prog Neuropsychopharmacol Biol Psychiatry 2002; 26: 407-9.
[133] Peng H, Kuang Y, Huang X. A control study of risperidone in combination with clozapine in treating refractory schizophrenia. J Mod Clin Med Bioeng. 2002; 7: 100-102.
[134] Procyshyn RM, Tse G, Sin O, *et al.* Concomitant clozapine reduces smoking in patients treated with risperidone. Eur Neuropsychopharmacol 2002; 12: 77-80.
[135] Raaska K, Raitasuo V, Neuvonen PJ. Therapeutic drug monitoring data: Risperidone does not increase serum clozapine concentration. Eur J Clin Pharmacol 2002; 58: 587-91.
[136] Senechal A, Landry P, Deschamps R, *et al.* Neutropenia in a patient treated with clozapine in combination with other psychotropic drugs. Encephale 2002; 28: 567-9.
[137] Wu L. A control study of risperidone and clozapine combination for the treatment of refractory schizophrenia. Health Psychol J. 2002; 10: 135-37.
[138] Yue H, Song L, Xu Y. A comparative trial of risperidone in the treatment of schizophrenia over two years. Shangai Arch Psychiatry. 2004; 16: 165-67.
[139] Anil Yagcioglu AE, Kivircik Akdede BB, Turgut TI, *et al.* A double blind controlled study of adjunctive treatment with risperidone in schizophrenic patients partially responsive to clozapine: Efficacy and safety. J Clin Psychiatry 2005; 66: 63-72.
[140] Josiassen RC, Joseph A, Kohegyi E, *et al.* Clozapine augmented with risperidone in the treatment of schizophrenia: A randomized, double-blind, placebo-controlled trial. Am J Psychiatry 2005; 162: 130-6.
[141] Honer WG, Thornton AE, Chen EY, *et al.* Clozapine alone *versus* clozapine and risperidone with refractory schizophrenia. N Engl J Med 2006; 354: 472-82.

[142] Freudenreich O, Henderson DC, Walsh JP, *et al.* Risperidone augmentation for schizophrenia partially responsive to clozapine: A double-blind, placebo-controlled trial. Schizophr Res 2007; 92: 90-4.

[143] Agelink MW, Kavuk I, Ak I. Clozapine with amisulpride for refractory schizophrenia. Am J Psychiatry 2004; 161: 924-5.

[144] Zink M, Knopf U, Henn FA, *et al.* Combination of clozapine and amisulpride in treatment-resistant schizophrenia: Case reports and review of the literature. Pharmacopsychiatry 2004; 37: 26-31.

[145] Kämpf P, Agelink MW, Naber D. Augmentation of clozapine with amisulpride: a promising therapeutic approach to refractory schizophrenic symptoms. Pharmacopsychiatry 2005; 38(1): 39-40.

[146] Lim S, Pralea C, Schnitt J, *et al.* Possible increased efficacy of low dose clozapine when combined with aripiprazole. J Clin Psychiatry 2004; 65: 1284-5.

[147] Ashton AK. Aripiprazole augmentation of clozapine in refractory schizophrenia. Psychiatry 2005, 2: 18-19.

[148] Ziegenbein M, Sieberer M, Calliess IT, *et al.* Combination of clozapine and aripiprazole: A promising approach in treatment-resistant schizophrenia. Aust N Z J Psychiatry 2005; 39: 840-1.

[149] Abu-Tair F, Kopitz J, Bergmann N. Clozapine augmented with aripiprazole i 5 patients with schizophrenia. J Clin Psychopharmacol 2006; 26(6): 669-71.

[150] Clarke LA, Lindenmayer JP, Kaushik S. Clozapine augmentation with aripiprazole for negative symptoms. J Clin Psychiatry 2006; 67: 675-6.

[151] Henderson DC, Kunkel L, Nguyen DD, *et al.* An exploratory open-label trial of aripiprazole as an adjuvant to clozapine therapy in chronic schizophrenia. Acta Psychiatr Scand 2006; 113: 142-7.

[152] Rocha FL, Hara C. Benefits of combining aripiprazole to clozapine: three case reports. Progr neuro-Psychopharnacol Biol Psychiatry 2006; 30(6): 1167-9.

[153] Ziegenbein M, Wittmann G, Kropp S. Aripiprazole augmentation of clozapine in treatment-resistant schizophrenia - a clinical observation. Clin Drug Investig 2006; 26(3): 117-24.

[154] Zink M, Knopf U, Kuwilsky A. management of clozapine-induced obsessive compulsive symptoms in a man with schizophrenia. Austr NZ J Psychiatry 2006,41(3): 293-4.

[155] Karunakaran K, Tungaraza TE, Harborne GC. Is clozapine-aripiprazole combination a useful regime in the management of treatment-resistant schizophrenia? J Psychopharmacol 2007; 21: 453-6.

[156] Mitsonis CI, Dimopoulos NP, Mitropoulos PA, *et al.* Aripiprazole augmentation in the management of residual symptoms in clozapine-treated outpatients with chronic schizophrenia: An open-label pilot study. Prog Neuropsychopharmacol Biol Psychiatry 2007; 31: 373-7.

[157] Chang JS, Ahn YM, Park HJ, *et al.* Aripiprazole augmentation in clozapine-treated patients with refractory schizophrenia: an 8-week, randomized, double blind, placebo-controlled trial. J Clin Psychiatry 2008; 69: 720-31.

[158] Benedetti A, Di Paolo A, Lastella M, *et al.* Augmentation of clozapine with aripiprazole in severe psychotic bipolar and schizoaffective disorders: a pilot study. Clin Pract Epidemiol Ment Health 2010; 6: 30-5.

[159] Fleischhacker WW, Heikkinen ME, Olia JP, *et al.* Effects of adjunctive treatment with aripiprazole on body weight and clinical efficacy in schizophrenia patients treated with

clozapine: a randomized, double-blind, placebo-controlled trial. Int J Neuropsychopharmacol 2010; 12: 1-11

[160] Barbui C, Accordini S, Nosè M, *et al.* Aripiprazole *versus* haloperidol in combination with clozapine for treatment-resistant schizophrenia in routine clinical care: a randomized, controlled trial. J Clin Psychopharmacol 2011; 31(3): 266-73.

[161] De Risio A, Pancheri A, Simonetti G, *et al.* Add-on of aripiprazole improves outcome in clozapine-resistant schizophrenia. Prog Neuropsychopharmacol Biol Psychiatry. 2011; 35: 1112-16.

[162] Muscatello MR, Bruno A, Pandolfo G, *et al.* Effect of aripiprazole augmentation of clozapine in schizophrenia: a double-blind, placebo-controlled study. Schizophr Res 2011; 127(1-3); 93-9.

[163] Kaye NS. Ziprasidone augmentation of clozapine in 11patients. J Clin Psychiatry 2003; 64: 215-6.

[164] Zink M, Mase E, Dressing H. Combination of ziprasidone and clozapine in treatment-resistant schizophrenia. Hum Psychopharmacol 2004; 19: 271-3.

[165] Zink M, Kuwilsky A, Krumm B, *et al.* Efficacy and tolerability of ziprasidone *versus* risperidone as augmentation in patients partially responsive to clozapine: a randomised controlled clinical trial. J Psychopharmacol. 2009; 23: 305-314.

[166] Ziegenbein M, Kropp S, Kuenzel HE. Combination of clozapine and ziprasidone in treatment-resistant schizophrenia: An open clinical study. Clin Neuropharmacol 2005; 28: 220-4.

[167] Ziegenbein M, Calliess IT. Clozapine and ziprasidone: A useful combination in patients with treatment-resistant schizophrenia. J Neuropsychiatry Clin Neurosci 2006; 18: 246-7.

[168] Reinstein MJ, Sirotovskaya LA, Jones LE, *et al.* Effect of clozapine-quetiapine combination therapy on weight and glycaemic control: Preliminary findings. Clin Drug Investig 1999; 18: 99-104.

[169] Diaz P, Hogan TP. Granulocytopenia with clozapine and quetiapine. Am J Psychiatry 2001; 158: 651.

[170] Gupta S, Sonnenberg SJ, Frank B. Olanzapine augmentation of clozapine. Ann Clin Psychiatry 1998; 10: 113-5.

[171] Rhoads E. Polypharmacy of 2 atypical antipsychotics. J Clin Psychiatry 2000; 61: 678-80.

[172] Barrett WW, Elsworth RB, Clark LD, *et al.* Study of the differential behavioral effects of reserpine, chlorpromazine, and a combination of these drugs in chronic schizophrenic patients. Dis Nerv Syst. 1957; 18(6): 209-215.

[173] Talbot DR. Are tranquilizer combinations more effective than a single tranquilizer? Am J Psychiatry. 1964; 121: 597-600.

[174] Chien CP, Cole JO. Depot phenothiazine treatment in acute psychosis: a sequential comparative clinical study. Am J Psychiatry. 1973; 130(1): 13-18.

[175] Nishikawa T. Prophylactic effects of neuroleptics in symptom-free schizophrenics: roles of dopaminergic and noradrenergic blockers. Biol Psychiatry. 1985; 11: 1161-66.

[176] Higashima M, Takeda T, Nagasawa T, *et al.* Combined therapy with low-potency neuroleptic levomepromazine as an adjunct to haloperidol for agitated patients with acute exacerbation of schizophrenia. Eur Psychiatry. 2004; 19(6): 380-81.

[177] Takhar J. Pimozide augmentation in a patient with drug-resistant psychosis previously treated with olanzapine. J Psychiatry Neurosci 1999; 24: 248-9.

[178] Raskin S, Durst R, Katz G, *et al.* Olanzapine and sulpride: A preliminary study of combination/augmentation in patients with treatment-resistant schizophrenia. J Clin Psychopharmacol 2000; 20: 500-3.

[179] Mujica R, Weiden P. Neuroleptic malignant syndrome after addition of haloperidol to atypical antipsychotic. Am J Psychiatry 2001; 158: 650-1.

[180] Abdullah N, Voronovitch L, Taylor S, *et al.* Olanzapine and haloperidol: Potential for neutropenia? Psychosomatics 2003; 44: 83-4.

[181] Tofler IT, Ahmed B. Atypical (olanzapine) plus conventional (fluphenazine) neuroleptic treatment associated with the neuroleptic malignant syndrome. J Clin Psychopharmacol 2003; 23: 672-4.

[182] Grover S, Sharan P, Gupta N. Aripiprazole worsens psychosis: a case report. Prim Care Companion J Psychiatry 2006; 8(6): 380-81.

[183] Gahr M, Gastl R, Kölle AM, *et al.* Successful treatment of schizophrenia with melperone augmentation in a patient with phenotypic CYP2D6 ultrarapid metabolization: a case report. J Med Case Rep 2012; 6: 49. doi: 10.1186/1752-1947-6-49.

[184] John V, Rapp M, Pies R. Aggression, agitation, and mania with olanzapine. Can J Psychiatry 1998; 43: 1054.

[185] Gaston RL, George M, Azhahan N. Diabetic control and atypical antipsychotics: a case report. J Med Case Rep 2008; 2: 155. doi: 10.1186/1752-1947-2-155.

[186] Lerner V, Chudakova B, Kravets S, *et al.* Combined use of risperidone and olanzapine in the treatment of patients with resistant schizophrenia: A preliminary case series report. Clin Neuropharmacol 2000; 23: 284-6.

[187] Chue P, Welch R, Snaterse M. Combination risperidone and quetiapine therapy in refractory schizophrenia. Can J Psychiatry 2001; 46: 86-7.

[188] Seger A, Lamberti JS. Priapism associated with polypharmacy. J Clin Psychiatry 2001; 62: 128.

[189] Hedges DW, Jeppson KG. New-onset seizure associated with quetiapine and olanzapine. Ann Pharmacother 2002; 36: 437-9.

[190] Jones GH. 'Clozapine effect' without the blood tests? Prog Neurol Psychiatry 2002; 6: 32.

[191] Bozikas VP, Deseri C, Pitsavas S, *et al.* Antiaggressive action of combined risperidone and quetiapine in a patient with schizophrenia. Can J Psychiatry 2003; 48: 426-7.

[192] Nelson MW, Reynolds RR, Kelly DL, *et al.* Adjunctive quetiapine decreases symptoms of tardive dyskinesia in a patient taking risperidone. Clin Neuropharmacol 2003; 26: 297-8.

[193] O'Shea M, Sazhin V, Collins A. Ventricular ectopics during crossover of atypical antipsychotics. Aust N Z J Psychiatry 2003; 37: 773-4.

[194] Minov C. Risk of QTc prolongation due to combination of ziprasidone and quetiapine. Psychiatr Prax 2004; 31: S142-4.

[195] Zink M, Henn FA, Thome J. Combination of amisulpride and olanzapine in treatment-resistant schizophrenic psychoses. Eur Psychiatry 2004; 19: 56-8.

[196] Duggal HS. Aripiprazole-olanzapine combination for treatment of schizophrenia. Can J Psychiatry 2004; 49: 151.

[197] Reeves RR, Mack JE. Worsening schizoaffective disorder with aripiprazole. Am J Psychiatry 2004; 161: 1308.

[198] DeQuardo JR. Increased efficacy with addition of clozapine to aripiprazole: Alternative explanations. J Clin Psychiatry 2005; 66: 396; author reply 396.

[199] Dunkley MJ, Reveley MA. Successful treatment of refractory schizophrenia with combined olanzapine and quetiapine in a patient with a prolactin secreting pituitary microadenoma. J Psychopharmacol 2005; 19: 97-101.

[200] Suzuki T, Uchida H, Watanabe K, *et al.* Effectiveness of antipsychotic polypharmacy for patients with treatment refractory schizophrenia: an open-label trial of olanzapine plus risperidone for those who failed to respond to a sequential treatment with olanzapine, quetiapine and risperidone. Hum Psychopharmacol 2008; 23(6): 455-63.

[201] Bork JA, Rogers T, Wedlund PJ, *et al.* A pilot study on risperidone metabolism: The role of cytochromes P450 2D6 and 3A. J Clin Psychiatry 1999; 60: 469-76.

[202] Margolese HC, Kolivakis TT, Turnier L, *et al.* Clinical improvement with quetiapine augmentation of combination atypical antipsychotic pharmacotherapy in treatment resistant schizophrenia and schizoaffective disorder. Presented at 39th Annual Meeting of the American College of Neuropsychopharmacology, San Juan, Puerto Rico, Dec. 10-14, 2000: 188.

[203] Potkin SG, Thyrum PT, Alva G, *et al.* The safety and pharmacokinetics of quetiapine when co-administered with haloperidol, risperidone, or thioridazine. J Clin Psychopharmacol 2002; 22: 121-30.

[204] McCue RE, Waheed R, Urcuyo L. Polypharmacy in patients with schizophrenia. J Clin Psychiatry 2003; 64: 984-9.

[205] Genç Y, Taner E, Candansayar S. Comparison of clozapine-amisulpride and clozapine-quetiapine combinations for patients with schizophrenia who are partially responsive to clozapine: A single-blind randomized study. Adv Ther 2007; 24: 1-13.

[206] Ramaswamy S, Vijay D, William M, *et al.* Aripiprazole possibly worsens psychosis. Int Clin Psychopharmacol 2004; 19: 45-8.

[207] Lerner V, Bergman J, Borokhov A, *et al.* Augmentation with amisulpride for schizophrenic patients nonresponsive to antipsychotic monotherapy. Clin Neuropharmacol 2005; 28: 66-71.

[208] Kane JM, Correll CU, Goff DC, *et al.* A multicenter, randomized, double-blind, placebo-controlled, 16-week study of adjunctivearipiprazole for schizophrenia or schizoaffective disorder inadequately treated with quetiapine or risperidone monotherapy. J Clin Psychiatry 2009; 70(10): 1348-57.

[209] Kuwilsky A, Krumm B, Englisch S, *et al.* Long-term efficacy and tolerability of clozapine combined with ziprasidone or risperidone. Pharmacopsychiatry 2010; 43(6): 216-20.

[210] Tiihonen J, Wahlbeck K, Löonqvist J, *et al.* Effectiveness of antipsychotic treatments in a nationwide cohort of patients in community care after first hospitalisation due to schizophrenia and schizoaffective disorder: observational follow-up study. BMJ, doi: 10.1136/bmj.38881.382755.2F (published 6 July 2006).

[211] Chan J, Sweeting M. Review: Combination therapy with non-clozapine atypical antipsychoticmedication: a review of current evidence. J Psychopharmacol 2007; 21(6): 657-64.

[212] Barnes TRE, Paton C. Antipsychotic polypharmacy in schizophrenia: benefits and risks. CNS Drugs 2011; 25 (5): 383-99.

[213] Mortimer AM. Update on the management of symptoms in schizophrenia: focus on amisulpride. Neuropsychiatr Dis Treat 2009; 5: 266-77.

[214] Topiwala A, Fazel S. The pharmacological management of violence in schizophrenia: a structured review. Expert Rev Neurother 2011; 11: 53-63.

[215] Ito H, Koyama A, Higuchi T. Polypharmacy and excessive dosing: psychiatrists' perception of antipsychotic drug prescription. Br J Psychiatry 2005; 187: 243-7.

[216] Gaebel W, Weinmann S, Sartorius N, *et al.* Schizophrenia practice guidelines: international survey and comparison. Br J Psychiatry 2005; 187: 248-55.

[217] Marder SR, Essock SM, Miller AL, *et al.* The Mount Sinai conference on the pharmacotherapy of schizophrenia. Schizophr Bull 2002; 28: 5-16.

[218] Taylor D, Paton C, Kapur S. The Maudsley prescribing guidelines. 10th ed. London: Informa Healthcare, 2009.

[219] Essock S, Schooler NR, Scott Stroup T, *et al.* Effectiveness of switching from antipsychotic polypharmacy to monotherapy. Am J Psychiatry 2011; 168: 702-708.

[220] Correll CU. Antipsychotic polypharmacy, part 2: why use 2 antipsychotics when 1 is not good enough? J Clin Psychiatry. 2008; 69: 860-61.

[221] Mellsop G, El-Badri S. Developing Classification in Psychiatry - Implications of 50 Years of Progress in Psychopharmacologic Therapeutics. Businnes Briefing: European Pharmaco Therapy, 2006. [Cited 2012 Jan 25]. Available from: http://www.touchbriefings.com/cdps/cditem.cfm?NID=1692#Psychiatry

[222] Leucht S, Arbter D, Engel RR, Kissling W, Davis JM. How effective are second-generation antipsychotic drugs? A meta-analysis of placebo-controlled trials. Mol Psychiatry. 2009; 14: 429-47.

[223] Weinberger DR, Lipska BK. Cortical maldevelopment, antipsychotic drugs, and schizophrenia: A search for common ground. Schizophr Res.1995; 16: 87-110.

[224] Zanger UM, Klein K. Pharmacogenetics of cytochrome P4502B6(CYP2B6): advances on polymorphisms, mechanisms, and clinical relevance. Front Genetics 2013; 24: 1-12.

[225] Pal D, Kwatra D, Minocha M, *et al.* Efflux transporters- and cytochrome P-450-mediatedinteractions between drugs of abuse and antiretrovirals. Life Sci. 2011; 23: 959-971.

[226] Dandara C, Lombard Z, Du Plooy I, *et al.* Genetic variants in *CYP* (*-1A2*, *-2C9*, *-2C19*, *-3A4* and *-3A5*), *VKORC1* and *ABCB1* genes in a black South African population: a window into diversity. Pharmacogenomics 2011; 12: 1663-1670.

[227] Huo R, Tang K, Wei Z, *et al.* Genetic Polymorphisms in CYP2E1: Association with Schizophrenia Susceptibility and Risperidone Response in the Chinese Han Population. PLoS ONE 2012; 7(5): e34809. doi: 10.1371/journal.pone.0034809.

[228] Gosh C, Marchi N, Desai NK, *et al.* Cellular localization and functional significance of CYP3A4 in the human epileptic brain. Epilepsia. 2011; 52: 562-571.

[229] Hiemke C, Shams M. Phenotyping and genotyping of drug metabolism to guide pharmacotherapy in psychiatry. Curr Drug Deliver 2013; 1: 46-53.

[230] Conca A, Schmidt E, Pastore M, *et al.* Therapeutic drug monitoring in Italian psychiatry. Pharmacopsychiatry 2011; 6: 259-262.

[231] Schaller G, Jacobi A, Rotter A, *et al.* Perazine elevates clozapine serum levels by inhibiting hepatic metabolism. Prog Neuropsychopharmacol Biol Psychiatry 2009; 33: 908-909.

[232] Fischer M, Unterecker S, Deckert J, *et al.* Elevated clozapine serum levels in combination with perazine. Psychopharmacology 2013; 226: 623-625.

[233] Grözinger M, Dragicevic A, Hiemke C, *et al.* Melperone is an inhibitor of the CYP2D6 catalyzed O-demethylation of venlafaxine. Pharmacopsychiatry. 2003; 36: 3-6.

[234] FDA, 2010. Information for Healthcare Professionals: Venlafaxine (marketed as Effexor) - Selective Serotonin Reuptake Inhibitors (SSRIs), Selective Serotonin-Norepinephrine Reuptake Inhibitors (SNRIs), 5-Hydroxytryptamine Receptor Agonists (Triptans). Retrieved, 26th March, 2013, from: http://www.fda.gov/drugs/drugsafety/postmarketdrug safetyinformationforpatientsandproviders/ucm125925.htm

[235] Rittmannsberger H, Werl R. Does aripiprazole protect from serotonin syndrome? Psychiatr Danub 2012; 24: 100-101.

Frontiers in CNS Drug Discovery, **2013**, *2*, 211-280

CHAPTER 7

The Role of Natural Products on the Discovery of New Drug Candidates for Neurogenerative Disorders

Flávia P.D. Viegas[1,2], Rodolfo do C. Maia[3], Roberta Tesch[3,4], Carlos A.M. Fraga[3,4] and Claudio Viegas-Jr.[*,1,2]

[1] LFQM - Laboratório de Fitoquímica e Química Medicinal, Instituto de Química, Universidade Federal de Alfenas (UNIFAL-MG), 37130-000, Alfenas, MG, Brazil; [2]Programa de Pós-Graduação em Química, Universidade Federal de Alfenas (UNIFAL-MG), 37130-000, Alfenas, MG, Brazil; [3]LASSBio-Laboratório de Avaliação e Síntese de Substâncias Bioativas, Faculdade de Farmácia, Universidade Federal do Rio de Janeiro (UFRJ), 21941-902, Rio de Janeiro, RJ, Brazil; [4]Programa de Pós-Graduação em Farmacologia e Química Medicinal, Instituto de Ciências Biomédicas, Universidade Federal do Rio de Janeiro (UFRJ), 21941-902, Rio de Janeiro, RJ, Brazil

Abstract: Neurodegenerative disorders such as Parkinson's disease (PD), Alzheimer's disease (AD), Huntington's disease (HD) and amyotrophic lateral sclerosis (ALS) are incurable pathologies with huge social and economic impacts closely related to the increasing of life expectancy in modern times. Although the clinical and neuropathological aspects of these debilitating disorders are distinct, they have a unified feature that is the characteristic pattern of neurodegeneration in anatomically or functionally related regions. All of them remain uncured and presently available treatments are only symptomatic and do not alter the course or progression of the underlying diseases. In this context, the search for new effective chemical entities, capable to act in diverse biochemical targets, with new mechanisms of action and low toxicity stands as a challenge to research groups and Pharmaceutical Industry. This scenery has been promising to the reemerging of modern natural products chemistry to provide active, sophisticated and complex new lead molecules to drug discovery and development. In this publication, we discuss some of the main contributions of the natural products chemistry including more than thirty plant species and the main pharmacological advances for the discovery of active constituents in plants, herbs and extracts prescribed by Traditional Medicine practices to treat senile neurodegenerative disorders, especially for AD and PD, in the period after the 2000s. Many of the recent reported data are resultant of studies carried out during the 90s decade, and the most important contributions are also cited, as well as the main advances in the

***Address correspondence to Claudio Viegas-Jr.:** LFQM - Laboratório de Fitoquímica e Química Medicinal, Instituto de Química, Universidade Federal de Alfenas (UNIFAL-MG), 37130-000, Alfenas, MG, Brazil; Tel: +55-35-32991466; Fax: +55-35-32991384; E-mail: cvjviegas@gmail.com

Atta-ur-Rahman & M. Iqbal Choudhary (Eds.)

pharmacological basis to understand the mechanisms of action and to explain the effects of some of these active compounds in the improvement on memory and cognition, in neurovascular function, and as neuroprotective agents.

Keywords: Neurodegenerative disorders, biodiversity, natural products, Alzheimer, Parkinson, drug discovery, medicinal chemistry.

1. INTRODUCTION

Natural products (NP) have been explored as medicines since ancient times, when human beings had only the nature as the source for the cure of their illness. After centuries of exploration as commercials, NP were closely related to the development of occidental and oriental civilizations, passing from simple commodities to medicines, starting materials and medicinal products with high value for therapeutical and industrial purposes related to public health. The World's history is very rich in examples of how NP were determinant in changing civilization's way of life. In science, especially in the medicinal chemistry field, they were responsible for great and revolutionary discoveries, *e.g.,* salicilates, penicillin, quinine, campthotecin and taxol [1]. After the 2nd World War, as a result of military efforts for the discovery of new weapons, technologies and drugs, organic chemistry experienced a period of great development with pharmaceutical and chemical industries changing their focus to massive investments on research of new synthetic chemical entities [1-3].

The advent of combinatorial chemistry and high throughput screening (HTS) established a feeling of associated-expectation about the potential of these techniques to disclose massive sources of innovative drug prototypes or new chemical entities (NCEs) with higher complexity/novel frameworks, being able to obtain hundred of thousands of new compounds in a short-time work reinforced the wane in NP exploitation as an approach for drug development and discovery [1,4]. Despite the high expectation around combinatorial chemistry and HTS, only in 2005 sorafenib was approved by FDA (U.S. Food and Drug Administration) for renal carcinoma in humans, as the first combinatorial NCE therapeutically available. Consequently, synthetic chemists realized that the combinatorial libraries lacked the complexity normally associated with bioactive natural products [5]. Despite of billions of dollars invested by pharmaceutical industry in the research and development of new bioactive chemical entities, the number of innovative and effective drug candidates that overcome pre-clinical and clinical phases is decreasing year by year [1,5].

As a consequence to this paradoxical scenery, modern natural products chemistry has been re-emerging as a promising and effective alternative to provide active, sophisticated and innovative lead molecules to drug discovery and development [6]. On the other hand, severe pathologies remain without cure (*e.g.,* AIDS, many types of cancer, CNS disorders) or with few available therapeutic alternatives (*e.g.,* malaria). Microorganisms are getting more and more resistant to known anti-infectious drugs and others are re-emerging more powerfully due to genetic mutations and evolution. In this context, neurodegenerative disorders are genuine examples of challenges to be faced, due to the huge social and economic impact that these incurable pathologies represent, worsen by the fact that better life conditions created by our development are continuously increasing the life expectancy and, consequently, the incidence of age-related illnesses will grow. These pathologies include common and debilitating disorders such as Parkinson's disease (PD), Alzheimer's disease (AD), Huntington's disease (HD) and amyotrophic lateral sclerosis (ALS). Although the clinical and neuropathological aspects of these disorders are distinct, they have a common and characteristic pattern of neuronal degeneration in anatomically or functionally related regions. To date, no cure is available for these diseases and the available therapies are symptomatic, being unable to change the course or progression of the underlying disease. The most effective symptomatic therapies are those for PD due to the availability of a large number of agents from several pharmacological classes that, in general, when skillfully applied, lead to an improvement of functional ability and life span [7].

In previous communications we reviewed the role of natural products from different chemical classes in the development of new anti-Alzheimer and anti-Parkinson drugs up to 2000s [8,9]. In recent years, we have observed a significant increase of interest to investigate antioxidative and anti-inflammatory effects of phenolic compounds from diverse sources that could act as neuroprotective agents in AD and PD. This interest is supported by many pathologic conditions associated with overproduction of reactive oxygen species (ROS) and reactive nitrogen species (RNS), such as superoxide anion, hydroxyl radicals, hydrogen peroxide, lipid peroxyl radicals, nitric oxide and peroxynitrite. These species are commonly generated in many cellular systems, through enzymatic and nonenzymatic reactions, but in excess these species can attack key proteins, lipids and DNA, affect signal transduction pathways, destroy membranes and subcellular organelles, and cause subsequent apoptosis and cell death. These secondary metabolites were initially identified as a defensive response of plants against stress from UV radiation, pathogens and physical damage, which may explain the different content of polyphenols in specific plant [8,9].

Herein, we aim to discuss some of the main contributions of the natural products chemistry and pharmacological advances for the discovery of active constituents in plants, herbs and extracts prescribed by traditional medicine practices to treat senile neurodegenerative disorders, especially for AD and PD, in the period after the 20th century. Many of the recent reported data are resultant of studies carried out during the nineties, and the most important contributions are also cited in this chapter, as well as the main pharmacological advances resulting in a better understanding of the molecular basis of these diseases. Also, the mechanisms of action by which some of these bioactive compounds promote the improvement of memory and cognition, neurovascular functions, and neuroprotection are discussed.

2. NATURAL PRODUCTS CHEMISTRY AND CENTRAL NERVOUS SYSTEM

The use of mind-altering substances, especially from plants, is a part of the human and civilizations history. Religious rituals, magic and alchemy demonstrations have always caught our attention. Particulary consideration was given to those able to alter conscience and sensory, as exemplified for hallucinogens that occupied much of the research's time over the decades to elucidate their properties, mechanism of action and therapeutic utility. More recently, the same plant products were considered in another priority level, trying to find beneficial properties to treat mental diseases and some psychic disorders. This new way of thinking about mind-active plants led to dramatic changes in wrong beliefs, such as that products originated directly from nature were much less toxic than synthetic drugs [10a].

As a consequence of this turning point, the pharmaceutical industry recognizes in the natural product chemistry a valorous business as more and more people were prone to prefer this alternative therapy. In the ninetees, a study conducted by Eisenberg and co-workers [11] showed that almost 34% of American citizens had made use of alternative therapies in the last year. In the same study, other data revealed that 72% Americans used unconventional therapy without their GP's knowledge. An extrapolation to the U.S. population suggests that, in 1990, Americans made an estimated 425 million visits to providers of unconventional therapy, number that exceeds the visits to all U.S. primary care physicians (388 million). From 23 to 28% of this group use this kind of drugs to Central Nervous System (CNS) symptoms, such as insomnia, headache, anxiety and depression, and 3% of those were based on herbal medicines [11].

Carlini and co-workers also discussed the therapeutic uses of several commonly medicinal herbs, including *Ephedra sinica*, *Paullinia sp.* (Guaraná) and *Illex paraguariensis* (South American erva-mate) as CNS stimulants and some adaptogens, that are nonspecific substances that are capable to develop a state of raised resistance, enabling the organism to adapt against stressful situations [10a].

Considering that neurodegenerative disorders such as schizophrenia, Parkinson's and Alzheimer's diseases are among those of the more dramatic social and economical modern challenges for medicine, with high impacts over public health systems around the world, anxiolytic plants have been described as effective adjuvants in the treatment and ameliorate health quality of such patients. As a possible alternative to the use of benzodiazepine synthetic drugs that exhibit a wide range of side effects in the therapeutics of neurodegenerative illnesses, plants such as *Passiflora incarnata* L., *Valleriana officinalis* L. and *Piper methysticum (kava-kava*) have been deeply studied to obtain chemical and pharmacological data for their use as CNS agents.

P. incarnata and other species of *Passiflora* genus are widely used all over American and European traditional medicine for their seemingly sedative and anxiolytic properties. Chemical investigations have indicated that flavonoids (*e.g.*, apigenin (**1**), vitexin (**2**), kampferol (**3**), chrysin (**4**)), harmane alkaloids (harman (**5**), harmalin (**6**), harmalol (**7**), Fig. **1**) are probably responsible for such observed therapeutic effects [10a, 12-14]. Subsequent pharmacological investigations suggested that effects on CNS of the active metabolites of these plants are not mediated by action on the benzodiazepine/GABA receptors.

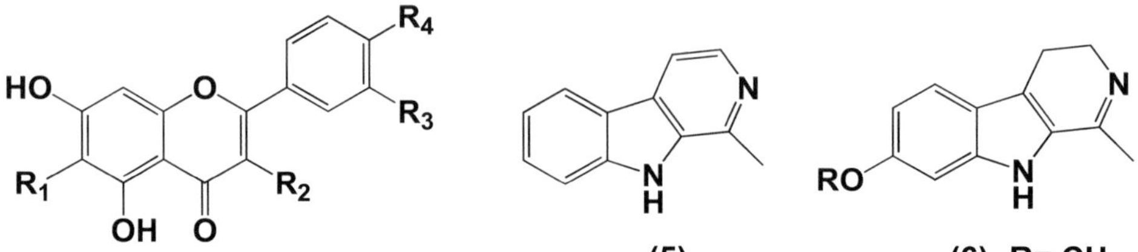

(5)

(6)- R= CH_3
(7)- R= H

(1)- R_1, R_2, R_3 = H, R_4= OH
(2)- R_1= OGlu, R_2, R_3 = H, R_4= OH
(3)- R_2= OH, R_1, R_3 = H, R_4= OH
(4)- R_1, R_2, R_3, R_4= H

Fig. (1). Flavonoids and some alkaloids present in CNS active *Passiflora* and *Piper* extracts.

On the Greek Islands and Oceania, *P. methysticum* (also known as Kava-kava) is used to prepare a beverage offered in welcoming ceremonies for important visitors [10a]. The lipid-soluble extract of this plant contains at least seven pyrones, called kavalactones, that were identified to be responsible for the pleasant warm and cheerful feelings, while reducing fatigue and anxiety [10b]. In the brain, it was demonstrated that these compounds, such as kavaine (**8**) and dihydrokavaine (**9**, Fig. **2**), may interact with a large number of targets, including dopaminergic, serotonergic, GABAergic and glutamatergic bioreceptors, and also inhibit Monoanine oxidase B (MAO B) and affect ion channels [10b].

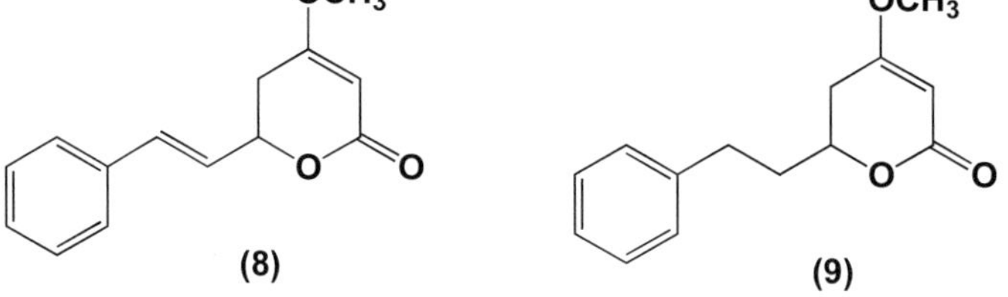

(8) (9)

Fig. (2). Kavaine (**8**) and dihydrokavaine (**9**), two bioactive kavalactones from *P. methysticum*.

"Ginseng" is usually related to the dried roots of several species from *Panax* genus (Araliaceae), but the most used member is *Panax ginseng, an indigenous species* from Korea and China. It is one of the most famous constituent of the ancient Chinese Traditional Medicine and is indicated as a general tonic, adaptogen and aphrodisiac. The precise quantity of *ginseng* consumption has not been established, but it occupies a permanent and prominent position in the herbal "best-sellers" list throughout the world [15]. The benefits of *ginseng*'s treatment are a current issue in the literature and several studies have confirmed its pharmacological effects such as CNS-stimulating, CNS-sedative, tranquilizing, antifatigue and hypotensive [15].

A diverse group of saponins and triterpenoid glycosides, so called ginsenosides, are the active constituents in root extracts of *Panax* species. Over 30 compounds, many of them occurring only in minor amounts, were identified and classified into three groups on the basis of the chemical structure of their triterpenoid sapogenins (aglycones): protopanaxadiol group (**10-19**), protopanaxatriol group (**20-25**) and oleanolic acid group (**26**) (Fig. **3**) [16,17].

The mechanisms of action of ginsenosides at CNS have been discussed by a number of studies and experimental data examining the supposedly underling ginseng's efficacy. The indication of ginseng in the treatment of neurodegenerative disorders is due to the belief of its properties to improve cognitive performance and general well-being. Recently, it have been shown that the effects of *ginseng* and its ginsenosides include increased cell survival, extension of neurite growth and rescuing of neurons from death in consequence of different insults either *in vivo* or *in vitro* [16]. Several studies reported in literature have pointed that neuroprotective properties of ginsenosides should be related to effects in protection of hippocampal neurons [18] and reduction of infarct area [19] after ischemia in rodents. Wen and co-workers, using a step-down passive avoidance task and subsequent neuron and synapse counts in the hippocampal CA1 neurons, evidenced that ginsenoside Rb_1 (**10**) significantly prolonged the response latency of ischemic gerbils and rescued a significant number of ischemic CA1 pyramidal neurons, whereas ginsenosides Rg_1 (**22**) and Ro (**26**) were ineffective [18]. In other studies, it was showed that compound **10**, together with ginsenosides Rg_3 (**15**) and **22**, were also capable to protect neurons from glutamate-induced neurotoxicity [20] and spinal neurons from excitotoxicity induced by glutamate and kainic acid and oxidative stress induced by H_2O_2 [21].

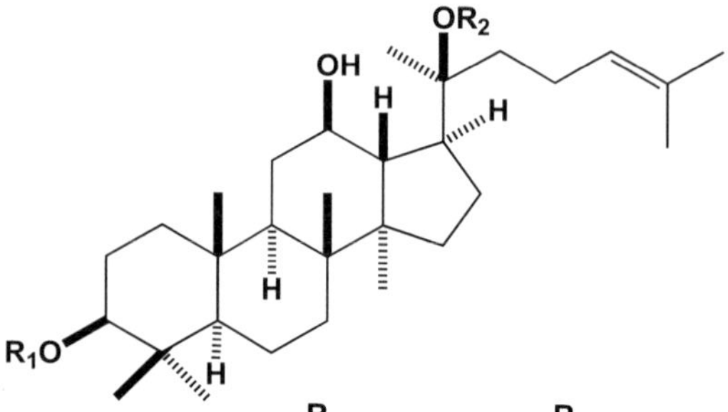

		R_1	R_2
(**10**) ginsenoside -	Rb_1:	-glc(2-1)glc	-glc(6-1)glc
(**11**)	Rb_2:	-glc(2-1)glc	-glc(6-1)arap
(**12**)	Rb_3:	-glc(2-1)glc	-glc(6-1)xyl
(**13**)	Rc:	-glc(2-1)glc	-glc(6-1)araf
(**14**)	Rd:	-glc(2-1)glc	-glc
(**15**)	Rg_3:	-glc(2-1)glc	-H
(**16**)	Rh_2:	-glc	-H
(**17**)	Rs_1:	-glc(2-1)glc(6)Ac	-glc(6-1)arap
(**18**)	Mc:	-H	-glc(6-1)araf
(**19**)	F_2:	-glc	-glc

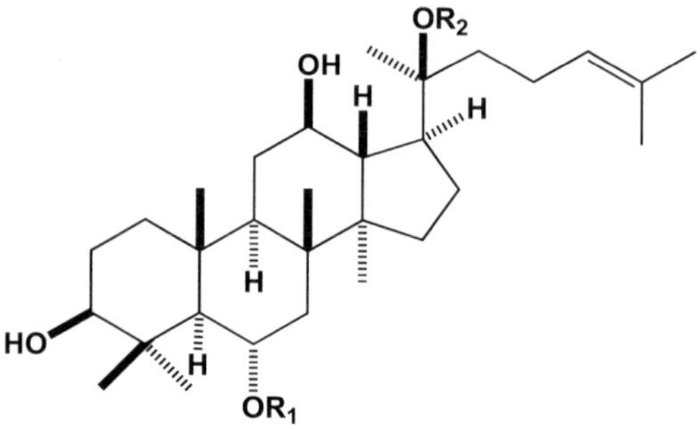

		R_1	R_2
(**20**) ginsenoside -	Re:	-glc(2-1)rha	-glc
(**21**)	Rf:	-glc(2-1)glc	-H
(**22**)	Rg_1:	-glc	-glc
(**23**)	Rg_2:	-glc(2-1)rha	-H
(**24**)	Rh_1:	-glc	-H
(**25**)	F_1:	-H	-glc

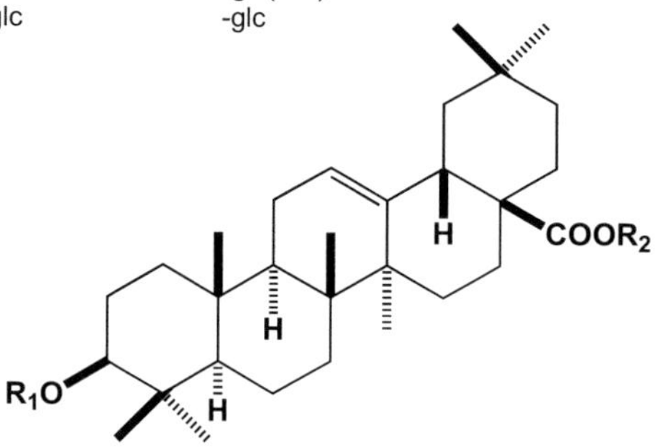

(**26**) ginsenoside - Ro: R_1= -glcUA(2-1), R_2= -glc

araf= α-L-arabinofuranosyl
arap= α-L-arabinopyranosyl
glc= β-D-glucopyranosyl
rha=α-L-rhamnopyranosyl
xyl= β-D-xylopyranosyl
glcUA= β-D-glucoronic acid

Fig. (3). Ginsenosides isolated from the roots of *Panax* species.

The biological characteristic responses for each ginsenoside are attributed to the differences in the type, position, and number of sugar moieties attached by the glycosidic bond at C-3 and C-6 [22]. This observation is critical for the evaluation of pharmacological properties, because the ginsenoside content in *ginseng* is varying depending on the *Panax* species, the plant age, the part of the plant used, the preservation method, the season of harvest and the extraction method [23, 24]. To prevent the huge variation in ginsenosides content across commercial available *ginseng* preparations, the most widely used standardized *ginseng* extract, for both research and commercial purposes, is G115, a concentrated aqueous extract of *P. ginseng* with an invariable 4% of ginsenosides, produced by Pharmaton at Switzerland [25].

In the last decade, Kennedy and co-workers [26-31] among other research groups [32] have published several papers about human studies involving acute administration of *ginseng*'s extract G115 [27,28]. All experiments were performed according to a randomized double blind placebo-controlled balanced crossover design, and in almost all cases 20 participants received three different single doses of the extract and a same dose of placebo in distinct occasions. In a first study, administration of 200, 400 and 600 mg of G115 was effective to improve the memory tasks, but the middle dose of 400 mg was the most pronounced [27]. In a second experiment, following the same protocol, another three doses of 320, 640 and 960 mg of a 100:60 combination of G115 and *G. biloba* standardized extract (GK501) were compared to a placebo [28]. The pattern of results were closely to that following single doses of G115 alone, but very different to those found in a previous study using single doses of GK501 [26]. In order to confirm second memory improvements, other studies were carried out, using different single doses of *ginseng, gingko* and a combination of both. Again, the best results were performed by single *ginseng* (400 mg) or in combination with *gingko*. Following 400 mg of G115 alone, there was also an evidence of improved "speed of memory" and "accuracy of attention" factors. Considering the above summarized examples of the *in vitro*, *in vivo* with species of *Passiflora, Panax* and *Gingko* its is possible to assume that traditional medicine herbs (*e.g., Ginseng*, *Gingko)* are able to alleviate neurodegenerative impairments, and particularly ginsenosides can modulate a number of physiological mechanisms and may improve indices of stress, fatigue and learning in rodents. However, from the Medicinal Chemistry point of view, in order to effectively design structurally optimized and less complex derivatives of the pure active principle of such extracts aiming the development of innovative, effective and safer new drugs, a better understanding of their mechanism of action and the identification of the structural features involved in their molecular recognition by target bioreceptors is fundamentally necessary.

3. ALZHEIMER'S AND PARKINSON'S DISEASES: SOME RECENT DATA ABOUT THEIR PATHOPHYSIOLOGY, TREATMENT AND THERAPEUTIC ALTERNATIVES

Neurodegenerative disorders are characterized by progressive and irreversible loss of neurons from specific regions of the brain. Parkinson's disease is a kind of prototypical neurodegenerative pathology where loss of neurons occurs from structures in the basal ganglia, resulting in abnormalities in the control of movements. Alzheimer's disease is another kind of neurodegenerative disorder resultant of a neuronal loss in hippocampal and cortical regions, leading to impairment in memory and cognitive abilities [33]. Despite these different pathophysiological features, AD and PD have a very particular specificity related to selectively vulnerability of specific types neurons affected in each case. In AD, neuronal injury is most severe in the hippocampus and neocortex neurons and the loss is not uniform but varies dramatically in different functional regions [34]. In contrast, PD is characterized by an extensive degeneration of dopaminergic neurons of the substantia nigra [35]. Excitotoxicity is though to be another factor that may contributes to neurodegenerative selective vulnerability. This term is used to describe the neuronal injury caused by excessive concentration of glutamate in the brain [36]. In normal amounts, this neurotransmitter is essential to brain function, and it is believed to mediate most excitatory synaptic transmission in the mammalian brain. If it is excessively released or accumulated in brain tissue, glutamate can lead to excitotoxic cell death, a process mediated by glutamate receptors, especially those of *N*-methyl-D-aspartate (NMDA) type [37]. Unlike other glutamate-gated ion channels, which primarily regulate the flow of Na^+, activated NMDA receptors-channels allow an excessive influx of Ca^{2+} that can then activate the installation of a destructive process.The effects of aging in neuronal injury could be close-related to the excitotoxic hypothesis, since capacity for oxidative metabolism decreases progressively, in consequence of cumulative mutations in mitochondrial genome [38].

Disturbances that impair the metabolic capacity of neurons will impact the ability of Mg^{2+} to block NMDA receptor-channel, which is membrane potential dependent, and predispose the excitotoxic injury. This feature is corroborated by observations that PD patients exhibit several defects in energy metabolism which are even greater than expected for their age, most notably a reduction in the function of complex I of the mitochondrial electron transport chain [39].

In the light of the multifactorial patterns of neural degeneration, the process of neural injury has been proposed to be viewed as the interaction of genetic and environmental influences with the intrinsic physiological characteristics of the affected population of neurons. These intrinsic factors may include susceptibility to excitotoxic injury, regional variation in capacity for oxidative metabolism and the production of toxic free radicals as products of cellular metabolism (Fig. **4**).

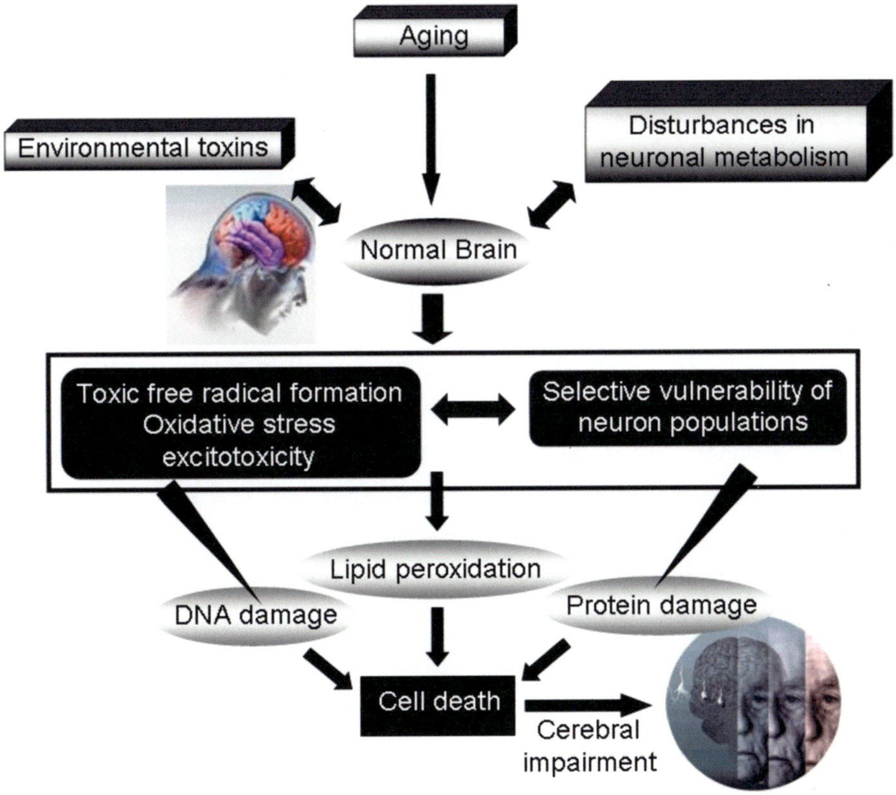

Fig. (4). Possible factors of selective neuronal vulnerability in neurodegenerative diseases (adapted from ref. [33]).

Alzheimer's disease was first described by Alois Alzheimer in 1907 and is characterized by a progressive lost of neurons from hippocampus and cortical area leading to impairment of memory and cognitive ability. It is the most common type of dementia among elderly people, affecting more than 4 million of Americans and 15-20 million people worldwide. Taking into account the great increase observed in longevity in the last decades, the projection is that these numbers may triplicate by 2050 [40]. Data from 2003 pointed that financial and social costs of AD in United States were staggering, accounting for about annual U$ 100 billion in medical and custodial expenses with an average required per patient of about U$ 27,000/year. In addition, the impact of the disease covers the caregivers that report stress in 80% and depression in 50% of the cases [41,42].

The physiopathology of AD is associated to a marked atrophy of the cerebral cortex and loss of cortical and subcortical neurons, with accumulation of amyloid plaques and neurofibrilary tangles.The early development of AD, an uncommon form of genetic-related AD, affects 30-40 aged people and comprises around 7% of familial AD patients (FAD In another way, the late onset AD is also related to epi-genetic and environmental factors that are known to play an important role in the sequential events that culminate in AD installation. Cardiovascular abnormalities, such as hypertension, diabetes, mini-stroke and artherosclerose are accumulating factors that increase the risk for AD [43].

There are sufficient evidences supporting that oxidative stress is associated to the early development of AD [44], and therefore search for new chemical entities and effective alternative therapies to combat the oxidative neuronal damage is a fact. Recent data clearly indicate that at least part of oxidative mechanism is contributed by the β-amyloid (Aβ) peptides, fragments of 39-43 amino acids released from the amyloid precursor protein (APP) through the action of β- and γ-secretases. The grouping of these Aβ oligomeric fragments can confer oxidative insult to neurons and glial cells and initiate changes in synaptic plasticity, a sequence of events occurring long before their deposition to form the amyloid plaques [45]. The mechanism involved in these peptides cytotoxicity is not clearly established. Although, there is evidence that they can act specifically on *N*-methyl-D-aspartic acid receptors (NMDA) and its activation is coupled to ROS production [46-48].Thus, NADPH oxidase may be involved in Aβ and NMDA-induced ROS production and activation of signaling pathways, including mitogen activated protein kinase (MAPK) and protein kinase C (PKC). These pathways leads to activation of cytosolic phospholipase A2 ($cPLA_2$) and release of arachidonic acid (AA) [49]. AA is not only a precursor for biosynthesis of prostaglandins, but is also known to serve as a retrograde transmitter in regulating synaptic plasticity [50]. Studies carried out by Kriem and co-workers also demonstrated $cPLA_2$ is involved in Aβ-induced apoptosis in neurons [51]. Furthermore, NADPH oxidase has been regarded as an important source of ROS that mediate the inflammatory responses in astrocytes and microglial cells in the brain [52].

Studies published on 70's decade by Davies [53], Bowen [54], Perry and collaborators [55] reported the discovery of a fairly selective deficit in cortical markers of cholinergic neurons in a number of AD patients [55]. Several subsequent studies identifiedthe specific regions affected by neuronal damage. By this hypothesis, the modulation of cholinergic transmission might offer a rational route to the symptomatic treatment of AD and in fact, this approach led to the design and optimization of the most currently available agents in clinical use [56].

Parkinson's disease (PD) is less common than AD, affecting nearly 2% of the U.S. population [57]. It is the second most prevalent age-related neurodegenerative disease, reaching more than 4 million people over the age 50 in the large population countries in 2005, number that is expected to increase nearly 9 million by 2030 [58]. The main physiological manifestations include tremors, bradykinesia, abnormal postural reflexes, muscle rigidity and akinesia, and the pathological landmarks include a progressive loss of dopaminergic neurons in the substantia nigra [59, 60]. Epidemiological studies classify PD cases into two classes, depending on whether the disease is hereditary (familial PD, FPD) or idiopathic PD (IPD), when the origin is unknown and possibly is due to exposure to environmental toxins [61, 62].

The brain is only 2-3% of the body mass, but it is responsible for the consumption of 20% of body oxygen [63]. Thus, cells in neuronal tissue are particularly susceptible to oxidative damage due to high levels of polyunsaturated fatty acids in their membranes and relatively low activity of endogenous antioxidant enzymes. Aging is associated to an increase of oxidative stress and the consequent accumulation of oxidatively damaged biomolecules which gradually weakens cognition. The increase of oxidative stress, summed up to decline of endogenous antioxidant metabolites, is important risk factor for older people to develop neurodegenerative diseases such as PD. In fact, dopaminergic neurons are able to oxidize neurotransmitter dopamine through MAO action or by autooxidation, resulting in the production of superoxide anion, hydrogen peroxide and hydroxyl radicals, which are able to promote permanent state of oxidative stress of dopaminergic neurons and an imbalance that may lead to reduced levels of endogenous antioxidants [59, 60, 64].

In addition, after an inflammatory response or excitotoxic insult, activation of microglia produces nitric oxide (NO), that in combination with ROS can also produce peroxynitrite anions to confer dopaminergic neurotoxicity [65,66]. Moreover, microglia activation is an important factor contributing to the inflammatory responses in PD, and its ability to produce high levels of ROS through NADPH oxidase is regarded as an important factor underlying the MPTP-induced dopaminergic neurodegeneration [67-69].

Many hypotheses are considered about PD's etiology, but oxidative stress remains the strongest leading theory [60], which relates PD risk with exposure to environmental factors including heavy metals and herbicides, such as 1-methyl-4-phenyl-1,2,3,6-tetrahydropyridine (MPTP, **27**) [70-72], rotenone (**28**), manganese [73, 74], 3,4-dimethoxyphenyl-ethylamine (DMPEA, **29**) [75] and 1,1'-dimethyl-4-4'-bipyridinium (Paraquat, **30**, Fig. **5**) [72, 76, 77] that selectively act over dopamine neurons, making their way to the substantia nigra and inducing apoptosis [65, 78]. Recent studies strongly suggests the direct involvement of Manganese exposure to PD's etiology, since it tends to accumulate in the same brain areas affected in patients presenting this disease, and it can induce a syndrome called manganism, which is closely resembled to PD. Postmortem studies revealed the subcellular deposition of cytoplasmatic Lewy bodies composed of aggregated protein, including α-synuclein [74], and also increased oxidation of proteins, lipids and DNA [59].

Among the several risk factors mentioned to be associated to PD development, age is the main one, followed by using well water, living on a farm, occupational use of herbicides, family history of PD and head trauma [79, 80]. Over 90% of the PD cases after the age 50, non-familial factors seem to be present. An increased risk for PD is correlated to environmental factors including herbicides containing paraquat, but there was no increased risk with occupational exposure to chemicals in general, such as heavy metals and minerals, and only 10% of the patients reported using any herbicide [80-82]. 6-Hydroxydopamine (6-OHDA, **31**, Fig. **5**) is a neurotoxin, a structural analog of dopamine and norepinephrine, able to cause damage in cathecholaminergic neurons and also induce activation of glial cells. This endogenous toxin can accumulate in the brain and upon transport to the neurons, **31** is oxidized like dopamine to generate free radicals and quinines. In addition, 6-OHDA inhibits mitochondrial complex I and produces superoxide and hydroxyl radicals through participation in the Fenton reaction [83].

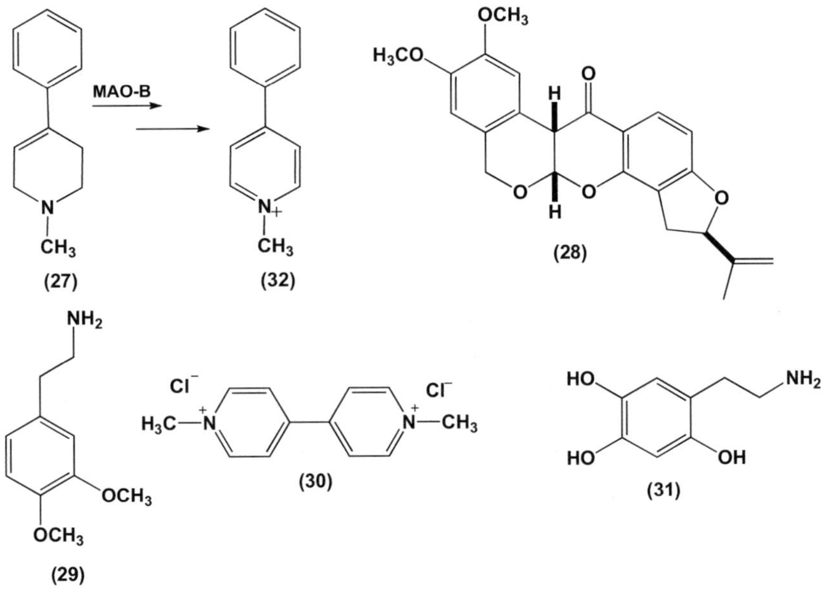

Fig. (5). Some environmental toxins related to the incidence of Parkinson's disease (PD).

It is noteworthy that the use of 6-OHDA to mimic the dopaminergic pathological features of the PD is the most widespread model for identifying therapeutic leads for the treatment of this disease [84]. 6-OHDA specifically affects catecholaminergic neurons in animals thus, being a useful tool for identifying new compounds that reduce the symptoms of PD. A disadvantage of the 6-OHDA model is that it lacks the ability to identify compounds modulating the non-dopaminergic features of the PD. However, useful alternatives to the 6-OHDA model have not yet emerged [85].

Some natural products presenting remarkable activity against the 6-OHDA toxicity have been described. The compounds stilbostemin B 3'-β-*D*-glucopyranoside (**32**), stilbostemin H 3'-β-*D*-glucopyranoside (**33**), and stilbostemin I 2''-β-*D*-glucopyranoside (**34**), isolated from the roots of *Stemona tuberosa*, all protected SH-SY5Y cells from 6-OHDA-induced toxicity at concentrations of 1 μM (Fig. **6**) [86].

Paeoniflorin (**35**), a compound isolated from the roots of *Paeonia lactiflora* with a very unique pinane moiety, decreased behavioral abnormalities induced by 6-OHDA when administered at 5 mg/kg in rats (Fig. **6**) [87]. Another interesting natural product is Cytisine (**36**), a quinolizidine alkaloid that was originally isolated from the seeds of *Sophora secundiflora*. This compound and its 5-bromo analog (**37**), but not its 3-bromo analog (**38**), were able to significantly reduce the striatal dopamine loss induced by 6-OHDA in rats at a dose of 2 mg/kg (Fig. **6**) [88]. These results are significant since it has been shown that a decrease in striatal dopamine levels is a key pathological feature of the 6-OHDA model of Parkinson's disease.

The metabolite isolated from the marine soft coral *Sinularia nanolobata*, Nanolobatolide (**39**), also reduced the 6-OHDA-related toxicity in SH-SY5Y neuronal cells at a concentration of 0.1 μM (Fig. **6**) [89]. A series of secoiridoid glycosides, isolated from the plant *Ligustrum japonicum*, attenuated the toxicity of 6-OHDA in human neuroblastoma cells. The metabolites (8*E*)-nuezhenide (**40**), (8*Z*)-nuezhenide (**41**), (8*Z*)-nuezhenide A (**42**) and oleonuezhenide (**43**) all protected SH-SY5Y cells against 6-OHDA induced toxicity at concentrations of 10 μM (Fig. **6**) [90].

In another example, Esculin (**44**) (Fig. **7**), a metabolite from *Fraxinus sieboldiana*, was also identified to be able to protect SH-SY5Y cells from dopamine-induced toxicity when applied to the cells at a concentration of 0.1 μM. This demonstrates that dopamine-induced toxicity can be used as an alternative to 6-OHDA to investigate the therapeutic potential of some compounds in the treatment of PD symptoms [91].

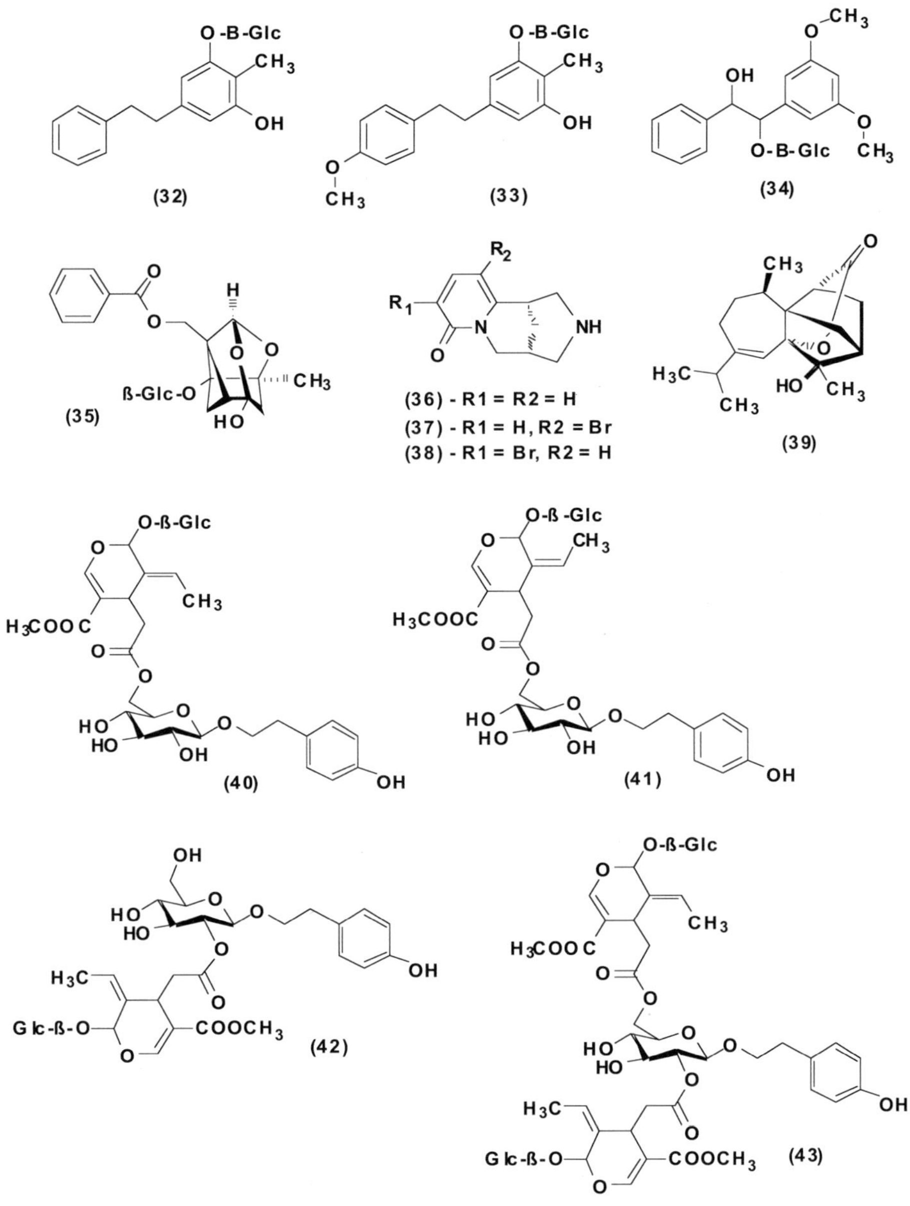

Fig. (6). Examples of natural products active in the 6-OHDA model of Parkinson's disease.

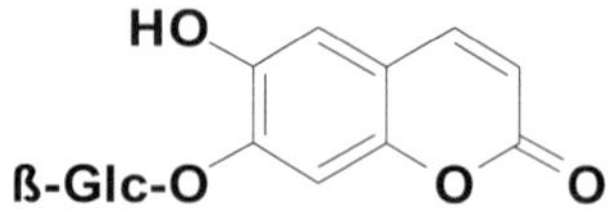

(44)

Fig. (7). Esculin (**44**), compound able to reduce the dopamine-induced toxicity in SH-SY5Y cells.

An interesting neuronal protection profile, through depression of the oxidative stress, was observed for (-)-epigallocatechin-3-gallate (**45**) (Fig. **8**) in the

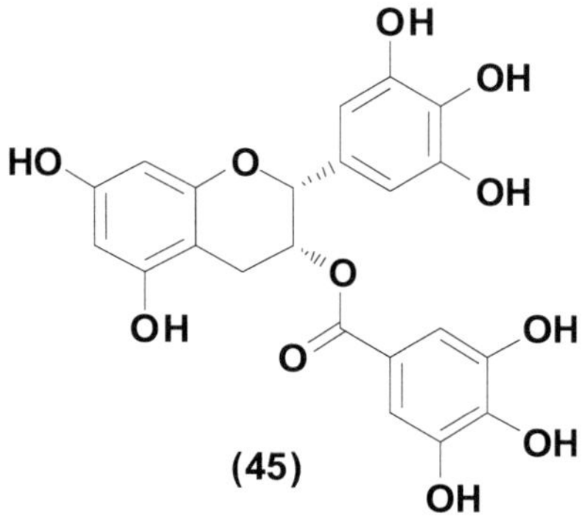

(45)

Fig. (8). Neuronal protector compound (-)-epigallocatechin-3-gallate (**45**).

6-OHDA PD cell model. It was demonstrated that 6-OHDA can cause neuronal death by disrupting the activity of signal transducers and activators of transcription-3 (STAT3). The administration of 1 μM of **45** completely prevented the STAT3 activity decline induced by 6-OHDA in SH-SY5Y cells. Additionally, it was seen that neuronal cell proliferation can be stimulated by treatment with **45**. These data clearly demonstrate that the protection of (-)-epigallocatechin-3-gallate (**45**) on neurons against oxidative stress-induced cell death may result from the re-stimulation of STAT3 signaling pathway [92].

Later on, other study investigated the involvement of inducible nitric oxide synthase (iNOS) in the neuroprotective activity of **45**. For this purpose, compound **45** was evaluated at 10 and 50 mg/kg in the 1-methyl-4-phenylpyridinium-(MPP+) induced oxidative stress model. This treatment reduced the neuronal death rate to less than 50%. The level of iNOS expression in the MPP+ group was

20% higher than that seen in the control group, but in the treated groups, iNOS expression was reduced to the level observed in the negative control group. The two doses of (-)-e pigallocatechin-3-gallate (**45**) were equally beneficial for cell rescue and no toxicity was observed with the higher dose. Inhibition of iNOS may be an important mechanism underlying the prevention of MPTP toxicity and can be an important mechanism mediating the neuroprotective effect observed for (-)-epigallocatechin-3-gallate (**45**) [93].

Baicalein (**46**) (Fig. **9**), a flavonoid obtained from the roots of the chinese medicinal herb *Scutellaria baicalensis*, has been shown to be a promising candidate for prevention or treatment of Parkinson's disease, due to its anti-apoptotic, pro-differentiation and anti-inflammatory action. In *in vitro* experiments, it was shown that baicalein (**46**) (at 0.5 μg/mL) could significantly attenuate the 6-OHDA-induced SH-SY5Y cell apoptosis in 66%, and also promote neurite outgrowth of PC12 cell. In *in vivo* experiments, baicalein (**46**) had no effect on apomorphine (APO)-induced rotations, but it could significantly reduce muscle tremor of 6-OHDA-lesioned rats [94].

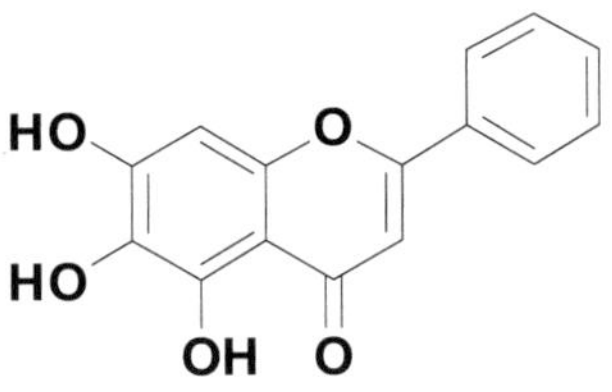

(46)

Fig. (9). The flavonoid bacalein (**46**), active in *in vivo* and *in vitro* models of PD.

MPTP (**27**) was discovered in 1982 as a contaminant of synthetic heroin, when several drug abusers in Northern California developed severe PD-like symptoms. Despite physiological manifestations similar to PD, these patients also shown, upon autopsy, damage to the dopaminergic system in the substantia nigra, but unlike PD, Lewis bodies was not present [83,95]. It is not neurotoxic itself, but its lipophilic properties assure the crossing through the blood-brain barrier, being readily metabolized by MAO-B into its corresponding piridinium ion derivative (MPP^+, **32**, Fig. **5**), a toxic metabolite [83,96].

Paraquat has been widely used as herbicide in the 20th and 21st centuries in agriculture fields such as cotton, to control weeds and grasses. Similarly to MPP^{+}, paraquat (**30**) also depletes dopaminergic neurons in substantia nigra and cause the symptoms of Parkinsonism [97-99] and epidemiological data have pointed an overlap between areas where paraquat is used and increased incidence of PD [100]. In fact, Kang and co-workers [101] demonstrated that **30** is more cytotoxic than MPP^{+}, and despite being a polar molecule it crosses the blood-brain barrier and accumulates in the brain [102]. Once in the brain, paraquat is selectively taken up into terminals of dopaminergic melanin-containing neurons in substantia nigra through the dopamine transporter, and produce ROS leading to malondialdehyde, protein carbonyls and DNA fragmentation [81, 87, 98, 102, 104-106]. In addition **30** can also be reduced by NADPH to give rise paraquat radicals and superoxide anions, inhibiting mitochondrial complex I and impairing energy metabolism through perturbation of mitochondrial respiratory chain [97-99, 101, 103].

Rotenone (**28**) is a naturally occurring complex ketone isolated from the roots of *Lonchocarpus* species. It is the most potent member of the cytotoxic rotenoids class and is widely used as insecticide. After exposure to rotenone, it is slowly and incomplete absorbed in the stomach and intestines, but once into the body, like MPTP, is very lipophilic and crosses the blood-brain barrier to distribute evenly throughout the brain [96]. In the brain, it can enter organelles including double-membrane encased mitochondria where it inhibits with high affinity complex-I of the mitochondrial electron transport chain leading to selective degeneration of dopaminergic neurons [96, 107, 108]. For these reasons dopaminergic cells are targeted for destruction and rotenone plays an important role as an environmental contributor to the etiology of PD in certain individuals.

The natural brassinosteroid 24-epibrassinolide (**47**) had its antioxidant and neuroprotective role examined in a mammalian neuronal cell line (Fig. **10**). The brassinosteroids are phytosterols recognized to promote stress tolerance of vegetables *via* modulation of the antioxidative enzyme cascade. However, their antioxidative effects on mammalian neuronal cells have never been examined previoulsy. Therefore, the ability of 24-epibrassinolide (**47**) to protect neuronal PC12 cells from 1-methyl-4-phenylpyridinium-(MPP+-) induced oxidative stress and consequent apoptosis in dopaminergic neurons was evaluated. The results demonstrated that **47** reduces the levels of intracellular reactive oxygen species and modulates superoxide dismutase, catalase, and glutathione peroxidase activities. Finally, it was identified that the antioxidative properties of **47** lead to the inhibition of MPP+-induced apoptosis by reducing DNA fragmentation as well as the Bax/Bcl-2 protein ratio and cleaved caspase-3 [109].

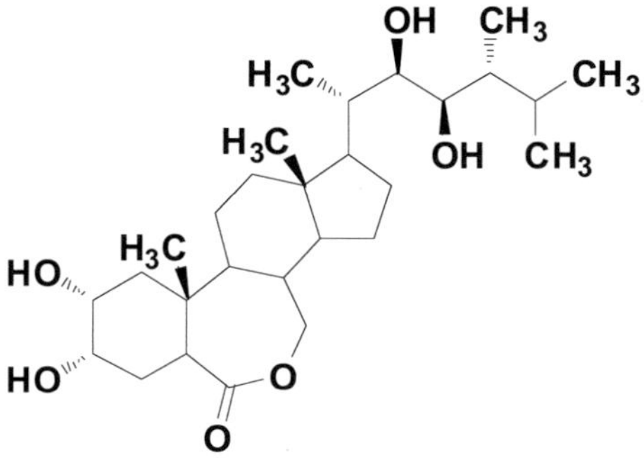

(47)

Fig. (10). Chemical structure of derivative 24-epibrassinolide (**47**), a natural brassinosteroid with antioxidant and neuroprotective properties.

It is well known that dopaminergic neurotoxins exhibit common characteristics, inhibiting either mitochondrial complex I or complex III in neurons. Moreover, not only oxidative stress in CNS, but activated microglia are also responsible for production of ROS, playing capital role in several neurodegenerative disorders including PD. Microglia behave as macrophages in the brain and are one of four major cell types in the CNS, acting against infections and removing debris in the brain [110, 111]. After brain damage or exposure to immune mediators such as IL-1β or TNF-α, activated microglia are responsible for production of cytokines, proteases, prostanoids, superoxide and nitric oxide [111]. In many instances, activation of microglia and generation of ROS coincide with neurochemical changes such as the decrease in dopamine synthesis [112], and a brief exposure to an insult can unleash a process of continuous neurodegeneration [113]. Thus, activation of microglia may play an important role in the initiation and progression of PD and enhance neurotoxicity elicited by neurotoxins [114, 115].

As stated before, oxidative processes involved in the injury of neuronal tissue and in the development of PD, and AD as well, plays an important role in the metabolism of molecular oxygen and the generation of superoxide anion as product such as NADPH oxidase. Similar to other immune cells, high levels of NADPH is also present in microglia, and recent studies with PD patients revealed that NADPH oxidase is up regulated in substantia nigra [60]. As already pointed for AD, several protein kinases, including MAPK and PKC have been implicated in activation of NADPH oxidase and therefore contribute to oxidative stress. MAPKs are highly conserved and ubiquitously expressed in all tissue, activating many enzymatic pathways and contributing to oxidative stress [116, 117]. To date, five MAPK families are known, including extracellular-regulated kinase (ERK) 1/2, JNK 1/2/3, p38α, β, γ, δ, ERK5, and ERK7 [116, 118-120]. MAPKs are involved in the expression of inducible nitric oxide synthase in macrophages and ultimately in inflammation [118]. PKC exist as more than 10 isoforms and are also ubiquitously expressed in mammalian brain tissue, being involved in regulation of ion channels and receptors, neurotransmitters release, and synaptic communication [121-125]. PKC-δ is a novel isoform of PKC that is calcium-independent and is expressed in many cell types, being involved in the mitochondrial-dependent pathway of apoptosis [126, 127]. It is also substrate for caspase, and cleavage by caspase-3 permanently activates PKC-δ, which have been evidenced to be related with phophorylation of cytosolic subunits and activation of NADPH oxidase [128-132].

Nitric oxide (NO) is another possible source of oxidative stress. It is produced from L-arginine which is converted to L-citrulline by nitric oxide synthase (NOS), by using NADPH and O_2 as co-factors [132-135]. There are three known isoforms of NOS, and they are classified in type 1 NOS (neuronal), type 2 NOS (immunologic) and type 3 NOS (endothelial). NOS1 and NOS3 are constitutive and require calcium and calmodulin for activity [132]. NOS2 type, an inducible isoform of NOS, was firstly discovered in macrophages where it is involved in host defense and requires *de novo* synthesis of the enzyme upon activation of transcriptional pathway by cytokines or lipopolysacharides (LPS) [132, 133]. Actually, this isoform is also present in many other cells including certain types of neurons, astrocytes and microglia [136, 137]. Depending on the concentration, type of cell and isoform expressed, NO exert different roles in the body, such as signaling molecule in a wide array of physiological events. Specifically in the brain, NO is involved in neurotransmitter release and reuptake, synaptic plasticity and gene expression [133-136, 138]. In addition, due to its vasodilatory properties, increased production may benefit the brain after injury [139], but in excess it may also cause stroke and PD [140]. Under many conditions, activated glia can simultaneously stimulate the production of NO, ROS and cytokines that togheter form the basis of neuroinflammatory responses [141]. One hypothesis for the role of NO in neurodegeneration is its capability to form adducts with mitochondrial enzymes and dysregulate mitochondrial function. On the other hand, another possibility of mechanisms associated to NO are inhibition of cytochrome oxidase, ribonucleotide reductase, superoxide dismutase, glyceraldehyde-3-phosphate, impairment of iron metabolism, generation of peroxynitrite, and hydroxyl radicals [135, 142]. These speculations have been supported by the observation of high levels of proinflammatory cytokines such as interleukin-1β (IL-1β) and interferon γ (IFNγ) in PD brains, which can induce iNOS in activated microglia [143, 144].

4. RECENT CONTRIBUTIONS OF NATURAL PRODUCTS CHEMISTRY AGAINST ALZHEIMER'S DISEASE

Acetylcholinesterase (AChE) enzyme inhibition is an important target for the management of AD and AChE inhibitors are currently the main drugs available for its management. An important class of natural products that have been described as AChE inhibitors are the coumarins. Structure-activity relationship studies have demonstrated that the coumarin moiety plays a pharmacophore role in the AChE inhibition, becoming an important scaffold when this activity is concerned [145]. Decursinol (**48**), a natural product present in the methanolic extract of *Angelica gigas*, was reported to exhibit a potent AChE inhibition with IC_{50} in the range of 0.28 μM (Fig. **11**) [146]. The hexane extract of the bark of *Mesua elegans* presents four different 4-phenylcoumarins (Fig. **11**), mesuagenin A, B, C and D, AChE inhibitory activity was observed for all of them with Mesuagenin B (**49**) being the most potent inhibitor with IC_{50} of 0.7 μM [147].

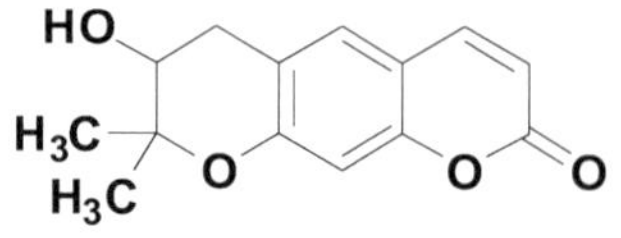

(48)

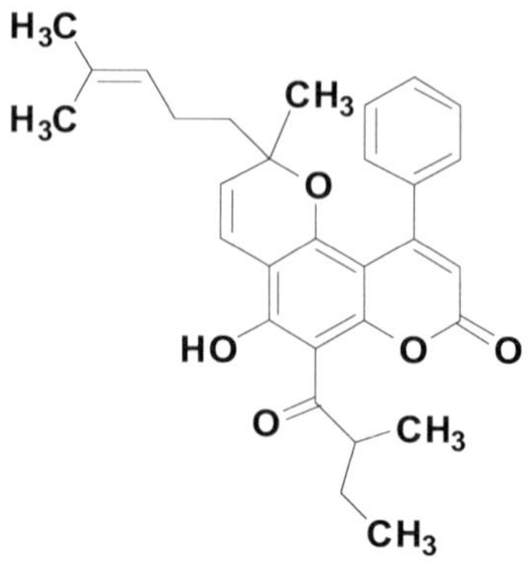

(49)

Fig. (11). Coumarin derivatives Decursinol (**48**) and Mesuagenin B (**49**).

Scopoletin (**50**) and its glucoside scopolin (**51**) (Fig. **12**), both derived from *Scopolia carniolica*, showed to have potent AChE inhibitory activity. In addition, *in vivo* experiments also revealed an increase in the extracellular ACh following their administration [148]. Furanocoumarins with AChE inhibitory activity were discovered in the hexane and dichloromethane extracts of *Citrus hystrix* fruits (Fig. **12**), the most potent being compounds (R)-(+)-6'-hydroxy-7'-methoxybergamottin (**52**) and (R)-(+)-6',7'-dihydroxybergamottin (**53**) which showed IC_{50} values of 11.2 ± 0.1 and 15.4 ± 0.3 μM, respectively [149].

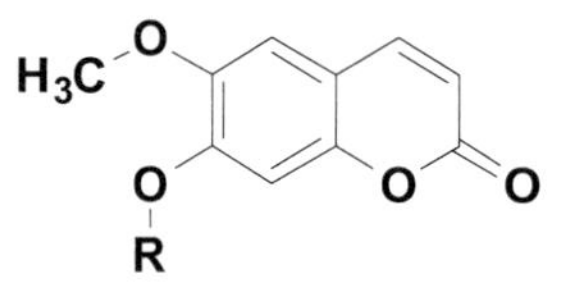

(50)- R = H
(51)- R = ß-D-glicopiranose

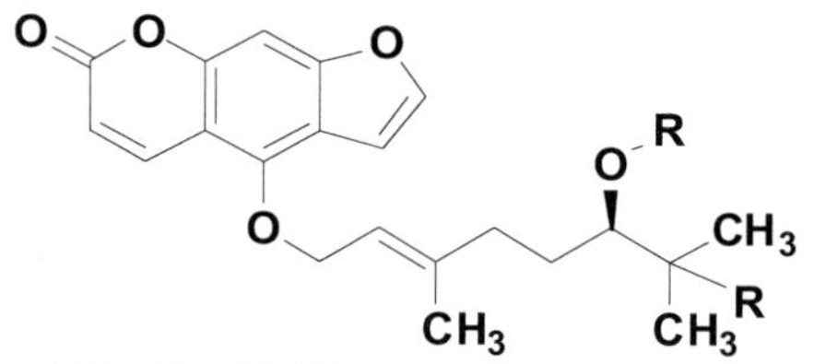

(52)- R = OCH$_3$
(53)- R = OH

Fig. (12). Coumarins from *Scopolia carniolica* with AChE inhibitory properties.

Further studies led Kim and co-worker to demonstrate that *ginseng*'s extract was able to attenuate significantly the activation of NMDA receptors and that the minor ginsenoside Rg_3 (**15**) was the most active metabolite [150]. In addition, a detailed *in vitro* study focused on the mechanism of action of the Rg_3-mediated inhibition on NMDA receptors, showed that the hippocampal neurons protection against NMDA insults was due to an interaction of **15** with the glycine-site at NMDA receptors [151].

Considering that most herbal medicines are orally administrated, their components may be biotransformed by the action of intestinal bacteria [152, 154], and therefore, the pharmacological actions of ginsenosides could be explained by their metabolites [153, 155]. This hypothesis was corroborated when Park and co-workers showed the protective effect in ischemia-reperfusion brain injury by Rh_2 (**56**), the main metabolite of Rg_3 (**15**) [156]. Furthermore, many studies have been conducted by using epimeric mixtures of 20(*R*)- and 20(*S*)-ginsenosides, but recent works have shown the stereo-specific modulation of this compounds on voltage- ou ligand-gated channels [157, 158].

For these reasons, Lee and co-workers [159] decide to evaluate the effects of purified forms of 20(*S*)-ginsenosides **10**, **15**, **22**, the three most commonly studied ginsenosides in the CNS and their effects on the NMDA receptors. To perform this study, the authors investigated the modulation of NMDA-induced [Ca^{2+}] increase promoted by compounds **10**, **15**, **22** and their main metabolites **54-59** (Fig. **13**). Compounds **10**, **22**, **54**, **58** and **59** presented very weak inhibitory profile (< 25% of inhibition), followed by compounds **55** and **57** (50% inhibition). However, the two compounds glycosylated only at C-3 position, **15** and **56**, produced the highest inhibitory effect among the nine ginsenosides evaluated. In one hand, stereospecificity of the NMDA-inhibitory effect was not significant between the epimers 20(*S*)-**15** (70 %) and 20(*R*)-**15** (63%), but on the other hand compound 20(*S*)-**56** was 6.7-fold more potent than its epimer. Due to the similar results observed for 20(*S*)-forms of **15** and **56**, they were tested on non-NMDA receptors, by using selective agonists of NMDA-receptors, AMPA (α-amino-3-hydroxy-5-methyl-4-isoxazolepropionic acid) and kainic acid. The mean percentage inhibition on NMDA receptors caused by compound 20(*S*)-**56** (10 μM) was significantly bigger than the inhibition on non-NMDA receptor agonists and this pattern of activity was common for both 20(*S*)-**15** and 20(*S*)-**56**. Based on the results of a NMDA dose-response assay, 20(*S*)-**56**-mediated inhibition showed to be unchanged by varying concentrations of NMDA, suggesting that this compound blocks NMDA receptors *via* a non-competitive mechanism with NMDA-binding site in hippocampal neurons. To speculate these data, one possibility could be the inhibition of NMDA receptors by 20(*S*)-**56** as a competitive antagonist at the glycine-binding site as ginsenoside **15** does. However, it seems not be the case, since the mechanisms by which **15** and **56** affects the target receptor is different, and the evidences suggests that **56** may modulate other regulatory sites of the NMDA receptor. Another data pointed to the possibility of compound **56** exert its regulatory effect in receptor sites such as polyamine-binding sites and sites within the channel lumen. However, based on diverse and experimental evidences, Lee and co-workers strongly believe that the polyamine-binding site may be the possible target for 20(*S*)-**56**-mediated inhibition on NMDA receptors [159].

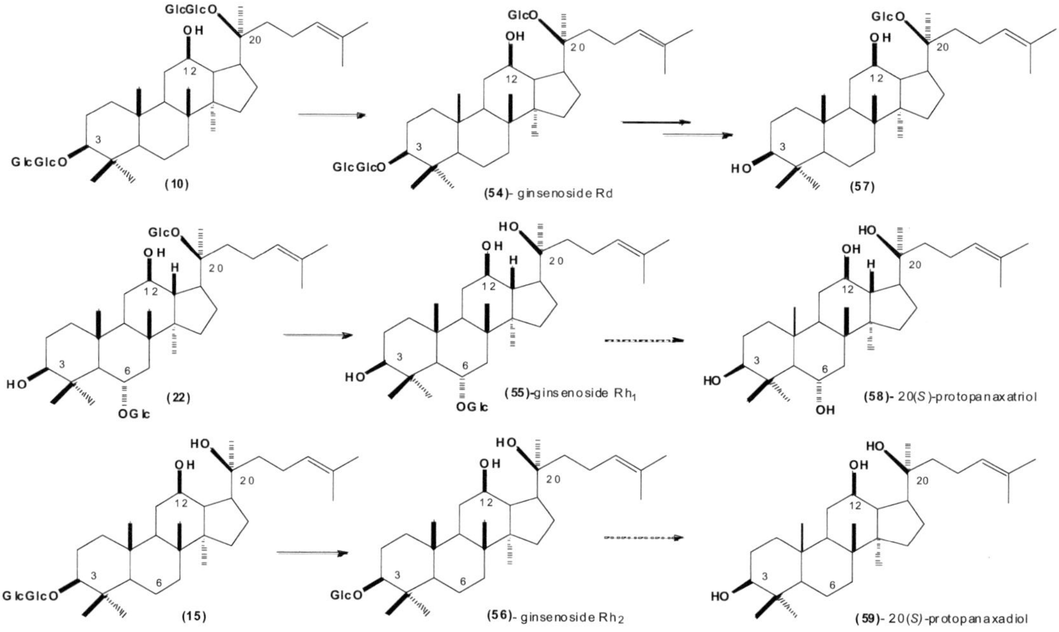

Fig. (13). Ginsenosides 20(*S*)-Rb$_1$ (**10**), 20(*S*)-Rg$_3$ (**15**), 20(*S*)-Rg$_1$ (**22**) and its main metabolites **54-59**.

Despite all these evidence data, they are not sufficient to rule out that **56** affects other regulatory sites that have not been yet examined, but the finding that this compound is an active compound is very important because its immediate metabolic precursor is one of the most active component of *Panax ginseng*. These data also corroborate that the **56**-mediated neuroprotective properties, should be resultant from NMDA receptors inhibition [159].

Based on all these data, the structure-activity relationshipsassociated with the modulation of NMDA receptors seems to be related to carbon-3 and carbon-20 positions of ginsenosides. The structural difference between **15** and **56** is the presence of a mono-glycosylated group at the C-3 position, and the change from *S* to *R* configuration at the C-20 position of **56** contributes to the lossof inhibitory profile, while there was no difference between 20-epimers of ginsenoside **15**. Then, the mono-glycosylated group at C-3 and the *S* configuration at C-20 positions seem to be essential for the binding to polyamine sites. Furthermore, these results also may suggest that the two glycine- and polyamine-binding sites, modulated by 20(*S*)-**15** and 20(*S*)-**56**, are located in an adjacent distanceof NMDA receptors [159], as have been confirmed by others research groups [160-162]. Based on these data, a detailed analysis on the different structural attributes of the main active ginsenosides, compounds **15** and **56**, makes clear to understand that **56** could fit in the polyamine-binding site, while compound **15**, with a more bulky side chain is binds better to the glycine-binding site [159].

Some other plants, used in Chinese and Indian traditional medicine for memory and cognitive improvements, have been chemically investigated, in order to determine the main active constituents and try to establish and clarify the pharmacological basis for such medicinal benefits. In traditional practices of medicine, plants have been used to enhance cognitive function and to alleviate other symptoms associated to AD, and in some cases the experience have shown that some constituents may not only act synergistically with other metabolites of the same plant, but may also raise the activity of compounds or counteract toxic effects of compounds form other plants [163]. This approach has been used in many prescriptions for cognitive disorders, including anticholinesterase (AChE), anti-inflammatory and antioxidant activities.

In the Ayurvedic Medicine (also known as Indian Traditional Medicine) *Celastrus paniculatus* Willd. (Celastraceae) have been used for intellect stimulation and sharpening the memory. Many studies with the seeds, seed oil had attested decreasing in noradrenaline, dopamine and 5-hydroxytriptamine (5-HT) in the brain of rats, which were correlated with as improvement in learning and memory processes [163, 164]. Furthermore, the antioxidant effect in CNS observed by the administration of aqueous seed extract, may explain the reputed benefits on memory [165].

Nevertheless, pharmacological studies using the seeds' methanolic extract of this plant do not showed any response over NMDA and δ-aminobutiric acid (GABA) receptors and nerve growth factor (NGF), suggesting that, if this herb really have the reputed properties, the active constituents must be identified in less polar solvent fraction. In another work, investigations on the flowers of *C. paniculatus* have shown anti-inflammatory activity in methanolic extract, which may have some relevance in the management of neurodegenerative disorders [166].

Centella asiatica (Umbelliferae) is an ancient prescription of Ayurvedic to restore youth, memory, and longevity and to treat rheumatic diseases, which also suggests its anti-inflammatory properties [163]. In China, this plant is also used for combating mental and physical exhaustion [167]. Several studies reported that its leaf essential oil contains mainly monoterpenes including bornyl acetate (**60**), α-pinene (**61**), β-pinene (**62**) and δ-terpinene (**63**) [167, 168], which were described to inhibit AChE [169, 171]. However, their inhibition potency is very weak when compared to alkaloid physostigmine (**64**, Fig. **14**), suggesting that they should not be therapeutically effective in cognitive disorders through this mechanism of action [163]. Other research groups showed that ethanolic extracts of *C. asiatica*, reputed to present anti-amnesic effects, have demonstred tranquillizing properties in rats, an activity attributed to the triterpene brahmoside, a glycoside of brahmic acid (**65**) [172, 173]. In addition, leaf extracts showed to be sedative, antidepressant and potentially cholinomimetic *in vivo* [172], suggesting that this plant may be appropriate for the treatment of symptoms of depression and anxiety of AD patients, and that may also influence positively thecognitive function through the modulation of cholinergic receptors [163].

On the other hand, other neurotransmitters, including dopamine, serotine and glutamate have been associated to the pathophysiology and progression of AD, and some drugs that modulate these neurotransmitter systems have shown some additional benefits in AD-related symptoms. Studies *in vivo* showed that the aqueous extract of the leaves of *C. asiatica* could modulate dopamine, 5-HT and noradrenaline systems in rat brain and improved learning and memory processes [173-176]. Glutamate may induce neuronal degeneration by overstimulation of NMDA receptor and some triterpenes from *C. asiatica* such as asiatic acid (**66**, Fig. **14**) and derivatives [177, 178] have been shown to protect cortical neurons from glutamate-induced injury *in vitro*, but further research regarding the clinical potential of these compounds may be warranted [178]. In another work, Barbosa and co-workers [179] quantified that asiaticoside (**67**) is present in 84% in the water extract and evaluated it effects against subtypes of phospholipases A_2 (PLA_2) in cerebellum from rats. PLA_2 are a family of key enzymes in the metabolism of phospholipids, and in the brain these enzymes preferentially cleave membrane phosphatidylcholine to release free arachidonic acid (AA) and lysophosphatidylcholine, which are important mediators for memory processing [180]. Stimulus-induced AA release is thought to be mediated mainly by secretory PLA_2 ($sPLA_2$) and by cytosolic PLA_2 ($cPLA_2$), whereas group VI Ca^{2+}-independent PLA_2 ($iPLA_2$) has been suggested to contribute to phospholipids remodeling [181]. Evaluation of dose-dependent effect of *C. asiatica* water extract on $iPLA_2$ and $cPLA_2$, showed 96% and 77% of maximal inhibitory activity (at 500 μg/mL), respectively. These results are particularly relevant due to previous observations that $iPLA_2$ is responsible for about 80% of all PLA_2 activity in the brain [179]. The effectiveness of *C. asiatica* water extract in the treatment of neurodegenerative disorders was confirmed by a number of studies reporting prevention of oxidative damage, improvement of antioxidant status in brain [182], improvement of acetylcholine synthesis by asiatic acid (**66**) [183], dose-dependent normalization of brain enzyme levels of malondialdehyde, catalase and glutathione, whereas derivatives of asiaticoside and asiatic acid showed a protective effect against β-amyloid-induced neurotoxicity [184, 185].

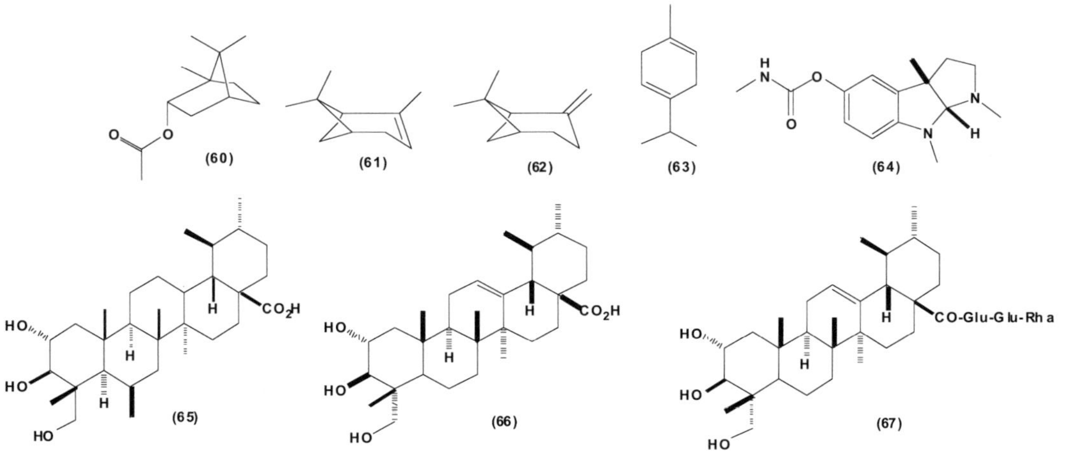

Fig. (14). Monoterpenoid acetycholinesterase inhibitors (**60-63**), brahmic acid (**65**), asiatic acid (**66**), asiaticoside (**67**) isolated from *C. asiatica*, and physostigmine (**64**).

Curcuma longa L. (Zimgiberaceae) has also been used as a counteract aging agent in Ayurvedic, and also for culinary purposes. Its rhizomes are very rich in curcumin (**68**), a compound with well described antioxidant, anti-inflammatory [186-189] and neuroprotective [190] properties. Considering the inflammatory process in CNS associated to AD physiology, substances able to inhibit these deleterious events could be of interest to the AD's therapy. Some compounds from *C. longa*, including **68**, demethoxycurcumin (**69**), bisdemethoxycurcumin (**70**) and calebin-A (**71**, Fig. **15**) were investigated and proved to be capable to protect PC12 cells from β-amyloid insult *in vitro* [191, 192] due to, in part, their antioxidant effect [193]. Anti-inflammatory activity of **68** had already been investigated and the results were suggestive for modulation of eicosanoid biosynthesis and inhibition of ciclooxigenase (COX)-1, COX-2 and lipoxygenase (LOX) [194-196]. Other activity that may be relevant in the management of AD is antidepressant and, for this reason, aqueous extract of *C. longa* was evaluated by oral administration in mice. The observed antidepressant activity was attributed to inhibition of brain monoamine oxidase (MAO) A [197].

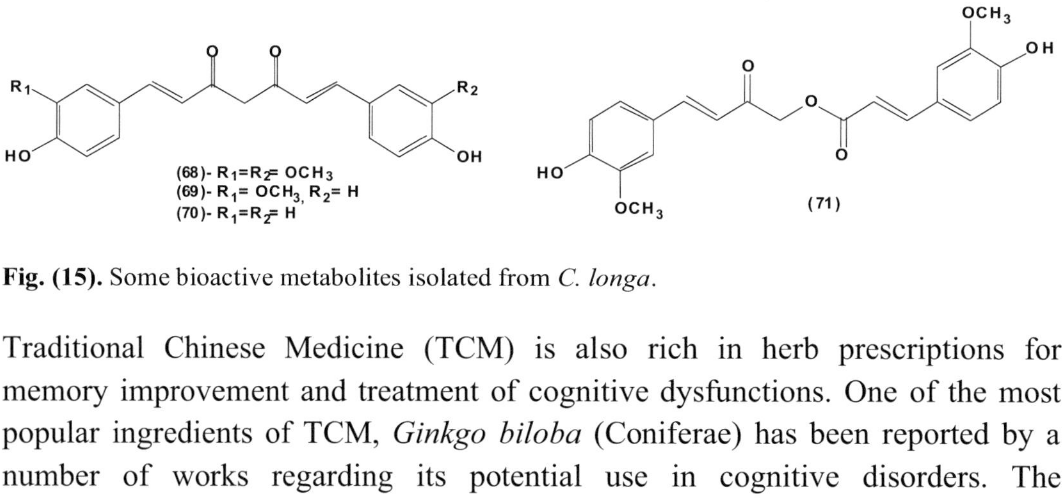

Fig. (15). Some bioactive metabolites isolated from *C. longa*.

Traditional Chinese Medicine (TCM) is also rich in herb prescriptions for memory improvement and treatment of cognitive dysfunctions. One of the most popular ingredients of TCM, *Ginkgo biloba* (Coniferae) has been reported by a number of works regarding its potential use in cognitive disorders. The standardized extract of *G. biloba* (EGb 761) has been investigated for CNS activities [198] relevant to the treatment of cognitive dysfunction, and there are evidences offavorable effects on cerebral circulation and neuronal cell metabolism [199-201] and also on muscarinic cholinergic system [202]. In addition, antioxidant properties were reported for this extract [203-205], which may be associated to neuroprotection against β-amyloid and nitric oxide (NO)-induced toxicity *in vitro* [206, 207] and could alsobe responsible their anti-apoptotic effects both *in vitro* and *in vivo* [208, 209]. Extract EGb 761 is known to contain 24% flavonol glycosides, 6% terpene trilactones (ginkgolides A (**72**), B (**73**), C (**74**) and bilobalide (**75**, Fig. **16**), about 7% proanthocyanidines, some organic acids among other common compounds. It is suggested that the cardio and neuroprotective effects of EGb 761 is associated with the free-radical scavenging and/or antioxidant properties of the extract, mainly promoted by their flavonoid constituents [206, 210-212]. Pietri and co-workers, investigating cardioprotective and antioxidant effects of terpenoid metabolites from *G. biloba* extracts (GBE) could conclude that bilobalide (**75**) is not able to scavenge free radicals in cell-free systems, but can inhibit production of reactive oxygen species in perfused heart tissue [213]. Based on these data, EGb 761 and **75**were further investigated and it was demonstrated to have potently protective effects against ischemia-induced reductions in mitochondrial gene expression and neuronal death [210].

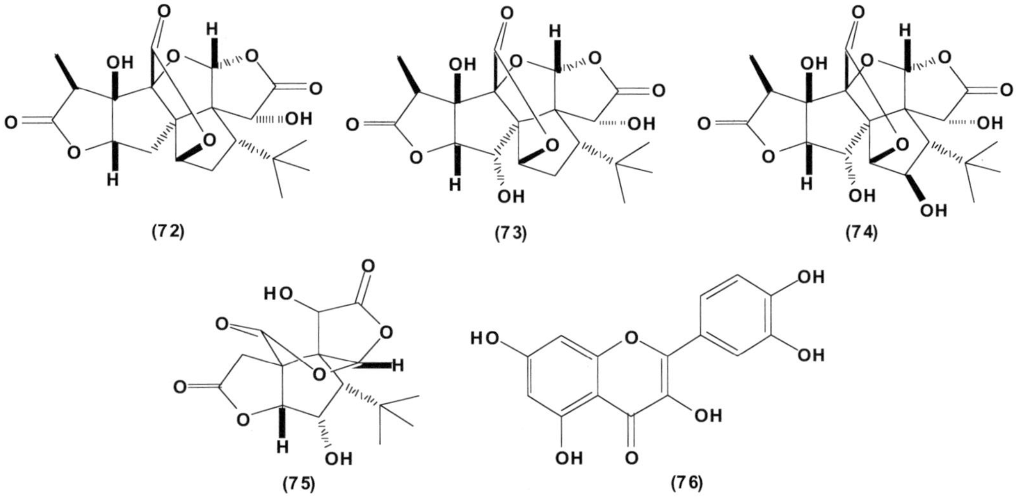

Fig. (16). Ginkgolides A (**72**), B (**73**), C (**74**), bilobalide (**75**) and quercetin (**76**) isolated from *G.biloba*.

In the last decade, several behavioral assays using GBEwere performed to evaluate cognitive and memory effects and it was observed that extracts were capable to attenuate scopolamine-induced amnesia in rats [214], enhance memory retention in both young and old rats [215], and improve short-term memory in mice [216].

Clinical studies, conducted in different research centers during the last decade [217-224], were also conclusive for the efficacy of using *G. biloba* extracts that produced modest improvement in cognitive function when administered to AD and non-AD-patients submitted to different protocol analysis.

Taking into account the numerous positive data available for *in vitro* and *in vivo* pharmacological investigations, involving a wide range of activities probably related to biotargets related to AD development, the use of GBE apparently supports the clinical improvements observed among AD patients. However, the identification of pure compounds responsible for these activities remain obscure, but it is suggested that some flavonoids could be responsible for vasodilatory properties [225] and ginkgolide B (**73**) that is a platelet-activating factor (PAF) antagonist could act on theinflammatory process associated to AD [226]. Interested in clarify the vasodilatory properties produced by GBE on the thoracic aorta isolated from rats and on the intracellular calcium level of cultured aortic endothelial cells, Kubota and co-workers confirmed that GBE and its major flavonoid ingredient, quercetin (**76**, Fig. **16**), produce vasodilation *via* NO in the aorta cells [225]. These findings suggest a possibility that GBE and **76** can activate undefined Ca^{2+} channels in endothelial cells and that the resultant increase in intracellular calcium level can activate NO-synthase and enhance the formation of NO, which may promote improvements in the local circulation. With reference to the numerous studies described in the literature, it is apparent that EGB can really be useful in the treatment of AD symptoms, however additional research must be taken to identify appropriate dosing regimens, potential benefits and unlike effects of long-term use and interactions with other medicines [163].

Huperzia serrata (Lycopodiaceae) is used in TCM to prepare "Qian Ceng Ta" which is prescribed to alleviate memory loss [122]. Huperzine A (**77**, Fig. **17**), a lycopodium alkaloid related to the quinolizidines isolated from *H. serrata*, is a reversible inhibitor of acetylcholinesterase (AChE) *in vitro* and *in vivo* [8, 9, 227-231], capable to improve memory retention processes in cognitively impaired rats [232], attenuate cognitive deficits in chronically hyperfused rats [233], and in gerbils following ischemia [234]. Clinical evaluation of **77** revealed a significant improvement of memory and behavior in AD patients, inhibiting AChE selectively with less toxic effects than the commercially available drugs donepezil and tacrine [235, 236]. Xiao and co-workers [237] suggested that AChE inhibition may not be the unique explanation for the clinical effects observed for **77**, as it has also been shown to be neuroprotective against β-amyloid peptide fragment 25-53 [237], oxygen-glucose deprivation [238], and free-radical-induced cytotoxicity [239].

Huperzine also showed to be an NMDA receptor antagonist in the cerebral cortex, and for instance a neuroprotector against glutamate [240, 241]. A mechanism of action based on the ability of **77** to inhibit the mitochondria-capase pathway has been proposed to explain its anti-apoptoticeffects [242].

Galanthamine (**78**, Fig. **17**) is an Amaryllidaceae alkaloid isolated from the Chinese *Lycoris radiata*, and from the European *Galanthus nivalis* L. and *Narcissus spp.* [243], that nowadays is one of the more important orally active drugs approved for the treatment of AD due to the improvement of cognitive function [244-245] resultant from selective AChE inhibition [246-248]. Further studies demonstrated that **78** are also able to stimulate alosterically nicotinic receptors [249-250], enhancing cholinergic function and memory of AD patients. This profile represents and advantage over other classical AChE inhibitor drugs. In 1960, Irwin and co-workers have already reported lycoramine (**79**, Fig. **17**) as another AChE inhibitor alkaloid isolated from *L. radiate* [251], but it does not have been subject to exhaustive pharmacological and clinical tests as galanthamine.

Magnolia officinalis (Magnoliacaceae) is another plant used in TCM in the treatment of nervous disturbances and anxiety. Phytochemical studies with its bark and stem led to isolation of biphenolic lignans, such as honokiol (**80**) and magnolol (**81**, Fig. **17**). These compounds showed to increase choline acetyltransferase (ChAT) and inhibit AChE activity *in vitro* and increase hippocampal ACh release *in vivo* [253]. Further studies have shown other relevant pharmacological properties of these compounds for the management of AD, including antioxidant activities [254-257], anxiolytic effects of **80** [258-259] and ability of **81** to potentiate GABAergic neurotransmission [260]. Magnolol (**81**) demonstrated additional neuroprotection against chemical hypoxic damage and necrotic cell death in cortical neuron-astrocyte cultures *in vitro* [261] and anti-inflammatory activity *in vitro* and *in vivo* by inhibition of COX and 5-LOX [262, 263]. So, these apparently multiple spectrum of actions of *M. officinalis*, especially its metabolites **80** and **81**, may justify further research to evaluate the therapeutic potential and the development of possible new anti-Alzheimer drugs.

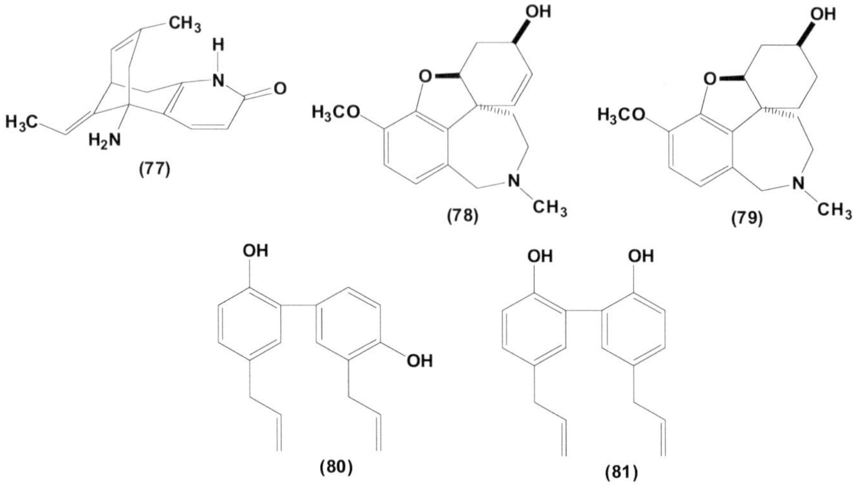

Fig. (17). Structures of AChE inhibitors huperzine (**77**), galanthamine (**78**), lycoramine (**79**), honokiol (**80**) and magnolol (**81**).

Pagliosa and co-workers investigated the *in vitro* AChE inhibitory effect of three isoquinoline alkaloids (**82-84**) (Fig. **18**) isolated from *Hippeastrum psittacinum* and *Hippeastrum vittatum.* However, despite these three alkaloidal metabolites are belonging to species of Amaryllidaceae, as well as galanthamine (**78**), only the alkaloid montanine (**82**) showed some inhibitory activity [252].

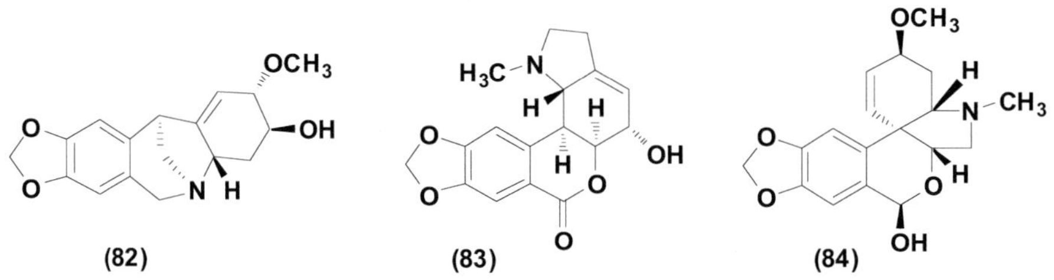

Fig. (18). Alkaloids isolated from species of the Amaryllidaceae family.

Polygala tenuifolia (Polygalaceae) is a Chinese herb described as memory and intelligence enhancer in TCM for about 2000 years and produces anextractknown as tenuigenin, which has been used to AD treatment. In order to examine these therapeutic effects, Jia and co-workers, tested tenuigenin (**85**) in the inhibition of Aβ secretion in neuroblastoma cells stably transfected with two amyloid precursor protein (APP) constructs: the APP695 cDNA (SH-SY5Y APP695) and the C-terminal 99 amino acid residues of APP plus the signal peptide (SH-SY5Y SPA4CT). The results demonstrated that compound **85** was capable to inhibit secretion of Aβ and C-terminal 99 amino acid residues of APP in SH-SY5Y APP695 cells, but did not change the Aβ and C99 levels in SH-SY5Y SPA4CT cells [264]. In addition, Fluorescence Resonance Energy Transfer (FRET) assays showed that **85** also inhibited the proteolytic activities of β-secretase on its substrate *in vivo*, without cytotoxic effects [264]. In another study, the extract of dried root of *P. tenuifolia,* called BT-11, was subject to pharmacological evaluation, showing that the 80% ethanol extract of BT-11 could improve learning and memory in scopolamine-induced amnesia model in rats [265]. Investigation of possible mechanism of cognitive enhancing and neuroprotection led the authors to identify AChE inhibition by BT-11, in a dose dependent manner, indicating that this plant might contain one or more unidentified anticholinesterase components. Other results indicate that BT-11 inhibits AChE in a non-competitive manner and that it can penetrate the blood-brain-barrier to promote cognitive improvement through elevating cholinergic neurotransmission. This effect was suggested to occur by blocking ACh hydrolysis and also protect neurons against glutamate, Aβ and amyloidogenic C-terminal fragments [265].

P. tenuifolia has also been used in Traditional Japanese Medicine (TJM) and is a component of a prescription containing 12 other herbs, so called Kami-utan-to (KUT), indicated for the treatment of psychoneurological diseases [163]. Likely it was described for BT-11, KUT exhibited a dose dependent up-regulated ChAT activity and increased NGF secretion *in vitro*, besides improved passive avoidance behavior and induced ChAT activity in the cerebral cortex of aged rats and in scopolamine-induced memory impaired rats [266, 267]. The cinnamic acid derivative sinapic acid (**86**), isolated from the roots of *P. tenuifolia*, was converted into its sodium carboxylate soluble salt, that showed to increase ChAT activity in the frontal cortex of brain-lesioned rats [266]. In 2004, Ikeya and co-workers reported that tenuifoliside B (**87**) and 3,6'-disinapoylsucrose (**88**), which are two acylated oligosaccharides present in the roots of *P. tenuifolia*, displayed cerebral protective effects on KCN-induced anoxia in mice, had a positive effect on the reversion of scopolamine-induced impairment of performance in passive avoidance task in rats and also enhanced oxotremorine-induced tremors in mice, suggesting that compound **87** could act as a cholinergic system enhancer [268]. Next, in a more detailed study involving compounds **86-88**, the authors suggested that the pharmacophoric sinapoyl subunit present in the structure of **87** and **88** could responsible for their cerebral protective and cognition-improving effects. An examination of the cerebral protective effects of **86** (10-100 mg/kg), showed the inhibition of KCN-induced hypoxia and scopolamine-induced memory impairment as evidenced also for compounds **87** (3-100 mg/kg) and **88** (10-100 mg/kg) (Fig. **19**). In addition, taking together a set of experimental data, including inhibition of hypobaric hypoxia-induced or bilateral carotid artery ligation-induced mortality, CO_2-induced memory impairment in mice, and forebrain lesion-induced cerebral cholinergic dysfunction, suggest a possibility of sinapinic acid not only could be an important structural moiety of the active compounds **87**and **88**, but also a candidate for a cerebral protective and cognition-improving drug [268, 269].

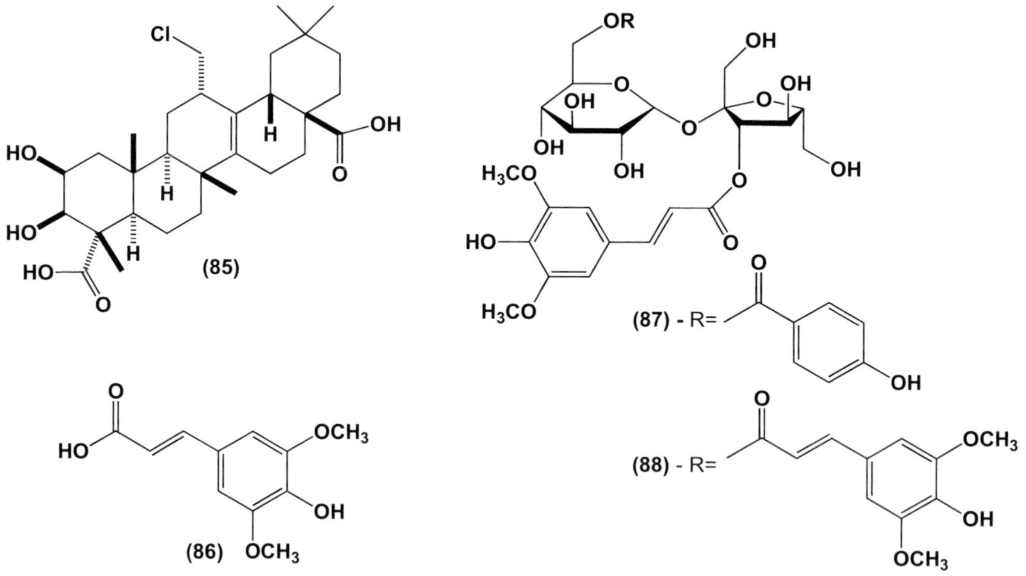

Fig. (19). Cerebral protective and cognition-improving metabolites, tenuigenin (**85**), sinapic acid (**86**), tenuifoliside B (**87**) and 3,6'-disinapoylsucrose (**88**), isolated from the roots of *P. tenuifolia*.

Salvia species, *Salvia lavandulaefolia* Vahl., *S. miltiorrhiza* Bung. (Labiatae) are prominent for their reputed beneficial effects on memory disorders, depression and cerebral ischaemia [163, 170]. Besides anticholinesterase activity, these plants have showed other activities relevant to AD treatment, including antioxidant, anti-inflammatory and estrogenic effects [270, 271]. Recently, many studies have been undertaken to scientifically investigate the traditional CNS-related properties of *S. lavandulaefolia*, focusing mainly the activity of the essential oil. The individual constituents of the essential oil *S. lavandulaefolia* (the monoterpenoids 1,8-cineole (**89**), linalool (**90**), α-pinene (**91**, Fig. **20**) and herb, including the phenolic monoterpenoid carvacrol (**92**), the flavone luteoline (**93**) and the phenolic rosmarinic acid (**94**) have been reported to be antioxidant [271, 276]. Rosmarinic acid displayed more potent radical scavenging activity than trolox, an α-tocoferol derivative used as reference [271-276]. In addition to the antioxidant effects, many isolated *Salvia* constituents demonstrate anti-inflammatory properties [277, 278]. Compounds **91-94** were characterized to be anti-inflammatory constituents of *S. lavandulaefolia.* α-Pinene (**91**, 0.2 nM) and geraniol (**95**, 0.2 nM) promoted eicosanoid inhibition in rat leucocytes [271], and compound **91** is also an inhibitor of the enzyme cyclooxygenase, activities that could be of particular relevance to anti-inflammatory treatment of AD [279].

Anticholinesterase activity, the main original activity sought in the research into the putative CNS beneficial effects of *S. lavandulaefolia*, was observed *in vitro* for the essential oil (human brain, IC_{50}= 0.07 mg/mL and bovine erythrocyte, IC_{50}= 0.03-0.05 mg/mL) [270] and was also confirmed *in vivo* [280]. In another work, Perry and co-workers, examined the*in vitro* human erythrocyte AChE inhibition by *S. lavandulaefolia* essential oil and some of its major constituents, *i.e.,* 1,8-cineole (**89**, 13%), α- (**91**) and β-pinene (**96**, 10-15%), camphor (**97**, 27%) and bornyl acetate (**98**, 10%, Fig. **20**). The IC_{50} value obtained for the essential oil was 0.03 μg/mL, while the IC_{50} values for constituents **89**, **91** and **97** were 0.67 mM, 0.63 mM and > 10 mM, respectively [281]. It was assumed that the anti-cholinesterase activity of the whole essential oil is resultant from synergistic antiChE effectsof the major monoterpenoid constituents [281, 282]. More recently, Savelev and co-workers, observed synergistic (**89**/**91** and **89**/caryophyllene epoxide (**99**)) and antagonistic (**89**/**97**) interactions between the antiChE constituents of *S. lavandulaefolia* essential oil, and concluded that theAChE inhibitory activity of this essential oil results from a response of an association of these complex interactions [282].

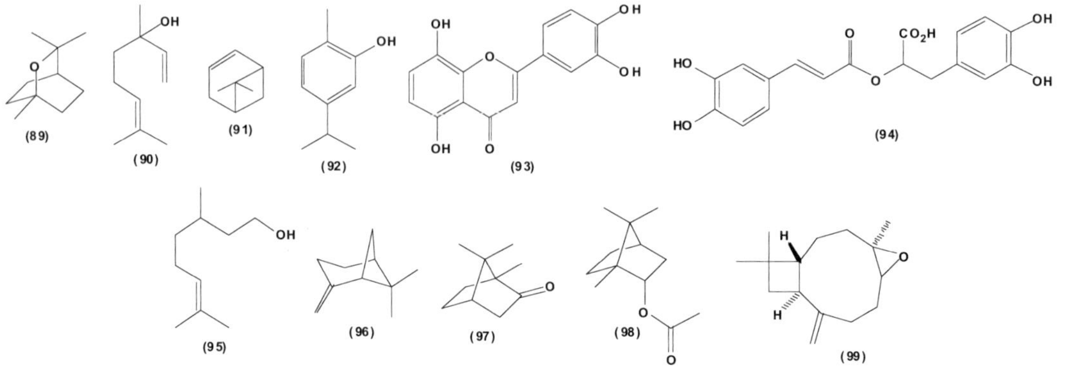

Fig. (20). Monoterpenoids and other CNS-active secondary metabolites isolated from *S. lavandulaefolia.*

S. miltiorrhiza is another medicinal *Salvia* species, prescribed in folk medicine to relief blood disorders, to stabilize heart and calm nerves (TCM) [163]. More recently, more careful investigations of this plant led to the identification of numerous pharmacological activities that could be relevant in CNS dysfunctions, including AD and cerebral vascular disease, including protective effect against cerebral ischemia, probably by regulation of substance P distribution in CNS [283] and inhibition of NO formation [284], and prevention of neuronal cell death by inhibition of pre-synaptic glutamate release [285].

Some other studies showed relevant antioxidant properties of the roots of *S. miltiorrhiza*, reducing lipoperoxidation during the metabolism of free fatty acids from the breakdown of lipid membranes during ischemia [286-289]. Chemical investigations led to the isolation of several quinones, such as dihydrotanshinone (**100**), tanshinone I (**101**), methylenetanshinone (**102**) and cryptotanshinone (**103**, Fig. **21**), provided of significant antioxidant activity [290, 291]. Moreover, other secondary metabolites of *S. miltiorrhiza* have also displayed important antioxidant effects, *e.g.*, salvianolic acids A (**104**) and B (**105**) [291, 292], rosmariquinone (**106**) among other phenolic compounds [287, 289, 291-294]. Some evidences of sedative and analgesic properties of *S. miltiorrhiza* stimulate Chang and co-workers to conduct a study of structure-activity relationship (SAR) with compound **106** and other analogue derivatives, which lead them to identify**106** as a central benzodiazepine receptor ligand [295]. These findings may suggest that **106** and other quinones present in the roots of *S. miltiorrhiza* could be responsible forthe tranquillizing effects observed and could be further developed as anxiolytic drugs for managing the behavioural disturbances often present in AD patients [163].

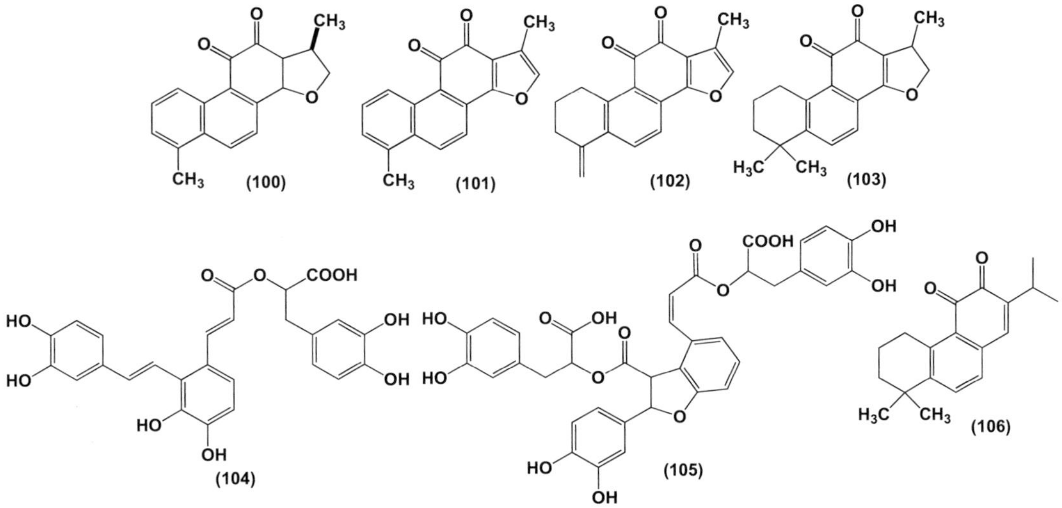

Fig. (21). CNS-active secondary metabolites isolated from *S. miltiorrhiza.*

Other plants used in TCM to prevent or treat impairments associated to neurodegenerative disorders that have their active compounds isolated and are under pharmacological investigation include *Coptis chinensis* (Ranunculaceae), *Crocus sativus* (Iridaceae) and *Evodia rutaecarpa* (Rutaceae) [163].

The methanolic extracts of *C. chinensis*, as well as its constituents, jatrorrhizine (**107**) and berberine (**108**), have shown to be MAO inhibitors, displaying antidepressant activity [296]. Besides **108**, some other alkaloids isolated from *C. chinensis*, such as coptisine (**109**) and palmatine (**110**, Fig. **22**), also demonstrated anti-ChE activities and showed NGF-enhancing activity in PC12 cells [297].

Crocus sativus (Iridaceae), commonly known as saffron in folk medicine was recently evaluated about their effects on memory and learning in animals.

Behavioural and electrophysiological studies have demonstrated that *C. sativus* extract improved ethanol-induced impairments of learning behaviours in mice and prevent ethanol-induced inhibition of hippocampal long-term potentiation, a form of activity-dependent synaptic plasticity that may underly learning and memory. Despite these CNS effects were most attributed to crocin (**111**), crocetin (**112**, Fig. **23**), the main secondary metabolite present in saffron extract, is also thought to be useful candidate to treatment for neurodegenerative disorders accompanying memory impairment [298].

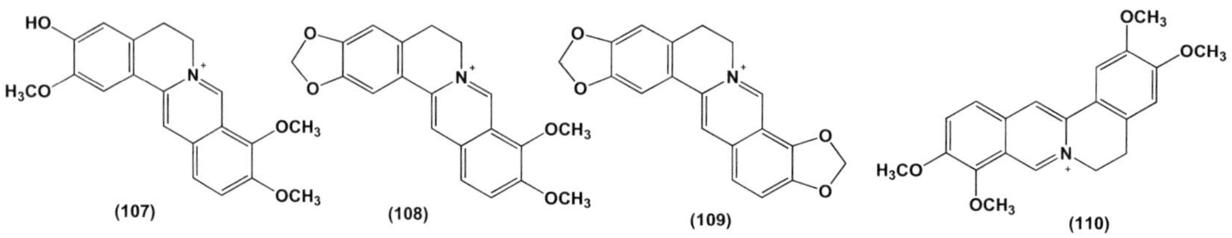

Fig. (22). CNS active alkaloids jatrorrhizine (**107**), berberine (**108**), coptisine (**109**) andpalmatine (**110**) isolated from *C. chinensis.*

Evodia rutaecarpa (Rutaceae) and dehydroevodiamine (**133**, Fig. **23**), an alkaloidal metabolite, inhibited AChE *in vitro* and reversed scopolanine-induced memory impairment in rats [299]. Morever, compound **133** promoted also an increase of cerebral blood flow *in vivo* [300].

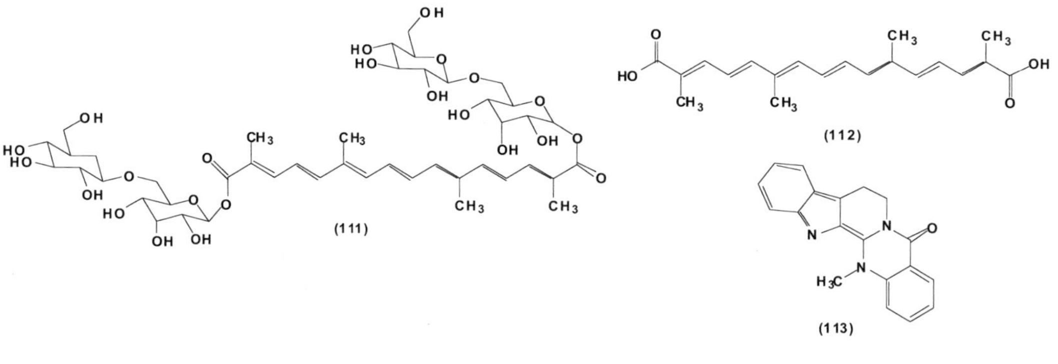

Fig. (23). CNS active metabolites crocin (**111**), crocetin (**112**) from *C. sativus* and dehydroevodiamine (**113**) an IAChE isolated from *E. rutaecarpa.*

In Oriental Traditional Medicine, the roots of *Sanguisorba officinalis* L. (Rosaceae), also known as *Sanguisorbae* radix (SR), have been used to treat diarrhea, chronic intestinal infections, duodenal ulcers and bleeding, due to its hemostatic, analgesic, anti-inflammatory, anti-allergic and anxiolytic properties [301]. Moreover, SR and its constituents have been reported to have antioxidant activity *in vitro* and *in vivo* [302-304]. To further investigate neuroprotective effect of SR, Nguyen and co-workers carried out a study using models of oxidative stress-induced toxicity and on ischemia-induced brain damage in rats [301]. It was confirmed at the first time that SR elicited neuroprotective activity (at 100 μM) against neuronal death induced by H_2O_2 in the MTT assay and that the addition of SR also decreased significantly the apoptotic neuronal death induced by H_2O_2 in a dose-dependent manner (at 10, 30 and 50 μg/mL). In this study, H_2O_2 elicited significant increases in $[Ca^{2+}]_i$ and glutamate release within a short time after treatment, which were blocked by SR. Therefore, it was suggested that SR could prevent Ca^{2+} entry through voltage-dependent Ca^{2+} channel (VDCC) and/or N-methyl-D-aspartate (NMDA)-receptor operated channels to inhibit neuronal death. Several compounds including triterpenes and flavonoids such as quercetin (**114**) and kaempferol (**115**, Fig. **24**), well known for their antioxidant properties, have been isolated from SR. In order to identify the possible constituents responsible for the neuroprotective activities observed for SR, gallic acid (**116**) and catechin (**117**, Fig. **24**) were isolated [301]. Catechin, but not gallic acid inhibited H_2O_2-induced neuronal death and other studies have indicated that flavonoids including cathechins reduce glutamate and AMPA induced $[Ca^{2+}]_i$ increase. It was presumed that inhibition by SR on $[Ca^{2+}]_i$ elevation might be due to these polyphenolic compounds, which could stabilize membranes in amanner that blocks Ca^{2+} influx *via* VDCC. It could be also suggested that radical oxigen species (ROS)-scavenging activity of SR possibly attributable to compound **117** played a critical role in neuronal survival, since **117** has been shown to have neuroprotective property directly associated with ROS-scavenging activity [301, 305, 306].

Curcumin (**118**, Fig. **25**), is the major yellow pigment extracted from the Indian turmeric spice, obtained from the rizome of *Curcuma longa* Linn. (Zingiberaceae). This polyphenolic compound is supported by the current literature to regulate numerous transcription factors, cytokines, protein kinases, adhesion molecules, redox status, enzymes associated to inflammatory process and to elicit anti-amyloidgenic neuroprotective properties [307-309]. Rajeswari and Sabesan investigated compound **118** and its main metabolite tetrahydrocurcumin (ThC, **119**, Fig. **25**) in a model of Parkinson's disease induced in mice by MPTP (1-methyl-4-phenyl-1,2,3,6-tetrahydropyridine), which is based on the increase of monoamino-oxidase (MAO) activity due to depletion of dopamine and DOPAC (3,4-dihydroxy phenyl acetic acid) [310]. Both compounds at the dose of 60 mg/kg reversed the reduction in striatal dopamine and DOPAC levels of mice after treatment with MPTP. In addition, when animals were treated by **118** or **119** alone, MAO-B was significantly decreased, being ThC (**119**) a much more potent inhibitor than curcumin (**118**) [310].

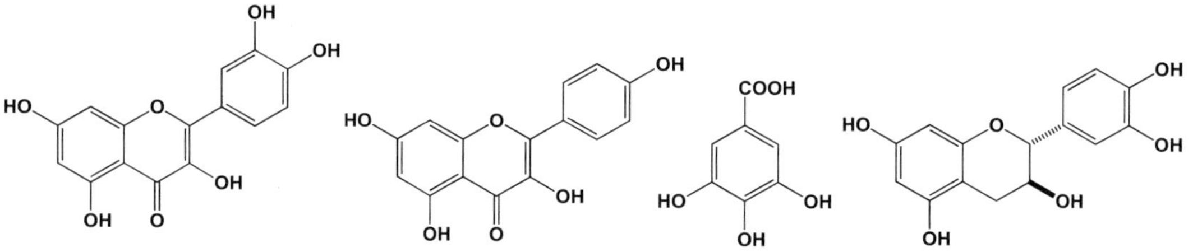

(114) (115) (116) (117)

Fig. (24). Gallic acid (**116**) and polyphenols (**114**, **115** and **117**) with antioxidant activities isolated from the roots of *S. officinalis*.

Furthermore, dietary curcumin also prevented Aβ-induced spatial memory deficits in the Morris water maze and postsynaptic density loss and reduced Aβ deposits [311]. To better evaluate whether **118** could affect AD-like pathology in Tg2576 mice, both low and high doses of **118** were administered andshowed to be able to reduce significantly oxidized proteins and interleukin-1β (IL-1β), a pro-inflammatory cytokine that appear elevated in the brains of these mice [312]. Besides its antiamyloid properties, compound **118** can also show antioxidant, anti-inflammatory and cholesterol lowering properties that play important role in ameliorating the deleterious consequences of AD. For this reasons, many other studies are in progress to evaluate its safety, tolerability and bioavailability [313].

Resveratrol (**120**, Fig. **26**), another polyphenolic compound of recent interest, was firstly isolated and identified in 1940 from *Veratrum grandiflorum* [314] and later from the roots of *Polygonum cuspidatum*, a plant used in traditional Oriental medicine [315]. Until 1992, it remained neglected when it was suggested that resveratrol was the active ingredient in wines causing reduction of serum lipids. From 1997, the interest by **120** was reinforced when it was shown that it could have chemopreventive activity [314, 315]. Thus, in recent years many studies have been conducted to evaluate therapeutic properties and possible mechanisms of action of resveratrol [314]. To date, many sources of **120** were identified, including skin of grapes, raspberries, mulberries, pistachios and peanuts, besides plants species such as *Arachis hypogaea, Rhizoma polygoni cuspidate, Yucca shidigera, Cassia quinquangulata, Rheum rhaponticum* among others [316, 317]. Resveratrol represents 5-10% of the biomass of grape skins and it is present in concentrations ranging from 0.05 to 25 mg/L in most red wines and grape juices [318]. Recent studies have attributed to compound **120** antiinflammatory, analgesic, antioxidant and anti-isquemic activities [317, 319, 320] and at this moment much efforts and attention have been devoted to stablish its properties and mechanisms of action in neurodegenerative diseases and aging [321].

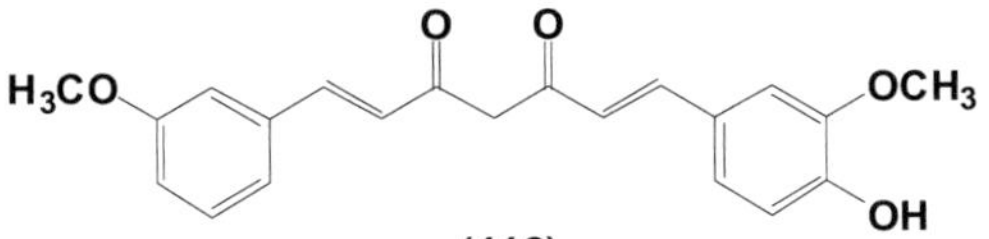

(118)

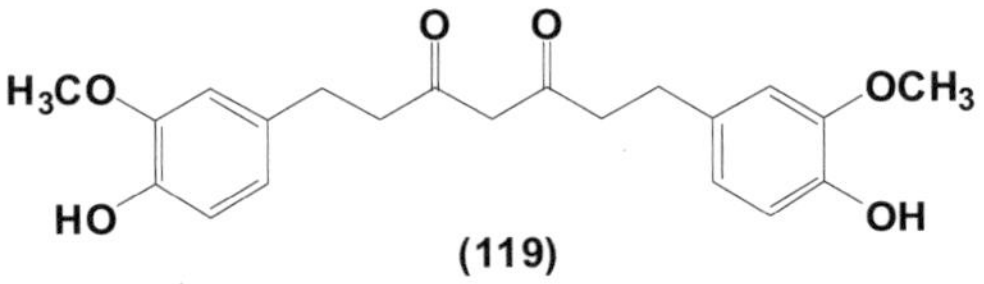

(119)

Fig. (25). Curcumin (**118**), isolated from *C. longa* and its main metabolite ThC (**119**).

Epidemiological studies have shown that moderate diary consumption of red wine can attenuate clinical manifestations produced by DA [322], which have been corroborated by the diminishing in the DA-related deterioration of spatial memory in mice [323], increasing in cells viability in cultures [324] and memory improvement in different behavioral tests [325]. Facing the pathological hallmarks of DA, treatment with **120** resulted in significantly inhibition of β-amyloid peptide polymerization [326], through a mechanism that not seems to be related to β-amyloid, once **120** do not act on the activity of β- and γ-secrctases, but indirectly stimulates the proteasomal degradation of β-amyloid peptides [327]. In 1999, Miloso and co-workers showed that **120** could activate ERK1/2 kinases in neuroblastoma cells [328] and more recently, Han and co-workers also reported that protective effects of **120** on β-amyloid protein-induced toxicity in cultured rat hippocampal cells are related to activation of PKC [329]. Other hypothesis for neuroprotective activity of **120** have taking into account its capability to enhance the intracellular free-radical scavenger glutathione, decrease malondialdehyde levels and suppress AChE activity [324]. In addition, Chen and co-workers have observed that the neurodegeneration induced by β-amyloid peptides depends on contributions from surrounding glia where nuclear factor κ-B (NF-κB) signaling activation plays an important role [330]. In support to these data, compound **120** significantly reduces the expression of genes modulated by NF-κB, such as iNOS, COX-2 and chatepsin, as well as NO and prostaglandine E_2 (PGE_2) metabolites [330, 331]. In spite of these many supporting data, there is no direct experimental evidence that the consumption of red wine or resveratrol itself beneficially AD. Considering that resveratrol is present in red wine in average amounts of 0.88 μM, which is 10-fold lower than the minimal effective concentration demonstrated to be necessary to elicits *in vivo* effects (10-40 μM) [314], many authors support that the properties attributed to **120** may be, in reality, due to other antioxidant-constituents present in red wine.

Taking into account the pathophysiology of PD, dopamine theory for explanation of cell death of nigrostriatal dopaminergic neurons consider that this cathecolamine can be oxidized spontaneously or by some enzyme as MAO-B or COX-2 to generate free radicals [332], then dopamine oxidation products can suffer polymerization to form a neurotoxin called neuromelanin [333]. In this regard, low doses of **120** (~5 μM) are capable to attenuate dopamine-induced cell death in neuroblastoma cells by activation of the antiapoptotic factor Bcl-2 and inhibition of caspase-3 [334]. Antoher theory suggests that the NO is involved in superoxide radicals generation and lipid peroxidation, leading to the release of arachidonic acid (AA). In fact, 0.1 mM of **120** was effective in the prevention of NO- and cyclic GMP-dependent inhibitory effect on AA incorporation into phophatidylinositol possibly by NOS inhibition [335]. In addition, Dore and co-workers postulated that the induction of heme-oxygenase by stilbenoid antioxidants, such as **120**, could lead to a protection against neuronal disorders [336].

Face to all these data, **120** have been considered the most effective polyphenol constituent in producing beneficial health effects of grape and red wine, such as protection against neurodegenerative diseases [337-340], evidenced by amelioration of oxidative damage in synaptic membranes in the brain induced by chronic alcohol consumption [338, 340] and prevention of chronic ethanol-induced increase in COX-2 *m*RNA expression in the rat brain [338]. Studies with PC-12 cells showed that compound **90** was more effective in protecting against oxidative damage than vitamins E and C combined [341] and also demonstrated neuroprotective effects in Parkinson's disease models resultant from alleviating oxidative damage induced by neurotoxins [341, 342a].

The multiple roles of resveratrol (**120**) as an antioxidant and life-promoting agent make it an attractive candidate for treatment of neurodegenerative disorders, and several studies have demonstrated its ability to protect neurons against Aβ-induced toxicity *in vitro* [46, 342b-e]. This effect was confirmed by the observation that combination of **120** with other polyphenolic compounds, such as catechin (**117**) can produce synergism in the evidenced protective effects [343-345]. Moreover, Ono and co-workers demonstrated that **120** can also inhibits formation and extension of Aβ fibrils and destabilizes the fibrilized Aβ [346, 347]. Despite the unknown mechanism related to the ability of **120** to minimize ROS production from NADPH oxidase, a number of studies have demonstrated its effects in the suppression of neuroinflammatory responses, attenuating iNOS and COX-2 expression [331, 348, 349].

Several preclinical studies have suggested that **120** may be useful in the protection of brain and spinal cord against traumatic neuronal injury, due to its ability to modulate different oxidative stress neuronal markers *in vivo* at the injury site. In brain, compound **120** decreases lactate dehydrogenase, xanthine oxidase, metalloproteinase 9, heme-oxygenase, and malondialdehyde levels, and it increases reduced glutathione levels induced by several types of injury [350, 351]. Moreover, **120** inhibits peroxisome proliferator-activated receptors α (PPARα) [352], decrease NFκB p65 expression involved in inflammation after ischemia-reperfusion injury [314], and in cultures it also inhibits postsynaptic glutamate receptors and voltage-activated K^+ channels [353]. All these effects combined lead to a decrease in anxiety, motor improvement, cognitive skills, attenuation of edema and cellular death as well as glial cell activation [354, 355]. Furthermore, some authors suggest that neuroprotection by resveratrol on memory improvement is mainly a result of its antioxidant properties [356, 357].

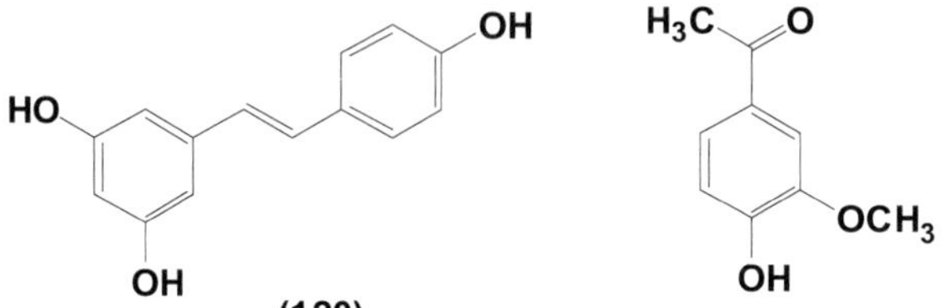

(120) **(121)**

Fig. (26). Resveratrol (**120**) andapocynin (**121**), plant-derived phenolic antioxidant and neuroprotective compounds.

Picrorhiza kurroa is a creeping plant native to the mountains of India, Nepal, Tibet and Pakistan used for centuries for treatment of various inflammatory diseases [358]. During an activity-guided study for immunomodulatory constituents from *P. kurroa*, apocynin (**121**, Fig. **26**) was discovered as a powerful antioxidant and anti-inflammatory compound, specifically blocking the activity of NADPH oxidase through interfering with the assembly of the cytosolic NADPH oxidase components with its membrane components [359]. Recent studies disclosed that brain cells constitutively express a superoxide-generating enzyme analogous to the NADPH oxidase in phagocytes [360]. NADPH oxidase-dependent production of superoxide radicals has been identified as the major contributor to oxidative and inflammatory responses in the brain under different injury conditions. Activation of NADPH oxidase in glial cells is linked to increased secretion of cytokines and other inflammatory factors [361] that may interact with nitric oxide from iNOS to form the toxic peroxynitrite, which is considered an important factor associated with neuronal death [362]. Besides suppression of NF-κB pathway and to prevent COX-2 expression in activated monocytes, apocynin (**121**) showed to be also effective against Aβ-induced microglial proliferation and lipopolysaccharide (LPS) and interferon γ-induced neuronal death [363-365]. However, an apparent limitation to the use of **121** for treatment of neurodegenerative disturbances is the high doses necessary to produce desired therapeutic effects [43].

Despite different neurodegenerative diseases are manifestations associated to complex diverse genetic and epi-genetic factors, there are strong evidences to believe that oxidative stress is a common factor playing a central role in the pathogenesis of these disorders. While many pathological conditions are associated to ROS production from mitochondria, more recent studies have unveiled an important role of ROS from NADPH oxidase. It seems that polyphenolic compounds such as catechin (**117**), curcumin (**118**), resveratrol (**120**), apocynin (**121**), epigallocatechin-gallate (**45**) not only exhibit potent antioxidantive properties for scavenging free radicals, but may also act on specific signaling pathways for regulating inflammatory responses, which supports the use of natural phenolic compounds as supplements in promoting general health and preventing age-related diseases in humans [43].

5. CONCLUDING REMARKS

Considering the diversity and complexity of genetic and epi-genetic factors underlying manifestations of neurodegenerative diseases, such as Alzheimer's and Parkinson's diseases, where many abnormal physiologic aspects should be considered as consequence of exposition to environmental toxins and risk factors associated to cardiovascular abnormalities, poor quality of life and dietary, and aging, there are many targets to be considered in the challenge to discover new effective drugs and mechanisms to treat these disorders or, at least, furnish better life conditions. In this context, new chemical entities capable to act in the selective inhibition of key enzymes such as AChE, NADPH oxidase, MAO-B, in the suppressing of β-amiloid protein deposits, degradation of microtubules to generate TAU fragments neurobrilary tangles and neuroinflammation are of capital importance for the development of novel and innovative therapeutical alternatives. Among many pathological conditions associated to emerge and evolution of AD and PD, there are sufficient reasons to believe that oxidative stress plays an important role in the installation of neuroinflammatory process, as consequence of ROS and NOS overproduction, lead to unbalance in mitochondrial function, abnormal apoptosis process and neuronal injury. As part of the efforts focused in the identification of new lead compounds, plants seems to be an interesting alternative due to the modern facilities to cultivate medicine promising species, to isolate and identify extracts, fractions and pure active metabolites and, of course, to have access to rapid, selective and effective pharmacological models to permit *in vitro* and *in vivo* evaluation of thousands of substances per day. However, despite of many studies that have been conducted in the last two decades, and many promise active compounds identified with diverse modes and sites of possible action, rational treatment of CNS disorders by plant constituents seems to be in infancy due to the complex chemistry and pharmacology of a plant extract, which contain a bewildering variety of chemical entities. In addition, many of these active compounds have been disclosed to be active as single molecules, but others seem to exert their pharmacologic properties as a result of synergy with other analogue metabolites. Recent advances in analytical chemistry, spectroscopic methods and in neuropharmacology have been decisive to the discovery of new molecules that can be promising candidates to new prototype compounds or have lead to identification of new structural frameworks and pharmacophoric subunits useful as models to the design of new innovative bioactive molecules.

After the 2nd world war, until recently, we had observed a very little attention given by the scientific community to the benefits, as accepted by the medicine, of the therapeutic usefulness of plants endowed with neuroactive properties, but in counterpart recently this view have been changed. Many reasons could be cited to explain this turned point, among them the wrong belief that plants, by originating directly from nature, must be less active toxic than synthetic compounds, and the recent strategies of Pharmaceutical Industry to look nature, and specially plants, as being a good bussiness as more and more people were prone for this unconventional form of therapy. In fact, by so many examples cited in this review, Chinese and Ayurveda Medicine have played an important role in the discovery of new active compounds and biological targets, and helping to understand many aspects related to the relief, treatment, and or prevention of neurodegenerative disordes. As we can conclude, due to this complex universe of research, many efforts are still necessary to complete understand the hallmarks of neurogenerative pathologies, their causes and modes of therapeutical intervention, but maybe the integration of natural chemistry, medicinal chemistry, pharmacology, biology and other associated disciplines could be the most promising way to drug discovery and ensures a greater chance to advance natural products and natural-based products into therapeutically useful drugs.

To reinforce this point of view, we can medidate about Schultes's words: "People whom we have to consider members of less-advanced societies have consistently looked to the Plant kingdom… for the betterment of life. Should we as chemists, pharmacologists and botanicals - with so many and varied means at our disposal - not take a lesson from them?" [366].

ACKNOWLEDGEMENTS

This work was supported by grants from INCT de Fármacos e Medicamentos (INOFAR, CNPq, Brazil, #573.564/2008-6) and PPSUS (FAPEMIG-MG, Brazil, #3336/06) and Universal Project (CNPq, Brazil, #471178/2007-1). The authors are also grateful for the fellowships granted by CAPES, CNPq, FAPERJ, FAPEMIG and PROBIC-UNIFAL.

CONFLICT OF INTEREST

The authors state that there is no conflict of interest.

REFERENCES

[1] Viegas CJ, Bolzani VS; Barreiro EJ. Os produtos naturais e a química medicinal moderna. Quim Nova 2006; 29(2): 326-37.

[2] Cragg GM, Newmann DJ, Snader KMJ. Natural products in drug discovery and development. J Nat Prod 1997; 60(1): 52-60.

[3] Cragg GM, Newmann DJ; Snader KMJ. Natural products as sources of new drugs over the period 1981-2002. J Nat Prod 2003; 66(7): 1022-37.

[4] Newmann DJ, Cragg G M. Natural products as sources of new drugs over the last 25 years. J Nat Prod 2007; 70: 461-77.

[5] Newmann DJ. Natural products as leads to potential drugs: an old process or the new hope for drug discovery? J Med Chem 2008; 51(9): 2589-99.

[6] Ojima I. Modern natural products chemistry and drug Discovery. J Med Chem 2008; 51(9): 2587-8.

[7] Standaert DG, Young AB. Treatment of Central Nervous System Degenerative Disorders. In: Hardamn JG, Limbird LE, Molinoff PB, Ruddon RW, Gilman AG, Eds. The

Pharmacological Basis of Therapeutics. 9nd ed. United States: McGraw Hill 1996; pp 503-519.

[8] Campos HC, Rocha M D, Viegas FPD, *et al.* The role of natural products in the Discovery of new drug candidates for the treatment of neurodegenerative disorders I: Parkinsons disease. CNS Neurol Disord Drug Targets 2011; 10: 239-50.

[9] Rocha RD, Viegas FPD, Campos HC, *et al.* The role of natural products in the Discovery of new drug candidates for the treatment of neurodegenerative disorders II: Alzheimer's Disease. CNS Neurol Disord Drug Targets 2011; 10: 251-70.

[10] (a) Carlini EA. Plants and the central nervous system. Pharmacol Biochem Behav 2003; 75(3): 501-12. b) Grunze H, Langosch J, Schirrmacher K, Bingmann D, Von Wegerer J, Walden J. Kava pyrones exert effects on neuronal transmission and transmembraneous cation currents similar to estabilished mood stabilizers-a review. Prog Neuropsychopharmacol Biol Psychiatry 2001; 25(8): 1555-70.

[11] Eisenberg DM, Kessler RC, Foster C, Norlock FE, Calkins DR, Delbanco TL. Unconventional medicine in the United States. Prevalence, costs, and patterns of use. N Eng J Med 1993; 328(4): 246-52.

[12] Speroni E, Billi R, Mercati V, Boncompagni E, Toja E. Sedative effects of crude extract of passiflora incarnata after oral administration. Phytoter Res 1996; 10: S92-4.

[13] Soleimani R, Younos C, Jarmouni S, Bousta D, Misslin R, Mortier F. Behavioural effects of Passiflora incarnata L. and its indole alkaloid and flavonoid derivatives and maltol in the mouse. J Ethnopharmacol 1997; 57(1): 11-20.

[14] Dhawan K, Kumar S, Sharma A. Anti-anxiety studies on extracts of Passiflora incarnata Linneaus. J Ethnopharmacol 2001; 78: 165-70.

[15] Kennedy DO, Scholey AB. Ginseng: potential for the enhancement of cognitive performance and mood. Pharmacol Biochem Behav 2003; 75: 687-700.

[16] Raddad K, Gille G, Liu L, Rausch WD. Use of ginseng in medicine with emphasis on neurodegenerative disorders. J Pharmacol Sci 2006; 100: 175-86.

[17] Dewick PM, Medicinal Natural Products: A Biosynthetic Approach. New York: John Wiley & Sons, 1997.

[18] Wen TC, Yoshimura H, Matsuda S, Lim JH, Sakanaka M. Ginseng root prevents learning disability and neuronal loss in gerbils with 5-minute forebrain ischemia Acta Neuropathol 1996; 91(1): 15-22.

[19] Zhang YG, Liu TP. Influences of ginsenosides Rb_1 and Rg_1 on reversible focal brain ischemia in rats. Acta Pharmacol Sin 1996; 17(1): 44-8.

[20] Kim YC, Kim SR, Markelonis GJ, Oh TH. Ginsenosides Rb1 and Rg3 protect cultured rat cortical cells from glutamate-induced neurodegeneration. J Neurosci Res 1998; 4: 426-32.

[21] Liao B, Newmark H, Zhou R. Neuroprotective effects of ginseng total saponin and ginsenosides Rb1 and Rg1 on spinal cord neurons *in vitro*. Exp Neurol 2002; 173: 224-34.

[22] Byun BH, Shin I, Yoon YS, Kim SI, Joe CO. Modulation of protein kinase C activity in NIH 3T3 cells by plant glycosides from Panax ginseng. Planta Medica1997; 63: 389-92.

[23] Liberti LE, Der Mardesian A. Evaluation of commercial ginseng product. J Pharm Sci 1978; 10: 1487-9.

[24] Phillipson JD, Anderson LA. Ginseng-quality, safety and efficacy? Pharm J 1984; 232: 161-5.

[25] Soldati F, Sticher O. HPLC separation and quantitative determination of ginsenosides from Panax ginseng, Panax quinquefolium and from ginseng drug preparations. 2nd communication. Planta Medica 1980; 39(8): 348-57.
[26] Kennedy DO, Scholey AB, Wesnes KA. The dose-dependent cognitive effects of acute administration of Ginkgo biloba to healthy young volunteers. Psychopharmacol 2000; 151: 416-23.
[27] Kennedy DO, Scholey AB, Wesnes KA. Dose dependent changes in cognitive performance and mood following acute administration of Ginseng to healthy young volunteers. Nutr Neurosci 2001; 4(4): 295-310.
[28] Kennedy DO, Scholey AB, Wesnes KA. Differential, dose dependent changes im cognitive performace following acute administration of a Ginkgo biloba/Panax ginseng combination to healthy young volunteers. Nutr Neurosci 2001; 4(5): 399-412.
[29] Kennedy DO, Scholey AB, Wesnes KA. Modulation of cognition and mood following administration of single doses of Ginkgo biloba, Ginseng and a Ginkgo/Ginseng combination to healthy young adults. Physiol Behav 2002; 75: 1-13.
[30] Kennedy DO, Scholey AB, Tildesley NTJ, Perry EK, Wesnes KA. Modulation of mood and cognitive performance following acute administration of Melissa officinalis (Lemon Balm). Pharmacol Biochem Behav 2002; 72(4): 953-64.
[31] Kennedy D, Scholey AB, Drewery L, Marsh R, Moore B, Ashton H. Electroencephalograph (EEG) effects of single doses of Ginkgo biloba and Panax ginseng in healthy young volunteers. Pharmacol Biochem Behav 2003; 75: 701-9.
[32] Wesnes KA, Ward T, McGinty A, Petrini O. The memory enhancing effects of a Ginkgo biloba/Panax ginseng combination in healthy middle aged volunteers. Psychopharmacology 2000; 152: 353-61.
[33] Standaert DG, Young AH. Treatment of Central Nervous System Degenerative Disorders. In: Goodman and Gilman's, Eds. The Pharmacological Basis of Therapeutics. 9nd ed. New York: McGraw Hill 1996; pp. 503-19.
[34] Arnold SE, Hyman BT, Flory J, Damasio AR, Van Hoesen GW. The topographical and neuroanatomical distribution of neurofibrillary tangles and neuritic plaques in the cerebral cortex of patients with Alzheimer's disease. Cereb Cortex 1991; 1: 103-16.
[35] Gibb WR. Neuropathology of Parkinson's disease and related syndromes. Neuro Clin 1992; 10: 361-76.
[36] Olney JW. Brain Lesions, Obesity, and Other Disturbances in Mice Treated with Monosodium Glutamate. Science 1969; 164: 719-21.
[37] Lipton SA, Rosenberg PA. Excitatory amino acids as a final common pathway for neurologic disorders. New Engl J Med 1994; 330: 613-22.
[38] Wallace DC. Mitochondrial Genetics: A Paradigm for Aging and Degenerative Diseases? Science 1992; 256: 628-32.
[39] Schapira AH, Mann VM, Cooper JM, Dexter D, *et al.* Anatomic and disease specificity of NADH CoQ1 reductase (complex I) deficiency in Parkinson's disease. J Neurochem 1990; 55: 2142-5.
[40] McKeel DW, Jr Price JL, Miller JP, Grant EA, Xiong C, Berg L. Neuropathologic criteria for diagnosing Alzheimer disease in persons with pure dementia of Alzheimer type. J Neuropathol Exp Neurol 2004; 63: 1028-37.
[41] Delagarza VW. Pharmacological treatment of Alzheimer's disease: An update. Am Family Phys 2003; 68(7): 1365-72.

[42] Small GW, Rabins PV, Barry PP, *et al*. Diagnosis and treatment of Alzheimer disease and related disorders. JAMA 1997; 278(16): 1363-71.
[43] Sun AY, Wang Q, Simonyi A, Sun GY. Botanical Phenolics and Brain Health. Neuromol Med 2008; 10: 259-74.
[44] Butterfield DA, Griffin S, Munch G, Pasinetti GM. Amyloid β-peptide and amyloid pathology are central to the oxidative stress and inflammatory cascades under which Alzheimer's disease brain exists. J Alzheimer's Disease 2002; 4: 193-201.
[45] Selkoe DJ. Alzheimer's disease results from the cerebral accumulation and cytotoxicity of amyloid β-protein. J Alzheimer Disease 2001; 3: 75-80.
[46] Snyder EM, Nong Y, Almeida CG, *et al*. Regulation of NMDA receptor trafficking by amyloid beta. Nat Neurosci 2005; 8: 1051-8.
[47] Kishida KT, Pao M, Holland SM, Klann E. NADPH oxidase is required for NMDA receptor-dependent activation of ERK in hippocampal area CA1. J Neurochem 2005; 94: 299-306.
[48] Kishida KT, Klann E. Sources and targets of reactive oxygen species in synaptic plasticity and memory. Antioxid and Redox Signal 2007; 9: 233-44.
[49] Shelat PB, Chalimoniuk M, Wang JH, *et al*. Amyloid beta peptide and NMDA induce ROS from NADPH oxidade and AA release from cytosolic phosphoslipase A2 in cortical neurons. J Neurochem 2008; 106(1): 45-55.
[50] Sang N, Chen C. Lipid signaling *and* synaptic plasticit. Neuroscientist 2006; 12: 425-34.
[51] Kriem B, Sponne I, Fifre A, *et al*. Cytosolic phospholipase A2 mediates neuronal apoptosis induced by soluble oligomers of the amyloid-β peptide. FASEB J 2005; 19: 85-7.
[52] Abramov AY, Canevari L, Duchen MR. β-Amyloid peptides induce mitocondrial dysfunction and oxidative stress in astrocytes and death of neurons through activation of NADPH oxidase. J Neurosc. 2004; 24: 565-75.
[53] Davies P, Maloney AJ. Selective loss of central cholinergic neurons in Alzheimer's disease. Lancet 1976; 2: 1403.
[54] Bowen DM, Smith CB, White P, Davison AN. Neurotransmitter-related enzymes and indices of hypoxia in senile dementia and other abiotrophies. Brain 1976; 99: 459-96.
[55] Perry EK, Gibson PH, Blessed G, Perry RH, Tomlinson BE. Choline acetyltransferase and glutamic acid decarboxylase activities in necropsy brain tissue. J Neurol Sci 1977; 34(2): 247-65.
[56] Hardy J. A hundred years of Alzheimer's disease research. Neuron 2006; 52: 3-13.
[57] Bushnell DM, Martin ML. Quality of life and Parkinson's disease: translation and validation of the US Parkinson's Disease Questionnaire (PDQ-39). Qual Life Res 1999; 8: 345-50.
[58] Dorsey ER, Constantinescu R, Thompson JP, *et al*. Projected number of people with Parkinson disease in the most populous nations, 2005 through 2030. Neurology 2007; 68: 384-6.
[59] Cardoso SM, Moreira PI, Agostinho P, Pereira C, Oliveira CR. Neurodegenerative pathways in Parkinson's disease: therapeutic strategies. Curr Drug Targets CNS Neurol Dis 2005; 4: 405-19.
[60] Miller RL, James-Kracke M, Sun GY, Sun AY. Oxidative and inflammatory pathways in Parkison's diease. Neurochem Res 2009; 34: 55-65.
[61] Dauer W, Przedborski S. Parkinson's disease: mechanisms and models. Neuron 2003; 39: 889-909.

[62] Samii A, Nutt JG, Ransom BR. Parkinson's disease. Lancet 2004; 363: 1783-93.
[63] Moreira PI, Siedlak SL, Aliev G, *et al.* Oxidative stress mechanisms and potential therapeutics in Alzheimer disease. J Neural Transm 2005; 112: 921-32.
[64] Beal M.F. Mitochondrial dysfunction and oxidative damage in Alzheimer's and Parkinson's diseases and coenzyme Q10 as a potential treatment. J Bioenerg Biomembr 2004; 36(4): 381-6.
[65] Abekawa T, Ohmori T, Koyama T. Effect of synthesus inhibition on striatal dopamine release and stereotyped behavior induced by a single administration of methamphetamine. Progress Neuro-Psychopharmacol Biol Psychiatry 1997; 21(5): 831-8.
[66] Gonzales-Hernandez T, Perez de la Cruz MA, Mantolan-Sarmiento B. Histochemical and immunohistochemical detection of neurons that produce nitric oxide: effect of diferente fixative parameters and immunoreactivity against non-neuronal NOS antisera. J Histochem Cytochem 1996; 44(12): 1399-413.
[67] Gao HM, Hong JS, Zhang W, Liu B. Synergistic dopaminergic neurotoxicity of the pesticide rotenone and inflammogen lipopolysaccharide: relevance to the etiology of Parkinson's disease. J Neurosci 2003; 23: 1228-36.
[68] Gao HM, Liu B, Zhang W, Hong JS. Critical role of microglial NADPH oxidase-derived free radicals in the *in vitro* MPTP model of Parkinson's disease. FASEB J 2003; 17: 1954-6.
[69] Mander PK, Jekabsone A, Brown GC. Microglia prolifer- ation is regulated by hydrogen peroxide from NADPH oxidase. J Immunol 2006; 176: 1046-52.
[70] Brooks AI, Chadwick CA, Gelbard HA, Cory-Slechta DA, Federoff HJ. Paraquat elicited neurobehavioral sindrome caused by dopaminergic neuron loss. Brain Res 1999; 823: 1-10.
[71] Liou HH, Tsai MC, Chen CJ, Jeng JS, Chang YC, Chen SY, Chen RC. Environmental risk factors and Parkinson's disease: A case-control study in Taiwan. Neurology 1997; 48 (6): 1583-8.
[72] Yang WL, Sun AY. Paraquat-induced cell death in PC12 cells. Neurochem Res1998; 23: 1387-94.
[73] Koshimura I, Imai H, Hidano T, *et al.* Dimethoxypheylethylamine and tatrahydropapaverine are toxic to the nigrostriatal system. Brain Res 1997, 773: 108-16.
[74] Benedetto A, Au C, Aschner M. Manganese-induced dopaminergic neurodegeneration: insights into mechanisms and genetics shared with Parkinson's disease. Chem Rev 2009; 109: 4862-84.
[75] Li X, Sun AY. Paraquat induced activation of transcription factor AP-1 and apoptosis in PC12 cells. J Neur Trans 1999; 106(1): 1-21.
[76] Yang W, Sun AY. Paraquat-induced free radical reaction in mouse brain microsomes. Neurochem Res 1998; 23: 47-53.
[77] Shober A. Classic toxin-induced animal models of Parkinson's disease: 6-OHDA and MPTP. Cell Tissue Res 2004; 318: 215-24.
[78] Lim ML, Mercer LD, Nagley P, Beart PM. Rotenone and MPP+ preferentially redistribute apoptosis-inducing factor in apoptotic dopamine neurons. Neuroreport 2007; 18: 307-12.
[79] Firestone JA, Smith-Weller T, Franklin G, Swanson P, Lonstreth WT, Checkoway H. Pesticides and risk of Parkinson disease: a population-based case-control study. Arch Neurol 2005; 62: 91-5.
[80] Semchuk KM, Love EJ, Lee RG. Parkinson's disease: a test of the multifactorial etiologic hypothesis. Neurology 1993; 43: 1173-80.

[81] Yang WL, Sun AY. Paraquat-induced free radical reaction in mouse brain microsomes. Neurochem Res 1998; 23: 47-53.
[82] Liou HH, Tsai MC, Chen CJ, *et al.* Environmental risk factors and Parkinson's disease: a case-control study in Taiwan. Neurology 1997; 48: 1583-8.
[83] Schober A. Classic toxin-induced animal models of Parkinson's disease: 6-OHDA and MPTP. Cell Tissue Res 2004; 318: 215-24.
[84] Jenner P. Functional models of Parkinson's disease: A valuable tool in the development of novel therapies. Ann Neurol 2008; 64: S16-29.
[85] Simola N, Morelli M, Carta A. The 6-Hydroxydopamine Model of Parkinson's Disease. Neurotoxic Res 2007; 11: 151-67.
[86] Lee KY, Sung SH, Kim YC. Neuroprotective Bibenzyl Glycosides of Stemona tuberosa Roots. J Nat Prod 2006; 69: 679-81.
[87] Liu DZ, Zhu J, Jin DZ, *et al.* Behavioral recovery following sub-chronic paeoniflorin administration in the striatal 6-OHDA lesion rodent model of Parkinson's disease. Ethnopharmacol 2007; 112: 327-32.
[88] Abin-Carriquiry JA, Costa G, Urbanavicius J, *et al. In vivo* modulation of dopaminergic nigrostriatal pathways by cytisine derivatives: Implications for Parkinson's disease. Eur J Pharmacol 2008; 589: 80-4.
[89] Tseng YJ, Wen ZH, Dai CF, Chiang MY, Sheu JH. Nanolobatolide, a new C_{18} metabolite from the Formosan soft coral *Sinularia nanolabata*. Org Lett 2009; 11: 5030-2.
[90] Sung SH, Kim ES, Lee KY, Lee MK, KimYC. A new neuroprotective compound of Ligustrum japonicum leaves. Planta Med 2006; 72: 62-4.
[91] Zhao DL, Zou LB, Lin S, Shi JG, Zhu HB. Anti-apoptotic effect of esculin on dopamine-induced cytotoxicity in the human neuroblastoma SH-SY5Y cell line Neuropharmacology 2007; 53: 724-32.
[92] Wang, L.; Xu, S.; Xu, X.; Chan, P.*J.* (-)- Epigallocatechin-3-Gallate protects SH-SY5Y cells against 6-OHDA-induced cell death through STST3 activation. Alzheimer's Disease 2009; 17: 295-304.
[93] Kim JS, Kim JM, JJ O, Jeon BS. Inhibition of inducible nitric oxide synthase expression and cell death by (−)-epigallocatechin-3-gallate, a green tea catechin, in the 1-methyl-4-phenyl-1, 2, 3, 6-tetrahydropyridine mouse model of Parkinson's disease. J Clin Neurosci 2010; 17: 1165-8.
[94] Mu X, He G, Cheng Y, Li X, Xu B, Du G. Baicalein exerts neuroprotective effects in 6-hydroxydopamine-induced experimental parkinsonism *in vivo* and *in vitro*. Pharmacol Biochem Behav 2009; 92: 642-8.
[95] Landrigan PJ, Sonawane B, Butler RN, Trasande L, Callan R, Droller D. Early environmental origins of neuro-degenerative disease in later life. Environ Health Perspect 2005; 113: 1230-3.
[96] Uversky, VN. Neurotoxicant-induced animal models of Parkinson's disease: understanding the role of rotenone, maneb and paraquat in neurodegeneration. Cell Tissue Res 2004; 318: 225-41.
[97] Thiruchelvam M, Richfield EK, Baggs RB, Tank AW, Cory-Slechta DA. The nigrostriatal dopaminergic system as a preferential target of repeated exposures to combined paraquat and maneb: implications for Parkinson's Disease. J Neurosci Res 2000; 20: 9207-14.

[98] Brooks AI, Chadwick CA, Gelbard HA, Cory-Slechta DA, Federoff HJ. Paraquat elicited neurobehavioral syndrome caused by dopaminergic neuron loss. Brain Res 1999; 823: 1-10.

[99] Yang WL, Sun AY. Paraquat-induced cell death in PC12 cells. Neurochem Res 1998; 23: 1387-94.

[100] Shimizu K, Matsubara K, Ohtaki K, Shiono H. Paraquat leads to dopaminergic neural vulnerability in organotypic midbrain culture. Neurosci Res 2003; 46: 523-32.

[101] Kang D, Miyako K, Kuribayashi F, Hasegawa E. Changes of energy metabolism induced by 1-methyl-4-phenylpyridinium (MPP+)-related compounds in rat pheochromocytoma PC12 cells. Arch Biochem Biophys 1997; 337: 75-80.

[102] Chun HS, Gibson GE, DeGiorgio LA, Zhang H, Kidd VJ, Son JH. Dopaminergic cell death induced by MPP(+), oxidant and specific neurotoxicants shares the common molecular mechanism. J Neurochem 2001; 76: 1010-21.

[103] Shimizu K, Matsubara K, Ohtaki K, Fujimaru S, Saito O, Shiono H. Paraquat induces long-lasting dopamine overflow through the excitotoxic pathway in the striatum of freely moving rats. Brain Res 2003; 976: 243-52.

[104] Peng J, Stevenson FF, Doctrow SR, Andersen JK. Superoxide dismutase/catalase mimetics are neuroprotective against selective paraquat-mediated dopaminergic neuron death in the substantial nigra: implications for Parkinson disease. J Biol Chem 2005; 280: 29194-8.

[105] Yang W, Tiffany-Castiglioni E. The bipyridyl herbicide paraquat produces oxidative stress-mediated toxicity in human neuroblastoma SH-SY5Y cells: relevance to the dopaminergic pathogenesis. J Toxicol Environ Health Part A 2005; 68(22): 1939-61.

[106] Thiruchelvam M, Prokopenko O, Cory-Slechta D, Richfield E, Buckley B, Mirochnitchenko O. Overexpression of superoxide dismutase or glutathione peroxidase protects against the paraquat + maneb-induced Parkinson Disease phenotype. J Biol Chem 2005; 280: 22530-9.

[107] Maguire-Zeiss KA, Short DW, Federoff HJ. Synuclein, dopamine and oxidative stress: co-conspirators in Parkinson's disease? Molecular Brain Research 2005; 134: 18-23.

[108] Kotake Y, Ohta S. MPP+ analogs acting on mitochondria and inducing neurodegeneration. Curr Med Chem 2003; 10: 2507-16.

[109] Carange J, Longpré F, Daoust B, Martinoli MG. 24-Epibrassinolide, a phytosterol from the brassinosteroid family, protects dopaminergic cells against MPP+-induced oxidative stress and apoptosis. J Toxicol 2011; Article ID 392859: 13 pages.

[110] Mander PK, Jekabsone A, Brown GC. Microglia proliferation is regulated by hydrogen peroxide from NADPH oxidase. J Immunol 2006; 176: 1046-52.

[111] Dringen R. Oxidative and antioxidative potential of brain microglial cells. Antioxid Redox Signal 2005; 7: 1223-33.

[112] Scheller C, Sopper S, Jenuwein M *et al.* Early impairment in dopaminergic neurotransmission in brains of SIV-infected rhesus monkeys due to microglia activation. J Neurochem 2005; 95(2): 377-87.

[113] Langston JW, Forno LS, Tetrud J, ReevesAG, Kaplan JA, Karluk D. Evidence of active nerve cell degeneration in the substantia nigra of humans years after 1-methyl-4-phenyl-1,2,3,6-tetrahydropyridine exposure. Ann Neurol 1999; 46: 598-605.

[114] Gao HM, Hong JS, Zhang W, Liu B. Distinct role for microglia in rotenone-induced degeneration of dopaminergic neurons. J Neurosci 2002; 22: 782-90.

[115] Casarejos MJ, Menendez J, Solano RM, Rodriguez-Navarro JA, Garcia de Yebenes J, Mena MA. Susceptibility to rotenone is increased in neurons from parkin null mice and is reduced by minocycline. J Neurochem 2006; 97: 934-46.
[116] Nishimoto S, Nishida E. MAPK signaling: ERK5 *versus* ERK1/2. EMBO Rep 2006; 7: 782-6.
[117] Bardwell L. Mechanisms of MAPK signaling specificity. Biochem Soc Trans 2006; 34: 837-41.
[118] Cuschieri J, Maier RV. Mitogen-activated protein kinase (MAPK).Crit Care Med 2005; 33: S417-19.
[119] Kaminska B. MAPK signaling pathways as molecular targets for anti-inflammatory therapy - from molecular mechanisms to therapeutic benefits. Biochim Biophys Acta 2005; 1754: 253-62.
[120] Uhlik, MT, Abell AN, Cuevas BD, Nakamura K, Johnson GL. Wiring diagrams of MAPK regulation by MEKK1, 2, and 3. Biochem Cell Biol 2004; 82: 658-63.
[121] Wagey R, Hu J, Pelech SL, Raymond LA, Krieger C. Modulation of NMDA-mediated excitotoxicity by protein kinase C. J Neurochem 2001; 78: 715-726.
[122] Ran X, Miao HH, Sheu FS, Yan D. Structural and Dynamic Characterization of a Neuron-Specific Protein Kinase C Substrate, Neurogranin. Biochemistry 2003; 42: 5143-50.
[123] Catarsi S, Drapeau P. Requirement for tyrosine phosphatase during serotonergic neuromodulation by protein kinase C. J Neurosci Res 1997; 17: 5792-7.
[124] Ahlemeyer B, Kolker S, Zhu Y, Hoffmann GF, Krieglstein J. Increase in glutamate-induced neurotoxicity by activated astrocytes involves stimulation of protein kinase C. J Neurochem. 2002; 82: 504-15.
[125] Battaini F. Protein kinase C isoforms as therapeutic targets in nervous system disease states. Pharmacol Res 2001; 44: 353-61.
[126] Gallagher HC, Murphy KJ, Foley AG, Regan CM. Protein kinase C delta regulates neural cell adhesion molecule polysialylation state in the rat brain. J Neurochem 2001; 77: 425-34.
[127] DeVries TA, Neville MC, Reyland ME. Nuclear import of PKCδ is required for apoptosis: identification of a novel nuclear import sequence. EMBO J 2002; 21: 6050-60.
[128] Leverrier S, Vallentin A, Joubert D. Positive feedback of protein kinase C proteolytic activation during apoptosis. Biochem J 2002; 368: 905-13.
[129] Anantharam V, Kitazawa M, Wagner J, Kaul S, Kanthasamy AG. Caspase-3-dependent proteolytic cleavage of protein kinase C is essential for oxidative stress-mediated dopaminergic cell death after exposure to methylcyclopentadienyl manganese tricarbonyl. J Neurosci Res 2002; 22(5): 1738-51.
[130] Bey E A, Xu B, Bhattacharjee A *et al.* Protein kinase C δ is required for p47phox phosphorylation and translocation in activated human monocytes. J Immunol 2004; 173: 5730-8.
[131] He R, Nanamor M, Sang H, Yin H, Dinauer MC, Ye RD. Reconstitution of chemotactic peptide-induced nicotinamide adenine dinucleotide phosphate (reduced) oxidase activation in transgenic COS-phox cells. J Immunol 2004; 173(12): 7462-70.
[132] Day BJ, Patel M, Calavetta L, Chang LY, Stamlet JS. A mechanism of paraquat toxicity involving nitric oxide synthase. PNAS 1999; 96(22): 12760-5.
[133] Duval DL, Miller DR, Collier J, Billings RE. Characterization of hepatic nitric oxide synthase: identification as the cytokine-inducible form primarily regulated by oxidants. Mol Pharmacol 1996; 50: 277-84.

[134] Margolis AS, Porasuphatana S, Rosen GM. Role of paraquat in the uncoupling of nitric oxide synthase. Biochim Biophys Acta 2000; 1524: 253-7.
[135] Guo Q, Tirosh O, Packer L. Inhibitory effect of α-lipoic acid and its positively charged amide analogue on nitric oxide production in RAW 264.7 macrophages. Biochem Pharmacol 2001; 61(5): 547-54.
[136] Shih CL, Chi SI, Chiu TH, Sun GY, Lin TN. Ethanol effects on nitric oxide production in cerebral pial cultures. Alcohol Clin Exp Res 2001; 25: 612-18.
[137] Connelly L, Madhani M, Hobbs AJ. Resistance to endotoxic shock in endothelial nitric oxide synthase (eNOS) knockout mice: a pro-inflammatory role for eNOS-derived NO. J Biol Chem 2005; 280: 10040-46.
[138] Xia J, Simonyi AS, Sun GY. Chronic ethanol and iron administration on iron content, neuronal nitric oxide synthase, and superoxide dismutase in rat cerebellum. Alcohol Clin Exp Res 1999; 23(4): 702-07.
[139] Gobbel GT, Chan TYY, Chan PH. Nitric Oxide- and Superoxide-Mediated Toxicity in Cerebral Endothelial Cells. J Pharmacol Exp Ther 1997; 282: 1600-07.
[140] Tomita M, Okuyama T, Ishikawa T, Hidaka K, Nohno T. The role of nitric oxide in paraquat-induced cytotoxicity in the human A549 lung carcinoma cell line. Free Radical Res 2001; 34(2): 193-202.
[141] Shin CY, Choi JW, Jang ES *et al.* Dehydroepiandrosterone inhibits the death of immunostimulated rat C6 glioma cells deprived of glucose. Brain Res 2001; 922(2): 267-75.
[142] Yamamoto F, Ohgari Y, Yamaki N, Kitajima S, Shimokawa O, Matsui H, Taketani S. The role of nitric oxide in delta-aminolevulinic acid (ALA)-induced photosensitivity of cancerous cells. Biochem Biophys Res Commun 2007; 353: 541-46.
[143] Goralski KB, Renton KW. Brain inflammation enhances 1-methyl-4-phenylpyridinium-evoked neurotoxicity in rats. Toxicol Appl Pharmacol 2004; 196: 381-89.
[144] Schroeder K, Sweet MJ, Hume DA. Signal integration between IFN gamma and TLR signaling pathways in macrophages. Immunobiology 2006; 211(6-8): 511-24.
[145] Anand P, Singh B, Singh N. A review on coumarins as acetylcholinesterase inhibitors for Alzheimer's disease. Bioorg Med Chem 2012; 20: 1175-80.
[146] Kang SY, Lee KY, Sung SH, Park MJ, Kim YC. Coumarins isolated from *Angelica gigas* inhibit acetylcholinesterase: structure−activity relationships. J Nat Prod 2001; 64: 683-85.
[147] Awang K, Chan G, Litaudon M, Ismail NH, Martin MT, Gueritte F. 4-Phenylcoumarins from *Mesua elegans* with acetylcholinesterase inhibitory activity. Bioorg Med Chem 2010; 18(22): 7873-77.
[148] Rollinger JM, Hornick A, Langer T, Stuppner H, Prast H. Acetylcholinesterase inhibitory activity of scopolin and scopoletin discovered by virtual screening of natural products. J Med Chem 2004; 47: 6248-54.
[149] Youkwan J, Sutthivaiyakit S, Sutthivaiyakit P. Citrusosides A-D and furanocoumarins with cholinesterase inhibitory activity from the fruit peels of *Citrus hystrix*. J Nat Prod 2010; 73: 1879-83.
[150] Kim S, Ahn K, Oh TH, Nah SY, Rhim H. Inhibitory effect of ginsenosides on NMDA receptor-mediated signals in rat hippocampal neurons. Biochem Biophys Res Commun 2002; 296: 247-54.

[151] Kim S, Kim T, Ahn K, Park WK, Nah SY, Rhim H. Ginsenoside Rg_3 antagonizes NMDA receptors through a glycine modulatory site in rat cultured hippocampal neurons. Biochem Biophys Res Commun 2004; 323: 416-24.

[152] Karikura M, Miyase T, Tanizawa H, Taniyama T, Takino Y. Studies on absorption, distribution, excretion and metabolism of ginseng saponins. VII. Comparison of the decomposition modes of ginsenoside-Rb1 and -Rb2 in the digestive tract of rats. Chem Pharm Bull 1991; 39: 2357-61.

[153] Bae EA, Han MJ, Choo MK, Park SY, Kim DH. Metabolism of 20(S)- and 20(R)-ginsenoside Rg3 by human intestinal bacteria and its relation to *in vitro* biological activities. Biol Pharm Bull 2002; 25(1): 58-63.

[154] Akao, T. Kanaoka, M.; Kabashi, K. Appearance of compound K, a major metabolite of ginsenoside Rb1 by intestinal bacteria, in rat plasma after oral administration-measurement of compound K by enzyme immunoassay. Biol Pharm Bull 1998; 21: 245-9.

[155] Hasegawa H, Sung JH, Matsumiya S, Uchiyama M. Main ginseng saponin metabolites formed by intestinal bacteria. Planta Med 1996; 62: 453-7.

[156] Park EK, Choo MK, Oh JK, Ryu JH, Kim DH. Ginsenoside Rh2 reduces ischemic brain injury in rats. Biol Pharm Bull 2004; 27: 433-6.

[157] Jeong SM, Lee JH, Kim JH, *et al.* Stereospecificity of ginsenoside Rg3 action on ion channels. Mol Cells 2004; 18: 383-9.

[158] Kang DI, Lee JY, Yang JY, *et al.* Evidence that the tertiary structure of 20(S)-ginsenoside Rg3 with tight hydrophobic packing near the chiral center is important for Na(+) channel regulation. Biochem Biophys Res Commun 2005; 333: 1194-201.

[159] Lee E, Kim S, Chung KC, *et al.* 20(S)-ginsenoside Rh_2, a newly identified active ingredient of ginseng, inhibits NMDA receptors in cultured rat hippocampal neurons. Eur J Pharmacol 2006; 536: 69-77.

[160] Kuryatov A, Laube B, Betz H, Kuhse J. Mutational analysis of the glycine-binding site of the NMDA receptor: structural similarity with bacterial amino acid-binding proteins. Neuron 1994; 12: 1291-300.

[161] Williams K, Kashiwagi K, Fukuchi J, Igarashi K. An acidic amino acid in the N-methyl-D-aspartate receptor that is important for spermine stimulation. Mol Pharmacol 1995; 48: 1087-98.

[162] Hirai H, Kirsch J, Laube B, Betz H, Kuhse J. The glycine binding site of the N-methyl-D-aspartate receptor subunit NR1: identification of novel determinants of co-agonist potentiation in the extracellular M3-M4 loop region. Proc Natl Acad Sci U.S.A. 1996; 93: 6031-6.

[163] Howes MJR, Houghton PJ. Plants used in Chinese and Indian traditional medicine for improvement of memory and cognitive function. Pharmacol Biochem Behav 2003; 75: 513-27

[164] Nalini K, Karanth KS, Rao A, Aroot AR. Effects of Celastruspaniculatuson passive avoidance performance and biogenic amine turnover in albino rats. J Ethnopharmacol 1995; 47: 101-8.

[165] Kumar MHV, Gupta YK. Antioxidant property of *Celastrus paniculatus* Willd.: a possible mechanism in enhancing cognition. Phytomedicine 2002; 9(4): 302-11.

[166] Dev S. Ethnotherapeutic and modern drug development: The potential of Ayurveda. Curr Sci 1997; 73(11): 909-28.

[167] Brinkhaus B, Lindner M, Schuppan D, Hahn EG. Chemical, pharmacological and clinical profile of the East Asian medical plant Centella asiática. Phytomedicine 2000; 7(5): 427-48.

[168] Asakawa Y, Matsuda R, Takemoto T. Mono and sesquiterpenoids from Hydrocotyle and Centella species. Phytochemistry 1982; 21(10): 2590-2.

[169] Miyazawa M, Watanabe H, Kameoka H. Inhibition of acetylcholinesterase activity by monoterpenoids with ap-menthane skeleton. J Agric Food Chem 1997; 45: 677-9.

[170] Perry NSL, Houghton PJ, Theobald A, Jenner P, Perry EK. In-vitro in- hibition of erythrocyte acetylcholinesterase by Salvia lavandulaefolia essential oil and constituent terpenes. J Pharm Pharmcol 2000; 52: 895-902.

[171] Ryan MF, Byrne O. Plant-insect coevolution and inhibition of acetylcholinesterase. J Chem Ecol 1988; *14*(10): 1965-75.

[172] Sakina MR, Dandiya PC. A psychoneuropharmacological profile of Centella asiatica extract. Fitoterapia 1990; 61(4): 291-6.

[173] Lake JT, Grossberg GT. Eichelman B: Neurochemical basis of aggressive behavior. Psychiatr Ann 1987; 17: 371-4.

[174] Lebert, F.; Pasquier, F.; Petit, H. Behavioral effects of trazodone in Alzheimer's disease. J Clin Psychiatry 1994; 55(12): 536-8.

[175] Simpson, P.M.; Foster, D. Improvement in organically disturbed behavior with trazodone treatment. J Clin Psychiatry 1986; 47: 191-3.

[176] Nalini, K.; Aroor, A.R.; Karanth, K.S.; Rao, A. Effect of Centella asiatica fresh leaf aqueous extract on learning and memory and biogenic amine turnover in albino rats. Fitoterapia 1992; 63(3): 232-7.

[177] Inamdar PK, Yeole RD, Ghogare AB, de Souza NJ. Determination of biologically active constituents in Centella asiática. J Chromatography A 1996; 742: 127-30.

[178] Lee MK, Kim SR, Sung SH, *et al.* Asiatic acid derivatives protect cultured cortical neurons from glutamate-induced excitotoxixity. Res Comm Mol Pathol Pharmacol 2000; 108(1-2): 75-86.

[179] Barbosa NR, Pitella F, Gattaz WF. Centella asiatica water extract inhibits iPLA2 and cPLA2 activities in rat cerebellum. Phytomedicine 2008; 15: 896-900.

[180] Farooqui AA, Yang HC, Rosemberger TA, Horrocks LA. Phospholipase A 2 and its role in brain tissue. J Neurochem 1997; 69: 889-901.

[181] Murakami M, Shimbara S, Kambe T, *et al.* The functions of five distinct mammalian phospholipase A2S in regulating arachidonic acid release. J Biol Chem 1998; 23: 14411-23.

[182] Subathra M, Shila S, Devi MA, Panneerselvam C. Emerging role of Centella asiática in improving age-related neurological antioxidante status. Exp Gerontol 2005; 40: 707-15.

[183] Kim SR, Koo KA, Lee MK, *et al.* Asiatic acid derivatives enhance cognitive performance partly by improving acetylcholine synthesis. J Pharm Pharmacol 2004; 56: 1275-82.

[184] Inhee MJ, Eun SJ, Hwan YS, *et al.* Protective effects of asiaticoside derivatives against beta-amyloid neurotoxicityJ. Neurosci Res 1999; 58: 417-25.

[185] Sang-Sup J, Chi-Hyoung Y, Doo-Yeon L, *et al.* Structure-activity relationship study of Asiatic acid derivatives against beta amyloid-induced neurotoxicity. Biorg Med Chem Lett 2000; 10: 119-21.

[186] Das KC, Das CK. Curcumin (diferuloylmethane), a singlet oxygen ($^1O_2$) quencher. Biochem Biophys Res Commun 2002; 295(1): 62-6.

[187] Miquel J, Bernd A, Sempere JM, Diaz-Alperi J, Ramirez A. The curcuma antioxidants: pharmacological effects and prospects for future clinical use. A review. Arch Gerontol Geriatr 2002; 34(1): 37-46.
[188] Priyadarsini KI. Free radical reactions of curcumin in membrane models. Free Radic Biol Med 1997; 23(6): 838-43.
[189] Scartezzini P, Speroni E. Review on some plants of Indian traditional medicine with antioxidant activity. J Ethnopharmacol 2000; 71(1-2): 23-43.
[190] Rajakrishman V, Viswanathan P, Rajasekharam KN, Menon VP. Neuroprotective role of curcumin from Curcuma longa on ethanol-induced brain damage. Phytother Res 1999; 13(7): 571-4.
[191] Kim DSHL, Kim JY. Total synthesis of Calebin-A, preparation of its analogues, and their neuronal cell protectivity against beta-amyloid insult. Bioorg Med Chem Lett 2001; 11(18): 2541-3.
[192] Park SY, Kim DSHL. Discovery of natural products from Curcuma longa that product cells from beta-amyloid insult: a drug discovery effort against Alzheimer's disease. J Nat Prod 2002; 65(9): 1227-31.
[193] Kim DSHL, Park SY, Kim JY. Curcuminoids from Curcuma longa L. (Zingiberaceae) that protect PC rat pheochromocytoma and normal human umbilical vein endothelial cells from beta A(1-42) insult. Neurosci Lett 2001; 303(1): 57-61.
[194] Ramsewak RS, DeWitt DL, Nair MG. Cytotoxicity, antioxidant and anti-inflammatory activities of Curcumins I-III from Curcuma longa. Phytomedicine 2000; 7(4): 303-8.
[195] Skrzypczak-Jankun E, McCabe NP, Selman SH, Jankun J. Curcumin Inhibits Lipoxygenase by Binding to its Central Cavity: Theoretical and X-ray Evidence. Int J Mol Med 2000; 6(5): 521-6.
[196] Srivastava KC, Bordia A, Verma SK. Curcumin, a major component of food spice turmeric (Curcuma longa) inhibits aggregation and alters eicosanoid metabolism in human blood platelets. Prostaglandins Leukot Essent Fatty Acids 1995; 52(4): 223-7.
[197] Yu ZF, Kong LD, Chen Y. Antidepressant activity of aqueous extracts of Curcuma longa in mice. J Ethnopharmacol 2002; 83(1-2): 161-5.
[198] Maurer K, Ihl R, Dierks T, Frölich L. Clinical efficacy of Ginkgo biloba special extract EGb 761 in dementia of the Alzheimer type. J Psychiatr Res 1997; 31(6): 645-55.
[199] Heiss WD, Zeiler K. Medikamentöse Beeinflussung der Hirndurchblutung. Pharmakoterapie 1978; 1: 137-44.
[200] Loffler T, Lee SK, Noldner M, Chatterjee SS, Hoyer S, Schliebs R. Effect of Ginkgo biloba extract (EGb761) on glucose metabolism-related markers in streptozotocin-damaged rat brain. J Neural Transm 2001; 108(12): 1457-74.
[201] Tea S, Celsis P, Clanet M, Marc-Vergnes J-P, Boeters U. Quanifizierte Parameter zum Nachwels von zerebraler Durchblutungs- und Stoffwechselsteigerung unter Ginkgo-biloba-Therapie. Therapiewoche 1987; 37: 2655-7.
[202] Kristofiková Z, Benesová O, Tejkalová H. Changes of high-affinity choline uptake in the hippocampus of old rats after long-term administration of two nootropic drugs (tacrine and Ginkgo biloba extract). Dementia 1992; 3: 304-7.
[203] Barth SA, Inselmann G, Engemann R, Heidemann HT. Influences of Ginkgo biloba on cyclosporin A induced lipid peroxidation in human liver microsomes in comparison to vitamin E, glutathione and N-acetylcysteine. Biochem Pharmacol 1991; 41: 1521-6.

[204] Marcocci L, Packer L, Droy-Lefaix M-T, Sekaki A, Gardès-Albert M. Antioxidant action of Ginkgo biloba extract EGb 761. Methods Enzymol 1994; 234: 462-75.
[205] Topic B, Tani E, Tsiakitzis K, *et al.* Enhanced maze performance and reduced oxidative stress by combined extracts of zingiber officinale and Ginkgo biloba in the aged rat. Neurobiol Aging 2002; 23(1): 135-43.
[206] Bastianetto S, Ramassamy C, Dore S, Christen Y, Poirier J, Quirion R. The Ginkgo biloba extract (EGb 761) protects hippocampal neurons against cell death induced by beta-amyloid. Eur J Neurosci 2000; 12(6): 1882-90.
[207] Bastianetto S, Zheng WH, Quirion R. The Ginkgo biloba extract (EGb 761) protects and rescues hippocampal cells against nitric oxide-induced toxicity. Involvement of its flavonoid constituents and protein kinase C. J Neurochem 2000; 74(6): 2268-77.
[208] Schindowski K, Leutner S, Kressmann S, Eckert A, Muller WE. Age-related increase of oxidative stress-induced apoptosis in mice prevention by Ginkgo biloba extract (EGb761). J Neural Transm 2001; 108(8-9): 969-78.
[209] Yao Z, Drieu K, Papadopoulos V. The Ginkgo biloba extract EGb 761 rescues the PC12 neuronal cells from β-amyloid-induced cell death by inhibiting the formation of β-amyloid-derived diffusible neurotoxic ligands. Brain Res 2001; 889 (1-2): 181-90.
[210] Chandrasekaran K, Mehrabian Z, Spinnewyn B, Drieu K, Fiskum G. Neuroprotective effects of bilobalide, a component of the Ginko biloba extract (EGb 761), in gerbil global brain ischemia. Brain Res 2001; 922: 282-92.
[211] Rapin JR, Zaibi M, Drieu K. *In vitro* and *in vivo* effects of an extract of Ginkgo biloba (EGb 761), ginkgolide B, and bilobalide on apoptosis in primary cultures of rat hippocampal neurons. Drug Dev Res 1998; 45: 23-9.
[212] Seif-El-Nasr M, El-Fattah AA. Lipid peroxide, phospholipids, glutathione levels and superoxide dismutase activity in rat brain after ischaemia: effect of ginkgo biloba extract. Pharmacol Res 1995; 32: 273-8.
[213] Pietri S, Maurelli E, Drieu, K, Culcasi M. Cardioprotective and anti-oxidant effects of the terpenoid constituents of Ginkgo biloba extract (EGb 761). J Mol Cell Cardiol 1997; 29: 733-42.
[214] Chopin P, Briley M. Effects of four non-cholinergic cognitive enhancers in comparison with tacrine and galanthamine on scopolamine-induced amnesia in rats. Psychopharmacology 1992; 106: 26-30.
[215] Petrov VD, Kehayov R, Belcheva S, *et al.* Memory Effects of Standardized Extracts of Panax ginseng (G115), Ginkgo biloba (GK 501) and their Combination Gincosan® (PHL-00701). Planta Med 1993; 59: 106-14.
[216] Stoll S, Scheuer K, Pohl O, Müller WE. Ginkgo Biloba Extract (EGb 761) Independently Improves Changes in Passive Avoidance Learning and Brain Membrane Fluidity in the Aging Mouse. Pharmacopsychiatry 1996; 29: 144-9.
[217] Hofferberth B. The efficacy of EGb 761 in patients with senile dementia of the Alzheimer type, a double-blind, placebo-controlled study on different levels of investigation. Hum Psychopharmacol 1994; 9: 215-22.
[218] Kanowski S, Hermann WM, Stephan K, Wierch W, Hörr R. Proof of efficacy of the Ginkgo biloba special extract EGb 761 in outpatients suffering from mild to moderate primary degenerative dementia of the Alzheimer type or multi-infarct dementia. Phytomedicine 1997; 4(1): 3-13.

[219] Le Bars PL, Katz MM, Berman N, Itil TM, Freedman AM, Schatzberg AF. A placebo-controlled, double-blind, randomized trial of an extract of Ginkgo biloba for dementia. J Am Med Assoc 1997; 278(16): 1327-32.

[220] Le Bars PL, Kieser M, Itil KZ. A 26-Week Analysis of a Double-Blind, Placebo-Controlled Trial of the Ginkgo biloba Extract EGb 761® in Dementia. Dement Geriatr Cogn Disord 2000; 11(4): 230-7.

[221] Le Bars PL, Velasco FM, Ferguson JM, Dessain EC, Kieser M, Hoerr R. Influence of the Severity of Cognitive Impairment on the Effect of the Ginkgo biloba Extract EGb 761® in Alzheimer's Disease. Neuropsychobiology 2002; 45(1): 19-26.

[222] Oken BS, Storzbach DM, Kaye JA. The efficacy of Ginkgo biloba on cognitive function in Alzheimer disease. Arch Neurol 1998; 55: 1409-15.

[223] Rai GS, Shovlin C, Wesnes KA. A double-blind, placebo controlled study of Ginkgo biloba extract ('Tanakan™') in elderly outpatients with mild to moderate memory impairment. Curr Med Res Opin 1991; 12(6): 350-5.

[224] Rigney U, Kimber S, Hindmarch I. The effects of acute doses of standardized Ginkgo biloba extract on memory and psychomotor performance in volunteers. Phytother Res 1999; 13: 408-15.

[225] Kubota Y, Tanaka N, Umegaki K, Takenaka H, Mizuno H, Nakamura K, Shinozuka K, Kunitomo M. Ginkgo biloba extract-induced relaxation of rat aorta is associated with increase in endothelial intracellular calcium level. Life Sci 2001; 69: 2327-36.

[226] Koltai M, Hosford D, Braquet PG. PAF-induced amplification of mediator release in septic shock: prevention or downregulation by PAF antagonists. J Lipid Mediat 1993; 6(1-3): 183-98.

[227] Skolnick, AA. Old Chinese herbal medicine used for fever yields possible new Alzheimer disease therapy. J Am Med Assoc 1997; 277(10): 776.

[228] Wang, Y-E.; Yue, D-X.; Tang, X-C. Anticholinesterase activity. Acta Pharmacol. Sin. 1986, 7(2), 110-13.

[229] McKinney M, Millar JH, Yamada F, Tuckmantel W, Kozikowski AP. Potencies and stereoselectivities of enantiomers of huperzine A for inhibition of rat cortical acetylcholinesterase. Eur J Pharmacol 1991; 203: 303-05.

[230] Laganiere S, Corey J, Tang X-C, Wülfert E, Hanin I. Acute and chronic studies with the anticholinesterase Huperzine A: effect on central nervous system cholinergic parameters. Neuropharmacol 1991; 30(7): 763-8.

[231] Ashani Y, Peggins JO, Doctor BP. Mechanism of inhibition of cholinesterases by huperzine A. Biochem Biophys Res Commun 1992; 184(2): 719-26.

[232] Lu W-H, Shou J, Tang X-C. Improving effect of huperzine A on discrimination performance in aged rats and adult rats with experimental cognitive impairment. Acta Pharmacol Sin 1988; 9(1): 11-15.

[233] Wang LM, Han YF, Tang XC. Huperzine A improves cognitive deficits caused by chronic cerebral hypoperfusion in rats. Eur J Pharmacol 2000; 398(1): 65-72.

[234] Zhou J, Fu Y, Tang XC. Huperzine A and donepezil protect rat pheochromocytoma cells against oxygen-glucose deprivation. Neurosci Lett 2001; 306: 53-6.

[235] Shu Y-Z. Recent natural products based drug development: a pharmaceutical industry perspective. J Nat Prod 1998; 61: 1053-71.

[236] Small GW, Rabins RV, Barry PP, *et al.* Diagnosis and Treatment of Alzheimer Disease and Related Disorders: Consensus Statement of the American Association for Geriatric

Psychiatry, the Alzheimer's Association, and the American Geriatrics Society. J Am Med Assoc 1997; 278 (16): 1363-71.

[237] Xiao XQ, Zhang HY, Tang XC. Huperzine A attenuates amyloid beta-peptide fragment 25-35-induced apoptosis in rat cortical neurons via inhibiting reactive oxygen species formation and caspase-3 activation. J Neurosci Res 2002; 67(1): 30-6.

[238] Zhou J, Zhang HY, Tang XC. Huperzine A attenuates cognitive deficits and hippocampal neuronal damage after transient global ischemia in gerbils. Neurosci Lett 2001; 313(3): 137-40.

[239] Xiao XQ, Yang JW, Tang XC. Huperzine A protects rat pheochromocytoma cells against hydrogen peroxide-induced injury Neurosci Lett 1999; 275: 73-6.

[240] Ved HS, Koenig ML, Dave JR, Doctor BP. Huperzine A, a potential therapeutic agent for dementia, reduces neuronal cell death caused by glutamate. Neuroreport 1997; 8(4): 963-8.

[241] Wang XD, Zhang JM, Yang HH, Hu GY. Modulation of NMDA receptor by Huperzine A in rat cerebral cortex. Acta Pharmacol Sin 1999; 20(1): 31-5.

[242] Zhou J, Tang XC. Huperzine A attenuates apoptosis and mitochondria-dependent caspase-3 in rat cortical neurons. FEBS Lett 2002; 526: 21-5.

[243] Bores GM, Huger FP, Petko W, *et al.* Pharmacological evaluation of novel Alzheimer's disease therapeutics: acetylcholinesterase inhibitors related to galanthamine. J Pharmacol Exp Ther 1996; 277: 728-38.

[244] Wilcock GK, Lilienfeld S, Gaens E. Efficacy and safety of galantamine in patients with mild to moderate Alzheimer's disease: multicentre randomised controlled trial. Galantamine International-1 Study Group. BMJ 2000; 321: 1445-9.

[245] Wilkinson D, Murray J. Galantamine: a randomized, double-blind, dose comparison in patients with Alzheimer's disease. Int J Geriatr Psychiatry 2001; 16(9): 852-7.

[246] Bickel U, Thomsen T, Weber W, Fischer JP, Bachus R, Nitz M. Pharmacokinetics of galanthamine in humans and corresponding cholinesterase inhibition. Clin Pharmacol Ther 1991; 50: 420-8.

[247] Fulton B, Benfield P. Galanthamine. Drugs Aging 1996; 9(1): 60-5.

[248] Harvey AL. The pharmacology of galanthamine and its analogues. Pharmacol Ther 1995; 68(1): 113-28.

[249] Pearson VE. Galantamine: a new alzheimer drug with a past life. Ann Pharmacother 2001; 35(11): 1406-13.

[250] Woodruff-Pak DS, Vogel RW, Wenk GL. Galanthamine: effect on nicotinic receptor binding, acetylcholinesterase inhibition and learning. Proc Natl Acad Sci USA 2001; 98(4): 2089-94.

[251] Irwin RL, Smith HJ. Cholinesterase inhibition by galanthamine and lycoramine. Biochem Pharmacol 1960; 3(2): 147-8.

[252] Pagliosa LB, Monteiro SC, Silva KB, *et al.* Effect of isoquinoline alkaloids from two Hippeastrum species on *in vitro* acetylcholinesterase activity. Phytomedicine 2010; 17: 698-701.

[253] Hou YC, Chao PD, Chen SY. Honokiol and magnolol increased hippocampal acetylcholine release in freely-moving rats. Am J Chin Med 2000; 28 (3-4): 379-84.

[254] Chen YL, Lin KF, Shiao MS, Chen YT, Hong CY, Lin SJ. Magnolol, a potent antioxidant from Magnolia officinalis, attenuates intimal thickening and MCP-1 expression after balloon injury of the aorta in cholesterol-fed rabbits. Basic Res Cardiol 2001; 96(4): 353-63.

[255] Kong CW, Tsai K, Chin JH, Chan WL, Hong CY. Magnolol Attenuates Peroxidative Damage and Improves Survival of Rats With Sepsis. Shock 2000; 13(1): 24-28.
[256] Lo YC, Teng CM, Chen CF, Chen CC, Hong CY. Magnolol and honokiol isolated from Magnolia officinalis protect rat heart mitochondria against lipid peroxidation. Biochem Pharmacol 1994; 47(3): 549-53.
[257] Chiu JH, Ho CT, Wei YH, Lui WY, Hong CY. *In vitro* and *in vivo* protective effect of honokiol on rat liver from peroxidative injury. Life Sci 1997; 61(19): 1961-71.
[258] Kuribara H, Kishi E, Hattori N, Yuzurihara M, Maruyama Y. Application of the elevated plus-maze test in mice for evaluation of the content of Honokiol in water extracts of magnolia. Phytother Res 1999; 13(7): 593-6.
[259] Kuribara H, Kishi E, Hattori N, Okada M, Maruyama Y. The anxiolytic effect of two oriental herbal drugs in Japan attributed to honokiol from Magnolia bark. J. Pharm Pharmacol 2000; 52(11): 1425-9.
[260] Squires RF, Ai J, Witt MR, *et al.* Honokiol and magnolol increase the number of [3H] muscimol binding sites three-fold in rat forebrain membranes *in vitro* using a filtration assay, by allosterically increasing the affinities of low-affinity sites. Neurochem Res 1999; 24(12): 1593-1602.
[261] Lee MM, Hseih MT, Kuo JS, Yeh FT, Huang HM. Magnolol protects cortical neuronal cells from chemical hypoxia in rats. Neuroreport 1998; 9(15): 3451-56.
[262] Wang JP, Hsu MF, Raung SL, Chen CC, Kuo JS, Teng CM. Anti-inflammatory and analgesic effects of magnolol. Naunyn Schmiedebergs Arch Pharmacol 1992; 346(6): 707-12.
[263] Wang JP, Ho TF, Chang LC, Chen CC. Anti-inflammatory Effect of Magnolol, Isolated from Magnolia officinalis, on A23187-induced Pleurisy in Mice. J Pharm Pharmacol 1995; 47(10): 857-60.
[264] Jia H, Jiang Y, Ruan Y, *et al.* Tenuigenin treatment decreases secretion of the Alzheimer's disease amyloid β-protein in cultured cells. Neurosci Lett 2004; 367: 123-8.
[265] Park CH, Choi SH, Koo J-W, *et al.* Novel cognitive improving and neuroprotective activities of Polygala tenuifolia Willdenow extract, BT-11. J Neurosci Res 2002; 70: 484-92.
[266] Yabe T, Iizuka S, Komatsu Y, Yamada H. Enhancements of choline acetyltransferase activity and nerve growth factor secretion by Polygalae radix-extract containing active ingredients in Kami-untan-to. Phytomedicine 1997; 4(3): 199-205.
[267] Yamada H, Yabe T. Anti-demetia actions of Kampo (japonese-herbal) medicines effects of Kampo medicines on central nervous system. Curr Top Phytochem 1997; 1: 157-68.
[268] Ikeya Y, Takeda S, Tunakawa M, *et al.* Cognitive Improving and Cerebral Protective Effects of Acylated Oligosaccharides in Polygala tenuifolia. Biol Pharm Bull 2004; 27(7): 1081-5.
[269] Karakida F, Ikeya Y, Tsunakawa M, *et al.* Cerebral Protective and Cognition-Improving Effects of Sinapic Acid in Rodents. Biol Pharm Bull 2007; 30(3): 514-19.
[270] Perry NSL, Bollen C, Perry EK, Ballard C. Salvia for dementia therapy: review of pharmacological activity and pilot tolerability clinical trial. Pharmacol Biochem Behav 2003; 75(3): 651-9.
[271] Perry NSL, Houghton PJ, Sampson J, *et al.* In-vitro activity of S. lavandulaefolia (Spanish sage) relevant to treatment of Alzheimer's disease. J Pharm Pharmacol 2001; 53(10): 1347-56.

[272] Adam K, Sivropoulou A, Kokkini S, Lanaras T, Arsenakis M. Antifungal Activities of *Origanum vulgare* subsp. *hirtum, Mentha spicata, Lavandula angustifolia*, and *Salvia fruticosa* Essential Oils against Human Pathogenic Fungi. J Agric Food Chem 1998; 46(5): 1739-45.

[273] Dorman HJP, Deans SG, Noble RC. Evaluation *in vitro* of plant essential oils as natural antioxidants. J Essent Oil Res 1995; 7(6): 645-51.

[274] Lu Y, Foo LY. Antioxidant activities of polyphenols from sage (Salvia officinalis). Food Chem 2001; 75(2): 197-202.

[275] Malencic DJ, Gasic O, Popovic M, Boza P. Screening for antioxidant properties of *Salvia reflexa* Hornem. Phytoter Res 2000; 14(7): 546-8.

[276] Zupko I, Hohmann J, Redei D, Falkay G, Janicsak G, Mathe I. Antioxidant Activity of Leaves of *Salvia* Species in Enzyme-Dependent and Enzyme-Independent Systems of Lipid Peroxidation and their Phenolic Constituents. Planta Med 2001; 67(4): 366-8.

[277] Howes M-JR, Perry NSL, Houghton PJ. Plants with traditional uses and activities, relevant to the management of Alzheimer's disease and other cognitive disorders. Phytother Res 2003; 17(1): 1-18.

[278] Maklad YA, Aboutabi EA, El-Sherei MM, Meselhy KM. Bioactivity studies of *Salvia transsylvanica* (Schur ex Griseb) grown in Egypt. Phytoter Res 1999; 13(2): 147-50.

[279] Zandi PP, Breitner JCS. Do NSAIDs prevent Alzheimer's disease? And, if so why? The epidemiological evidence. Neurobiol Aging 2001; 22(6): 811-17.

[280] Perry NSL, Houghton PJ, Jenner P, Keith A, Perry EK. *Salvia lavandulaefolia* essential oil inhibits cholinesterase *in vivo*. Phytomedicine 2002; 9(1): 48-51.

[281] Perry NSL, Houghton PJ, Theobald A, Jenner P, Perry EK. In-vitro inhibition of human erythrocyte acetylcholinesterase by *Salvia lavandulaefolia* essential oil and constituent terpenes. J Pharm Pharmacol 2000; 52(7): 895-902.

[282] Savelev S, Okello E, Perry NS, Wilkins RM, Perry EK. Synergistic and antagonistic interactions of anticholinesterase terpenoids in *Salvia lavandulaefolia* essential oil. Pharmacol Biochem Behav 2003; 75(3): 661-68.

[283] Kuang P, Wu W, Liu J, Zhang F, Pu CJ. The effect of radix *Salviae Miltiorrhizae* (RSM) on substance P in cerebral ischemia--animal experiment. Trad Chin Med 1991; 11(2): 123-27.

[284] Kuang P, Tao Y, Tian Y. Effect of radix *Salviae miltiorrhizae* on nitric oxide in cerebral ischemic-reperfusion injury. J Trad Chin Med 1996; 16(3): 224-27.

[285] Kuang P, Xiang J. Effect of radix *Salviae miltiorrhizae* on EAA and IAA during cerebral ischemia in gerbils: a microdialysis study. J Trad Chin Med 1994; 14(1): 45-50.

[286] Kuang P, Tao Y, Tian Y. Radix *Salviae miltiorrhizae* treatment results in decreased lipid peroxidation in reperfusion injury J Trad Chin Med 1996; 16(2): 138-42.

[287] Liu GT, Zhang TM, Wang BE, Wang YW. Protective action of seven natural phenolic compounds against peroxidative damage to biomembranes. Biochem Pharmacol 1992; 43(2): 147-52.

[288] Zhao B, Jiang W, Zhao Y, Hou J, Xin W. Scavenging effects of *Salvia miltiorrhiza* on free radicals and its protection for myocardial mitochondrial membranes from ischemia-reperfusion injury. Biochem Mol Biol Int 1996; 38(6): 1171-82.

[289] Weng XC, Gordon MH, Antioxidant activity of quinones extracted from tanshen (*Salvia miltiorrhiza* Bunge). J Agric Food Chem 1992; 40(8): 1331-36.

[290] Zhang K, Bao Y, Wu P, Rosen RT, Ho C. Antioxidative components of tanshen (*Salvia miltiorhiza* Bung). J Agric Food Chem 1990; 38(5): 1194-97.
[291] Du GH, Qiu Y, Zhang JT. Salvianolic acid B protects the memory functions against transient cerebral ischemia in mice. J Asian Nat Prod Res 2000; 2(2): 145-152.
[292] Guanhua D, Juntian Z. Protective effects of salvianolic acid A against impairment of memory induced by cerebral ischemia-reperfusion in mice. Chin Med J (Engl) 1997; 110(1): 65-8.
[293] Huang YS, Zhang JT. Antioxidative effect of three water-soluble components isolated from *Salvia miltiorrhiza in vitro* Acta Pharmacol Sin 1992; 27(2): 96-100.
[294] Kang HS, Chung HY, Jung JH, Kang SS, Choi JS. Antioxidant effect of *Salvia miltiorrhiza*. Arch Pharm Res 1997; 20(5): 496-500.
[295] Chang HM, Chui KY, Tan FWL, Yang Y, Zhong ZP. Structure-activity relationship of miltirone, an active central benzodiazepine receptor ligand isolated from *Salvia miltiorrhiza* Bunge (Danshen). J Med Chem 1991; 34(5): 1675-92.
[296] Kong LD, Cheng CH, Tan RX. Monoamine oxidase inhibitors from rhizoma of *Coptis chinensis*. Planta Med 2001; 67(1): 74-6.
[297] higeta K, Ootaki K, Tatemoto H, Nakanishi T, Inada A, Muto N. Potentiation of nerve growth factor-induced neurite outgrowth in PC12 cells by a *Coptidis Rhizoma* extract and protoberberine alkaloids. Biosci Biotechnol Biochem 2002; 66(11): 2491-94.
[298] Abe K, Saito H. Effects of saffron extract and its constituent crocin on learning behaviour and long-term potentiation. Phytother Res 2000; 14(3): 149-152.
[299] Park CH, Kim S, Choi W, *et al.* Novel anticholinesterase and antiamnesic activities of dehydroevodiamine, a constituent of *Evodia rutaecarpa*. Planta Med 1996; 62(5): 405-9.
[300] Haji A, Momose Y, Takeda R, Nakanishi S. Increased feline cerebral blood flow induced by dehydroevodiamine hydrochloride from *Evodia rutaecarpa*. J Nat Prod 1994; 57(3): 387-9.
[301] Nguyen TTH, Cho SO, Ban JY, *et al.* Neuroprotective effect of *Sanguisorbae radix* against oxidative stress-induced brain damage: *in vitro* and *in vivo*. Biol Pharm Bull 2008; 31(11): 2028-35, and references cited in.
[302] Yokozawa T, Chen CP, Tanaka T. Direct scavenging of nitric oxide by traditional crude drugs. Phytomedicine 2000; 6(6): 453-63.
[303] Yokozawa T, Chen CP, Tanaka T, Kitani K. Effects of sanguiin H-6, a component of *Sanguisorbae radix*, on lipopolysaccharide-stimulated nitric oxide production. Biochem Pharmacol 2002; 63(5): 853-58.
[304] Yokozawa T, Chen CP, Tanaka T, Kitani K. A study on the nitric oxide production-suppressing activity of sanguisorbae radix components. Biol Pharm Bull 2000; 23(6): 717-22.
[305] Mandel SA, Avramovich-Tirosh Y, Reznichencko L, *et al.* Multifunctional activities of green tea catechins in neuroprotection. Modulation of cell survival genes, iron-dependent oxidative stress and PKC signaling pathway. Neurosignals 2005; 14(1-2): 46-60.
[306] Yazawa K, Kihara T, Shen H, Shimmyo Y, Niidome T, Sugimoto H. Distinct mechanisms underlie distinct polyphenol-induced neuroprotection. FEBS Lett 2006; 580(28-29): 6623-28.
[307] Khanna S, Park H-A, Sen CK, *et al.* Neuroprotective and antiinflammatory properties of a novel demethylated curcuminoid. Antoxidant Redox Signal 2009; 11(3): 449-68.

[308] Chan MM, Huang HI, Fenton MR, Fong D. *In vivo* inhibition of nitric oxide synthase gene expression by curcumin, a cancer preventive natural product with anti-inflammatory properties. Biochem Pharmacol 1998; 55(12): 1955-62.

[309] Ono K, Hasegawa K, Naiki M, Yamada J. Curcumin has potent anti-amyloidogenic effects for Alzheimer's beta-amyloid fibrils *in vitro*. Neurosci 2004; 75(6): 742-50.

[310] Rajeswari A, Sabesan M. Inhibition of monoamine oxidase-B by the polyphenolic compound, curcumin and its metabolite tetrahydrocurcumin, in a model of Parkinson's disease induced by MPTP neurodegeneration in mice. Inflammopharmacology 2008; 16(2): 96-9.

[311] Frautschy SA, Hu W, Kim P, *et al.* Phenolic anti-inflammatory antioxidant reversal of Abeta-induced cognitive deficits and neuropathology. Neurobiol Aging 2001; 22(6): 993-1005.

[312] Lim HJ, Chu T, Yang F, Beech W, Frautschy SA, Cole GM. The curry spice curcumin reduces oxidative damage and amyloid pathology in an Alzheimer transgenic mouse. J Neurosci 2001; 21(21): 8370-77.

[313] Ringman JM, Frautschy SA, Cole GM, Masterman DL, Cummings JL. A potential role of the curry spice curcumin in Alzheimer's disease. Curr Alzheimer Res 2005; 2(2): 131-36.

[314] Rocha-González HI, Ambriz-Tututi M, Granados-Soto V. Resveratrol: a natural compound with pharmacological potential in neurodegenerative diseases. CNS Neurosci Ther 2008; 14(3): 234-47, and references cited in.

[315] Nonomura S, Kanagawa H, Makimoto A. Chemical Constituents of Polygonaceous Plants. I. Studies on the Components of Ko-J O-Kon. (polygonum cuspidatum sieb. et zucc.). Yakugaku Zasshi 1963; 83: 988-90.

[316] Tokusoglu O, Unal MK, Yemis F. Determination of the Phytoalexin Resveratrol (3,5,4'-Trihydroxystilbene) in Peanuts and Pistachios by High-Performance Liquid Chromatographic Diode Array (HPLC-DAD) and Gas Chromatography−Mass Spectrometry (GC-MS) J Agric Food Chem 2005; 53(12): 5003-09.

[317] Baur JA, Sinclair DA. Therapeutic potential of resveratrol: the *in vivo* evidence. Nat Rev Drug Discov 2006; 5(6): 493-506.

[318] Ribeiro de Lima MT, Waffo-Téguo P, Teissedre PL, *et al.* Determination of Stilbenes (*trans*-Astringin, *cis*- and *trans*-Piceid, and *cis*- and*trans*-Resveratrol) in Portuguese Wines. J Agric Food Chem 1999; 47(7): 2666-70.

[319] Frémont L. Biological effects of resveratrol. Life Sci 2000; 66(8): 663-73.

[320] Granados-Soto V. Pleiotropic effects of resveratrol. Drug News Perspect 2003; 16(5): 299-307.

[321] Ramassamy C. Emerging role of polyphenolic compounds in the treatment of neurodegenerative diseases: a review of their intracellular targets. Eur J Pharmacol 2006; 545(1): 51-64.

[322] Orgogozo JM, Dartigues JF, Lafont S, *et al.* Wine consumption and dementia in the elderly: a prospective community study in the Bordeaux area. Rev Neurol (Paris) 1997; 153(3); 185-92.

[323] Wang J, Ho L, Zhao Z, *et al.* Moderate consumption of Cabernet Sauvignon attenuates Abeta neuropathology in a mouse model of Alzheimer's disease. FASEB J 2006; 20(13): 2313-20.

[324] Jang JH, Surh YJ. Protective effect of resveratrol on beta-amyloid-induced oxidative PC12 cell death. Free Radic Biol Med 2003; 34(8): 1100-10.

[325] Kim D, Nguyen MD, Dobbin MM, *et al.* SIRT1 deacetylase protects against neurodegeneration in models for Alzheimer's disease and amyotrophic lateral sclerosis. EMBO J 2007; 26(13): 3169-79.
[326] Rivière C, Richard T, Quentin L, Krisa S, Mérillon JM, Monti JP. Inhibitory activity of stilbenes on Alzheimer's beta-amyloid fibrils *in vitro*. Bioorg Med Chem 2007; 15(2): 1160-67.
[327] Marambaud P, Zhao H, Davies P. Resveratrol promotes clearance of Alzheimer's disease amyloid-beta peptides. J Biol Chem 2005; 280(45): 37377-382.
[328] Miloso M, Bertelli AA, Nicolini G, Tredici G. Resveratrol-induced activation of the mitogen-activated protein kinases, ERK1 and ERK2, in human neuroblastoma SH-SY5Y cells. Neurosci Lett 1999; 264(1-3): 141-44.
[329] Han YS, Zheng WH, Bastianetto S, Chabot JG, Quirion R. Neuroprotective effects of resveratrol against beta-amyloid-induced neurotoxicity in rat hippocampal neurons: involvement of protein kinase C. Brit J Pharmacol 2004; 141(6): 997-1005.
[330] Chen J, Zhou Y, Mueller-Steiner S, *et al.* SIRT1 protects against microglia-dependent amyloid-beta toxicity through inhibiting NF-kappaB signaling. Biol Chem 2005; 280(48): 40364-74.
[331] Kim YA, Lim SY, Rhee SH, *et al.* Resveratrol inhibits inducible nitric oxide synthase and cyclooxygenase-2 expression in beta-amyloid-treated C6 glioma cells. Int J Mol Med 2006; 17(6): 1069-75.
[332] Singh N, Pillay V, Choonara YE. Advances in the treatment of Parkinson's disease. Prog Neurobiol 2007; 81(1): 29-44.
[333] Jellinger K, Kienzl E, Rumpelmair G, *et al.* Neuromelanin and nigrostriatal dopamine neuron degeneration. J Neurochem 1993; 60(5): 1976-77.
[334] Lee MK, Kang SJ, Poncz, M, Song KJ, Park KS. Resveratrol protects SH-SY5Y neuroblastoma cells from apoptosis induced by dopamine. Exp Mol Med 2007; 39(3): 376-84.
[335] Chalimoniuk M, Glowacka J, Zabielna A, Eckert A, Strosznajder JB. Nitric oxide alters arachidonic acid turnover in brain cortex synaptoneurosomes. Neurochem Int 2006; 48(1): 1-8.
[336] Dore S. Unique properties of polyphenol stilbenes in the brain: more than direct antioxidant actions; gene/protein regulatory activity. Neurosignals 2005; 14(1): 61-70.
[337] Esposito E, Rotillo D, Di Matteo, V, Di Giulio C, Cacchio M, Algeri S. A review of specific dietary antioxidants and the effects on biochemical mechanisms related to neurodegenerative processes. Neurobiology of Aging 2002; 23(3): 719-35.
[338] Simonyi A, Woods D, Sun AY, Sun GY. Grape polyphenols inhibit chronic ethanol-induced COX-2 mRNA expression in rat brain. Alcohol Clin Exp Res 2002; 26(3): 352-57.
[339] Sun GY, Xia J, Draczynska-Lusiak B, Simonyi A, Sun AY. Grape polyphenols protect neurodegenerative changes induced by chronic ethanol administration. Neuroreport 1999; 10(1): 93-6.
[340] Sun GY, Xia J, Xu J, Allenbrand B, Simonyi A, Rudeen PK. Dietary supplementation of grape polyphenols to rats ameliorates chronic ethanol-induced changes in hepatic morphology without altering changes in hepatic lipids. J Nutr 1999; 129(10): 1814-19.
[341] Chanvitayapongs S, Draczynska-Lusiak B, Sun AY. Amelioration of oxidative stress by antioxidants and resveratrol in PC12 cells. Neuroreport 1997; 8(6): 1499-1502.

[342] (a) Alvira D, Yeste-Velasco M, Folch J, Verdaguer E, Canudas AM, Pallas M. Comparative analysis of the effects of resveratrol in two apoptotic models: inhibition of complex I and potassium deprivation in cerebellar neurons. Neuroscience 2007; 147(3): 746-56. b) Baur JA, Sinclair DA. Therapeutic potential of resveratrol: the *in vivo* evidence. Nat Rev Drug Discov 2006; 5(6): 493-506. c) Han YS, Zheng WH, Bastinetto S, Chabot JG, Quirion R. Neuroprotective effects of resveratrol against beta-amyloid-induced neurotoxicity in rat hippocampal neurons: involvement of protein kinase C. Br J Pharmacol 2004; 141(6): 997-1005. d) Chen J, Zhou Y, Mueller-Steiner S, Chen LF, Kwon H, Yi S, Mucke L, Gan L. SIRT1 protects against microglia-dependent amyloid-beta toxicity through inhibiting NF-kappaB signaling. J Biol Chem 2005; 280(48): 40364-74. e) Anekonda TS. Resveratrol-a boon for treating Alzheimer's disease? Brain Res Rev 2006; 52(2): 316-26.

[343] Gelinas S, Martinoli MG J. Neuroprotective effect of estradiol and phytoestrogens on MPP+-induced cytotoxicity in neuronal PC12 cells. Neurosci Res 2002; 70(1): 90-6.

[344] Conte A, Pellegrini S, Tagliazucchi D. Effect of resveratrol and catechin on PC12 tyrosine kinase activities and their synergistic protection from beta-amyloid toxicity. Drugs Exp Clin Res 2003; 29(5-6): 243-55.

[345] Conte A, Pellegrini S, Tagliazucchi D. Synergistic protection of PC12 cells from beta-amyloid toxicity by resveratrol and catechin. Brain Res Bull 2003; 62(1): 29-38.

[346] Ono K, Naike H, Yamada M. The development of preventives and therapeutics for Alzheimer's disease that inhibit the formation of beta-amyloid fibrils (fAbeta), as well as destabilize preformed fAbeta. Curr Pharm Des 2006; 12(33): 4357-75.

[347] Ono K, Yamada M. Antioxidant compounds have potent anti-fibrillogenic and fibril-destabilizing effects for alpha-synuclein fibrils *in vitro*. J Neurochem 2006; 97(1): 105-15.

[348] Bi XL, Yang JY, Dong YX, *et al.* Resveratrol inhibits nitric oxide and TNF-alpha production by lipopolysaccharide-activated microglia. Int Immunopharmacol 2005; 5(1): 185-93.

[349] Kim YA, Kim GY, Park KY, Choi YH. Resveratrol inhibits nitric oxide and prostaglandin E2 production by lipopolysaccharide-activated C6 microglia. J Med Food 2007; 10(2): 218-24.

[350] Gao D, Zhang X, Jiang X, Peng Y, *et al.* Resveratrol reduces the elevated level of MMP-9 induced by cerebral ischemia-reperfusion in mice. Life Sci 2006; 78(22): 2564-70.

[351] Ates O, Cayli S, Altinaz E, *et al.* Neuroprotection by resveratrol against traumatic brain injury in rats. Mol Cell Biochem 2007; 294(1-2): 137-44.

[352] Inoue H, Jiang XF, Katayama T, Osada S, Umesono K, Namura S. Brain protection by resveratrol and fenofibrate against stroke requires peroxisome proliferator-activated receptor alpha in mice. Neurosci Lett 2003; 352(3): 203-6.

[353] Gao ZB, Hu GY. Trans-resveratrol, a red wine ingredient, inhibits voltage-activated potassium currents in rat hippocampal neurons. Brain Res 2005; 1056(1): 68-75.

[354] Sinha K, Chaudhary G, Gupta YK. Protective effect of resveratrol against oxidative stress in middle cerebral artery occlusion model of stroke in rats. Life Sci 2002; 71(6): 655-65.

[355] Wang Q, Xu J, Rottinghaus GE, *et al.* Resveratrol protects against global cerebral ischemic injury in gerbils. Brain Res 2002; 958(2): 439-47.

[356] Kumar P, Padi SS, Naidu PS, Kumar A. Effect of resveratrol on 3-nitropropionic acid-induced biochemical and behavioural changes: possible neuroprotective mechanisms. Behav Pharmacol 2006; 17(5-6): 485-92.

[357] Kumar A, Naidu PS, Seghal N, Padi SSV. Neuroprotective effects of resveratrol against intracerebroventricular colchicine-Induced Cognitive impairment and oxidative stress in rats. Pharmacology 2007; 79(1): 17-26.

[358] Stolk J, Hiltermann TJ, Dijkman JH, Verhoeven AJ. Characteristics of the inhibition of NADPH oxidase activation in neutrophils by apocynin, a methoxy-substituted catechol. Am J Respir Cell Mol Biol 1994; 11(1): 95-102.

[359] Infanger DW, Sharma RV, Davisson RL. NADPH oxidases of the brain: distribution, regulation, and function. Antioxid Redox Signal 2006; 8(9-10): 1583-96.

[360] Dringen R. Oxidative and antioxidative potential of brain microglial cells. Antioxid Redox Signal 2005; 7(9-10): 1223-33.

[361] Brown GC. Mechanisms of inflammatory neurodegeneration: iNOS and NADPH oxidase.Biochem Soc Trans 2007; 35(Pt 5): 1119-121.

[362] Barbieri SS, Cavalca V, Eligini S, *et al.* Apocynin prevents cyclooxygenase 2 expression in human monocytes through NADPH oxidase and glutathione redox-dependent mechanisms. Free Radic Biol Med 2004; 37(2): 156-65.

[363] Li M, Pisalyaput K, Galvan M, Tenner AJ. Macrophage colony stimulatory factor and interferon-gamma trigger distinct mechanisms for augmentation of beta-amyloid-induced microglia-mediated neurotoxicity. J Neurochem 2004; 91(3): 623-33.

[364] Jekabsone A, Mander PK, Tickler A, Sharpe M, Brown GC. Fibrillar beta-amyloid peptide Abeta1-40 activates microglial proliferation *via* stimulating TNF-alpha release and H2O2 derived from NADPH oxidase: a cell culture study. J Neuroinflam 2006; 3(24): 1-13.

[365] Shibata H, Katsuki H, Okawara M, Kume T, Akaike A. c-Jun N-terminal kinase inhibition and alpha-tocopherol protect midbrain dopaminergic neurons from interferon-gamma/lipopolysaccharide-induced injury without affecting nitric oxide production. J Neurosci Res 2006; 83(1): 102-9.

[366] Schultes RE. The virgin field in psychoactive plant research. Bol Mus Emilio Goeldi Ser Bot 1990; 6 (1): 7-82.

CHAPTER 8

Flavonoids – Their Preventer and Therapeutic Applications Against Parkinson's Disease

Elena González-Burgos and Maria P. Gómez-Serranillos*

Department of Pharmacology, Faculty of Pharmacy, University Complutense, Madrid, Spain

Abstract: Parkinson´s disease (PD) is a major public health problem worldwide that affects millions of people, increasingly prevalent as the population ages. This disease, the most common human neurodegenerative motor disorder, is characterized by a progressive decrease in striatal dopamine content of dopaminergic neurons in the substantia nigra pars compacta. Converging pathogenic factors such as oxidative stress, inflammation, mitochondrial impairment and altered calcium homeostasis, among others, have been described as biochemical mechanisms of neurodegeneration in PD. Presently, quite a few natural flavonoids with potential antioxidants and signaling properties have been investigated and are still in progress to identify hopefully preventive neuroprotective compounds to forestall clinical progression of PD.

Flavonoids are the most abundant plant polyphenolic substances (over 4000 different ones) and they are found in main dietary sources (fruits, vegetables and plant-derived beverages). Chemically, this group of natural products shares a 2-phenylbenzopyran as basic structure (C_6-C_3-C_6), and it is further subdivided into different classes (*i.e.* flavones, flavanones, flavonols anthocyanins, flavan-3-ols). Related to their structural characteristics, flavonoids can transfer a hydrogen atom to scavenge reactive oxygen species (ROS), chelate metal ions (*i.e.* iron, copper) and stabilize unpaired electrons by resonance. Structural differences found among individual types of flavonoids as well as glycosylation patterns determine the biological activities of these promising chemoprotective compounds. As neuroprotective agents, flavonoids have been reported to act as direct ROS scavengers, modulate the endogenous enzymatic and non-enzymatic antioxidant defense system and activate and regulate different pro-survival pathways.

This chapter, based on highlighted research articles, focuses on the multiple neuroprotection mechanisms of natural flavonoids in PD, covering the most recent preclinical *in vitro* and *in vivo* PD animal models' studies and clinical trials and providing an overview and challenges that may be helpful for future research.

Keywords: Flavonoids, Parkinson's disease, neuroprotection, antioxidants.

***Address correspondence to Maria P. Gómez-Serranillos:** Department of Pharmacology, Faculty of Pharmacy, University Complutense, Madrid, Spain; +34 913941767; Fax: + 34 91 394 17 26;
E-mail: pserra@farm.ucm.es

Atta-ur-Rahman & M. Iqbal Choudhary (Eds.)

FLAVONOIDS

Flavonoids are secondary metabolites of polyphenolic natural product classes widely distributed in both food (*i.e.* fruits and vegetables) and non-food plants; over 4,000 different flavonoids have been identified [1].

The common chemical structure of flavonoids consists of 15 carbon atoms ($C_6C_3C_6$). They have two aromatic rings named as A and B-ring connected by a linear three carbon bridge (C-ring) (flavan nucleus) [2]. The basic skeleton of a flavonoid is shown in Fig. (**1**).

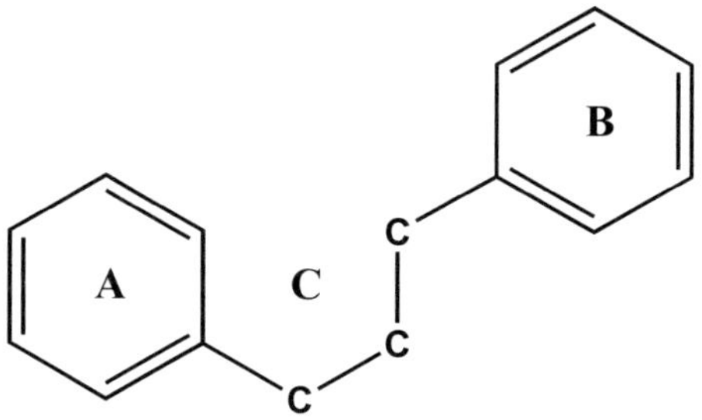

Fig. (1). Basic skeleton of flavonoids.

The aromatic B-ring could be attached to C-ring through its 2 or 3 carbon position [2].

The C-ring could be an acyclic form such as in chalcones; a heterocyclic five-member such as in the case of aurones; or a heterocyclic six-member (in most of flavonoids types including flavones, flavanones and isoflavones, among others) [2].

Moreover, depending on the degree of unsaturation of C-ring, three skeleton types have been differentiated: 2(3)-phenylbenzopyrone, 2-phenylbenzopyran and flavylium [2,3] (see Fig. **2**).

Flavonoids may be further classified into different subclasses according to the oxidation state of C-ring, the position of B-ring, and the type of the substituent that the C-ring has: **flavones**, **flavonols**, **flavanones**, **isoflavones**, **aurones**, **chalcones**, **flavanols** (catechins and proanthocyanidins) and **anthocyanidins**

[2,3]. The general structure of these types of flavonoids is shown in the Fig. (**3**) and some representative examples of each one are given.

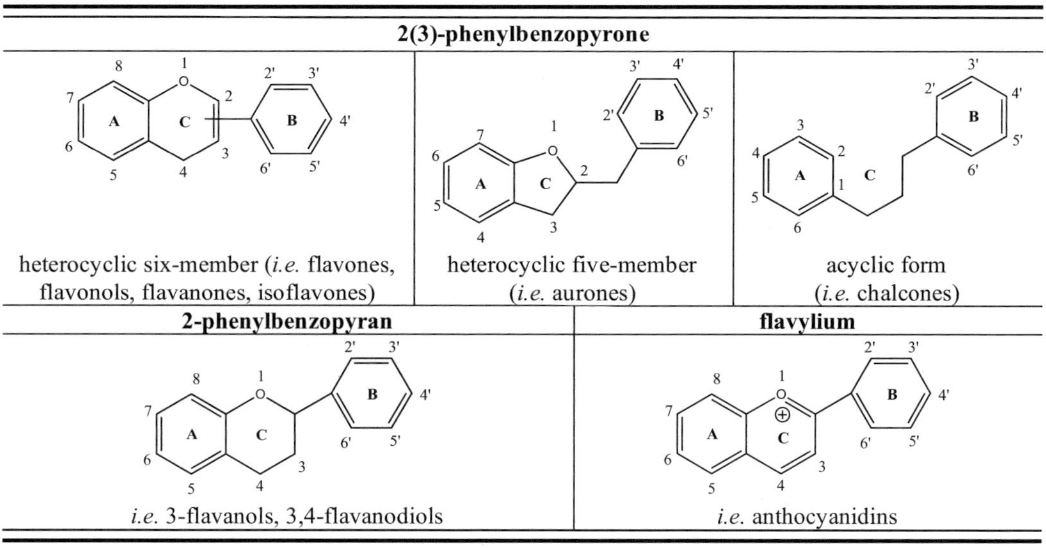

Fig. (2). Flavonoids types depending on the degree of unsaturation of C-ring.

Structurally, **flavones** include a double bond between C2 and C3 and a 4-oxo group in C ring. **Flavonols** have also a double bond between C2 and C3, in addition to a 3-hydroxy and a 4-oxo groups in the C ring. In the **flavanones** and **flavonols** structures, there is no double bond in the chromane ring. The structural difference between these two flavonoids types lies in the chemical substituents: flavanones have a 4-oxo group in the C ring whereas flavanols have a hydroxyl group at the 3 position. Furthermore, flavanols can form polymers (proanthocyanidins). The **isoflavones** have its C ring connected to the C_3 position as a differential structural feature with the other flavonoids. They have also a double bond between C2 and C3 and a 4-oxo functional group in the chromane ring. **Anthocyanidins** have double bond between C2 and C3 and between C3 and C4 in the C ring. **Aurones** differ from the other flavonoids in presenting a 5-membered ring instead of the 6-membered ring in the C-ring. **Chalcones** also do not have a 6-membered ring in the C-ring if not an enone group that links A-ring with B-ring [2,3].

FLAVONES

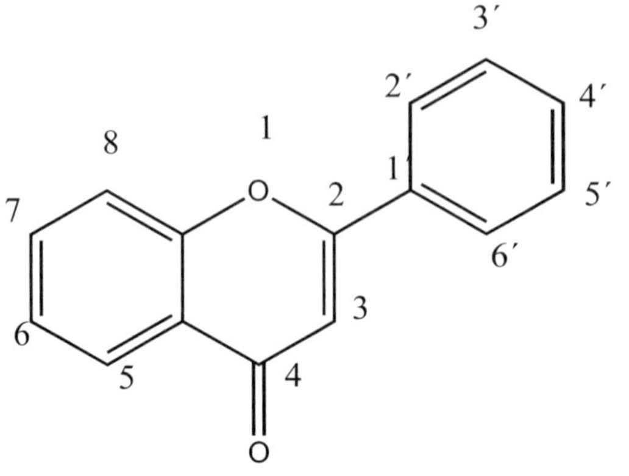

Apigenin (4′,5,7-trihydroxyflavone)
Luteolin (3′,4′,5,7-tetrahydroxyflavone)
Tangeritin (4′,5,6,7,8-pentamethoxyflavone)
Baicalein (5,6,7-trihidroxyflavone)
Scutellarein (5,6,7,4′-tetrahydroxyflavone)

FLAVONOLS

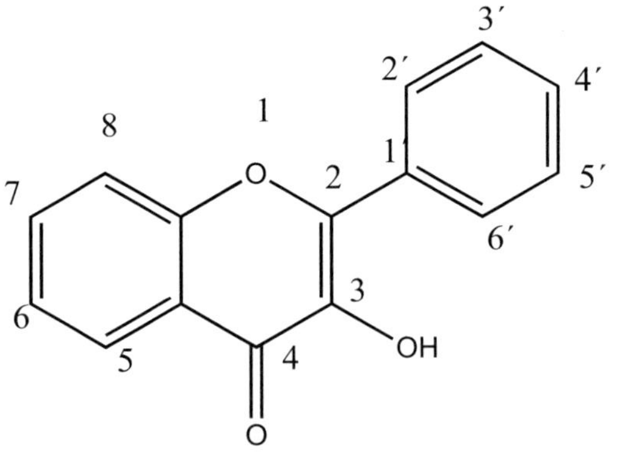

Quercetin (3,3',4',5,7-pentahydroxy-2-phenylchromen-4-one)
Kaempferol (3,4',5,7-tetrahydroxy-2-phenylchromen-4-one)
Myricetin (3,3',4',5',5,7-hexahydroxy-2-phenylchromen-4-one)
Isorhamnetin (3,5,7-trihydroxy-2-(4-hydroxy-3-methoxyphenyl)chromen-4-one)
Morin (2-(2,4-dihydroxyphenyl)-3,5,7-trihydroxychromen-4-one)

(Fig. 3) contd…..

FLAVANONES

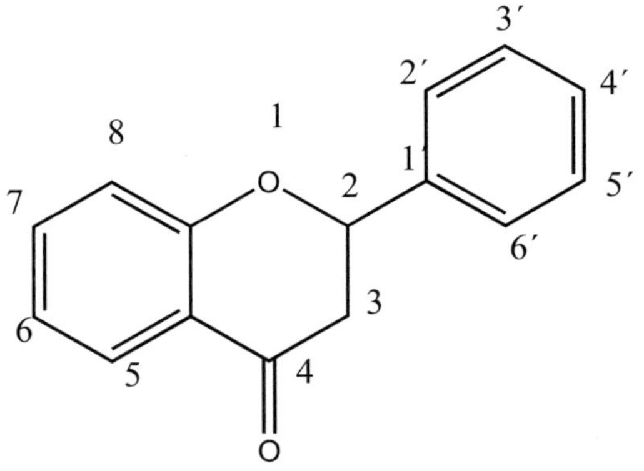

Naringenin (5,7-dihydroxy-2-(4-hydroxyphenyl)chroman-4-one)
Hesperetin (2,3-dihydro-5,7-dihydroxy-2-(3-hydroxy-4-methoxyphenyl)-4H-1-benzopyran-4-one)
Eriodictyol (2-(3,4-Dihydroxyphenyl)-5,7-dihydroxy-4-chromanone)
Butin (2-(3,4-Dihydroxyphenyl)-7-hydroxy-2,3-dihydrochromen-4-one)

ISOFLAVONES

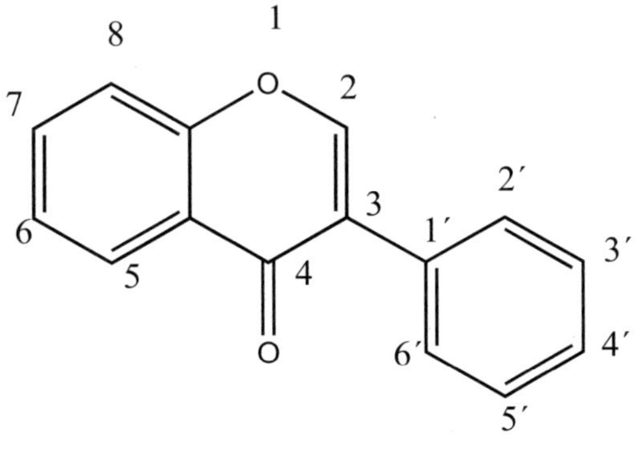

Genistein (5,7-Dihydroxy-3-(4-hydroxyphenyl)chromen-4-one)
Daidzein (7-Hydroxy-3-(4-hydroxyphenyl) chromen-4-one)
Glycitein (7-Hydroxy-3-(4-hydroxyphenyl)-6-methoxy-4-chromenone)

(Fig. 3) contd…..

AURONES

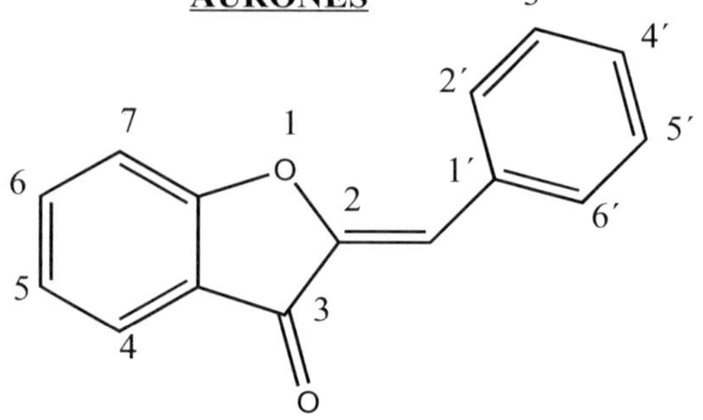

Auresidin (2-[(3,4-dihydroxyphenyl)methylidene]-4,6-dihydroxy-1-benzofuran-3-one)
Leptosidin (2-[(3,4-dihydroxyphenyl)methylidene]-6-hydroxy-7-methoxy-1-benzofuran-3-one)

CHALCONES

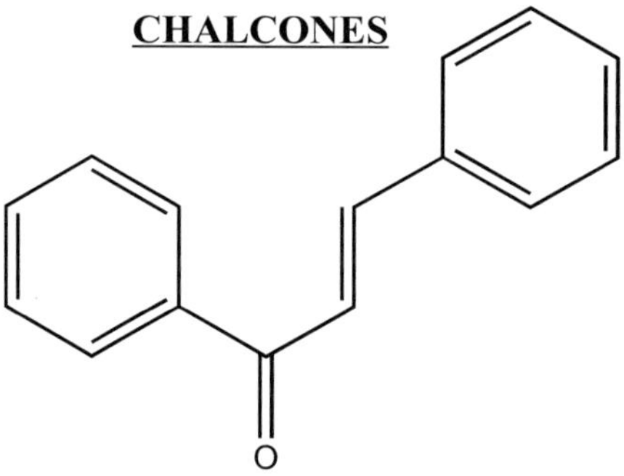

Flavokavain (1-(2-Hydroxy-4,6-dimethoxy-phenyl)-3-phenyl-propenone)

FLAVANOLS

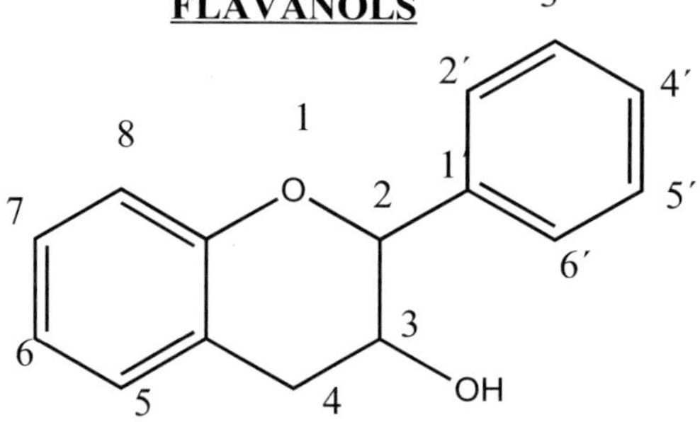

Catechin (2-(3,4-dihydroxyphenyl)-3,4-dihydro-2H-chromene-3,5,7-triol)
Epicatechin (3,3',4',5,7-Pentahydroxyflavane, (2R,3R)-2-(3,4-Dihydroxyphenyl)-3,4-dihydro-1(2H)-benzopyran-3,5,7-triol)
Epigallocatechin (3,3',4',5,5',7-Hexahydroxyflavane, (-)-cis-2-(3,4,5-Trihydroxyphenyl)-3,4-dihydro-1(2H)-benzopyran-3,5,7-triol)
Gallocatechin (2-(3,4,5-Trihydroxyphenyl)-3,4-dihydro-1(2H)-benzopyran-3,5,7-triol)
Fisetinidol (2alpha-(3,4-Dihydroxyphenyl)-3,4-dihydro-2H-1-benzopyran-3beta,7-diol)
Mesquitol (3,4-Dihydro-2alpha- (3,4-dihydroxyphenyl) -2H-1-benzopyran-3beta,7,8-triol)

(Fig. 3) contd.....

ANTHOCYANIDINS

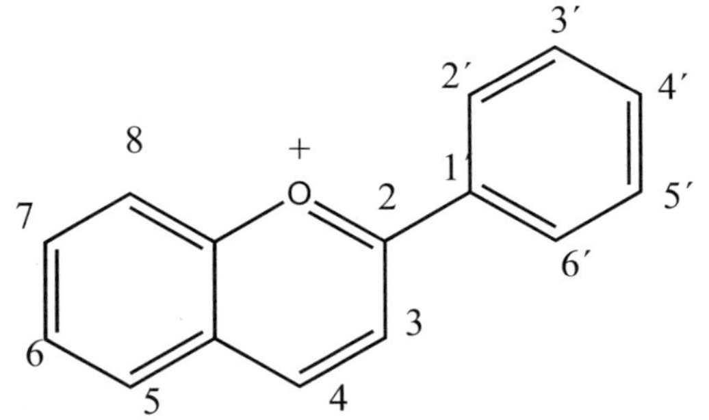

Cyanidin (2-(3,4-Dihydroxyphenyl) chromenylium-3,5,7-triol)
Delphinidin (2-(3,4,5-trihydroxyphenyl)chromenylium-3,5,7-triol)
Pelargonidin (2-(4-Hydroxyphenyl)chromenylium-3,5,7-triol)
Malvidin (3,5,7-trihydroxy-2-(4-hydroxy- 3,5-dimethoxyphenyl)chromenium)
Peonidin (2-(4-Hydroxy-3-methoxyphenyl)chromenylium-3,5,7-triol)

Fig. (3). Chemical structures of the subclasses of flavonoids. Some examples of each subclass are given.

Flavonoids are structurally characterized by presenting one or more hydroxyl groups (normally at the positions of 3,5,7,3′,4′and 5′). These hydroxyl groups are commonly found as sulphated, methylated, acetylated and prenylated forms. The position and the presence of these different chemical substituents lead to flavonoids are the most ubiquitous groups of plant phenolics [3].

Flavonoids can be found in nature as aglycone (without an attached sugar) and as glycosides (with an attached sugar substituent such as glucose, rhamnose, galactose, arabinose and glucorhamose). The sugar substituent can be attached to –OH groups of aglycone at 3 and 7 positions (O-glycosides) or to carbons at 6-C or 8-C positions (C-glycosides). Most flavonoids exist as glycosides except for flavonols (catechins and proanthocyanidins) [3].

Flavonoids constitute the majority of the flower and fruits pigments. Flavonols, flavones, chalcones and aurones are responsible for yellow colors -hence its name derives from the Latin word *flavus* that means yellow-, and anthocyanidins are for the red, the purple and the blue ones. In anthocyanidins, the type and the degree of substitutions as well as the value of pH determine its color. As example, anthocyanidins occur as red pigments in acidic conditions and as blue pigments in basic conditions [4].

Moreover flavonoids are responsible for other organoleptic properties including the bitterness and the astringency found in many foods such as chocolate, tea and wine, among others [5]. Protoanthocyanidins, which are flavanol polymers, are the main group of flavonoids contributing to these organoleptic properties. The different degrees as both bitter and astringent depend on several structural features such as the degree of polymerization, the specific chiral polarization configurations and the type and position of the monomeric flavanols units that comprise the polymer [5-7]. As example, the sensation of astringency will be higher and the bitterness lower, the higher degree of proanthocyanidin polymerization [8]. As another example, dimer B6 (catechin-4,6-catechin) is found to be more bitter and astringent than dimer B3 (catechin-4,8-catechin) and dimer B4 (catechin-4,8-epicatechin) [7].

In plants, flavonoids perform multiple roles in both defense and plant reproduction. The bright color (yellow, blue and red) of flowers and fruits, provided by flavonoids, attract pollinators and seed disperses involved in the reproductive processes [8]. Moreover, flavonoids protect the photosynthetic tissues of plants from the harmful effects of UV-B radiation. Under UV-B radiation exposition, flavonoids are able to absorb light from 280-315 nm (UV-B wavelength) and changes in their synthesis are induced to increase the content of flavonoids including flavone and flavonol-types [1]. Furthermore, they take part of the natural defense system, protecting plants from both insects and mammalian herbivores [8].

Biosynthesis of Flavonoids

Combinations of the shikimate pathway and the acetate pathway lead to the biosynthesis of flavonoids (Fig. **4**) [9, 10].

The phenylpropane unit of flavonoids (C6-C3; ring B and chromane ring) derives from the amino acid phenylalanine (shikimate pathway) whereas the C6 unit (ring A) comes from three units of malonyl-CoA (acetate pathway) [9, 10].

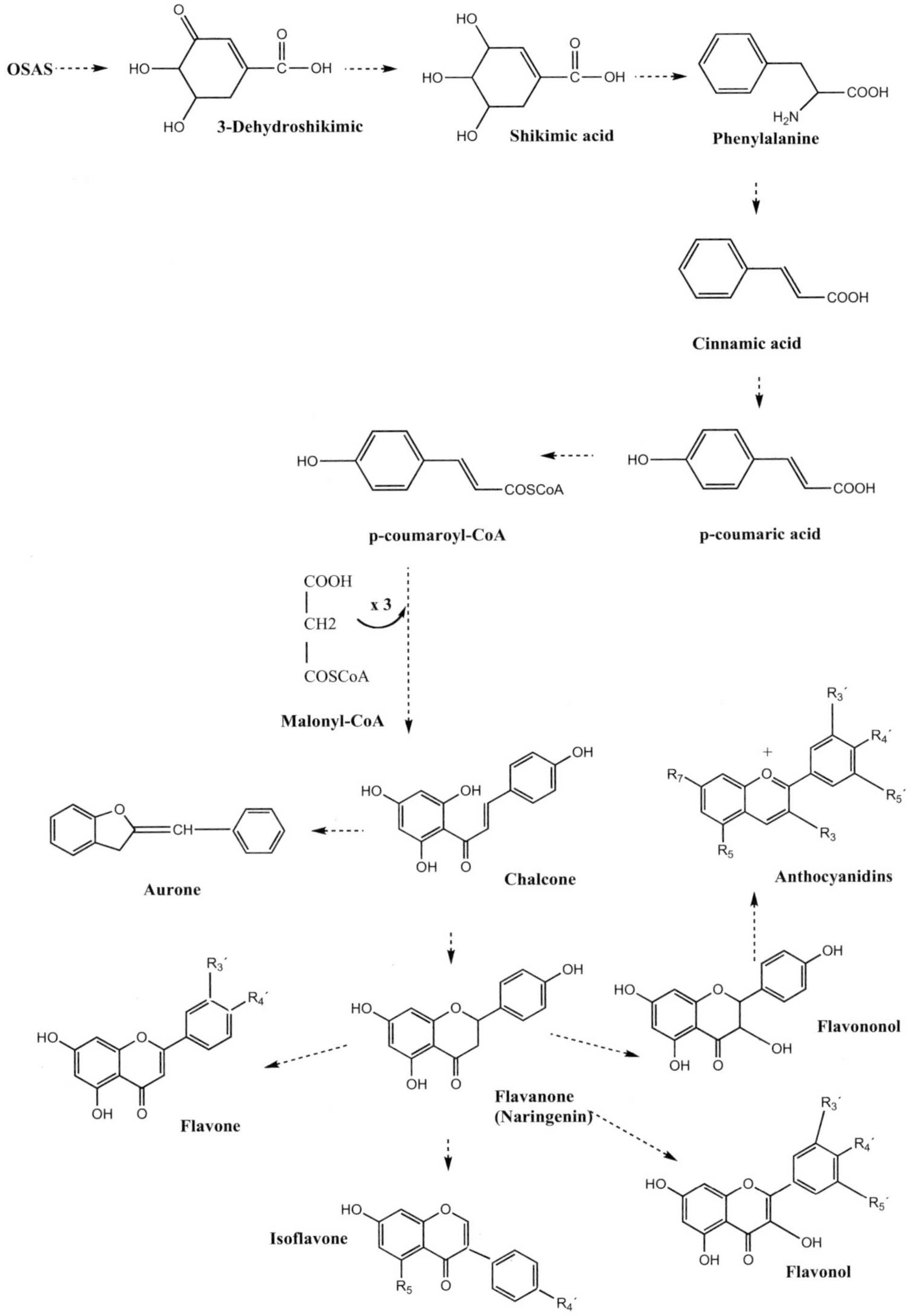

Fig. (4). Biosynthesis of flavonoids.

The condensation of one molecule of 4-coumaroyl-CoA (shikimate pathway) and three molecules of malonyl-CoA (acetate pathway) catalyzed by the enzyme chalcone synthase yields to the common intermediate of flavonoids synthesis named as 4,2′,4′,6′ tetrahydroxychalcone. Then, the chalcone isomerizes to the flavanone, being this structural type flavonoid the precursor of other flavonoids such as isoflavones, flavonols, flavones and anthocyanidins [9, 10].

Distribution of Flavonoids in Nature

Flavonoids are widely distributed in the plant kingdom. As we have commented previously, flavonoids provide the bright colors (yellow, blue, purple and red) to flowers and fruits of many different plants belonging to a wide range of plant families including Lamiaceae, Rutaceae, Leguminosae, Asteraceae, Fabaceae and Umbelliferae [8].

Flavones such as apigenin, luteolin and baicalein occur commonly as both aglycones and glycosides (generally as 7-,3′-and 4′-O-glycosides and 6-,8-C-glycosides in vacuoles of cells). As C-glycosides and O-glycosides, flavones are widely presented from green algae to higher plants. On the other hand, different species of the genus *Prunus*, *Betula* and *Alnus*, among others, contain flavones as aglycones [11,12].

Most of the identified flavonols (*i.e.* quercetin, kaempferol, myricetin, *etc.*) are found in the outer and aerial tissues (skin and leaves) of plants as O-glycosides (mainly 3-,7-,3′-4′-glycosides) from Bryophytes to higher plants. The most common glycosides encountered on flavonols are glucose and rhamnose, but other sugars including arabinose, galactose, xylose and glucuronic acid have been also identified. The third part of all sorts of flavonols occurs as aglycones such as in some species of the genus Betula and Artemisia [13,14]. The content in flavonols is highly dependent on the light. Hence, the concentration of flavonols will be higher when the higher sunlight exposition.

The plant families Rutaceae, Leguminosae and Compositae contain high amounts and variety of flavanones (*i.e.* naringenin, butin, hesperetin, *etc.*), mainly, as aglycones and O-glycosides [13,15].

Isoflavonoids (*i.e.* genistein, daidzein, glycitein) are commonly found as aglycones in the rhizomes, roots, wood, bark and seeds of different families of angiosperms such as Leguminosae and Iridaceae. Less common but not rare it is to find isoflavonoids in Gymnosperms, Bryophytes and Marine coral [13,14].

Aurones such as auresidin and leptosidin have been mainly identified in the Leguminosae and Compositae families as aglycones and O-glycosides. Moroever, the families Aspleniaceae (Pteridophytes) and Conocephalaceae, Fumariaceae and Marchantiaceae (Btyophytes) contain aurones as phytochemical constituents [15,16].

Most of the anthocyanidins including malvidin, cyanidin, pelargonidin and delphinidin, among others, are widespread distributed in higher plants (both angiosperms and gymnosperms) except in some families of the order Caryophyllales such as Cactaceae, Didiereaceae and Phytolaccaceae [17]. Other anthocyanidins including luteolinidin, apigeninidin and 3-deoxyanthocyanidins are more frequent in lower plants than in higher plants [18]. Most of the anthocyanidins occur as glycosides and they are responsible for the colors of many fruits, vegetables, cereal grains, and flowers [17].

Chalcones are commonly found in angiosperms taking part of the yellow pigments of the flowers. Three-quarters of the chalcones which occur in nature are aglycones and one-quarter are O-glycosides (in the literature has been only described one case of a C-glycoside chalcone, particularly, C-glucosylisoliquiritigenin found in *Cladrastis platycatpa* of the Leguminosae family) [15].

Among the different types of food, fruits, vegetables, whole grains and beverages including wine, tea and chocolate have high flavonoid content.

The green leafs spices including celery, parsley and capsicum pepper contain high amounts of flavones glycosides such as apigenin and luteolin. On the other hand, the skin of citrus fruit, and particularly the essential oil of mandarin are rich in polymethoxylated flavones such as tangeretin, nobiletin and sinensetin [19,20].

The citrus fruit contain high amounts of flavanones in the white spongy portion and in the membranes that separate the segments. Flavanones intake is up to 5 times higher in the whole fruit than in a glass of orange juice. Among the different citrus fruit and flavanones, grapefruits are rich in naringenin, lemons in eriodictyol and oranges in hesperetin [19,20].

It is estimated that the habitual intake of dietary flavonoids is about 23 mg/day, being quercetin the most abundant one (60 to 75% of total flavonoids content) [21]. Fruits, vegetables and beverages including broccoli, onions, leek, curly kale, blueberries, red wine and tea are flavonols-rich foods (Table **1**). Among this flavonoid-type, quercetin is the major dietary compound and it is commonly contained in onions (0.3 mg/g fresh weight), tea (10–25 mg/mL) and peel apple (1 mg/g fresh weight) [19,20,22,23].

The major source of the isoflavones such as genistein, daidzein and glycitein are found in high amounts in plants of the family Leguminosae, and predominantly in soy (genistein and daidzein represent approximately 1 mg/g dry soy bean) [19,20].

Table 1. Flavonoids in Food

Flavonoids Type	Food Sources	References
Flavones	Green leafs spices (*i.e.* celery, parsley and capsicum pepper); skin of citrus and the essential oil of mandarin	[19,20]
Flavanones	Citrus fruit (*i.e.* grapefruits, lemons, oranges)	[19,20]
Flavonols	Fruits, vegetables and beverages (*i.e.* broccoli, onions, leek, curly kale, blueberries, red wine and tea)	[19-23]
Isoflavones	Soya beans, legumes	[19,20]
Flavonols	Tea, apricots, chocolate, red wine, apples	[19,24]

Tea, both black and green, are beverages with high amounts of flavonols. The content in flavonols in this social drink is both time and temperature-dependent. The polymers thearubigems (7–15% by dry weight) and the dimers theaflavins (4% by dry weight) are found mainly in black tea whereas catechins, epigallocatechin, epigallocatechin-3-gallate, epicatechin-3-gallate and epicatechin are predominantly in green tea. Epigallocatechin-3-gallate represents more than 40% of the total polyphenolic content in green tea [24].

Table 2. Examples of Medicinal Plants Rich in Flavonoids

Botanical Name	Family	Type of Flavonoids Contained	References
Ficaria verna Huds.	Ranunculaceae	Kaempferol, quercetin, vitexin, orientin, isovitexin, disoorientin	[25]
Prunus serotina Ehrh	Rosaceae	Quercetin, kaempferol, isorhamnetin	[26]
Astragali Radix	Fabaceae	Ononin, calycosin and formononetin	[27]
Glycine max	Leguminosae	Genistein, daidzein, genistin, daidzin, malonylgenistin, acetylgenistin, malonyldaidzin	[28]
Caucalis platycarpos	Apiaceae	Luteolin-7-O-glucoside, apigenin-7-O-glucoside, luteolin, quercetin-3-O-galactoside, quercetin-3-O-rhamnoside, apigenin, chrysoeriol	[29]
Sophora flavescens	Leguminosae	Kushenol U, kurarinone, sophoraflavanone G, leachianone A, kuraridin, kushenol A	[30]
Rhodiola rosea	Crassulaceae	Gossypetin-di-O-glucoside, OH-gossypetin-7-O-rha-8-O-glu, Herbacetin-di-O-glucoside, Kaempferol-3-O-glu-7-O-glu, Quercetin-3-O-rha-7-O-glu, Gossypetin-di-O-glucoside or O-diglucoside, Gossypetin-7-O-rha-8-O-glu = rhodiolgidin, Gossypetin-3-O-glu-7-O-xylo/ara, Herbacetin-8-O-xylo-3-O-glu = rhodalidin, Herbacetin-7-O-rha-8-O-glu = rhodionidin, Herbacetin-3-O-glu -7-O-xylo/ara, Gossypetin-7-O-rha = rhodiolgin, Quercetin-3_/4_-rha, Herbacetin-7-O-rha = rhodionin	[31]
Reseda luteola	Resedaceae	Luteolin, luteolin-7-glucoside and luteolin-30,7-diglucoside	[32]
Adinandra nitida	Theaceae	epicatechin, rhoifolin, apigenin, quercitrin, camellianin A, camellianin B	[33]
Morettia philaena	Brassicaceae	kaempferol, kaempferol 3-O-β-glucopyranoside, kaempferol3, 7di-O-β-glucopyranoside, kaempferol3-O-β-sophoroside-7-O-β-glucopyranoside, quercetin, quercetin 3-O-β-glucopyranoside, quercetin 3-O-β-gentobioside, orientin, isoorientin	[34]
Kaempferia parviflora	Zingiberaceae	5,7-dimethoxyflavone, 5,7,4-trimethoxyflavone; 5-hydroxy-7-methoxyflavone; 5- hydroxy-3,7-dimethoxyflavone; 3,5,7-trimethoxyflavone; 5-hydroxy-3,7,4-trimethoxyflavone; 5-hydroxy-7,4-dimethoxyflavone; 5-hydroxy-3,7,3,4-tetramethoxyflavone; 3,5,7,4- tetramethoxyflavone; 5,7,3,4-tetramethoxyflavone; 3,5,7,3,4-pentamethoxyflavone	[35]
Chuquiraga spinosa	Asteraceae	quercetin-3-O-glucuronide, quercetin-3-O-rutinoside, quercetin-3-O-glucoside, kaemperol-3-O-glucuronide, kaemperol-3-O-rutinoside, kaempherol-3-O-glucoside, isorhamnetin-3-O-glucuronide, isorhamnetin-3-O-rutinoside and isorhamnetin-3-O-glucoside	[36]
Scutellaria baicalensis	Lamiaceae	5,2-Dihydroxy-6,7,8-trimethoxy flavone; 5,7-Dihydroxy-6-methoxy flavone; 5,2-Dihydroxy-6,7,8,6-tetramethoxy flavone; 5,7-Dihydroxy flavone; 5,7-Dihydroxy-6,8-dimethoxy flavone; 5,2-Dihydroxy-7,8,6-trimethoxy flavone; 5,5,6,6,7,7-Hexahydroxy-8,8-biflavone; 5,6,7-Trihydroxy flavone; 5,7,8-Trihydroxy flavone, baicalein-6-O-glucuronide; Wogonin-7-O-glucoside; Chrysin-6-C-glucosyl-8-C-arabonoside; Scutellarein-7-O-glucuronide	[37]

Apricots (250 mg/kg fresh weight), chocolate (up to 600 mg/L), red wine (up to 300 mg/L) and apples (65% of total polyphenol content) contain also large quantities of catechins. The skins and seed of grapes are rich in protoanthcyanidins [19,24].

PARKINSON´S DISEASE; A BRIEF OVERVIEW

Parkinson's disease was named after the English physician, Dr. James Parkinson, who first described it in 1817. Parkinson´s disease is a chronic and neurodegenerative disease characterized by a gradual and progressive loss of dopaminergic neurons, affecting the brain area that coordinates the muscle tone, movement and activity [38,39].

Dopaminergic neurons, which are located in the pars compacta of the substantia nigra, produce the neurotransmitter dopamine. When there is a depletion of dopamine, manifested in Parkinson´s disease as a degeneration and death of dopaminergic neurons in the striatum, there is a motor system incoordination and decontrol (rigidity, tremor, slowness of movement…) [39].

Parkinson´s disease is the second most common neurodegenerative disorder in the world. It affects both men and women (being much more common in men) of all races and all continents. The major percent of people suffer from Parkinson´s disease are over 60 years. It is estimated that more than 4.5 million people worldwide suffer from this disease, and it is expected to increase to some 9 million in the next 25 years [40,41].

The etiology is still unknown although two factors have been involved as main causes in the pathogenesis of Parkinson´s disease [42]:

- Endogenous and exogenous dopaminergic neurotoxins that inhibit the complex I of the mitochondrial electron transfer complex in the substantia nigra.

- Oxidative stress in dopaminergic neurons. The overproduction of reactive oxygen species (ROS) or the failure of endogenous antioxidant system (enzymatic and non-enzymatic type) may lead to a disturbance of intracellular pro-oxidant/antioxidant homeostasis. Then, harmful ROS may cause direct oxidative injury to cellular constituents such as lipids, DNA and proteins, altering its structure and function.

The symptoms of Parkinson´s disease include [43]:

- ❖ Motor Symptoms:

- – Tremor: rhythmic, oscillations movements of face, legs, arms, hands…
- – Bradykinesia: slowness of spontaneous and automatic movements.
- – Rigidity: muscle stiffness in neck, trunk and limbs that may cause pain.
- – Postural instability that may cause falls.

- ❖ Neuropsychiatric symptoms: depression, anxiety, apathy and psychosis, sleep disturbances, mild cognitive impairment and dementia.
- ❖ Automatic dysfunction: problems with urination, constipation, erectile dysfunction), hyperhidrosis, malnutrition…

Hoehn and Yahr established different 5 stages for the progression of Parkinson´s disease [44]:

- – Stage 1. Signs and symptoms on one side of the body.
- – Stage 2. Signs and symptoms on both sides of the body without impairment of balance.
- – Stage 3. Postural instability.
- – Stage 4. Severe disability although the patient can walk and stand unassisted.

– Stage 5. Requires constant cares. The patient lye in the bed or in the wheelchair. Only of 15% of patients reach the final stages of the disease.

Oxidative Stress in Parkinson´s Disease

The involvement of oxidative stress in the progressive neurodegeneration that occurs in the substantia nigra in Parkinson's disease has been demonstrated in numerous studies of the postmortem human brain and in studies with experimental models. The term "oxidative stress" defines a pathological condition resulting from the production of excessive amounts of reactive oxygen species (ROS) which can not be compensated by the antioxidant system of the organism (enzymatic and non-enzymatic). It was found that the levels of reactive oxygen species (ROS) in the pars compacta of the substantia nigra are much higher in PD patients than in people without this disease. These ROS derive mainly from the metabolism of dopamine itself [39,45].

The oxidative deamination of dopamine catalyzed by the enzymes monoamine oxidases A and B (MAO A and MAO B), leads to the formation of H_2O_2 [46]. This H_2O_2 produces hydroxyl radical *via* a Fenton-type reaction; this reaction is favored by high levels of Fe^{2+} in the substantia nigra (the ratio of the levels of Fe^{2+}: Fe^{3+} is 2:1 for Parkinson´s patients and 1:2 for people without such pathology) [47].

Dopamine can also auto-oxidized, resulting in the formation of reactive quinones and semiquinones with the consequent production of superoxide anion, hydroxyl radical and H_2O_2 [48].

From a biochemical point of view, the most significant changes observed in the substantia nigra that show oxidative stress and mitochondrial dysfunction conditions in patients suffer from Parkinson´s disease were: high levels of 4-hydroxy-2-nonenal (HNE), high levels of 8-hydroxy-2'-deoxyguanosine and 8-hydroxyguanine [49,50], a decreased in mitochondrial complex I activity which is accompanied by a decrease in ATP levels, abnormal calcium homeostasis and loss of membrane potential [51] and reduced levels of GSH that are significant from the earliest stages of the disease (30-40% reduction) and they are not accompanied by an increase in the oxidized form of glutathione [52,53]. It has been observed patients suffer from Parkinson's that this decrease in GSH levels is not due to a failure in the synthesis process since the activity of the enzyme γ-glutamyl transpeptidase is significantly increased. The release of excessive amounts of the dipeptide cysteinylglycine (CysGly) by the action of this enzyme, and the subsequent action of dipeptidases, yield to the amino acid cysteine. This amino acid, instead of being used in the synthesis of GSH, can react with dopamine quinones, forming **5**-S-cisteinil-dopamine. This compound can in turn be converted in dihidrobenzotiazine derivatives which are irreversible inhibitors of mitochondrial complex I [54].

The present chapter aims to review the *in vitro*, *ex vivo* and *in vivo* studies on flavonoids as potential preventive and therapeutic agents in Parkinson´s disease.

FLAVONOIDS AND STRUCTURE-ANTIOXIDANT ACTIVITY

Previous structure-antioxidant activity studies have identified several key features for explaining the radical scavenging, the metal ion chelation and the enhancement of antioxidant defense system properties of flavonoids.

The hydroxyl groups presented on the aromatic ring, and mainly on the B-ring, determine the free radical scavenging activity of flavonoids. Flavonoids act as good scavenger compounds through hydrogen atom transfer (HAT) and electron transfer (ET) mechanism [55,56].

The hydrogen atom transfer consist of transferring to free radical a hydrogen atom from the hydroxyl group, converting free radical into a less harmful substance and the aromatic ring into the oxidized $ArO^{\bullet}$ [55,56].

$$ArOH + R^{\bullet} \longrightarrow ArO^{\bullet} + RH$$

The electron transfer mechanism consists of the donation of an electron to the free radical, resulting in a cation radical $ArOH.^{+}$ and in an anion $R^{\bullet}$ (both less harmful that the scavenged free radical) [55,56].

$$ArOH + R^{\bullet} \longrightarrow ArO^{+\bullet} + R^{\bullet}$$

The odd electron on the aromatic rings ($ArO^{\bullet}$ and $ArO^{+\bullet}$) is stabilized by resonance through the conjugation with the benzene ring [55,56].

The higher the number of hydroxyl groups, the higher the peroxyl and the hydroxyl scavenging activities for flavones and flavanones [57]. Moreover, the position of hydroxyl groups also influence in the antioxidant activity of flavonoids. Hence, the scavenging ability of flavonoids is higher for those compounds with a 3′,4′-catechol in the B-ring (*i.e.* catechin and luteolin) that those don′t [58].

In addition to the hydroxyl groups, the presence the presence of 2,3 unsaturation together with an oxo function at position 4 in the C ring are also important structural features for their scavenging properties [55,56].

Moreover, flavonoids have the ability to bind metal ions such as iron and cupper which participate in different reactions to produce free radicals. The 4-carbonyl, 3-hydroxy and 5-hydroxy groups of the C-ring of flavonoids are responsible for the iron chelation [59].

PARKINSON′S DISEASE AND FLAVONOIDS AS ANTIOXIDANT COMPOUNDS (TABLES 3 AND 4)

Among the different mechanisms involved in the neuroprotective effect of flavonoids, we will focus in this chapter on the antioxidant defense ones.

Different classic toxin-induced *in vitro* and *in vivo* Parkinson′s diseases models have been employed for the experimental investigations of the neuroprotective therapeutic activity exhibited by flavonoids. Among Parkinson′s disease neurotoxicant mimetics are found 1-methyl-4-phenyl-1,2,3,6-tetrahydropyridine (MPTP), 6-hydroxydopamine (6-OHDA) and rotenone which destroy dopaminergic neurons in the substantia nigra of the brain, causing the appearance of similar symptoms to those of Parkinson′s disease. In addition to these neurotoxicant mimetics, other chemical compounds have been employed simulating oxidative stress-related events such as hydrogen peroxide and metal ions [39,45].

Few investigations have examined the potential protective effect of individual flavonoids as antioxidants in Parkinson´s disease models of oxidative stress. Most of these studies have been focused in flavones such as luteolin, flavonols such as quercetin and kaempferol and flavonols such as catechin and epigallocatechin.

Next, it is compiled a series of studies, based on the structural type, of flavonoids with potential application in oxidative stress involved in the Parkinson´s disease.

Flavones

Four flavones, named as luteolin, apigenin, 7,8-dihydroxyflavone and baicalein have been investigated for their antioxidant activity in Parkinson´s disease models. The mechanism of action of flavones include free radical scavenging activity and capacity of activate the endogenous defense system.

Luteolin, one of the most common flavonoids, has been identified as a potential neuroprotective agent against different oxidative stress inductors and on different nervous system cells type. Hence, luteolin restored redox equilibrium by inhibiting ROS production and by increasing the enzymatic system in both primary culture cortical neruons and astrocytes under oxidative stress conditions H_2O_2 and IL-1 beta-induced, respectively [60,61].

Apigenin showed an antioxidant activity in a pretreatment experimental model in hippocampal neurons kainic acid-induced toxicity through the scavenging of intracellular reactive oxygen species and the prevention of intracellular GSH depletion [62].

The **7,8-dihydroxyflavone** has also appeared as a potential promising therapeutic compound against the oxidative stress induced cell damage through antioxidant activity. Using hydrogen peroxide, menadione and glutamate as oxidative stress inductors, Chen *et al.* demonstrated that this flavone confers neuroprotection to the hippocampal HT-22 cell line by inhibiting ROS generation and increasing glutathione levels [63].

Pre- and post- treatments with **baicalein** (5,6,7-trihydroxyflavone), isolated from the stems and leaves of *Scutellaria baicalensis*, inhibited the ROS levels increment such as superoxide and NO when dopaminergic neurons were stimulated *in vitro* with the lipopolysaccharide as oxidant insult [64].

Flavonols

Quercetin, kaempferol and quercitrin have demonstrated to possess potential antioxidant properties in *in vitro* and *in vivo* models through free radical scavenging and endogenous defense system activation mechanisms. Quercetin is the flavonol and one of the flavonoids type more deeply investigated.

Quercetin, a flavonols widely distributed in the nature, has also been shown to have antioxidant activity. Gélinas and Martinoli suggested that quercetin attenuates MPP^+-induced oxidative stress *via* direct antioxidant mechanisms. Quercetin prevents *in vitro* the cell death in dopaminergic neurons caused by the accumulation of reactive oxygen species-elicited oxidative damage [65].

The nuclear transcription factor Nrf2 plays an important role in the ability of quercetin to protect CNS cells from oxidative damage. Through Nrf2 activation, quercetin modulated the intracellular redox targeting the GSH redox system and consequently, prevented from hydrogen peroxide induces *in vitro* death of neuronal cells [66].

Wagner *et al.* evaluated the potential protective antioxidant activity of quercetin, rutin and quercitrin by being these three flavonoids administered at a concentration of 10 μg/mL before MgHg injection (5 μM) as oxidative insult. The analysis of rat cortical brain slices demonstrated that **quercetin** and **quercitrin**, but not rutin, are mitochondrial-targeted neuroprotective compound by reducing the formation of ROS and the peroxidation of lipids that occurs in this organelle [67].

The study of several flavonoids from *Hypericum perforatum* revealed that the antioxidant properties of **quercetin** as well as of **kaempferol** are responsible, at least in part, from the oxidative damage to cell structures. Both compounds reduced the lipid peroxidation and prevented the loss of mitochondrial membrane potential that occurs as a consequence of the exposure to 100 μM kainate plus 100 μM N-methyl-D-aspartate in neuronal cells [68]. In an experimental model consisted on rat cortical cells under N-methyl-D-aspartate (NMDA)-induced toxicity, kaempferol exerted a neuroprotective effect acting as a lipid peroxidation inhibitor [69].

Anthocyanidins

Among anthocyanidins, four compounds named as cyanidin-3-O-glucoside, delphinidin-3-O-glucoside, petunidin-3-O-glucoside and pelargonidin act as potential antioxidants *via* activation of endogenous defense system and signaling pathway as well as *via* ROS inhibition.

The pretreatment with the following anthocyanidins **cyanidin-3-O-glucoside**, **delphinidin-3-O-glucoside**, and **petunidin-3-O-glucoside**, isolated from *Glycine max*, assisted in preventing ROS damage hydrogen peroxide-induced in the human brain neuroblastoma SK-N-SH cells *via* enhancement of HO-1 activity, free radical scavenging effects and inhibiting activation of ASK1-JNK/p38 signaling pathway [70].

The beneficial health properties of the oral anthocyanidin-type **pelargonidin** under oxidative stress conditions in a Parkinson´s disease model have been recently demonstrated. In this novelty study, the administration of pelargonidin *via* oral has shown to reduce the lipid peroxidation produced by 6-OHDA as revealed the thiobarbituric acid reactive substances (TBARS) assay [71].

Isoflavonoids

Yu *et al*. characterized the antioxidant properties of several isoflavonoids isolated from *Astragalus mongholicus*: formononetin, ononin, 9, 10-dimethoxypterocar-pan-3-O-beta-D-glucoside, calycosin and calycosin-7-O-glucoside. For this purpose, PC12 cells as neuronal model and xanthine (XA)/ xanthine oxidase (XO) as injury substance. Of all the studied isoflavonoids, **formononetin**, **calycosin** and **calycosin-7-O-glucoside** resulted potent antioxidant compounds by increasing the endogenous antioxidant enzymatic system, and particularly, the activity and the expression of superoxide dismutase and glutathione peroxidase [72].

Chalcones

The chalcone **isoliquiritigenin**, isolated from *Glycyrrhiza uralensis*, has been reported to attenuate 6-OHDA-induced stress injury, protecting Parkinson´s disease-related dopaminergic cells from the apoptotic cell death caused by oxidative stress *via* ROS inhibition [73].

Flavanones

The flavanone **fusin**, found in *Rhus verniciflua*, provides an antioxidant protective effect on the SK-N-SH human neuroblastoma cell line when it is applied as co-treatments and pretreatments prior to 6-OHDA. The action mechanism of this class of flavonoid consisted of the inhibition of the endogenous ROS generation and the rise in intracellular calcium caused by 6-OHDA [74].

Other flavanone, **naringenin** conferred *in vitro* protection to dopaminergic cells challenged with 6-OHDA as shown to the restoration of redox imbalance. On the other hand, in this study, quercetin and fisetin which have been previously shown to possess strong antioxidant effects were inactive in this Parkinson´s experimental model [75].

Flavonols

Previous reports have investigated the anti-oxidant stress activity of the flavonols **epigallocatechin-3-gallate**, which is one of the major compounds and the most biologically active catechin found in green tea. Schroeder *et al.* evaluated the beneficial effects of this flavonoid-type against different types of oxidative insults to primary cultures of rat cerebellar granule neurons. The co-incubation of epigallocatechin-3-gallate with the insults demonstrated that the investigated flavonoid, acting as free radical scavenger, protected neurons from apoptosis triggered by mitochondrial oxidative stress [76]. Moreover, in another study conducted using animal mice and non-human primates models for investigating the antioxidant mechanisms of epigallocatechin-3-gallate, it has been reported that this flavonoid possesses iron chelating scavenging properties, preventing the accumulation of iron and alpha-synuclein in the substantia nigra pars compacta [77]. Because the oxidative stress and iron accumulation are involved in the pathogenesis of Parkinson´s disease, the combination of both direct and the indirect antioxidant properties (free radical scavenging, iron chelating and enhancement of the enzymatic and non-enzymatic anti-oxidant defense systems) of the epigallocatechin-3-gallate makes this compound a potential and promising therapeutic agent for patients who suffer from Parkinson´s disease.

In another report, with the aim to improve the stability and bioavailability of epigallocatechin-3-gallate, the potential protective effect of a pro-drug (fully acetylated epigallocatechin-3-gallate) has been studied in a Parkinsonism mimic cellular model 6-OHDA-induced in retinoic acid (RA)-differentiated neuroblastoma SH-SY5Y cells. It has been shown that exposure to SH-SY5Y cells to 25 μM 6-OHDA for 24 h resulted in an increase of both caspase-3 activity and lactate dehydrogenase release. The pretreatment with the pro-drug of epigallocatechin-3-gallate (from 0.1 to 10 μM for 30 min) restored the oxidative equilibrium. This report shows that improving the galenic properties of epigallocatechin-3-gallate and maintaining its antioxidant properties can get a promising neuroprotective agent for the therapeutic of Parkinson´s disease [78].

Table 3. Antioxidant Mechanisms of Action of Flavonoids with Interest for the Treatment of Parkison´s Disease

Antioxidant Mechanism of Action	Flavonoids
Free radical scavenging	apigenin, baicalein, cyanidin-3-O-glucoside, delphinidin-3-O-glucoside, 7,8-dihydroxyflavone, epigallocatechin-3-gallate, fusin, isoliquiritigenin, kaempferol, luteolin, pelargonidin, petunidin-3-O-glucoside, quercetin, quercitrin.
Transition metal chelation	epigallocatechin-3-gallate
Activation of endogenous defense system	apigenin, calycosin, calycosin-7-O-glucoside, cyanidin-3-O-glucoside, delphinidin-3-O-glucoside, 7,8-dihydroxyflavone, epigallocatechin-3-gallate, formononetin, luteolin, petunidin-3-O-glucoside, quercetin
Activation of signaling pathway	cyanidin-3-O-glucoside, delphinidin-3-O-glucoside, petunidin-3-O-glucoside.

From a global point of view, most of the studies performed for evaluating the antioxidant activity of flavonoids in Parkinson´s disease models have been *in vitro* type using both primary cell cultures and cell lines. The action mechanisms that

Table 4. Examples of Flavonoids with Pharmacological Interest for the Treatment of Parkison´s Disease

Compound	Type of Flavonoid	Origin	Type of Study	Effect	References
7,8-dihydroxyflavone	flavone	commercial	*In vitro*	Inhibiting ROS generation and increasing glutathione levels	[63]
cyanidin-3-O-glucoside	anthocyanidins	*Glycine max*	*In vitro*	Enhancement of HO-1 activity, free radical scavenging effects and inhibiting activation of ASK1-JNK/p38 signaling pathway	[70]
delphinidin-3-O-glucoside	anthocyanidins	*Glycine max*	*In vitro*	Enhancement of HO-1 activity, free radical scavenging effects and inhibiting activation of ASK1-JNK/p38 signaling pathway	[70]
epigallocatechin-3-gallate	flavanol	Green tea	*In vitro* *In vivo*	Free radical scavenger, decrease caspase-3 activity, decrease LDH activity, increase the phosphorylation level of Akt, iron chelating scavenging activity	[76-78]
kaempferol	flavonol	*Hypericum perforatum* *Ginkgo biloba*	*In vitro*	Lipid peroxidation reduction, prevention of the loss of mitochondrial membrane potential	[68,69]
luteolin	flavone	*Perilla frutescens*	*In vitro*	Inhibition ROS generation, restored enzymatic and non-enzymatic system, increased mitochondria activity, reducing the expression of proinflammatory cytokines and chemokines	[60]
petunidin-3-O-glucoside	anthocyanidins	*Glycine max*	*In vitro*	Enhancement of HO-1 activity, free radical scavenging effects and inhibiting activation of ASK1-JNK/p38 signaling pathway	[70]
quercetin	flavonol	commercial *Hypericum perforatum*	*In vitro* *In vivo*	Modulation of the GSH redox system, lipid peroxidation reduction, prevention of the loss of mitochondrial membrane potential, ROS inhibition	[65-68]

(Table 4) contd.....

Compound	Type of Flavonoid	Origin	Type of Study	Effect	References
apigenin	flavone	*Cirsium japonicum* *Chrysanthemum boreale*	*In vitro* *In vivo*	Scavenging of intracellular reactive oxygen species, prevention of intracellular GSH depletion	[62]
quercitrin	flavonol	commercial	*In vivo*	ROS inhibition and lipid peroxidation reduction	[68]
baicalein	flavone	*Scutellaria baicalensis*	*In vitro*	ROS inhibition	[64]
fusin	flavanone	*Rhus verniciflua*	*In vitro*	Inhibition of the endogenous ROS generation, inhibition the rise in intracellular calcium	[74]
naringenin	flavanone	commercial	*In vitro*	Restoration of redox imbalance	[75]
formononetin	isoflavonoid	*Astragalus mongholicus*	*In vitro*	Increasing the endogenous antioxidant enzymatic system (SOD, GPx)	[72]
calycosin	isoflavonoid	*Astragalus mongholicus*	*In vitro*	Increasing the endogenous antioxidant enzymatic system (SOD, GPx)	[72]
calycosin-7-O-glucoside	isoflavonoid	*Astragalus mongholicus*	*In vitro*	Increasing the endogenous antioxidant enzymatic system (SOD, GPx)	[72]
isoliquiritigenin	chalcone	*Glycyrrhiza uralensis*	*In vitro*	ROS inhibition	[73]

predominate in these studies are free radical scavenging activity and the activation of endogenous defense system. Moreover, in the treatment of central nervous system diseases, the passage of active compounds to the brain represents an important step for the therapeutically action. In this regard, experimental animal studies have been shown that several flavonoids such as epicatechin and quercetin and their metabolites are transport across the blood-brain barrier after oral administration [79-81]. Furthermore, most of the flavonoids employed in these investigations have been isolated from medicinal plants including *Glycine max*, *Hypericum perforatum*, *Ginkgo biloba*, and *Astragalus mongholicus*, among others, which are traditionally employed for Central Nervous System disorders (Table **2**). Combining flavonoids found in the diet and in medicinal plants with potential antioxidant properties and able to penetrate in the brain are key strategies for the prevention and treatment of Parkinson´s disease. However, all studies are very preliminary and further *in vivo* and clinical studies are required for strong demonstrating their therapeutic implications in this neurodegenerative disease.

CONCLUSIONS

Flavonoids, in a broad perspective, are a wide group of 4,000 phenolic compounds found virtually in all plants, being responsible for the flower and fruit pigmentation.

Flavonoids, is one of the most studied group of natural products, having demonstrated significant effects on human health for their antioxidant, antiinflammatory, venotonic and vascular protective effects.

In the last recent years, the potential effect as antioxidants of flavonoids in Parkinson´s disease, present in dietary and medicinal plants, have been investigated. Despite the high number of compounds identified (more than 4,000), very few compounds have been studied including quercetin, luteolin, baicalein and cyaniding-3-O-glucoside. Therefore, continuing research in the role of individual flavonoids as antioxidants is required and may yield further insights into its therapeutic role in the prevention and treatment of Parkinson´s disease. Moreover, since most of the studies are *in vitro*, it is necessary to perform *in vivo* and clinical assays that support the potential role demonstrated for these compounds.

ACKNOWLEDGEMENTS

None declared.

CONFLICT OF INTEREST

The authors state that there is no conflict of interest.

REFERENCES

[1] Harborne JB, Williams CA. Advances in flavonoid research since 1992, Phytochemistry 2000;55:481–504.
[2] Corradini E, Foglia P, Giansanti P, Gubbiotti R, Samperi R, Lagana A. Flavonoids: chemical properties and analytical methodologies of identification and quantitation in foods and plants. Nat Prod Res. 2011; 25:469-95.
[3] Sandhar HK, Kumar B, Prasher S, Tiwari P, Salhan M, Sharma P. A review of phytochemistry and pharmacology of flavonoids. Int Pharm Sci 2011; 1: 25-41.
[4] He F, Mu L, Yan GL, Liang NN, Pan QH, Wang J, Reeves MJ, Duan CQ. Biosynthesis of anthocyanins and their regulation in colored grapes. Molecules. 2010; 15:9057-91.
[5] Peleg H, Gacon K, Schlich P, Noble AC. Bitterness and astringency of flavan-3-ol monomers, dimers and trimmers. J. Sci. Food Agric. 1999;79: 1123-28.
[6] Lesschaeve I, Noble AC. Polyphenols: factors influencing their sensory properties and their effects on food and beverage preferences. Am J Clin Nutr. 2005;81:330S-5S.
[7] Kallithraka S, Bakker J, Clifford MN. Evaluation of bitterness and astringency of (_)-catechin and (_)-epicatechin in red wine and in model solution. J Sensory Stud 1997;12:25–37.
[8] Samanta A, Das G, Das SK. Roles of flavonoids in plants. Int J Pharm Sci Tech 2011;6:12-35.
[9] Knaggs R. The biosynthesis of shikimate metabolites. Nat Prod Rep 2001;18: 334-55.
[10] Ward RS. The synthesis of lignans and neolignans. Chem Soc Rev 1982;11:75-125.
[11] Iwashina T, Kadota Y, Ueno T, Ootani S. Foliar flavonoid composition in Japanese Cirsium species (Compositae), and their chemotaxonomic significance. J Jap Bot 1995; 70: 280-90.
[12] Iwashina T. Detection and distribution of chrysanthemin and idaein in autumn leaves of plants by high performance liquid chromatography. Ann Tsukuba Bot Gard. 1996;15: 1-18.
[13] Jay M. 1994. C-Glycosylflavonoids. In J.B. Harborne, ed., The Flavonoids: Advances in Research Since 1986. Chapman and Hall, London, pp. 57-93.
[14] Iwashina T, Ootani S. Three flavonol allosides from *Glaucidium palmatum*. Phytochemistry 1990; 29:3639- 41.
[15] Iwashina, T. The structure and distribution of the flavonoids in plants. J Plant Res 2000;113: 287-99.
[16] Giannasi DE. The flavonoid systematics of the genus Dahlia (Compositae). Mem. New York Bot. Gard 1975. 26 1-125.
[17] Piattelli M, Minale L. Pigments of Centrospermae- ll. Distribution of betacyanins. Phytochemistry 1964;3: 547-57.
[18] Bendz G, Mlrtensson 0. Moss pigments II. The anthocyanins of *Bryum rutilans* Brid. and *Bryum weigelii* Spreng. Acta Chem. Scand. 1963;17: 266.
[19] Manach C, Scalbert A, Morand C, Rémésy C, Jimenez L. Polyphenols: food sources and bioavailability. Am J Clin Nutr 2004;79:727-47
[20] Tomas-Barberan FA, Clifford MN. Dietary hydroxybenzoic acid derivatives and their possible role in health protection. J Sci Food Agric 2000;80:1024 –32.
[21] Mullie P, Clarys P, Deriemaeker P, Hebbelinck M. Estimation of daily human intake of food flavonoids. Plant Foods Hum Nutr. 2007;62:93-8.
[22] Guyot S, Le Bourvellec C, Marnet N, Drilleau JF. Procyanidins are the most abundant polyphenols in dessert apples at maturity. LWT-Food Sci. Technol. 2002; 35: 289-91.

[23] Guyot S, Marnet N, Sanoner P, Drilleau JF. Variability of the polyphenolic composition of cider apple (*Malus domestica*) fruits and juices J Agric Food Chem. 2003; 51, 6240-47.

[24] Baptista JAB, Tavares JFD, Carvalho RCB. Comparison of polyphenols and aroma in red wines from Portuguese mainland *versus* Azores Islands. Food Res Int 1998; 31:729-41.

[25] Tomczyk M, Gudej J. Quantitative analysis of flavonoids in the flowers and leaves of *Ficaria verna* Huds. Z Naturforsch C. 2003;58:762-4.

[26] Olszewska M. Quantitative HPLC analysis of flavonoids and chlorogenic acid in the leaves and inflorescences of *Prunus serotina* Ehrh. Acta Chromatographica. 2007;19:253-69.

[27] Lv YW, Hu W, Wang YL, Huang LF, He YB, Xie XZ. Identification and determination of flavonoids in astragali radix by high performance liquid chromatography coupled with DAD and ESI-MS detection. Molecules. 2011;16:2293-303.

[28] Caligiani A, Palla G, Maietti A, Cirlini M, Brandolini V. 1H NMR fingerprinting of soybean extracts, with emphasis on identification and quantification of isoflavones. Nutrients. 2010;2:280-9.

[29] Plazonić A, Bucar F, Males Z, Mornar A, Nigović B, Kujundzić N. Identification and quantification of flavonoids and phenolic acids in burr parsley (*Caucalis platycarpos* L.), using high-performance liquid chromatography with diode array detection and electrospray ionization mass spectrometry. Molecules. 2009;14:2466-90.

[30] S. J. Kim, S. M. Kim, M. C. Kim, S. W. Kang, B. H. Um. Fast identification of flavonoids in the roots of *Sophora flavescens* by on-flow LC-NMR. Med Plant Res. 2010;4:2452-9.

[31] Petsalo A, Jalonen J, Tolonen A. Identification of flavonoids of *Rhodiola rosea* by liquid chromatography-tandem mass spectrometry. J Chromatogr A. 2006;1112:224-31.

[32] Petsalo A, Jalonen J, Tolonen A. Identification of flavonoids of *Rhodiola rosea* by liquid chromatography-tandem mass spectrometry. J Chromatogr A. 2006;1112:224-31.

[33] Zhang J, Yang J, Duan JC, Liang Z, Zhang LH, Huo YS, Zhang YK. Quantitative and qualitative analysis of flavonoids in leaves of *Adinandra nitida* by high performance liquid chromatography with UV and electrospray ionization tandem Mass spectrometry detection. Anal Chim Acta 2005;532:97-104.

[34] Kawashty SA, Hussein SR, Marzouk MM, Ibrahim LF, Helal MMI, El Negomy SIM. Flavonoid constituents from *Morettia philaena* (Del.) DC. and their antimicrobial activity. J Appl Sci Res, 2012;8:1484-9.

[35] Sutthanut K, Sripanidkulchai B, Yenjai C, Jay M. Simultaneous identification and uantitation of 11 flavonoid constituents in *Kaempferia parviflora* by gas chromatography. J Chromatogr A. 2007;1143:227-33.

[36] Landa A, Casado R, Calvo MI. Identification and quantification of flavonoids from *Chuquiraga spinosa* (Asteraceae). Nat Prod Commun. 2009;4:1353-5.

[37] Liu G, Rajesh N, Wang X, Zhang M, Wu Q, Li S, Chen B, Yao S. Identification of flavonoids in the stems and leaves of *Scutellaria baicalensis* Georgi. J Chromatogr B Analyt Technol Biomed Life Sci. 2011;879:1023-8.

[38] Pandey S. Parkinson's disease: recent advances. J Assoc Physicians India. 2012 ;60:30-32.

[39] Jenner P. Oxidative stress in Parkinson's disease. Ann. Neurol. 2003; 53, S26–S36.

[40] Elbaz A, Moisan F. Update in the epidemiology of Parkinson's disease. Curr Opin Neurol. 2008; 21, 454–60.

[41] Muangpaisan W, Mathews A, Hori H, Seidel D. A systematic review of the worldwide prevalence and incidence of Parkinson's disease. J Med Assoc Thai. 2011; 94, 749-55.

[42] Gazewood JD, Richards DR, Clebak K. Parkinson disease: an update. Am Fam Physician. 2013, 87, 267-273.

[43] Ziemssen T, Reichmann H. Non-motor dysfunction in Parkinson's disease. Parkinsonism Relat Disord. 2007;13: 323-32.

[44] Reichmann H. Clinical criteria for the diagnosis of Parkinson's disease. Neurodegener Dis. 2010;7, 284-290.

[45] Zhou C, Huang Y, Przedborski S. Oxidative stress in Parkinson's disease: a mechanism of pathogenic and therapeutic significance. Ann New York Acad Sci. 2008;1147, 93-104.

[46] Ahmad FF, Cowan DL, Sun AY. Free radical generation from dopamine through the action of monoamine oxidase (MAO). Society of Neuroscience Abstract. 1990; 350, 9.

[47] Götz ME, Double K, Gerlach M, Youdim MB, Riederer P. The relevance of iron in the pathogenesis of Parkinson's disease. Ann N Y Acad Sci. 2004;1012, 193-208.

[48] Asanuma M, Miyazaki I, Ogawa N. Dopamine- or L-DOPA induced neurotoxicity: the role of dopamine quinone formation and tyrosinase in a model of Parkinson's disease. Review. Neurotox Res. 2003;5: 165–76.

[49] Alam ZI, Jenner A, Daniel SE, Lees AJ, Cairns N Marsden CD, Jenner P, Halliwell B. Oxidative DNA damage in the parkinsonian brain; a selective increase in 8-hydroxyguanine in substantia nigra? J Neurochem. 1997,69:1196–203.

[50] Zhang J, Perry G, Smith MA, Robertson D, Olson SJ, Graham DJ, Montine TJ. Parkinson's disease is associated with oxidative damage to cytoplasmic DNA and RNA in substantia nigra neurons. Am J Pathol. 1999;154:1423–29.

[51] Schulz JB, Beal MF. Mitochondrial dysfunction in movement disorders. Curr Opin Neurol. 1994;7: 333-39.

[52] Sofic E, Lange KW, Jellinger K, Riederer P.. Reduced and oxidized glutathione in the substantia nigra of patients with Parkinson's disease. Neurosci Lett. 1992;142: 128-30.

[53] Sian J, Dexter DT, Lees AJ, Daniel S, Jenner P, Marsden CD. Glutathione-related enzymes in brain in Parkinson's disease. Ann Neurol. 1994;36:356-61.

[54] Schultz JB, Kindeanau J, Dichgans J. Glutathione, oxidative stress and neurodegeneration. Eur J Biochem. 2000;267:4904-11.

[55] Leopoldini M, Russo N, Toscano M. The molecular basis of working mechanism of natural polyphenolic antioxidants. Food Chemistry. 2011; 125: 288–306.

[56] Heim KE, Tagliaferro AR, Bobilya DJ. Flavonoid antioxidants: chemistry, metabolism and structure-activity relationships. J Nutr Biochem. 2002, 13;572-84.

[57] Cao G, Sofic E, Prior RL. Antioxidant and prooxidant behavior of flavonoids: structure-activity relationships. Free Radic Biol Med 1997;22:749–60.

[58] Van Acker SABE, De Groot MJ, van den Berg, DJ, Tromp MNJL, den Kelder GDO, van der Vijgh WJF, Bast, A. A quantum chemical explanation of the antioxidant activity of flavonoid. Chem Res Toxicol. 1996;9:1305–12.

[59] Dušan M, Vesna K. Investigation of metal-flavonoid chelates and the determination of flavonoids *via* metal-flavonoid complexing reactions. J Serb Chem Soc. 2007, 72: 921-939

[60] Zhao G, Yao-Yue C, Qin GW, Guo LH. Luteolin from *Purple perilla* mitigates ROS insult particularly in primary neurons. Neurobiol Aging. 2012;33:176-86.

[61] Sharma V, Mishra M, Ghosh S, Tewari R, Basu A, Seth P, Sen E. Modulation of interleukin-1beta mediated inflammatory response in human astrocytes by flavonoids: implications in neuroprotection. Brain Res Bull. 2007;73:55-63.

[62] Han JY, Ahn SY, Kim CS, Yoo SK, Kim SK, Kim HC, Hong JT, Oh KW. Protection of apigenin against kainate-induced excitotoxicity by anti-oxidative effects. Biol Pharm Bull. 2012;35:1440-6.

[63] Chen J, Chua KW, Chua CC, Yu H, Pei A, Chua BH, Hamdy RC, Xu X, Liu CF. Antioxidant activity of 7,8-dihydroxyflavone provides neuroprotection against glutamate-induced toxicity. Neurosci Lett. 2011;499:181-5.

[64] Li FQ, Wang T, Pei Z, Liu B, Hong JS. Inhibition of microglial activation by the herbal flavonoid baicalein attenuates inflammation-mediated degeneration of dopaminergic neurons. J Neural Transm. 2005;112:331-47.

[65] Gélinas S, Martinoli MG. Neuroprotective effect of estradiol and phytoestrogens on MPP+-induced cytotoxicity in neuronal PC12 cells. J Neurosci Res. 2002;70:90-6.

[66] Arredondo F, Echeverry C, Abin-Carriquiry JA, Blasina F, Antúnez K, Jones DP, Go YM, Liang YL, Dajas F. After cellular internalization, quercetin causes Nrf2 nuclear translocation, increases glutathione levels, and prevents neuronal death against an oxidative insult. Free Radic Biol Med. 2010;49:738-47.

[67] Wagner C, Vargas AP, Roos DH, Morel AF, Farina M, Nogueira CW, Aschner M, Rocha JB. Comparative study of quercetin and its two glycoside derivatives quercitrin and rutin against methylmercury (MeHg)-induced ROS production in rat brain slices. Arch Toxicol. 2010;84:89-97.

[68] Silva B, Oliveira PJ, Dias A, Malva JO. Quercetin, kaempferol and biapigenin from *Hypericum perforatum* are neuroprotective against excitotoxic insults. Neurotox Res. 2008;13:265-79.

[69] Sloley BD, Urichuk LJ, Morley P, Durkin J, Shan JJ, Pang PK, Coutts RT. Identification of kaempferol as a monoamine oxidase inhibitor and potential neuroprotectant in extracts of *Ginkgo biloba* leaves. J Pharm Pharmacol. 2000;52:451-9.

[70] Kim SM, Chung MJ, Ha TJ, Choi HN, Jang SJ, Kim SO, Chun MH, Do SI, Choo YK, Park YI. Neuroprotective effects of black soybean anthocyanins *via* inactivation of ASK1-JNK/p38 pathways and mobilization of cellular sialic acids. Life Sci. 2012;90:874-82.

[71] Roghani M, Niknam A, Jalali-Nadoushan MR, Kiasalari Z, Khalili M, Baluchnejadmojarad T. Oral pelargonidin exerts dose-dependent neuroprotection in 6-hydroxydopamine rat model of hemi-parkinsonism. Neurosci Lett. 2010;469:360-4.

[72] Hwang CK, Chun HS. Isoliquiritigenin isolated from licorice *Glycyrrhiza uralensis* prevents 6-hydroxydopamine-induced apoptosis in dopaminergic neurons. Biosci Biotechnol Biochem. 2012;76(3):536-43.

[73] Yu DH, Bao YM, An LJ, Yang M. Protection of PC12 cells against superoxide-induced damage by isoflavonoids from *Astragalus mongholicus*. Biomed Environ Sci. 2009; 22:50-4.

[74] Park BC, Lee YS, Park HJ, Kwak MK, Yoo BK, Kim JY, Kim JA. Protective effects of fustin, a flavonoid from *Rhus verniciflua* Stokes, on 6-hydroxydopamine-induced neuronal cell death. Exp Mol Med. 2007;39:316-26.

[75] Zbarsky V, Datla KP, Parkar S, Rai DK, Aruoma OI, Dexter DT. Neuroprotective properties of the natural phenolic antioxidants curcumin and naringenin but not quercetin and fisetin in a 6-OHDA model of Parkinson's disease. Free Radic Res. 2005;39:1119-25.

[76] Schroeder EK, Kelsey NA, Doyle J, Breed E, Bouchard RJ, Loucks FA, Harbison RA, Linseman DA. Green tea epigallocatechin 3-gallate accumulates in mitochondria and

displays a selective antiapoptotic effect against inducers of mitochondrial oxidative stress in neurons. Brain Res Bull. 2010;82:279-83.

[77] Mandel S, Maor G, Youdim MB. Iron and alpha-synuclein in the substantia nigra of MPTP-treated mice: effect of neuroprotective drugs R-apomorphine and green tea polyphenol (-)-epigallocatechin-3-gallate. J Mol Neurosci. 2004;24:401-16.

[78] Chao J, Lau WK, Huie MJ, Ho YS, Yu MS, Lai CS, Wang M, Yuen WH, Lam WH, Chan TH, Chang RC. A pro-drug of the green tea polyphenol (-)-epigallocatechin-3-gallate (EGCG) prevents differentiated SH-SY5Y cells from toxicity induced by 6-hydroxydopamine. Neurosci Lett. 2010;469:360-4.

[79] Paulke A, Schubert-Zsilavecz M, Wurglics M. Determination of St. John's wort flavonoid-metabolites in rat brain through high performance liquid chromatography coupled with fluorescence detection. J Chromatogr B Analyt Technol Biomed Life Sci. 2006, 832, 109-113.

[80] Talavéra S, Felgines C, Texier O, Besson C, Gil-Izquierdo A, Lamaison JL, Rémésy C. Anthocyanin metabolism in rats and their distribution to digestive area, kidney, and brain. J Agric Food Chem. 2005, 53, 3902-3908.

[81] Abd El Mohsen MM, Kuhnle G, Rechner AR, Schroeter H, Rose S, Jenner P, Rice-Evans CA. Uptake and metabolism of epicatechin and its access to the brain after oral ingestion. Free Radic Biol Med. 2002;33:1693-702.

312 *Frontiers in CNS Drug Discovery*, **2013**, *2*, 312-333

CHAPTER 9

Essential Polyunsaturated Fatty Acids as New Treatments for Neurodegenerative Diseases

Cai Song*

Research Institute for Marine Nutrition and Drugs, Guangdong Ocean University, China; Department of Psychology and Neurosciences, Dalhousie University, Canada

Abstract: Inflammation plays an important role in the onset and progress of neurodegenerative diseases. Inflammation may trigger or exacerbate neuronal apoptosis and death through glucocorticoid secretion, oxidative stress, and changes in neurotransmission. Therefore, the use of anti-inflammatory drugs might diminish the cumulative effects of inflammation in the brain. Indeed, some epidemiological studies showed that sustained use of anti-inflammatory drugs or natural products may prevent or slow down the progression of neurodegenerative diseases.

Among several new products, omega (n)-3 fatty acids have anti-inflammatory and neuroprotective effects with few side effects. Essential polyunsaturated fatty acids (PUFA), including n-3 and 6 fatty acids can change brain and immune functions. The effects may be *via* modulating 1) membrane structure and fluidity; 2) the interaction between genes and proteins; 3) channel and receptor functions; 4) neurotransmitter release and long-term potentiation process, 5) the function of glial cells in the brain and 6) cellular and humoral inflammatory responses and more. Many studies have demonstrated that n-3 and n-6 fatty acids cooperate and compete with each other to maintain the homeostasis. Over intake of n-6 fatty acids may induce inflammation and neurodegeneration, while n-3 fatty acids have been tried clinically and experimentally to treat patients with neurodegenerative diseases or to explore therapeutic mechanisms in animal models.

More interestingly, the combination of n-3 and n-6 fatty acids at different ratios showed the enhancement of anti-inflammation, neuroprotection or gene and protein modulation.

This chapter will (1) review the new findings from studies in relationship between inflammation and neurodegenerative disease, mainly Alzheimer's disease (AD); (2) introduce the important role of PUFA in the brain and the immune system; (3) discuss clinical trials of n-3 fatty acids used for treatments of neurodegeneration and (4) explore/summarize possible mechanisms by which PUFA can be used for treatment of neurodegeneration. In addition, the limitation of current studies and further research directions will be raised.

***Address correspondence to Cai Song:** Research Institute for Marine Nutrition and Drugs, Guangdong Ocean University, China; Tel: 86-18275795829; email: cai.song@dal.ca

Keywords: Inflammation, neurodegeneration, microglia, astrocytes, cytokines, neurotransmitters, memory deficit, apoptosis, macrophages, T-lymphocytes.

INTRODUCTION

In the past decade, increasing evidence has demonstrated that inflammation plays an important role in the etiology of many CNS (central nerve system) diseases and neurodegeneration. Inflammation may trigger or promote neurodegeneration through several ways, including glial cell activation, proinflammatory cytokine releases, inflammation-induced dysfunction of the hypothalamic-pituitary adrenal axis (HPA) and glucocorticoid secretion, oxidative stress, and/or increased filtered macrophages or T-lymphacytes in the brain [1,2]. In addition, epidemiological studies have reported that Alzheimer's disease (AD) or Parkinson's disease (PD) patients who took non-steroid anti-inflammatory drugs (NSAID) showed reduced incidence and risk for the disease [3,4]. These data strongly suggest that anti-inflammatory drugs or natural products should be developed as a new generation of treatments for neurodegenerative diseases. Several candidates that showed anti-inflammatory effects have recently been studied, such as microlia inhibitor, NSAID and unsaturated essential omega (n)-3 fatty acids [4, 5]. Due to almost no side-effects and highly effective, n-3 fatty acids have received high attention. Thus, this chapter will first review the new findings from studies in relationship between inflammation and neurodegenerative diseases; secondly at will introduce the important role of polyunsaturated n-3 fatty acids (PUFAs) in the brain and the immune system; third, evaluate clinical trials of n-3 fatty acids in the treatments of neurodegenerative diseases and finally, explore and discuss the possible mechanism by which n-3 fatty acids treated these diseases by experimental results. In addition, the limitation of current studies and further research directions will be raised.

THE ROLE OF INFLAMMATION IN NEURODEGENERATION

The Influence of Immune System on the Brain

Nowadays, stress, anxiety, environment pollution, imbalance nutrition, ageing and drug abuse cause more inflammatory/autoimmune diseases. Peripheral inflammation consists of a response in the cytokine network, an acute phase response in the liver and activation of complement cascades. Activated macrophage can produce proinflammatory cytokines, *e.g.*, interleukin (IL)-1β, IL-6 IL-18 and tumor necrosis factor (TNF)-α, are primary inflammatory mediators, which are also called M1 response. M1 response can promote a Thelper-1 (Th1)-related response, which induces inflammatory and autoimmune activities *via* releasing interferon (IFN)-α and TNF-α. M2 macrophages are immunoregulatory and are involved in Th2-like responses, such as releasing Th2 cytokines IL-4, IL-5 and IL-10. The latter have anti-inflammatory functions. IL-1 and other related pro-inflammatory cytokines trigger inflammatory response, produce reactive oxygen and nitrogen species (ROS / RNS) and stimulate positive acute phase proteins, such as haptoglobin and C-reactive protein (CRP) [6]. These immune mediators not only modulate the immune system but also regulate brain functions. The immune system *via* cytokines, acute phase proteins, activated macrophages or T-lymphocytes that pass the brain-blood barrier into the brain affects neurotransmission, neuronal survival and apoptosis, neuroendocine function, which consequently result in behavioral abnormalities, including memory deficit, depression and anxiety [7,8]. Our and other's previous studies have demonstrated that IL-1β and peripheral inflammation can activate glial cells then trigger neuroinflammation [57]. Both microglia and astrocytes after activation can release inflammatory mediators and neurotoxic substances. Increased evidence seems to suggest that microglia produce proinflammatory cytokines, complements and ROS, which may injure neurons and induce apoptosis, while astrocyte activation also produces anti-inflammatory cytokines, chemokines and neurotrophins, which may nourish, support and repair neurons (this is already on a text book, is general knowledge) [9]. There are many cytokine receptors on the neurons. Our and other's previous studies have reported that periphery or centre administrations of pro- and anti-inflammatory cytokines differently change neurotransmitter synthesis and metabolism [10,11]. Moreover, most proinflammatory cytokines can stimulate the HPA axis to produce CRF that by stimulating the pituitary to secrete ACTH release adrenal hormone. Excessive secretion of the stress hormone has been found to cause hippocampus atrophy, neuron apoptosis and memory impairment [12].

Inflammation Related Changes in Neurodegenerative Diseases

Increasing evidence from clinical and experimental studies has shown that elevated neuroinflammatory response occurs in the brain of patients with Alzheimer's disease (AD), Parkinson's disease (PD) and other neurodegenerative diseases.

As mentioned above, microglia mediate neuroinflammation and can be triggered by Aβ. Aβ deposition and enhanced microglial activation are hallmarkers of AD. Olsson and co-workers [13] compared microglial markers between AD and controls, then investigated the relationship between mild cognitive impairment and microglial activity in AD patients and vascular dementia. In 96 AD patients, 65 healthy controls, and 170 patients with the cognitive impairment, microglial makers YKL-40 and sCD14 in cerebrospinal fluid (CSF) were measured from baseline and over 5-7 years. YKL-40, but not sCD14, was significantly elevated in AD compared with healthy controls. Furthermore, YKL-40 and sCD14 were increased in cognitive impaired patients who converted to vascular dementia, but not to AD according to NINCDS-ADRDA. However, when stratified according to CSF levels of tau and Aβ42, YKL-40 was elevated in those with an AD-indicative profile compared with stable mild cognitive impairment with a normal profile. Thus, these microglial markers may be useful as safety markers for monitoring CNS inflammation and microglia activation in clinical trials. On the other hand, a clinical trial (in 9 immunized AD and 8 unimmunized AD patients) studied the effects of Aβ42 immunization on microglial activation and the relationship with Aβ42 load [14]. The patients with immunization showed a decreased Aβ42 load when compared non-immunization. More interesting finding was that Aβ42 immunization increased CD 68 level and microglial phagocytic activity when the plaques were accumulated, but both were decreased below that observed in unimmunized AD when plaques have been cleared. The results suggest that the differences in microglial activation in the cortex were due to the presence of AD pathology. In consistent with increased macroglial activity, increased concentrations of proinflammatory cytokines have been reported since 20 years ago [58]. In the blood, hippocampus and cortex of AD patients, the concentrations of IL-1β, IL-6, TNF-α, CRP and T-helper 1 related inflammatory markers were increased. By contrast, other cytokines such as IL-1 receptor antagonist (IL-1RA),

IL-4, IL-10, and transforming growth factor (TGF)-β, which can suppress both proinflammatory cytokine production and their action, were decreased [15]. For example, 237 AD patients and 245 healthy controls, a clinical investigation measured interferon-γ (IFN-γ) T+874A, cytoplasmic phospholipase A_2(cPLA2), and cyclooxygenase-2 (COX-2) G-765C polymorphisms. The results showed that the expression of COX-2 G/G genotype was significantly increased in the AD, when compared with the control group but there was no significant correlation between IFN-γ or cPLA2 genotypes and AD [16]. Another clinical experiment demonstrated that in the cortex of AD patients, microglial activity, acute phase protein and proinflammatory cytokines are all increased [17]. Furthermore, the study showed that a neuroinflammatory response in the cerebral neocortex parallels the early stages of AD pathology and precedes the late stage, tau-related pathology [17]. Genetic evaluations revealed that some IL-1 phenotypes are significantly related to the high risk of AD [18].

Experimental studies from animal models further revealed the mechanism by which inflammation induces neurodegeneration. In transgenic models of AD, the role of microglia on neurogenesis has been studied. Microglial inhibitor tetracycline derivative minocycline was used to inhibit microglial activity in doubly transgenic mice expressing mutant human amyloid precursor protein (APP) and mutant human presenilin-1 (PS1). Minocycline increased the survival of new dentate granule cells in APP/PS1 mice indicated by more BrdU+/NeuN+ cells as compared to vehicle-treated transgenic littermates. Meantime, learning and memory performance were also markedly improved in a hippocampus-dependent learning task. These results suggest that modulation of microglial function with minocycline can protect hippocampal neurogenesis in the presence of Aβ pathology [53]. Similar to this experiment, a study from another direction investigated the microglia-driven apoptosis and the Aβ deposits triggered generation of new microglial cells in the neocortex of TgCRND8 mice. In 7-month-old transgenic mouse model of AD (TgCRND8) mice the Aβ-associated glial reaction was accompanied by an intense immunoreactivity of both TNF-α and inducible nitric oxide synthase. The expressions of apoptosis related genes also altered such as increased immunoreactivity of the pro-apoptotic protein Bax and a decrease in levels of the anti-apoptotic protein Bcl-2. Cortical and hippocampal neurons in TgCRND8 mice also displayed higher immunoreactivity and higher nuclear expression of the transcription factor NF-kB than controls. These findings indicate that Aβ deposits is related to brain-resident microglia population, and induce overproduction of inflammatory mediators that enhance pro- and anti-apoptotic cascades [19].

The other immune-like cells in the brain, astrocytes maintain the internal homeostasis of the CNS and are fundamentally involved in neuropathological processes, including AD [59]. Astrocytes can produce anti-inflammatory cytokines, regulate glutamate metabolism, produce neurotrophins, which are the most important neuroprotective and neurosupportive functions in the brain. To explore the neuroprotective role of astrocytes in AD pathogenesis, astrocyte activation-glial fibrillary acid protein (GFAP) and vimentin (Vim) related protein were deleted in transgenic mice expressing mutant human amyloid precursor protein and presenilin-1 (APP/PS1). The gene deletions increased amyloid plaque load at 8 and 12 months of age. Moreover, GFAP and Vim gene deletion resulted in a marked increase in dystrophic neuritis, 2- to 3-fold higher than wide type mice, even after normalization for amyloid load. These results suggest that astrocyte activation limits plaque growth and attenuates plaque-related dystrophic neurites [20].

In a triple transgenic mouse model of AD (3 × Tg-AD), the astrocytic cytoskeletal changes within the prefrontal cortex were studied by measuring the surface area and volume of GFAP-positive profiles in relation to the build-up and presence of Aβ, and compared the results with those found in non-transgenic control animals at different ages. 3 × Tg-AD animals showed clear astroglial cytoskeletal atrophy, which appeared at an early age and remained throughout the disease progression at 9, 12 and 18 months old. This atrophy was independent of Aβ accumulation, as only a few GFAP-positive cells were localized around Aβ aggregates, which suggests no direct relationship with Aβ toxicity [21]. However, the changes in astrocyte function may contribute to the decline in cognitive impairment.

Due to entorhinal cortex is fundamental for cognitive functions, astroglial morphology and the surface and volume of the GFAP profiles were measured in the entorhinal cortex of triple transgenic mouse model. A significant reduction in both the surface and volume of GFAP-labelled profiles was found in 3xTg-AD animals from very early ages (1 month) when compared with non-transgenic controls, which was sustained for up to 12 months. The appearance of Aβ depositions at 12 months of age did not trigger astroglial hypertrophy; nor did it result in the close association of astrocytes with senile plaques. The results demonstrated that the AD progressive cognitive impairment can be associated with an early reduction of astrocytic arborization and shrinkage of the astroglial domain, which may affect synaptic connectivity within the entorhinal cortex and between the entorhinal cortex and other brain regions [22]. However, some neurotoxic effects from astrocytes have been reported during neuroinflammation. At cellular level, adult human astrocytes were stimulated with IFN-γ and examined the resultant conditioned medium (CM) for toxicity against differentiated human neuroblastoma SH-SY5Y cells. Cell death was measured by lactate dehydrogenase release assay. Then various treatments were studied by determining the distribution of the toxic components. Removal of IL-6 by a specific antibody reduced IFN-γ-induced toxicity by 22%. Blockade of proteases with an inhibitor cocktail reduced it by a further 22%. When oxygen-free radical production was blocked with NADPH oxidase inhibitors, the toxicity was reduced by 15.4%. When prostaglandin production was blocked by cyclooxygenase inhibitors, the toxicity of the CM was reduced by 14.5%. When glutamate was removed by treatment with glutamate decarboxylase, the toxicity was reduced by 10.3%. When the inhibitors were added together to the astrocyte culture, the total toxicity of the CM was reduced by 91%. These results demonstrated that activated astrocytes release a specific combination of neurotoxic compounds. Even though acute and cellular experiment could not mimic a chronic neurodegenerative disease, the finding suggests that an appropriate combination of anti-inflammatory agents may improve neurodegenerative diseases [23]. As well, activated astrocytes could produce S100B, which has been reported as a pathological marker of AD [24] and PD [25]. S100B promotes the development and maturation of mammalian brains. However, prolonged or extensive S100B exposure can lead to neurodegeneration. S100B plays important role in the development and plasticity of the serotonergic neurotransmitter system, and in the cascade of glial changes associated with neuroinflammation. Both of these processes are therefore accelerated towards degeneration, such as AD and Down syndrome (DS). In these diseases, increased S100B has been reported [26]. In a S100B over-expressing transgenic mice, similar to AD and DS, the animals showed a profound change in serotonin innervation. By 28 weeks of age, there was a significant loss of serotonergical terminals in the hippocampus. The transgenic animals also showed neuroinflammatory changes analogous with AD and DS. These include decreased numbers of mature, stable astroglial cells, increased numbers of activated microglial cells and increased microglial expression of the cell surface receptor RAGE. Eventually, the S100B transgenic animals show neurodegeneration and the appearance of hyperphosphorylated tau structures, which are also seen in late stage DS and AD [27].

Moreover, Song and team have reported that in a chronic IL-1-induced neuroinflammation model, changes in cognitive behavior, neurotransmission, microglia and astrocytes, brain pro- and anti-inflammatory cytokines and neurotrophic system are similar to those observed in AD patients or AD models. For example increased in microglial CD11b expressions, which associated with elevated concentrations of proinflammatory cytokines, decreased astrocyte GFAP expression, which associated with decreased expressions of BDNF and NGF neurotrophins and their receptors. In the water or radial maze, animals showed impaired memory, which was correlated with lower acetylcholine release or lower concentration of NA during memory retrieval [28,52]. IL-1RA, microglia inhibitor, COX2 inhibitor or glucocorticoid receptor antagonist markedly attenuated IL-1-induced the changes [29,52].

With regards to PD, fast increasing evidence has demonstrated that idiopathic PD represents a complex interaction between the inherent vulnerability of the nigrostriatal dopaminergic system, a possible genetic predisposition, and exposure to environmental toxins including inflammatory triggers. Indeed, chronic neuroinflammation is consistently associated with the pathophysiology of PD. Activation of microglia and increased levels of pro-inflammatory mediators such as TNF-α, IL-1β and IL-6, ROS and eicosanoids has been reported in the post-mortem analysis of the substantia nigra from PD patients and in animal models of PD [30]. Moreover, nigrostriatal dopaminergic neurons are more vulnerable to pro-inflammatory and oxidative mediators than other cell types because of their low intracellular glutathione concentration. Systemic inflammation has also been suggested to contribute to neurodegeneration in PD, as lymphocyte infiltration has been observed in brains of PD patients and in animal models of PD. In the dopamine degeneration related brain areas, such as the substantia nigra and striatum, contain 6 times higher microglia than other brain regions, which indicates that inflammation play a key role in this diseases. Consistent with this special phenomenon, increased inflammatory cytokines and responses have been reported in PD patients. For example, in 60 PD patients and 24 matched controls without neurodegenerative and inflammatory disorders, the levels of cytokines, TNF-α, IL-1β, IL-6 and IL-10 were higher in serum of PD patients when compared to the control group. There are also correlations in serum of PD group: between IL-10 and IL-12, IL-6 and IL-1ß [31]. More interesting, an epidemiological study conducted a register-based nested case-control study in Sweden to examine infections of the CNS and sepsis in relation to PD. The study included 18,648 patients and 93,240 matched controls. PD patients were more likely to have a previous hospitalization for CNS infections than controls, while subjects with multiple CNS infections at least 5 years before the index date had higher PD occurrence than those without CNS infections, but there was no correlation between PD and sepsis [32]. It is more obvious that inflammation as a trigger or contributor of amyotrophic lateral sclerosis (ALS) and multiple sclerosis (MS) has been extensively reported.

THE FUNCTION OF OMEGA-3 FATTY ACIDS IN THE CNS AND IMMUNE SYSTEM

As mentioned above, inflammation has been associated with neurodegenerative diseases, and elevated level of pro-inflammatory markers is consistently found in patients with AD, PD or other neurodegenerative diseases. Thus, the increasing concerns have been drawn to the development of anti-inflammatory agents in the treatment of neurodegenerative diseases. Compelling evidence indicated that PUFAs have anti-inflammatory effects [28, 29, 33].

PUFAs are dietary lipids, which can be only synthesized from dietary precursors. PUFAs include omega (n)-3 α-linolenic (ALA), docosahexaenoic acid (DHA) and eicosapentaenoic acid (EPA), while n-6 linoleic fatty acids (LA), gamma-linolenic acid (GLA) and arachidonic acid (AA). These fatty acids are important lipid components of cell membranes, which can influence the structure and fluidity of membranes and regulate the interaction between proteins and genes. The change in PUFAs concentrations in the membranes significantly related to neuronal, glial and immune cell functions [5, 37].

The difference between n-3 fatty acids and n-6 fatty acids is the location of their double bonds in the fatty acid carbon chain. Because n-6 fatty acids metabolite eicosanoids are the precursor of inflammatory mediators, superfluous intake of n-6 fatty acids may trigger inflammation and some inflammation-induced diseases and an increasing intake of n-6 fatty acid can interfere the metabolism and synthesis of DHA and EPA. On the other hand, n-3 fatty acids has competitive interactions with the n-6 fatty acids, which have influence on the relative storage, mobilization, conversion and action of the n-3 and n-6 eicosanoid precursors [54,55]. Thus, n-3 fatty acids derived PUFAs have been demonstrated to inhibit inflammatory activity and depressive disorders. However, most western diets are enriched inn-6 fatty acids, which have a reverse effect on human health, and are associated with inflammation and some inflammation-induced diseases.

PUFAs are able to across the blood-brain barrier and have actions on specific binding sites in the brain. The roles of n-3 fatty acids in the brain include the regulation of cell membrane fluidity, neurotransmitter transmission, membrane bound enzymes and cellular signal transduction [34-36]. The incorporation of n-3 and n-6 fatty acids in neuronal membranes can increase its fluidity, thus enhancing neurotransmission and facilitating signal transduction pathways [34-36,56]. In the past decade, many studies have demonstrated the mechanism by which n-3 fatty acids inhibit inflammation, improve brain function and treat psychiatric diseases. Epidemiological evidence has established that ingestion of n-3 PUFAs, such as in fish oils, have profound effects on many human disorders and diseases, including affective disorders [60].

CHANGES IN N-3 FATTY ACIDS IN NEURODEGENERATION

The deficit of n-3 PUFAs has been associated with neurodegenerative diseases. For example, societies that consume a small amount of n-3 PUFAs appear to have a higher prevalence of neurodegenerative disorder. For example, a clinical investigation was to determine whether plasma PUFAs predict the risk of incident dementia in a cohort of elderly from Bordeaux, France, independently of their depressive status. Of 1214 non-demented participants were followed up for 4 years, in which 65 people developed dementia. A higher plasma EPA concentration was associated with a lower incidence of dementia, independently of depressive status and after adjustment for age, education, apolipoprotein E epsilon4 allele, diabetes, and baseline plasma vitamin E and triacylglycerol. The relations between DHA, total n-3 PUFAs, and incident dementia did not remain significant in multivariate models. Higher ratios of AA to DHA and of n-6 to n-3 fatty acids were related to an increased risk of dementia, particularly in depressive subjects [38]. Because hippocampus and amygdale atrophy and degeneration are the hall marker of AD, another clinical investigation checked whether plasma levels of EPA or DHA predict atrophy of medial temporal lobe (MTL) gray matter regions in older subjects. A total of 281 community dwellers from France, aged 65 years or older, had plasma fatty acid measurements at baseline and underwent MRI examinations at baseline and at 4 years. The association between plasma EPA and DHA and the change of MTL gray matter volume was determined at 4 years. In the patients, higher atrophy of the right amygdala was associated with greater 4-year decline in semantic memory performances and more depressive symptoms. However, plasma EPA, but not DHA, was associated with lower gray matter atrophy of the right hippocampal/parahippocampal area and of the right amygdala. Specially, a higher plasma EPA at baseline was related to smaller gray matter loss per year in the right amygdale [38]. As well, differences in plasma and brain fatty acid profiles between AD, mild cognitive impairment, and those with no cognitive impairment were analyzed. The finding showed that DHA was lower in the phosphatidylserine of the mid-frontal cortex and superior temporal cortex in AD compared to no cognitive impairment [39].

On the other hand, animals chronically fed n-3 fatty acid deficient diet showed memory deficit and other neurodegenerative changes. At 4 weeks of age, hypercholesterolemic (ICR) mice were subjected to a very low level of n-3 fatty acids through two generations. At the 1st generation, male mice with n-3 fatty acid deficient were provided with an experimental diet containing four kinds of lipids (safflower oil: Saf, DHA connecting triacylglycerols: DHA-TG, DHA connecting phospholipids: DHA-PL, soybean phospholipids: Soy-PL) for 5 weeks. Another group of ICR mice were obtained and fed a commercial diet as a control. The learning and memory abilities of the mice were evaluated by the avoidance procedure. The learning and memory ability level was significantly better in mice fed the DHA-PL diet than in those fed the Saf and Soy-PL diets, and was the same level as the control. The DHA levels of phosphatidylethanolamine in the brain were significantly higher in the mice fed the two types of DHA-containing diets than in those fed the Saf and Soy-PL diets. There was not significantly different between DHA-TG and DHA-PL. The dimethylacetal levels in the brain were significantly higher in the mice fed the DHA-PL diet than in those fed the Saf and DHA-TG diets [40]. In another cognitive tests, ICR mouse pups were fed an n-3 fatty acid deficient diet starting from the 2nd day of life. There was a 51% loss of total brain DHA in mice with the deficient diet when compared with a diet sufficient in n-3 fatty acids. The n-3 fatty acid-deficient mice demonstrated impaired learning in the reference-memory version of the Barnes circular maze as they spent more time and made more errors in search of an escape tunnel. These results suggest that the dietary DHA connecting phospholipids could improve memory learning, and may be related to the both the DHA and plasmalogen levels in the brain [56].

However, in 58 normal and 114 AD patients, the fatty acid compositions in the frontal, temporal and parietal neocortex were evaluated. Significant reductions of stearic acid (18:0) were found for in the frontal and temporal cortex and AA in the temporal cortex in AD, and increases in oleic acid in frontal and temporal cortex and palmitic acid (16:0) in parietal cortex. The mean values of DHA were not significantly different. Fatty acid composition was not related to APOE genotype, age, gender or post-mortem delay [41]. Even more surprising, a new investigation evaluated the association of erythrocyte membrane total n-3 PUFAs, DHA, EPA, and blood mercury with the incidence of dementia and AD in human subjects of the Canadian Study of Health and Aging (CSHA) with adjustment for confounders including apolipoprotein E epsilon4 (APOE epsilon4) status. The cohort study contained 663 persons aged older or equal 65 years old, conducted from 1991 to 2002. In adjusted Cox regression models with age as the time scale, there were no associations between total n-3 PUFAs, DHA, or EPA and dementia or AD. In contrast, a mercury concentration in the highest quartile was associated with a reduced risk of dementia. However, significant risk reductions were limited to subjects with concentrations of both n-3 PUFAs and mercury that were above the median. There was no modification of risk by APOE epsilon status. No associations between n-3 PUFAs and dementia or AD were found. The results regarding mercury may indicate a spurious association [42].

So far, most studies on relationship between n-3 fatty acids and brain function are in AD and depression areas. Recently, a clinical investigation purified frontal cortex lipid rafts and analyzed lipid composition from normal human subjects and patients with early motor stages of PD and with incidental PD. It was found that lipid rafts from PD and iPD cortices exhibit dramatic reductions in their contents of n-3 and n-6 long-chain polyunsaturated fatty acids, especially DHA and AA. In opposite, saturated fatty acids were significantly higher in both PD patients than those in control brains [43].

However, in 249 Japanese PD patients, a case-control study examined the relationship between dietary intake of individual fatty acids and the risk of PD onset within 6 years. Controls were 368 inpatients and outpatients without a neurodegenerative disease. Higher consumption of AA and cholesterol were related to an increased risk of PD. Consumption of total fat, saturated fatty acids, monounsaturated fatty acids, n-3 polyunsaturated fatty acids, ALA, EPA, DHA, n-6 PAUFs, and LA and the ratio of n-3 to n-6 fatty acid intake were not associated with PD [44]. These results are consistent with the inflammation theory of neurodegenerative disease, including PD since AA is the precursor of inflammatory mediators.

N-3 FATTY ACIDS IN THE TREATMENTS OF NEURODEGENERATIVE DISEASES

Above evidence indicates that n-3 fatty acids may be an effective treatment for neurodegenerative diseases. Thus, clinical and experimental investigations have been carried out. A clinical trial determined the effects of 6 months of dietary supplementation with an n-3 fatty acid preparation rich in DHA on global gene expressions in peripheral blood mononuclear cells of human subjects. Blood samples were obtained from 11 patients receiving a mixed 1.7 g of DHA and 0.6 g EPA and five placebo, expressions of approximately 8000 genes were assessed by gene array. Significant changes were confirmed by real-time PCR. At 6 months, the group intake n-3 fatty acids displayed significant rises of DHA and EPA plasma concentrations, while up- and down-regulation of nine and ten genes, respectively, was noticed. Many of these genes are involved in inflammation regulation and neurodegeneration, *e.g.,* up-regulating CD63 (regulation of inflammation), NAIP (apoptosis inhibitory proteins), MAN2A1 (linked to a systemic autoimmune disease) and CASP4 (an apoptosis-related cysteine protease), and down-regulating LOC399491 (a protein in the neuropeptide signaling pathway) and SORL1 (regulates processing of amyloid precursor protein), ANAPC5 (controls cell cycle progression by targeting a number of cell cycle regulators) and RHOB (a Rho-related GTP-binding protein with GTPase activity). These changes were correlated to increases of plasma DHA and EPA levels in the blood [45].

Since decreases in plasma DHA are associated with cognitive decline in healthy elderly adults and in patients with AD, effects of DHA administration on cognitive functions in healthy older adults with ageing-related cognitive decline (ARCD) were determined in total 485 healthy subjects, aged ≥55 by a randomized, double-blind, placebo-controlled, clinical study at 19 U.S. clinical sites. Subjects were randomly assigned to 900 mg/d of DHA orally or matching placebo for 24 weeks. The primary outcome was a visuospatial learning and episodic memory test. Intention-to-treat analysis demonstrated significantly less errors in learning and memory with DHA *versus* placebo at 24 weeks. DHA supplementation was also associated with improved immediate and delayed Verbal Recognition Memory scores, but not working memory or executive function tests. Plasma DHA levels doubled and correlated with improved memory scores in the DHA group. There was no reported treatment-related serious adverse events in DHA treated group [46]. Another 24-week, randomized, double-blind placebo-controlled study was carried out to test the feasibility of using 1080 mg of EPA and 720 mg of DHA monotherapy in people with cognitive impairment. 23 participants with mild or moderate AD and 23 with mild cognitive impairment were randomized to receive n-3 and placebo (olive oil). The treatment group showed better improvement on the Clinician's Interview-Based Impression of Change Scale (CIBIC-plus) than those in the placebo group over the 24 week follow-up. There was no significant difference in the cognitive portion of the AD Assessment Scale change during follow-up in these two groups. However, the n-3 fatty acids group showed significant improvement in AD Assessment Scale compared to the placebo group in participants with mild cognitive impairment. Higher proportions of EPA on RBC membranes were also associated with better cognitive outcome [47].

Many studies in animal AD models further revealed more mechanism by which n-3 fatty acids treat AD-like pathological changes. In the 3xTg-AD model of mice, the effect of DHA on the physiology of entorhinal cortex neurons was explored. It was shown that DHA consumption improved object recognition, preventing deficits observed in old 3xTg-AD mice. Moreover, 3xTg-AD mice displayed seizure-like akinetic episodes, was largely prevented by DHA. Furthermore, patch-clamp recording revealed that 3xTg-AD EC neurons displayed (i) loss of cell capacitance, suggesting reduced membrane surface area; (ii) increase of firing rate *versus* injected current (F-I) curve associated with modified action potentials, and (iii) over-activation of glutamatergic synapses, without changes in synaptophysin levels. DHA consumption increased cell capacitance and decreased F-I slopes, thereby preventing the opposite alterations observed in 3xTg-AD mice. These results indicate that cognitive performance and basic physiology of entorhinal cortex neurons depend on DHA intake in a mouse model of AD [48].

As the accumulation of the Aβ generated by β- and γ-secretase processing of the amyloid precursor protein (APP), the intake of the PUFA DHA has been associated with decreased Aβ deposition and a reduced risk in AD in several epidemiological trials. DHA reduces amyloidogenic processing by decreasing β- and γ-secretase activity, whereas the expression and protein levels of BACE1 and presenilin1 remain unchanged. In addition, DHA increases protein stability of α-secretase resulting in increased nonamyloidogenic processing. Besides the known effect of DHA to decrease cholesterol de novo synthesis, cholesterol distribution in plasma membrane could be altered. In the presence of DHA, cholesterol shifts from raft to non-raft domains, and this is accompanied by a shift in γ-secretase activity and presenilin1 protein levels. Taken together, DHA directs amyloidogenic processing of APP toward nonamyloidogenic processing, effectively reducing Aβ release. Some experiments also pointed out that DHA has a typical pleiotropic effect; such as mediated Aβ reduction is not the consequence of a single major mechanism but is the result of combined multiple effects [49].

It seems more conflict results from clinical investigations. A randomized, double-blind, placebo-controlled trial of DHA supplementation in individuals with mild to moderate AD (Mini-Mental State Examination scores, 14-26) was conducted in 3 years (between November 2007 and May 2009) at 51 US clinical research sites of the AD Cooperative Study. Participants were randomly assigned to algal DHA at a dose of 2 g/d or to identical placebo. Duration of treatment was 18 months. Supplementation with DHA compared with placebo did not slow the rate of cognitive and functional decline in patients with mild to moderate AD [50].

With regards to n-3 fatty acids in the treatment of PD, there seems no clinical trial yet. However, experimental studies have demonstrated some neuroprotective effect of n-3 fatty acids, specially EPA on PD like pathological changes. As mentioned above, glial cells and their triggered inflammation play an important role in PD. Glial cell line derived neurotrophic factor (GDNF) and neurturin (NTN) are very potent trophic factors for PD. To evaluate the neuroprotective effects of GDNF and NTN by investigating their immunostaining levels after administration of DHA in a model of PD, MPTP neurotoxin that induces dopaminergic neurodegeneration was used to create the experimental PD model. Dopaminergic neuron numbers were clearly decreased in MPTP animals, but showed an increase in MPTP+DHA group. As a result of this, DHA administration protected dopaminergic neurons as shown by tyrosine hydroxylase immunohistochemistry. In the MPTP+DHA group, GDNF, NTN immunoreactions in dopaminergic neurons were higher than that of the MPTP group [51].

As mentioned above, chronic IL-1β administration induced neuroinflammation model exhibited many changes that were similar to those observed in AD patients. Our team has carried out several studies to evaluate the effect of EPA on behavioral, neurotransmission, neuroinflammation, neurotrophin expression and glucocorticoid secretions.

In our lab, IL-1β-induced memory impairment in Morris water maze and 8-arm radio maze was attenuated by another n-3 fatty acid EPA treatment [52,53]. In subchronic IL-1-induced neuroinflammation model, microdialysis revealed that IL-1 significantly reduced noradrenaline and ACh release during memory retrieval phase, but increased glutamate release, which could be reversed by EPA. In this model, EPA treatment also largely attenuated IL-1-induced decreases in the expressions of NGF and normalized glucocoticoid levels [52].

THE LIMITATIONS AND FUTURE RESEARCHES

After reviewing above findings, it can be summarized that n-3 fatty acids could improve memory impairment and attenuate neurodegeneration-like changes, such as neurotransmitter dysfunction, neuronal apoptosis, deficiency in neurotrophins, neuroinflammation and oxidative stress. However, there were also conflicting results. Because many studies used different research protocols, different resources of n-3 fatty acids, subjects with various conditions and sampling at different seasons. As well, dissimilar study designs, including differences in study duration, time period of measurement and number of participants, as well as used different dosages and ratios between PUFAs. These factors could significantly affect results. Except for many studies that analyzed the profile of PAFUs in AD models, there were few investigations reported changes in the composition of PAFUs in the brain or blood of other neurodegenerative diseases. In the clinical trials, few other neurodegenerative diseases have been treated with n-3 fatty acids. Another important factor has been ignored in the most studied was that patients or animals have different type and speed of metabolism for n-3 fatty acids. N-3 fatty acids through oral administration could be metabolized by many enzymes in the body. What was the final substance getting into the brain and how these fatty acids interact in the body and brain are unknown. For example, EPA has been considered as a precursor of DHA, but EPA was more effective to treat depression than DHA. Our team has found that chronic and oral feeding animals with EPA markedly increased docosapentaenoic acid (DPA), another precursor of DHA but not DHA concentrations in the brain, which was associated with significant improvement in cognitive functions and anti-inflammatory effects (unpublished data). These limitations should be future invested.

ACKNOWLEDGEMENTS

None declared.

CONFLICT OF INTEREST

The author states that there is no conflict of interest.

REFERENCES

[1] Margaret M. Esiri. The interplay between inflammation and neurodegeneration in CNS disease. Journal of Neuroimmunology 2007; (184): 4-16.

[2] Lucas SM, Rothwell NJ, Gibson RM. The role of inflammation in CNS injury and disease. Br J Pharmacol 2006; 147 Suppl 1: S232-40.

[3] Zandi PP, Anthony JC, Hayden KM, Mehta K, Mayer L, Breitner JC. Reduced incidence of AD with NSAID but not H2 receptor antagonists: the Cache County Study. Neurology 2002; 59(6): 880-6.

[4] Gagne JJ, Power MC. Anti-inflammatory drugs and risk of Parkinson disease: a meta-analysis. Neurology 2010; 74(12): 995-1002.

[5] Song C, Zhao S. Omega-3 fatty acid eicosapentaenoic acid. A new treatment for psychiatric and neurodegenerative diseases: a review of clinical investigations. Expert Opin Investig Drugs 2007; 16(10): 1627-38.

[6] Miller GE, Chen E, Sze J, Marin T, Arevalo JM, Doll R, Ma R, Cole SW. A functional genomic fingerprint of chronic stress in humans: blunted glucocorticoid and increased NF-kappaB signaling. Biol Psychiatry 2008; 64(4): 266-72.

[7] Yan Q. Translational implications of inflammatory biomarkers and cytokine networks in psychoneuroimmunology. Methods Mol Biol. 2012; 934: 105-20.

[8] Haroon E, Raison CL, Miller AH. Psychoneuroimmunology meets neuropsychopharmacology: translational implications of the impact of inflammation on behavior. Neuropsychopharmacology. 2012; 37(1): 137-62.

[9] Song C, Wang H. Cytokines mediated inflammation and decreased neurogenesis in animal models of depression. Prog Neuropsychopharmacol Biol Psychiatry 2011; 35(3): 760-8.

[10] Leonard BE. The HPA and immune axes in stress: the involvement of the serotonergic system. Eur Psychiatry 2005; 20 Suppl 3: S302-6.

[11] Song C, Horrobin DF, Leonard BE. The comparison of changes in behavior, neurochemistry, endocrine, and immune functions after different routes, doses and durations of administrations of IL-1beta in rats. Pharmacopsychiatry 2006; 39(3): 88-99.

[12] Chen Y, Rex CS, Rice CJ, Dubé CM, Gall CM, Lynch G, Baram TZ. Correlated memory defects and hippocampal dendritic spine loss after acute stress involve corticotropin-releasing hormone signaling. Proc Natl Acad Sci U S A 2010; 107(29): 13123-8.

[13] Olsson B, Hertze J, Lautner R, Zetterberg H, Nägga K, Höglund K, Basun H, Annas P, Lannfelt L, Andreasen N, Minthon L, Blennow K, Hansson O. Microglial markers are elevated in the prodromal phase of Alzheimer's disease and vascular dementia. J Alzheimers Dis. 2013; 33(1): 45-53.

[14] Zotova E, Holmes C, Johnston D, Neal JW, Nicoll JA, Boche D. Microglial alterations in human Alzheimer's disease following Aβ42 immunization. Neuropathol Appl Neurobiol 2011, 37(5): 513-24.

[15] Rubio-Perez JM, Morillas-Ruiz JM. A review: inflammatory process in Alzheimer's disease, role of cytokines. Scientific World Journal 2012; 2012: 756357.

[16] Fehér A, Juhász A, Rimanóczy A, Kálmán J, Janka Z. Association study of interferon-γ, cytosolic phospholipase A2, and cyclooxygenase-2 gene polymorphisms in Alzheimer disease. Am J Geriatr Psychiatry 2010; 18(11): 983-7.

[17] Eikelenboom P, van Exel E, Hoozemans JJ, Veerhuis R, Rozemuller AJ, van Gool WA. Neuroinflammation - an early event in both the history and pathogenesis of Alzheimer's disease. Neurodegener Dis 2010; 7(1-3): 38-41.

[18] Griffin WS, Mrak RE. Interleukin-1 in the genesis and progression of and risk for development of neuronal degeneration in Alzheimer's disease. J Leukoc Biol 2002; 72(2): 233-8.

[19] Luccarini I, Grossi C, Traini C, Fiorentini A, Ed Dami T, Casamenti F. Aβ plaque-associated glial reaction as a determinant of apoptotic neuronal death and cortical gliogenesis: a study in APP mutant mice. Neurosci Lett 2012; 506(1): 94-9.

[20] Kraft AW, Hu X, Yoon H, Yan P, Xiao Q, Wang Y, Gil SC, Brown J, Wilhelmsson U, Restivo JL, Cirrito JR, Holtzman DM, Kim J, Pekny M, Lee JM. Attenuating astrocyte activation accelerates plaque pathogenesis in APP/PS1 mice. FASEB J 2013; 27(1): 187-98.

[21] Kulijewicz-Nawrot M, Verkhratsky A, Chvátal A, Syková E, Rodríguez JJ. Astrocytic cytoskeletal atrophy in the medial prefrontal cortex of a triple transgenic mouse model of Alzheimer's disease. J Anat 2012; 221(3): 252-62.

[22] Yeh CY, Vadhwana B, Verkhratsky A, Rodríguez JJ. Early astrocytic atrophy in the entorhinal cortex of a triple transgenic animal model of Alzheimer's disease. ASN Neuro 2011; 3(5): 271-9.

[23] Lee M, McGeer E, McGeer PL. Neurotoxins released from interferon-gamma-stimulated human astrocytes. Neuroscience 2013; 229: 164-75.

[24] Craft JM, Watterson DM, Frautschy SA, Van Eldik LJ Aminopyridazines inhibit beta-amyloid-induced glial activation and neuronal damage *in vivo*. Neurobiol Aging 2004; 25(10): 1283-92.

[25] Wilhelm KR, Yanamandra K, Gruden MA, Zamotin V, Malisauskas M, Casaite V, Darinskas A, Forsgren L, Morozova-Roche LA. Immune reactivity towards insulin, its amyloid and protein S100B in blood sera of Parkinson's disease patients. Eur J Neurol 2007; 14(3): 327-34.

[26] Lu J, Esposito G, Scuderi C, Steardo L, Delli-Bovi LC, Hecht JL, Dickinson BC, Chang CJ, Mori T, Sheen V. S100B and APP promote a gliocentric shift and impaired neurogenesis in Down syndrome neural progenitors. PLoS One 2011; 6(7): e22126.

[27] Shapiro LA, Bialowas-McGoey LA, Whitaker-Azmitia PM. Effects of S100B on serotonergic Plasticity and Neuroinflammation in the Hippocampus in Down Syndrome and Alzheimer's Disease: Studies in an S100B Overexpressing Mouse Model. Cardiovasc Psychiatry Neurol 2010; 2010: 153657.

[28] Song C, Horrobin DF. Omega-3 fatty acid ethyl-eicosapentaenoic acid but not soybean oil attenuates memory impairment induced by central IL-1beta-administration. J. Lipid Res 2004; 45: 1112-1121.

[29] Song C, Phillips AG, Leonard BE, Horrobin DF. Omega-3 fatty acid and RU 486 reverse IL-1-induced memory impairment in rats: a glucocorticoid involved mechanism. Mol. Psychiatry 2004 9: 630-638,.

[30] Qian L, Flood PM, Hong JS. Neuroinflammation is a key player in Parkinson's disease and a prime target for therapy. J Neural Transm 2010; 117(8): 971-9.

[31] Koziorowski D, Tomasiuk R, Szlufik S, Friedman A. Inflammatory cytokines and NT-proCNP in Parkinson's disease patients. Cytokine 2012; 60(3): 762-6.

[32] Fang F, Wirdefeldt K, Jacks A, Kamel F, Ye W, Chen H. CNS infections, sepsis and risk of Parkinson's disease. Int J Epidemiol 2012; 41(4): 1042-9.

[33] Song C, Li XW, Leonard BE, Horrobin DF. Effects of dietary n-3 or n-6 fatty acids on interleukin-1beta-induced anxiety, stress and inflammatory responses in rats. J. Lipid Res 2003; 44: 1984-1991,.

[34] Ramakrishnan U. Fatty acid status and maternal mental health. Child Nutrition 2011; 7 (Suppl. 2): 99-111.

[35] Gupta S, Knight AG, Gupta S *et al.*: Saturated long-chain fatty acids activate inflammatory signaling in astrocytes. Journal of Neurochemistry 2012; 120: 1060-1071.

[36] Weylandt KH, Chiu CY, Gomolka B *et al.*: Omega-3 fatty acids and their lipid mediators: Towards an understanding of resolvin and protectin formation Omega-3 fatty acids and their resolvin/protectin mediators. Prostaglandins & other Lipid Mediators 2012; 97(3-4),73-82.

[37] Hjorth E, Zhu M, Toro VC, Vedin I, Palmblad J, Cederholm T, Freund-Levi Y, Faxen-Irving G, Wahlund LO, Basun H, Eriksdotter M, Schultzberg M. Omega-3 Fatty Acids Enhance Phagocytosis of Alzheimer's Disease-Related Amyloid-β42 by Human Microglia and Decrease Inflammatory Markers. J Alzheimers Dis. 2013; 35(4): DOI- 10.3233/JAD-130131.

[38] Samieri C, Féart C, Letenneur L, Dartigues JF, Pérès K, Auriacombe S, Peuchant E, Delcourt C, Barberger-Gateau P. Low plasma eicosapentaenoic acid and depressive symptomatology are independent predictors of dementia risk. Am J Clin Nutr 2008; 88(3): 714-21.

[39] Cunnane SC, Schneider JA, Tangney C, Tremblay-Mercier J, Fortier M, Bennett DA, Morris MC. Plasma and brain fatty acid profiles in mild cognitive impairment and Alzheimer's disease. J Alzheimers Dis 2012; 29(3): 691-7.

[40] Hiratsuka S, Koizumi K, Ooba T, Yokogoshi H. Effects of dietary docosahexaenoic acid connecting phospholipids on the learning ability and fatty acid composition of the brain. J Nutr Sci Vitaminol (Tokyo). 2009 Aug; 55(4): 374-80.

[41] Fraser T, Tayler H, Love S. Fatty acid composition of frontal, temporal and parietal neocortex in the normal human brain and in Alzheimer's disease. Neurochem Res 2010; 35(3): 503-13.

[42] Kröger E, Verreault R, Carmichael PH, Lindsay J, Julien P, Dewailly E, Ayotte P, Laurin D. Omega-3 fatty acids and risk of dementia: the Canadian Study of Health and Aging. Am J Clin Nutr 2009; 90(1): 184-92.

[43] Fabelo N, Martín V, Santpere G, Marín R, Torrent L, Ferrer I, Díaz M. Severe alterations in lipid composition of frontal cortex lipid rafts from Parkinson's disease and incidental Parkinson's disease. Mol Med 2011; 17(9-10): 1107-18.

[44] Miyake Y, Sasaki S, Tanaka K, Fukushima W, Kiyohara C, Tsuboi Y, Yamada T, Oeda T, Miki T, Kawamura N, Sakae N, Fukuyama H, Hirota Y, Nagai M; Fukuoka Kinki

Parkinson's Disease Study Group. Dietary fat intake and risk of Parkinson's disease: a case-control study in Japan. J Neurol Sci 2010; 288(1-2): 117-22.

[45] Vedin I, Cederholm T, Freund-Levi Y, Basun H, Garlind A, Irving GF, Eriksdotter-Jönhagen M, Wahlund LO, Dahlman I, Palmblad J. Effects of DHA-rich n-3 fatty acid supplementation on gene expression in blood mononuclear leukocytes: the OmegAD study. PLoS One 2012; 7(4): e35425.

[46] Yurko-Mauro K, McCarthy D, Rom D, Nelson EB, Ryan AS, Blackwell A, Salem N Jr, Stedman M; MIDAS Investigators. Beneficial effects of docosahexaenoic acid on cognition in age-related cognitive decline. Alzheimers Dement. 2010 Nov; 6(6): 456-64.

[47] Chiu CC, Su KP, Cheng TC, Liu HC, Chang CJ, Dewey ME, Stewart R, Huang SY. The effects of omega-3 fatty acids monotherapy in Alzheimer's disease and mild cognitive impairment: a preliminary randomized double-blind placebo-controlled study. Prog Neuropsychopharmacol Biol Psychiatry 2008; 32(6): 1538-44.

[48] Arsenault D, Julien C, Tremblay C, Calon F. DHA improves cognition and prevents dysfunction of entorhinal cortex neurons in 3xTg-AD mice. PLoS One 2011; 6(2): e17397.

[49] Grimm MO, Kuchenbecker J, Grösgen S, Burg VK, Hundsdörfer B, Rothhaar TL, Friess P, de Wilde MC, Broersen LM, Penke B, Péter M, Vígh L, Grimm HS, Hartmann T. Docosahexaenoic acid reduces amyloid beta production *via* multiple pleiotropic mechanisms. J Biol Chem 2011; 286(16): 14028-39.

[50] Quinn JF, Raman R, Thomas RG, Yurko-Mauro K, Nelson EB, Van Dyck C, Galvin JE, Emond J, Jack CR Jr, Weiner M, Shinto L, Aisen PS. Docosahexaenoic acid supplementation and cognitive decline in Alzheimer disease: a randomized trial. JAMA 2010; 304(17): 1903-11.

[51] Tanriover G, Seval-Celik Y, Ozsoy O, Akkoyunlu G, Savcioglu F, Hacioglu G, Demir N, Agar A. The effects of docosahexaenoic acid on glial derived neurotrophic factor and neurturin in bilateral rat model of Parkinson's disease. Folia Histochem Cytobiol 2010; 48(3): 434-41.

[52] Taepavarapruk P, Song C. Reductions of acetylcholine release and nerve growth factor expression are correlated with memory impairment induced by interleukin-1beta administrations: effects of omega-3 fatty acid EPA treatment. J Neurochem 2010; 112(4): 1054-64.

[53] Biscaro B, Lindvall O, Tesco G, Ekdahl CT, Nitsch RM. Inhibition of microglial activation protects hippocampal neurogenesis and improves cognitive deficits in a transgenic mouse model for Alzheimer's disease. Neurodegener Dis 2012; 9(4): 187-98.

[54] Ibrahim A, Mbodji K, Hassan A *et al*. Anti-inflammatory and anti-angiogenic effect of long chain n-3 polyunsaturated fatty acids in intestinal microvascular endothelium. Clinical Nutrition 2011; 30: 678-687.

[55] Pascoe MC, Crewther SG, Carey LM, Crewther DP. What you eat is what you are -- a role for polyunsaturated fatty acids in neuroinflammation induced depression? Clin Nutr 2011; 30(4): 407-15.

[56] Fedorova I, Hussein N, Di Martino C, Moriguchi T, Hoshiba J, Majchrzak S, Salem N Jr. An n-3 fatty acid deficient diet affects mouse spatial learning in the Barnes circular maze. Prostaglandins Leukot Essent Fatty Acids 2007; 77(5-6): 269-77.

[57] Song C. The effect of thymectomy and IL-1 on memory: implications for the relationship between immunity and depression. Brain Behav Immun. 2002; 16: 557-68.

[58] Bonaccorso S, Lin A, Song C, Verkerk R, Kenis G, Bosmans E, Scharpe S, Vandewoude M, Dossche A, Maes M. Serotonin-immune interactions in elderly volunteers and in patients with Alzheimer's disease (DAT): lower plasma tryptophan availability to the brain in the elderly and increased serum interleukin-6 in DAT. Aging 1998; 10: 316-23.

[59] Bhat R, Crowe EP, Bitto A, Moh M, Katsetos CD, Garcia FU, Johnson FB, Trojanowski JQ, Sell C, Torres C. Astrocyte senescence as a component of Alzheimer's disease. PLoS One 2012; 7: e45069.

[60] Song C. Essential Fatty Acids as Potential Anti-inflammatory Agents in the Treatment of Affective Disorders. In : Modern Trends in Pharmacopsychiatry (edit. Leonard B, Halaris A). John Wiley, England (2012).

Frontiers in CNS Drug Discovery, 2013, *2*, 334-380

CHAPTER 10

Application of Monoterpenoids and their Derivatives Against CNS Disorders

Alla V. Pavlova, Konstantin P. Volcho* and Tatyana G. Tolstikova

Novosibirsk Institute of Organic Chemistry, Siberian Branch of the Russian Academy of Science, Novosibirsk, Russia

Abstract: Monoterpenoids and their derivatives play an important role in the creation of new bioactive substances including drugs. Many of these compounds possess substantial CNS activities such as antinociceptive, neuroprotective, anticonvulsant. In the past decades, interest in investigating the possibility of using monoterpenoids for the development of new drugs has increased significantly due to improvement of both chemical methods of modification of natural compounds, and a substantial deficit of breakthrough research to create drugs to treat diseases associated with central nervous system. The review covers the literature on monoterpenoids and their derivatives exhibit various types of CNS activities published up to early 2012.

Keywords: Essential oils, monoterpenoids, analgesic activity, anticonvulsant activity, neuroprotective activity, inhibition of acetylcholinesterase activity, anti-Alzheimer's disease activity, antiparkinsonian activity, anxiolytic-like effect, mecamylamine.

INTRODUCTION

Essential oils (EOs) are secondary metabolites that plants usually synthesize for combating infections or parasitic agents or generate in response to stress conditions. EOs are aromatic components obtained from different plant parts such as flowers, buds, seeds, leaves, and fruits [1].

The therapeutic use of essential oils and/or hydrolates has a long tradition. The pharmacological and/or psychological properties of odorants are nowadays

***Address correspondence to Konstantin P. Volcho:** Novosibirsk institute of Organic Chemistry, Siberian Branch of the Russian Academy of Science, Novosibirsk, Russia; Tel: +7-3833308870; Fax: +7-3833309752; E-mail: volcho@nioch.nsc.ru

Atta-ur-Rahman & M. Iqbal Choudhary (Eds.)

acknowledged and in many cases the combination of both plays an important role [2]. They are used as an adjunct in, folk medicine, Chinese medicine, alternative medicine, aromatherapy and massages, as well as in the cosmetics and perfume industries, in food flavorings and cleaning products. Plant-derived EOs exhibit a variety of biological properties. Most of the properties (including anxiolytic, anticonvulsant, antinociceptive, anti-inflammatory, *etc.*) substantially affect the central nervous system (CNS). Meanwhile, the chemical composition of EOs varies in a wide range depending on the time and place the plant raw material was collected, weather conditions, *etc.*, which considerably complicates the use of EOs in medical practice.

Many effects of EOs are attributed to monoterpenes, which are the major chemical components of essential oils [2, 3]. Monoterpenes represent a large group of naturally occurring organic compounds whose basic structure consists of two linked isoprene units [4]. Monoterpene derivatives containing heteroatoms (typically oxygen atoms) are known as monoterpenoids. The small molecular size of monoterpenes and most monoterpenoids is an important criterion, which allows them to easily penetrate through the blood–brain barrier. Monoterpenoids are often responsible for the CNS activity exhibited by EOs. The availability of many monoterpene types (usually in their optically active form) and wide possibilities for functionalization make them attractive initial compounds for designing new drugs.

Despite the large amount of data available on biological activity of monoterpenoids, until now, no reviews summarizing the results obtained on monoterpene exhibiting pharmacological activity on the CNS have been published. Hence, we decided to improve the situation by publishing this review and to combine the literature data on the effect of monoterpenes and their derivatives on the CNS. The review has been structured with respect to types of pharmacological activities, allowing one to trace the "structure–activity" regularities in a number of cases.

Two types of compounds, cannabinoids and mecamylamine, are the best-studied among the monoterpenoid derivatives; they have already been used in medical practice.

The pharmacological activity and the mechanisms of action of phytocannabinoids (most of which belong to monoterpene derivatives containing an aromatic fragment) have been rather thoroughly described in the literature. Cannabinoids are hydrocarbon compounds which can be grouped into three classes: endogenous (naturally occurring cannabinoids of the human body), plant (derivatives of marijuana found in the hemp plant *Cannabis sativa*), and synthetic (artificially synthesized by pioneering companies) [5]. Since the first endocannabinoid, anandamide, was discovered in 1992, the amount of data on physiological role of the endocannabinoid system and its role in the pathology has considerably increased. Intensive pharmacological studies based on these data have after a very short period of time resulted in the development of powerful selective agents targeted to the endogenous cannabinoid system. This has opened new perspectives in understanding and treatment of a number of significant diseases and pathological conditions, such as pain, neurodegeneration, anxiety disorders, and addiction to psychoactive drugs [6-8].

A number of recent reviews are devoted to different aspects of the CNS activity of phytocannabinoids [9-12]; hence, this group of compounds was eliminated from consideration in this study.

A separate section is devoted to mecamylamine, a monoterpenoid-based drug. Mecamylamine possesses potential pharmacotherapy in a variety of neuropsychiatric disorders such as mood disorders, nicotine dependence, schizophrenia, cocaine and alcohol dependence, Alzheimer's disease, Tourette's syndrome, autism and epilepsy [13, 14].

ANALGESIC (ANTINOCICEPTIVE) AND ANTI-INFLAMMATORY ACTIVITIES

Pain is defined by the International Association for the Study of Pain as an unpleasant sensory and emotional experience associated with actual or potential tissue damage [15]. Pain is the most common reason that individuals seek medical attention for. It can be divided into two types: acute pain and chronic pain [16]. The currently available and most widely prescribed are non-steroidal anti-inflammatory drugs (NSAIDs), opioids and synthetic drugs with narcotic properties targeting different components of the peripheral and central nervous system. These drugs have significant side effects (non-steroidal anti-inflammatory drugs – gastric disorders; opioids – tolerance and dependence) that limit their use, especially in chronic [17]. It is very evident that natural products have been and continue to be a valuable source of novel compounds that have the potential to serve as analgesic agents or as lead molecules for the development of such [16].

The compounds with the *p*-menthane framework are the most abundant natural monocyclic monoterpenoids. *D*-Limonene [*R*-(+)-isomer] is a monoterpene prevailing in essential oils of various plants, such as *Lippia alba*, *Artemisia dracunculus* L., and in other aromatic plants species, being a typical representative of this series of monoterpenoids [18, 19]. Studies with essential oils containing (+)-limonene as one of prevalent compounds or with pure limonene have demonstrated its anti-inflammatory and analgesic activities [20]. J.F. Amaral *et al.* have established that (+)-limonene at doses of 25 and 50 mg/kg, intraperitoneally, significantly reduced the number of acid-induced writhes. The analgesic mechanism of action of (+)-limonene can probably involve inhibition of the synthesis and/or a release of inflammatory mediators that promote pain in the nervous terminations, similarly to the indomethacin and the other NSAIDs suggesting a peripheral analgesic action [3]. Moreover, its antinociception action is probably unrelated to the stimulation of classical opioid receptors [3].

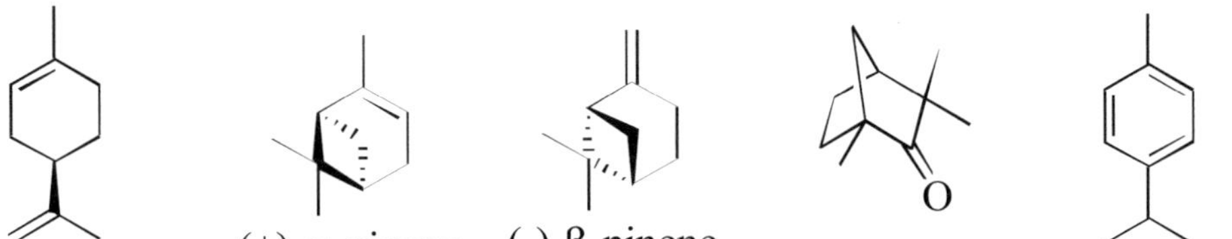

(+)-limonene (+)-α-pinene (-)-β-pinene (-)-fenchone *p*-cymene

(+)-α-Pinene and (–)-fenchone are the major constituents of *Foeniculum vulgare*; they exhibit antinociceptive activity in mice and have no sedative effect on the central nervous system in animals [21]. (–)-β-Pinene exerted supraspinal antinociceptive action in rats and reversed the antinociceptive effect of morphine in a degree equivalent to that of naloxone, presumably acting as a partial agonist through the μ-opioid receptors [22].

p-Cymene is a monoterpene biological precursor of carvacrol and one of the main constituents of the essential oil from species of *Protium*, with more than 80% of these species found in the Amazon region [23]. *p*-Cymene (100 mg/kg, i.p.) proved to have antinociceptive activity in mice that does not interfere with motor coordination of animals, and this pharmacological action may modulate both neurogenic and inflammatory pain. The antinociceptive action of *p*-cymene involves the opioid system [24]. *p*-Cymene at a dose of 50 and 100 mg/kg, i.p. inhibited leukocyte migration induced by carrageenan. A putative mechanism explaining this activity may include inhibition of the synthesis of inflammatory mediators whose involvement in cell migration is well established [4].

Myrcene, a monoterpene presented in essential oils of many medicinal and aromatic plants, exerts analgesia by acting at both central and peripheral sites as evidenced by an increase in reaction time of mice to thermal stimuli in the hot plate test and the decrease in the number of writhes to chemical stimuli in the acetic acid test. The analgesic effect induced by myrcene (20 and 40 mg/kg, s.c.) can be reversed by pretreatment with naloxone in both tests suggesting the mediation of endogenous opioids in its mechanism. It also implies that presynaptic α2-adrenoceptors are involved in its antinociceptive action [25].

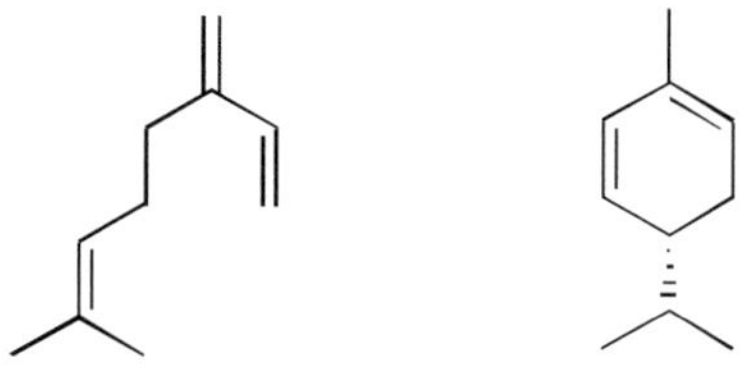

myrcene (-)-α-phellandrene

Monoterpene α-phellandrene found in *Curcuma zedoaria* Christm., *Eucaliptus dives* Schauer., *Matricaria chamomilla* L. and *Zingiber officinale* Roscoe shows analgesic and anti-inflammatory properties [26, 27]. Oral administration of the monoterpene α-phellandrene (3.125, 6.25 and 12.5 mg/kg) exerted pronounced antinociception when assessed in chemical-induced nociception models and mechanical hypernociception in rodents. Some of the possible mechanisms of action involve the opioid system *via* K^{+}_{ATP} channels, the glutamatergic system *via* the *L*-arginine/NO pathway, and an interaction of the monoterpene with the cholinergic (muscarinic receptors) and adrenergic (α2-receptors) systems [27].

Oxygen-containing monoterpenoids occur widely in nature and are used as flavors and fragrances. Menthol is the best-known oxygen-containing monoterpenoid extracted from the essential oil of the genus *Mentha* of the *Lamiaceae* family. Menthol can also be extracted or synthesized from other essential oils such as citronella oil, eucalyptus oil and Indian turpentine oil.

Menthol is a cyclic monoterpene alcohol with three asymmetric carbon atoms; therefore, it occurs as four pairs of optical isomers named (+)-menthol and (–)-menthol, (+)-neomenthol and (–)-neomenthol, (+)-isomenthol and (–)-isomenthol, and (+)-neoisomenthol and (–)-neoisomenthol. Among the optical isomers, (–)-menthol is the one that occurs most widely in nature and is endowed with the peculiar property to be a fragrance and flavor compound. For this reason it is widely used as flavoring for toothpaste, other oral hygiene products, and chewing gums [28].

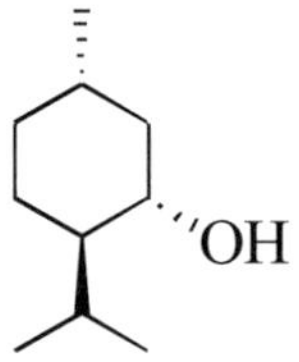

(+)-menthol

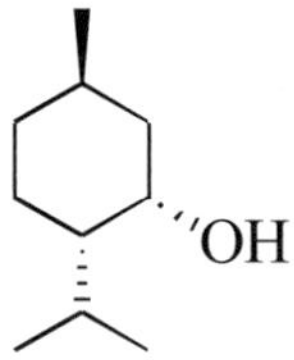

(+)-neomenthol

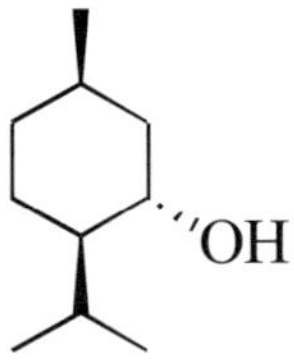

(+)-isomenthol

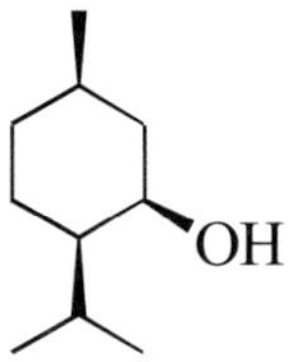

(+)-neoisomenthol

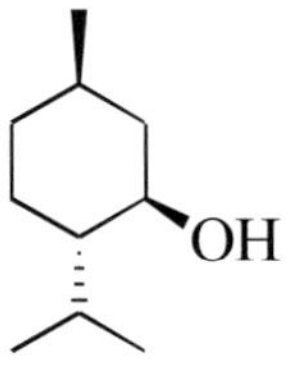

(-)-menthol

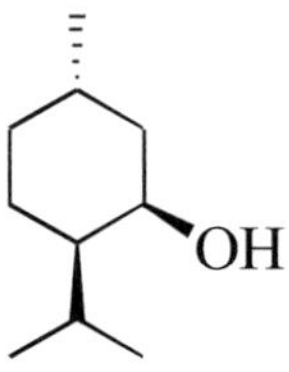

(-)-neomenthol

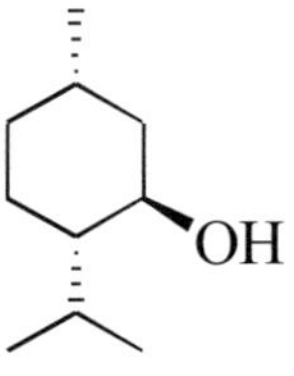

(-)-isomenthol

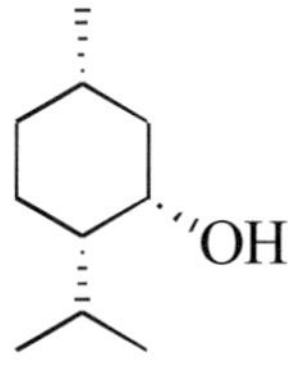

(-)-neoisomenthol

Menthol is the primary activator of the cold- and menthol-sensitive TRPM8 channels [29]. It facilitates glutamate release from sensory neurons by increasing intracellular Ca^{2+} level *via* the activation of TRPM8, leading to modulation of peripheral nociception [30, 31]. (–)-Menthol at a dose of 10 μM per mouse intracerebroventricularly and 10 ml/kg per os can induce analgesia through the activation of the central κ-opioid system [32]. Analgesia induced by (–)-menthol in the mouse hot-plate and abdominal constriction tests is obtained without any visible changes in the normal behavior of animals. Menthol, as a topical irritant, may also cause analgesia by reducing the sensitivity of cutaneous pain fibers [33].

When comparing the optical isomers of menthol, a significant effect of the absolute configuration of this compound on pharmacological activity was found; namely, (–)-menthol was capable of increasing the pain threshold, whereas (+)-menthol was completely devoid of any analgesic effect [32]. At the same time both isomers exhibit equivalent anesthetic activity [34].

Menthol enhances the effect of other analgesics; in particular, its synergetic action when used with methyl salicylate has been demonstrated [35].

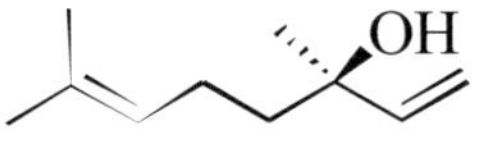

(-)-linalool

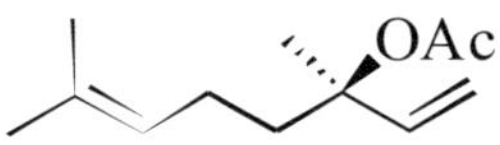

(-)-linalyl acetate

(–)-Linalool is a naturally occurring chiral monoterpene compound commonly found as a major volatile component of the essential oils of various aromatic plant species such as *Citrus bergamia* Risso, *Melissa officinalis* L., *Rosmarinus officinals* L., *Cymbopogon citratus* DC, and *Mentha piperita* L. [36, 37]. Likewise, essential oils containing (–)-linalool play a prominent role as flavoring agents in the food industry, as fragrances for the perfume industry and in drug formulations by the pharmaceutical industry [38]. It has been shown that (–)-linalool possesses anti-inflammatory and antinociceptive activities in several experimental models [37]. (–)-Linalool at a doses 50 and 200 mg/kg, i.p., displays significant antinociceptive effects in models of chronic pain in mice. (–)-Linalool reduced mechanical hypersensitivity induced by the neuropathic pain model (partial sciatic nerve ligation) as well as the mechanical and cold hypersensitivity caused by a chronic inflammatory model (Complete Freund's Adjuvant – induced persistent inflammation) [39]. The mechanism by which the anti-inflammatory effect occurs remains to be determined, although several observations suggest a possible involvement of NMDA receptors [40]. The antinociceptive effect of (–)-linalool involves peripheral and spinal sites of action and seems to be mediated by interaction with ionotropic glutamatergic-dependent mechanisms, *via* NMDA receptors [41]. Moreover, mechanisms of the antinociceptive action of (–)-linalool may include the stimulating effect on M2 muscarinic, opioid or dopamine D2 receptors [37]. The reduction of NO production/release is also responsible, at least partially, for the molecular mechanisms of (–)-linalool antinociceptive effect, probably through the mechanisms where cholinergic and glutamatergic systems are involved [42].

Linalyl acetate is the principal component of many essential oils known to possess several biological activities attributable to this monoterpenoid compound. Linalyl acetate plays a major role in the anti-inflammatory activity displayed by some essential oils containing it [40]. Linalyl acetate also possesses analgesic and anti-inflammatory activities and has sedative effect on the central nervous system [43].

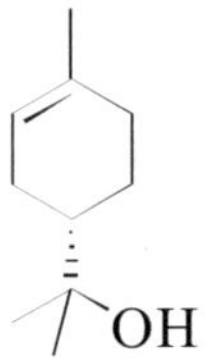

(-)-α-terpineol

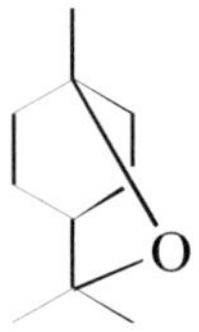

1,8-cineole

α-Terpineol is a volatile monoterpene alcohol, a major component of the essential oils of various plant species, such as *Ravensara aromatica, Melaleuca qinquenervia, Myrtus communis, Laurus nobilis, Croton sonderianus and Eucalyptus globulus*, which are widely used in folk medicine and aromatherapy [44]. α-Terpineol (100 mg/kg, i.p.) has a central analgesic effect, as evidenced by the prolonged delay in response time when mice were subjected to a nociceptive stimulus during the hot plate test [45]. α-Terpineol (25, 50 and 100 mg/kg, i.p.) possesses anti-inflammatory and antihypernociceptive properties. These effects seem to be associated with the ability of α-terpineol to inhibit the cytokine cascade generated by carrageenan and/or to decrease the production of inflammatory mediators as well as to inhibit NO release [44].

1,8-Cineole also known as eucalyptol or cajeputol is a terpene oxide and is the principal constituent of most *Eucalyptus* oils (~75%), *Rosmarinus* (~40%), *Psidium* (40–60%) and many other essential oils. It is often employed by the pharmaceutical industry in drug formulations, as a percutaneous penetration enhancer and for its decongestant and antitussive effects as well as in aromatherapy as a skin stimulant in the form of skin baths [46]. 1,8-Cineole possesses moderate antiexudant and cytotoxic properties and pronounced analgesic and antitumor activities [22]. 1,8-Cineole (50, 100 and 200 mg/kg, i.p.), produces anti-inflammatory and antinociceptive effects, which are dose-independent. The antinociceptive activity of 1,8-cineole was almost equivalent to that of morphine in rats at both spinal and supraspinal levels, while in mice it was exhibited at the supraspinal level only and was less prominent [47]. 1,8-Cineole inhibited not only the carrageenan oedema and an increased capillary permeability, but also the granuloma formation. The mechanism by which 1,8-cineole exerts its anti-inflammatory action is not clear [46].

Citronellol, a monoterpene alcohol, is a naturally occurring monoterpene compound prevalent in essential oils of various aromatic plant species, such as *Cymbopogon citratus*, *C. winterianus* and *Lippia alba* [48]. Citronellol at doses of 25, 50 and 100 mg/kg, i.p. is effective in various pain models, with its action probably mediated *via* the inhibition of peripheral mediators (such as TNF-a and NO synthesis) as well as central inhibitory mechanisms (opioid central receptors), which could be related to the strong antioxidant effect observed *in vitro* [49]. Citronellol possesses CNS depressant and hypnotic properties. Additionally, citronellol was effective as an anti-inflammatory and analgesic compound in various pain models, probably mediated *via* inhibition of prostaglandin synthesis as well as *via* central inhibitory mechanisms (opioid system) [50].

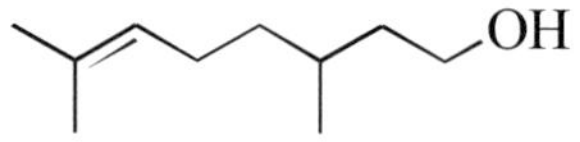

citronellol

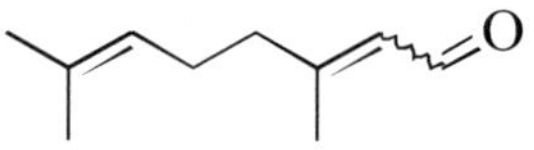

citral

Citral is a monoterpene that occurs naturally in herbs, plants and citrus fruits. It is a natural mixture of the isomeric acyclic aldehydes geranial (*trans*-citral, citral A) and neral (*cis*-citral, citral B). Due to its intense lemon aroma and favors, citral is widely used as an additive in food, cosmetics and detergents [51]. Citral (50, 100 and 200 mg/kg, i.p.) is endowed with peripheral antinociceptive property as well as anti-inflammatory activity. The precise mechanism of anti-inflammatory activity is currently being under investigation, but it could possibly be related to the arachidonic acid cascade and/or modulation of pro-inflammatory molecule production [52]. The antinociceptive action induced by citral could be due to the inhibition of TRPA1 channels, but it is also possible that other mechanisms might be involved [53]. The combined use of naproxen and citral has fewer gastrointestinal and renal side-effect profiles than the use of naproxen alone [54].

(*R*)-(+)-Pulegone is a monoterpene found in essential oils from plants of the *Labiatae* family. In nature, pulegone occurs in both (+)- and (–)-forms. Dextrorotatory pulegone is obtained from oils from *Mentha pulegium*, *M. longifolia*, and others. Levorotatory pulegone is the major constituent of *Agastache formosanum* oil [55, 56]. (*R*)-(+)-Pulegone (31.3 – 125 mg/kg intraperitoneally) dose-dependently inhibited both phases of the formalin test in a manner similar to that of morphine. The antinociceptive effect of the compound was observed by an increase in the reaction time of the mice subjected to the hot plate test [57].

The analgesic activity of enantiomeric hydroxy ketones of the *p*-methane series (+)- and (–)-**1** synthesized using (+)- and (–)-α-pinenes as starting compounds was studied [58]. Hydroxy keton **1** at a dose of 10 mg/kg exhibited a pronounced analgesic activity in the acetic acid writhing test in mice regardless of its absolute configuration. Meanwhile, it was demonstrated in the hot plate test that the direction of its action is determined by the enantiomeric composition: the (–)-isomer (–)-**1** displays analgesic activity; whereas its optical antipode, on the contrary, induces hyperalgesia [59].

The synthesis of diol (–)-**2** was also based on monoterpene α-pinene [60]. Compound (–)-**2** at a dose of 10 mg/kg exhibits a pronounced analgesic activity in the acetic acid writhing test in mice [61].

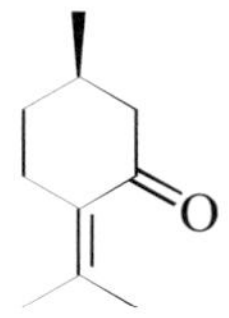

(+)-pulegone

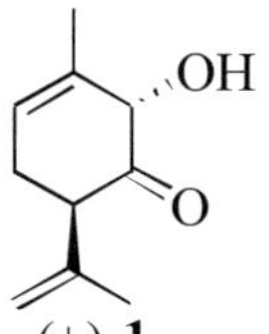

(+)-**1**

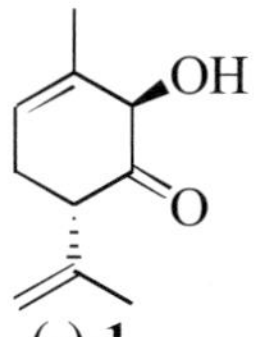

(-)-**1**

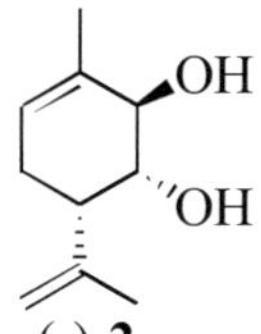

(-)-**2**

Heterocyclic compounds **3a-c** were prepared *via* the interaction between the monoterpenoid with the pinane skeleton, verbenol epoxide, with aromatic aldehydes containing various substituents at the *para*-position [62]. Compounds **3a** (R=F), **3b** (R=Cl), and **3c** (R=NO_2) at a dose of 10 mg/kg were shown to exhibit a reliable analgesic activity in the acetic acid writhing test in mice.

The investigation of the dose-dependent effect of compound **3b** in this test has shown that its ED_{50} is 4.5 mg/kg; *i.e.*, its activity in the acetic acid writhing test is considerably higher than that of all the reference drugs (sodium salicylate and diclofenac). As opposed to **3a** and **3b**, compound **3c** at a dose of 10 mg/kg exhibits reliable analgesic activity in the hot plate test as well [63].

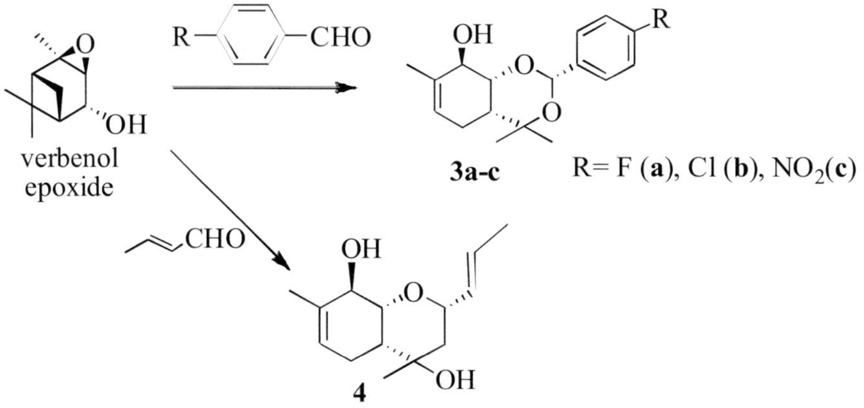

The reaction between verbenol epoxide and crotonic aldehyde yielded the heterocyclic compound **4** having a different skeleton type compared to that in compounds **3a-c** [60]. Compound **4** at doses of 5 and 10 mg/kg in the acetic acid writhing test in mice exhibits a pronounced analgesic activity comparable to that of sodium diclofenac. ED_{50} of compound **4** in this test is 4.2 mg/kg; the range of therapeutic effect ($IS_{50}=LD_{50}/ED_{50}$) of this compound is over 238, which considerably exceeds the identical index of the reference drugs [64].

The reactions between verbenol epoxide or diol **2** and vanillin enabled synthesizing the compound (2*S*,4a*R*,8*R*,8a*R*)-**5** with an acceptable yield [65]. At a dose of 10 mg/kg, this compound shows a marked analgesic activity in the acetic acid writhing test but is almost never active in the hot plate test. On the contrary, its enantiomer, compound (2*R*,4a*S*,8*S*,8a*S*)-**5** at a dose of 10 mg/kg shows a high analgesic activity in the hot plate test and a considerably lower activity in the acetic acid writhing test [66]. The use of a mixture of these two enantiomers at a ratio corresponding to the enantiomeric composition of commercially available verbenone allows one to design an agent that would exhibit significant activities in both tests.

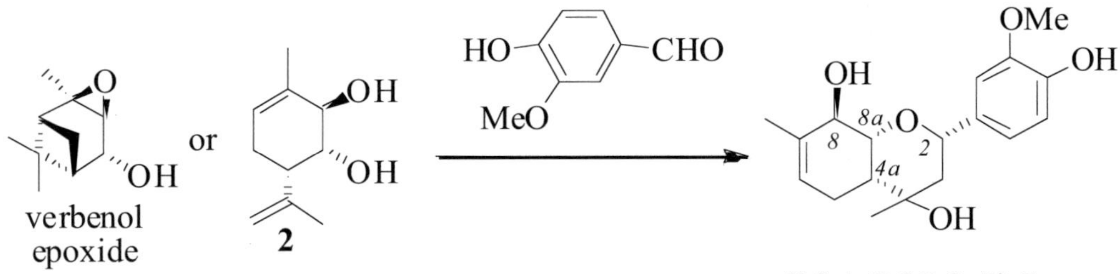

(2*S*,4a*R*,8*R*,8a*R*)-**5**

Thus, a number of monoterpenes, their oxygen-containing derivatives, and heterocyclic products based on them show a significant analgesic activity in various animal models. Some of these compounds are promising to be used to design new efficient low-toxicity analgesic drugs. The absolute configuration of these compounds typically has a crucial effect on the existence of analgesic activity.

ANTICONVULSANT ACTIVITY

Anticonvulsant drugs are primarily developed for the treatment of epilepsy, a neurological condition that affects ~50 million people worldwide. They reduce seizure frequency by suppressing neuronal excitability *via* various molecular targets in the synapse, including voltage-gated ion channels, voltage-gated sodium channels, $GABA_A$ (γ-aminobutyric acid type A) receptors and glutamate receptors [67].

γ-Aminobutyric acid (GABA) is one of the most important inhibitory neurotransmitters in the central nervous system. Its principal action consists in activating ionotropic $GABA_A$ receptors, leading to an inward flow of Cl^- and the hyperpolarizing postsynaptic response [68]. More than a third of the brain neurons use GABA for synaptic communication [69]. Identified over 50 years ago, GABA is the most abundant inhibitory neurotransmitter in the mammalian brain, where it is widely distributed [70]. GABA-mediated signaling has also been implicated in the regulation of nearly all the key developmental steps, from cell proliferation to circuit refinement. Considering that nearly all organisms, ranging from bacteria to humans, can synthesize GABA, it would be surprising if multiple functions for GABA had not evolved [71].

The GABAergic system is implicated in the path mechanism of many diseases of the CNS (*e.g.* epilepsy or mood disorders). One of the theories that attempt to explain the main causes of epilepsy assumes that this disorder may appear as a result of disturbances of the naturally existing balance between the concentrations of inhibitory and excitatory neurotransmitters in the CNS [72]. A reduction in the concentrations of GABA and of the glutamic acid decarboxylase has been implicated not only in the symptoms associated with epilepsy but also with several other neurological diseases such as schizophrenia, Huntington's chorea, Parkinson's disease, Alzheimer's disease, senile dementia, motion disorders, *etc.* [73]. However, GABA is not a good candidate for an antiepileptic drug because of the lack of the blood-brain-barrier penetration. The essential oils were deemed to display anticonvulsant activity when they had shown effects in one or more different seizure model, including the maximal electroshock model, the pentylenetetrazole (PTZ) seizures model, the pilocarpine model and the prolonged PTZ-kindling model [74].

Systemic administration of menthol (300 μM) selectively enhances tonic inhibition mediated by high-affinity, slowly desensitizing $GABA_A$ receptors in CA1 pyramidal neurons of rat hippocampus, leading to inhibition of *in vitro* neuronal excitability and *in vivo* network hyper-excitability of the hippocampus [75]. Menthol (50 μM) acts as a potent positive allosteric modulator of $GABA_A$ receptors *via* similar sites of action as the intravenous anesthetic, propofol. The enhancement of inhibitory neurotransmission by menthol and its analogs may confer important neuroactive properties, such as sedation and anesthesia [76].

When studying the effect of absolute configuration, it was found out that only (+)-menthol (100 μM), among the five stereoisomers analyzed, was active, stimulating the binding of an allosteric $GABA_A$ receptor ligand in a dose-response manner. (+)- And (–)-neomenthols were considered inactive because they were able to increment the binding only at a very high concentration (1000 μM) and because the dose-response curves could not be fitted to the data [77].

Terpinen-4-ol is a volatile monoterpenoid alcohol and the component of the essential oils of several plants such as *Alpinia zerumbet*, *Tanacetum cadmeum*, *Melaleuca alternifolia* and other aromatic plant species [78]. Pretreatment of mice with (–)-terpinen-4-ol at the doses of 100, 200 and 300 mg/kg, i.p., significantly increased the latency of convulsions, close to that of diazepam (4 mg/kg), a standard anticonvulsant drug. The anticonvulsant activity presumably mediated through its interaction with GABA receptors [79].

Racemic α-terpineol, a terpinen-4-ol isomer, at doses of 100 and 200 mg/kg was effective to induce a significant increase in the latency in PTZ-induced convulsions and in preventing tonic convulsions showing dose-dependent protection, at dose of 400 mg/kg, i.p., it afforded 100% protection [80].

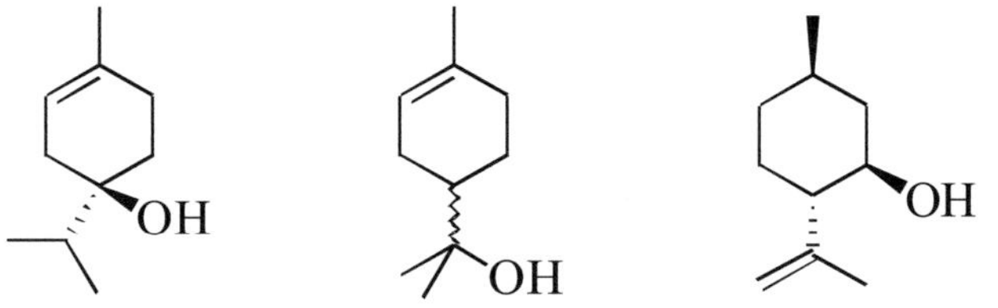

(-)-terpinen-4-ol *rac*-α-terpineol (-)-isopulegol

Isopulegol is a monoterpene alcohol of *p*-menthane family, intermediate in the synthesize of (–)-menthol, and it is present in the essential oils of various plants species, such as *Eucalyptus citriodora* Hook and *Zanthoxylum schinifolium* [81]. Isopulegol significantly prolonged the latency for development of PTZ-induced convulsions (at doses higher than 200 mg/kg) and death (at both 100 and 200 mg/kg, i.p.) in mice. Thus, isopulegol exhibits anticonvulsant and bioprotective effects against PTZ-induced convulsions. Such actions are possibly related to positive modulation of $GABA_A$ receptors and to antioxidant properties [82].

Diol **2** at a dose as low as 0.5 mg/kg shows a high anticonvulsant activity; its therapeutic index in the pentylenetetrazole (PTZ)-induced convulsion test is considerably higher than that of the currently used anticonvulsant drugs [83].

Moreover, this monoterpenoid at a dose of 10 mg/kg, p.o., has a significant anticonvulsant effect in the nicotine-induced convulsion and the arecoline-induced tremor tests. The anticonvulsant activity of compound **2** can presumably be associated with its effect on the neuromediatory (GABAergic and *N*, *M*-chlolinergic) systems participating in the regulation of the convulsive response [84]. The presence of unbound hydroxyl groups and the 8,9-double bond in diol **2** are important prerequisites for manifestation of the anticonvulsant properties, which was demonstrated by the synthesis and investigation of the pharmacological activity of compounds **6** and **7**, which are not active [84]. The combination of high activity, low toxicity, the absence of any effects on the psycholocomotor activity and of potentiation of action of hypnotic agents makes compound **2** promising for the development of a novel antiepileptic drug.

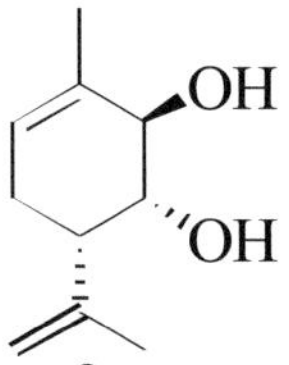

2

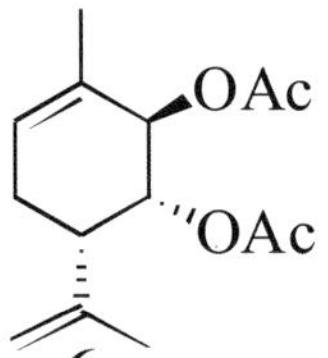

6

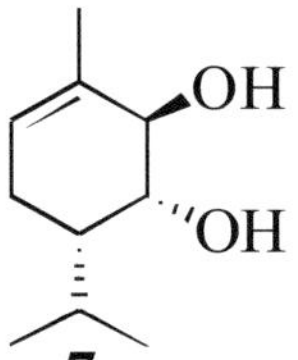

7

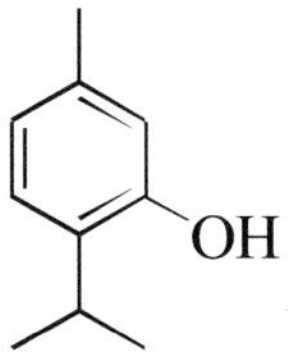

thymol

Thymol is an aromatic monoterpene that occurs as a component of many essential oils. It is widely used in dental practice and in anesthetic halothane preparations due to its anti-microbial and antioxidant properties [85]. Thymol (0–1 μM) was capable of enhancing the GABA action at concentrations lower than those exhibiting direct activity in the absence of GABA. This effect was inhibited by competitive and noncompetitive $GABA_A$ receptor antagonists, suggesting the direct interaction with the $GABA_A$ receptor [86].

Carvone is a monoterpene ketone found as the main active component of various essential oils, such as *Mentha spicata* L., *Anethum graveolens* L., *Carum carvi* L. and *Lippia alba.* It is obtained through lead distillation and occurs naturally as enantiomers (+)- and (−)-carvone [87]. Pretreatment of mice with (+)-carvone at a dose of 200 mg/kg, i.p., significantly increased the latency of PTZ- and picrotoxin-induced convulsions, close to that of diazepam. (–)-Carvone had no effect on the onset of convulsions [88]. Cyano-carvone, a synthetic derivative of carvone, possesses anticonvulsant activity probably due to the modulation of the cholinergic system and reduction of neuronal oxidative stress mainly through free radical scavenger [89]. α,β-Epoxy-carvone at a dose of 300 or 400 mg/kg, i.p., protected against convulsions induced chemically by PTZ by 75% and 87.5%, respectively, and was efficient in preventing the tonic convulsions induced by maximal electroshock at doses of 200, 300 or 400 mg/kg, i.p., resulting in 25%, 25% and 100% protection, respectively. α,β-Epoxy-carvone possesses anticonvulsant activity probably due to the modulation of the GABAergic system and reduction of neuronal excitability mainly through the voltage-dependent Na^+ channels [90].

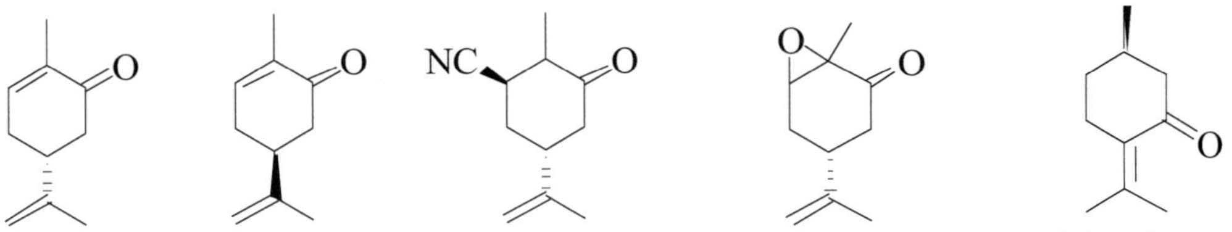

(-)-carvone (+)-carvone cyano-carvone α,β-epoxy-carvone (+)-pulegone

(*R*)-(+)-Pulegone (300 mg/kg i.p.) significantly increased the latency of PTZ-induced convulsions and had an effect similar to that of diazepam, a standard anticonvulsant drug [57].

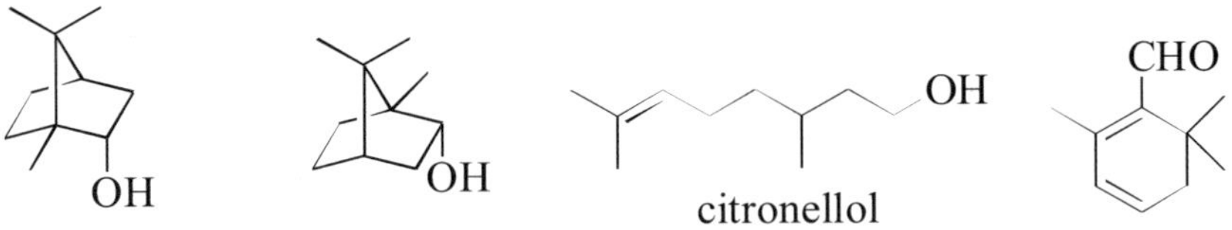

(+)-borneol (-)-borneol citronellol safranal

(+)-Borneol is a bicyclic monoterpene found in several species of *Artemisia* and *Dipterocarpaceae*, also present in the essential oils of numerous medicinal plants, including *Valeriana officinalis, Matricaria chamomilla, Lavandula officinalis* [91, 92]. Valerian extracts have been previously shown to prevent GABA re-uptake, to bind at the GABA and benzodiazepine sites of the $GABA_A$ receptor, and to facilitate GABA transport to the brain [93]. Additionally, lavender essential oil mildly potentiates the effects of GABA on $GABA_A$ receptors [94]. Menthol, borneol acts as a potent positive allosteric modulator at $GABA_A$ and glycine receptors [95]. (+)- And (–)-borneols produce a notable enhancement of the actions of GABA at recombinant $\alpha_1\beta_2\gamma_{2L}$ $GABA_A$ receptors, as well as a moderate direct action at these receptors. The comparison of the activities of enantiomers (+)- and (–)-borneols indicates that the presence and orientation of the hydroxyl group may be important for monoterpene activity at $\alpha_1\beta_2\gamma_{2L}$ $GABA_A$ receptors. (+)-Borneol generated the greatest direct action of the compounds tested at $\alpha_1\beta_2\gamma_{2L}$ $GABA_A$ receptors, producing up to 89% of the maximal GABA response in a concentration-dependent and reversible manner, with a threshold concentration of 300 μM. (–)-Borneol produced a slightly lower response, up to 84% and isoborneol produced 51% of the maximal GABA response The modulatory effects of (+)-borneol at low GABA concentrations were at least equivalent to those of anaesthetic etomidate and much greater than those of diazepam and 5α-pregnan-3α-ol-20-one. The efficacy of each enantiomer varied markedly with concentration of GABA present [96].

Citronellol (100, 200 and 400 mg/kg, i.p.) significantly increased, in a dose-dependent manner, the time for convulsion onset (defined here as the latency which means the time to begin the first complete clonic convulsion) in the PTZ model in mice, the maximal effect was observed using citronellol at a dose of 400 mg/kg [97]. Citronellol possesses significant anticonvulsant activity probably due to the reduction of neuronal excitability mainly through the voltage-dependent Na^+ channels; the GABAergic neurotransmitter system might also be involved [98].

Safranal, the main component of essential oil of *Crócus*, is formed from picrocrocin *via* hydrolysis during drying and storage of saffron [99]. Safranal is the main constituent of the essential volatile oil responsible for the characteristic odor and aroma of saffron [100]. Safranal has a protective effect in both the clonic and tonic phases of PTZ-induced seizures; the $GABA_A$ -benzodiazepine receptor complex may play an important role in the effects of drug; however, further investigations using $GABA_A$ selective antagonist should be conducted [101].

A number of derivatives of pinane amino acids **8-10** were synthesized from monoterpenes (+)- and (–)-α-pinenes [102]. Amino ester (–)-**9** exhibits a high anticonvulsant activity *in vivo* in the PTZ-induced convulsions and nicotine toxicity tests in mice at 10 mg/kg dose *per os*; it's LD_{50} is higher than 1000 mg/kg. Moreover, compound **9** at the studied dosage exerts a slight sedative effect on locomotor activity [103].

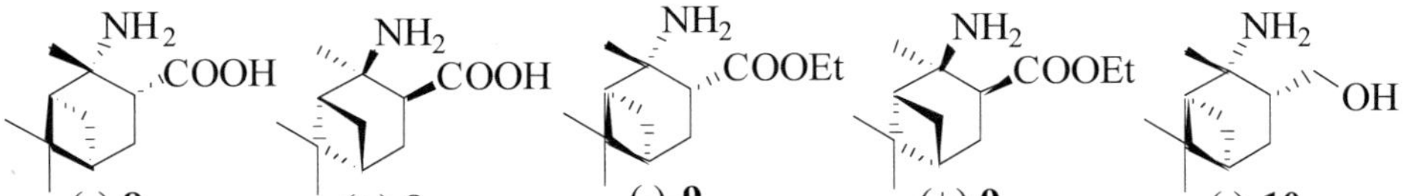

(-)-8 (+)-8 (-)-9 (+)-9 (-)-10

The transition from the amino ester (–)-**9** to its hydrogenated derivative, amino alcohol (–)-**10**, results in a noticeable decrease in anticonvulsant activity in both models; whereas amino acid (–)-**8** increases mortality among animals in both tests, exhibiting the opposite effect [102]. The absolute configuration of the compounds under study is of great significance. As opposed to amino ester (–)-**9**, its enantiomer (+)-**9** potentiates the action of PTZ, thus enhancing the development of convulsions. Compound (+)-**8** exhibited the same effect.

NEUROPROTECTIVE ACTIVITY

Any pathophysical mechanisms are triggered by various ethiological factors or biological events; therefore, a large number of neurologic disorders of different evolution (acute, chronic) are degenerative. Despite the fact that etiologic agents are not homogeneous, the same processes result in disruption of cell function and cell death. The neuroprotective therapy is aimed to block these pathogenetic processes. Neuroprotectors are the agents preventing the neuronal damage in brain caused by a pathogenic factor. The effect of these agents is supposed to eliminate or reduce the pathophysiological and biochemical disruptions in a neural cell. A few monoterpenoids have been known for their neuroprotective activity. As neurological disorders and neurodegenerative diseases, such as a stroke, Alzheimer's disease, and Parkinson's disease tend to become more frequent, the role of neuroprotective agents becomes more important [104].

It was found that α- and γ-terpinenes (10 μM) possess the significant neuroprotective activity on ischemia model involving human neuroblastoma SH-SY5Y [98].

Borneol exhibits neuroprotective effects against OGD/R (oxygen glucose deprivation/reperfusion), which is achieved through multifunctional cytoprotective pathways. The mechanisms of this reversal from OGD/R may be involved in the alleviation of intracellular ROS (reactive oxygen species) and nitric oxide synthase/NO-mediated pathway, the reduction of inflammatory factor release, the inhibition of IκBα degradation, the blockage of NF-κB p65 nuclear translocation, and depression of caspase-related apoptosis [105].

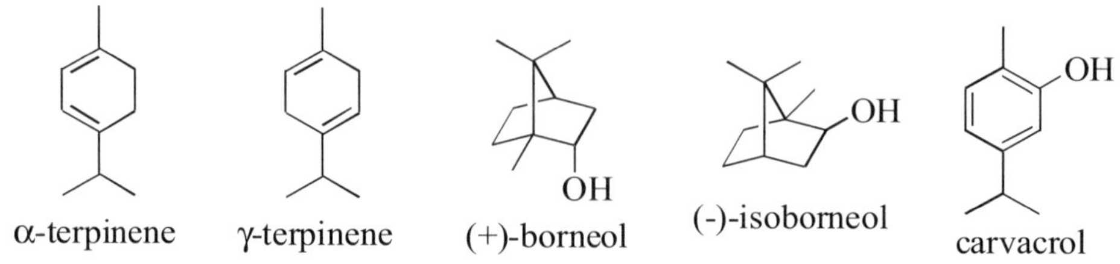

Borneol can increase the concentrations of sodium ferulate in plasma and in part in the brain [106]. Sodium ferulate is used in the therapy of free radical-related syndromes such as neurodegenerative disorders and protected mice against learning and memory deficits induced by centrally administered β-amyloid [107]. Unfortunately, sodium ferulate undergoes marked first-pass effects that limit its bioavailability and it is quickly metabolized in the liver [108]. Sodium ferulate (100-400 mg/kg, p.o.) in combination with borneol (10 mg/kg, p.o.) significantly enhances neuroprotective effects in brain I/R (ischemia/reperfusion) mice, which may in part be due to maintenance of the integrity of the blood-brain barrier and the restoration of the redox system [109].

rac-Isoborneol-mediated cytoprotection is due, at least in part, to inhibition of the oxidative stress resulting from the mitochondrial apoptotic pathway [110].

Carvacrol, a monoterpene phenol, is naturally occurring in various plants belonging to the *Lamiaceae* family. It is abundant in the essential oil fraction of oregano and thyme [111]. Carvacrol at doses of 25 and 50 mg/kg intraperitoneally provides neuroprotection on infarct volume and neuronal apoptosis in a focal MCAO (middle cerebral artery occlusion) mouse model [112].

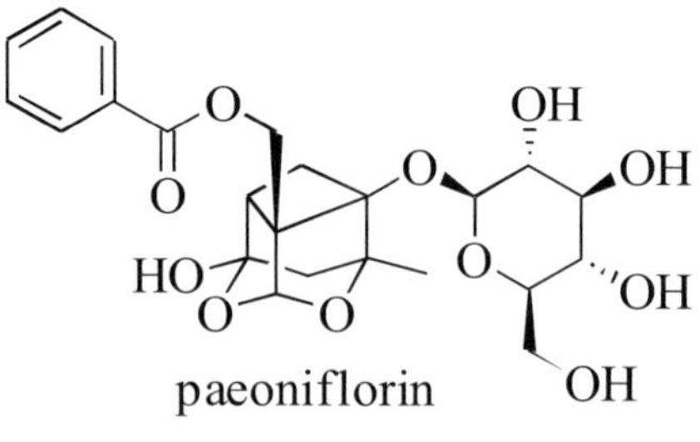

Paeoniflorin, monoterpenoid glucoside and the characteristic main principal bioactive component of *P. alba* Radix, has been reported to exhibit many pharmacological effects [113]. Paeoniflorin at doses of 2.5 and 5 mg/kg, s.c., had a potent neuroprotective effect on dopaminergic neurons in the MPTP mouse model of PD [114]. The neuroprotective effects of paeoniflorin might be mediated though its modulation of neuroinflammation by activation of the adenosine A1 receptors [116]. Paeoniflorin (10 and 50 μM) treatment could also protect against NMDA-induced cell death in PC12 cells. The protective effect of paeoniflorin was mediated by Ca^{2+} antagonism [115].

INHIBITION OF ACETYLCHOLINESTERASE ACTIVITY

The principal role of acetylcholinesterase (AChE) is the termination of nerve impulse transmission at the cholinergic synapses by rapid hydrolysis of acetylcholine (ACh). The inhibition of AChE serves as a strategy for the treatment of Alzheimer's disease (AD), senile dementia, ataxia, myasthenia gravis and Parkinson's disease [116]. Essential oils have gained importance thanks of their AChE inhibitory activity.

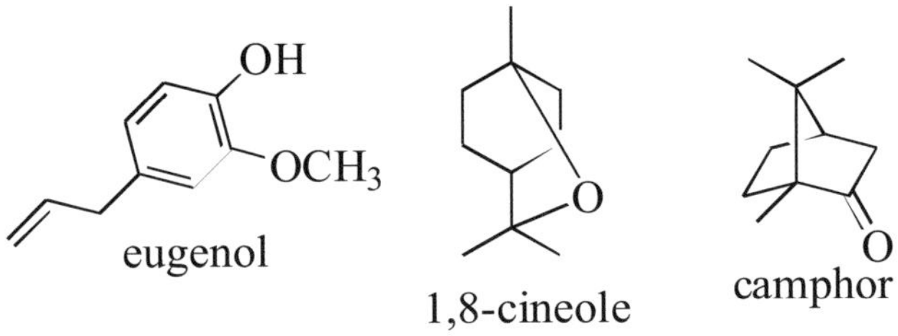

S. Dohi with co-authors [117] studied the AChE inhibitory activity of the main components of essential oils and found that the individual components of the oils, including a novel AChE inhibitor, contributed up to 25% of the observed AChE inhibitory activity. Eugenol had the highest contribution ratio among the active components, and it accounted for 25% of the observed inhibitory activity of the *O. sanctum* oil. The contribution ratio of 1,8-cineole accounted for over 6% of the inhibitory activity of the *L. officinalis* oil [117]. High 1,8-cineole and low camphor contents in the oil may increase its anticholinesterase activity. *Salvia fruticosa* may be ideal for AChE inhibition with a high level of 1,8-cineole up to 75% and low camphor content in a range of 0.8–30.3% [118]. The concentration-dependent inhibition of electric eel AChE was calculated for 1,8-cineole. The IC_{50} value for 1,8-cineole was 6 mM [119].

Four essential oil components showed substantial inhibition of AChE activity: carvacrol, 1,8-cineole, myrtenal and verbenone. Myrtenal exhibited a comparatively strong AChE inhibition potential, with IC_{50} = 0.17 μM, and might therefore be considered to be an interesting lead compound. The interaction of carvacrol with AChE is most likely based on the phenolic hydroxyl group, which binds to proteins, leading to a conformational change and therefore a loss of function [120].

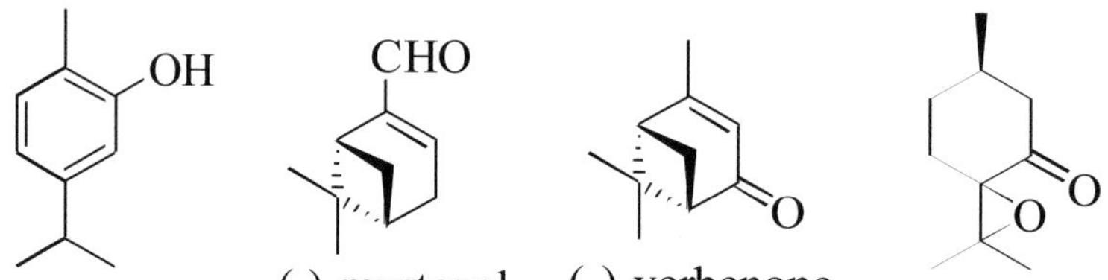

carvacrol (-)-myrtenal (-)-verbenone pulegone epoxide

The monoterpenoid epoxide, pulegone-1,2-epoxide, identified as the major insecticidal compound isolated from the medicinal plant *Lippia steochadifolia* was found to inhibit eel AChE as well as other cholinesterases (horse serum cholinesterase, house fly head cholinesterases, and head and thorax cholinesterases from the Madagascar roach) *in vitro* [121].

M. Miyazawa with co-authors studied the anticholinesterase activity of 17 kinds of monoterpenoids with the *p*-menthane skeleton and 17 kinds of bicyclic monoterpenoids; as a result, they ascertained the structure–activity dependence [122].

The monoterpenoid ketones showed stronger inhibition compared to that exhibited by the alcohols. Thus, (+)-pulegone was found to be a strong inhibitor of AChE activity. (–)- And (+)-carvones showed slightly weaker inhibition than (+)-pulegone. The presence of conjugated double bonds is related to the strength of inhibition of AChE. The presence of an isopropenyl group decreases the strength of inhibition of AChE. As shown in some of the comparative results between enantiomers, the (–)-form was a slightly more potent inhibitor than the (+)-form, such as for (–)- and (+)-carvones [122].

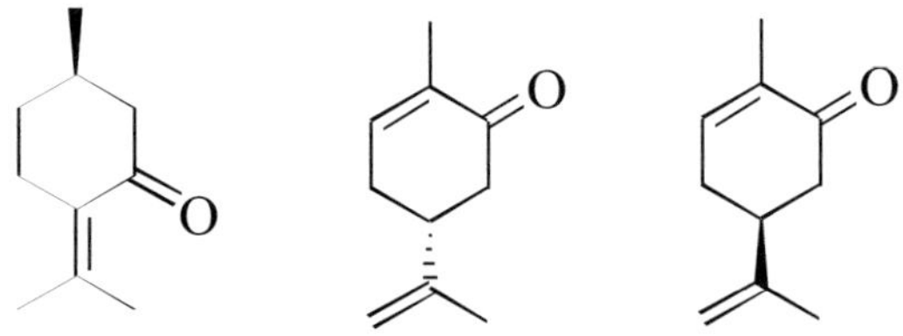

(+)-pulegone (-)-carvone (+)-carvone

The hydrocarbon compounds showed identical inhibitory activity with the terpene alcohols. Specifically, α-pinene showed the strongest inhibition next to (+)-pulegone. The position of C=C double bonds is related to the strength of inhibition of AChE.

The compounds with an allylic methyl group show more potent inhibitory activity ((–)-verbenol and (–)-verbenone, (+)-2- and (+)-3-carenes). The oxygenated compounds with a camphane skeleton were weak inhibitors of AChE ((+)- and (–)-fenchones). As was shown, (–)-fenchone was a slightly more potent inhibitor than (+)-fenchone [123].

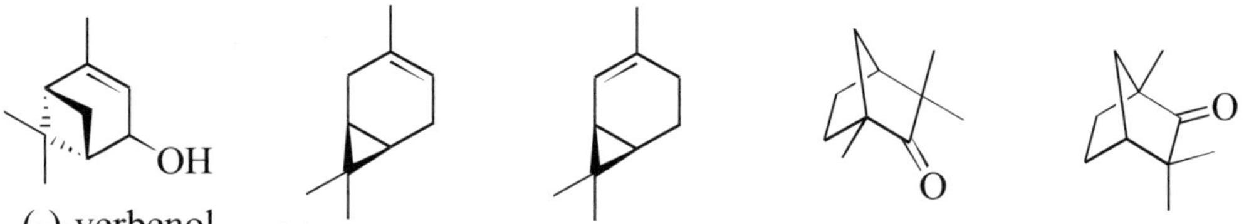

(-)-verbenol (+)-3-carene (+)-2-carene (-)-fenchone (+)-fenchone

ANTI-ALZHEIMER'S DISEASE ACTIVITY

Alzheimer's disease (AD) is one of the most well-known neurodegenerative diseases and is responsible for 50–60% of patients with dementia. The prevalence rate of AD is positively correlated with age, and AD occurs in ≥40% of the elderly population over 85 years old. Patients with AD develop a decline in cognitive function and find it difficult to remember recent events during the early stage (short-term memory loss) [124]. Treatment of AD includes the symptomatic therapy using acetylcholinesterase (AChE) inhibitors, modulators of *N*-methyl-*D*-

aspartic acid (NMDA) receptors, neuroprotectors, *etc.* Among many natural products, the terpenoids including monoterpenoids are the largest and the most diverse group of naturally occurring organic compounds, which increases the chance that a terpenoid will be identified as having activity against AD.

1,8-Cineole and α-pinene are considered to be the most active AChE inhibitory components of *S. lavandulifolia* oil although other oil constituents may inhibit AChE, perhaps synergistically. Limonene and perillyl alcohol, the components of *Citrus* (Rutaceae) essential oils, improve scopolamine-induced memory impairment, which is suggested to be due to AChE inhibition (observed *in vitro*) [125].

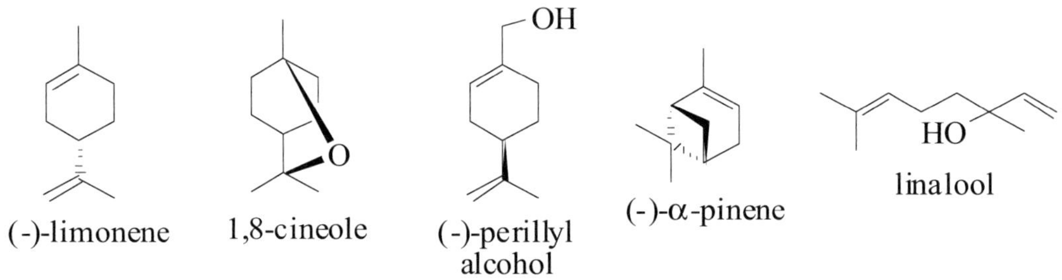

rac-Linalool (1.0 and 3.0 μM) demonstrated an inhibition of potassium-stimulated (but not basal) glutamate release, and antagonism to NMDA receptors [126]. Moreover, it was found that linalool has an inhibitory effect on the [^{3}H]glutamate binding. Increasing linalool concentrations indicate that the inhibitory effect on the [^{3}H]glutamate binding is dose-dependent, being abolished with 6.5 mM linalool [127].

ANTIPARKINSONIAN ACTIVITY

Parkinson's disease (PD) is the second most common neurodegenerative disorder after Alzheimer's disease. The worldwide prevalence is estimated to be 200 per 100 000 population [128]. Parkinson's disease (PD) is characterized by progressive loss of dopamine neurons and terminals from the nigrostriatal pathway and by a slow onset of motor symptoms [129]. Common parkinsonian symptoms are rest tremor, bradykinesia, rigidity, and loss of postural reflexes.

Gait disturbances are among the most common problems in Parkinson's disease [130].

It has been recently discovered that compound **2** (20 mg/kg) possesses a high antiparkinsonian activity expressed in the elimination of oligokinesia in C57Bl/6 mice caused by single or systematic injections of the neurotoxin MPTP (1-methyl-4-phenyl-1,2,3,6-tetrahydropyridine) [131]. It was shown that **2** (70% enantiomeric excess (*ee*)) enhanced the inhibitory effect of high doses of levodopa (1.0 mmol/kg (200 mg/kg)) and thereby potentiated the dopaminergic system. Moreover, in the arecoline tremor test, which makes it possible to estimate the effect on muscarinic cholinergic receptors, the compound decreased the duration of arecoline-induced tremor, exhibiting an *M*-anticholinergic activity. The combination of these properties is probably responsible for the antiparkinsonian activity of **2**.

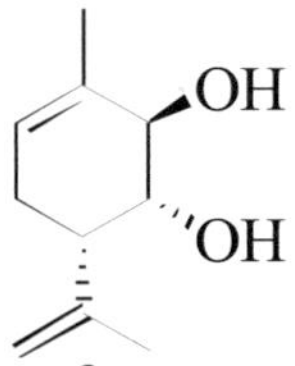

2

Compound **2** almost completely prevents the development of catalepsy caused by haloperidol, which is demonstrated by a notable decrease in the catalepsy duration in animals, the duration of haloperidol time course, and the percent of cataleptic animals [132]. The low acute toxicity of compound **2**, the LD_{50} of which amounts to 4250 mg/kg (p.o.), should also be mentioned [84]. Because of this combination of traits, further study of the antiparkinsonian activity of this substance holds much promise.

It is known, the absolute configuration of chiral compounds tends to be critical for the manifestation of various biological activities. Compound **2** has three asymmetric centers and, hence, eight stereoisomers. All these stereoisomers with high (no less than 93% *ee*) optical purity were synthesized and the antiparkinsonian activity of the stereoisomers of compound **2** was studied on a model with administration of MPTP neurotoxin to mice of C57Bl/6 line [132].

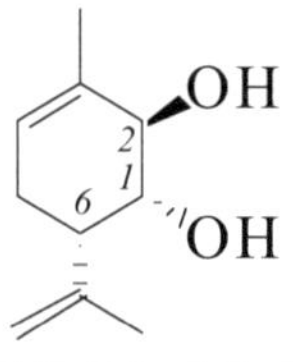

(1*R*,2*R*,6*S*)-**2**

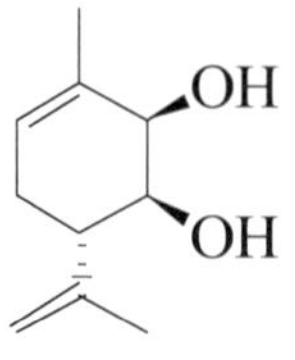

(1*S*,2*R*,6*S*)-**2**

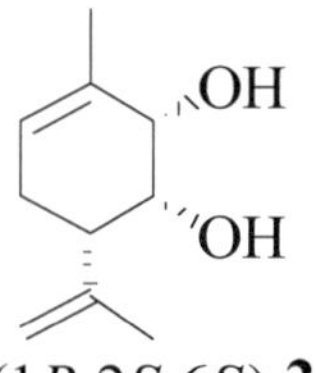

(1*R*,2*S*,6*S*)-**2**

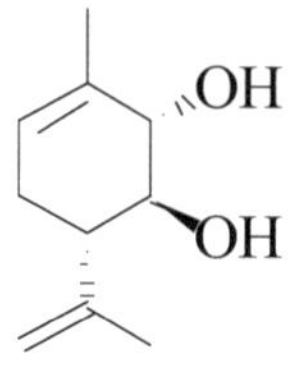

(1*S*,2*S*,6*S*)-**2**

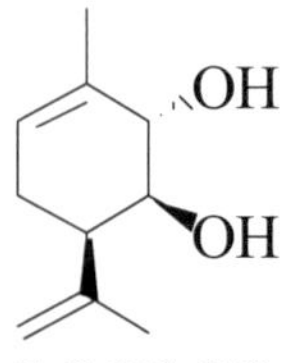

(1*S*,2*S*,6*R*)-**2**

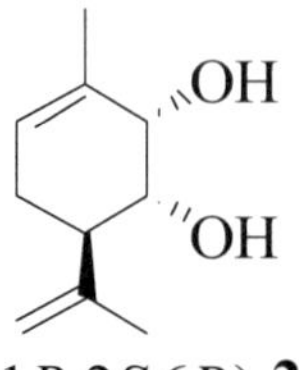

(1*R*,2*S*,6*R*)-**2**

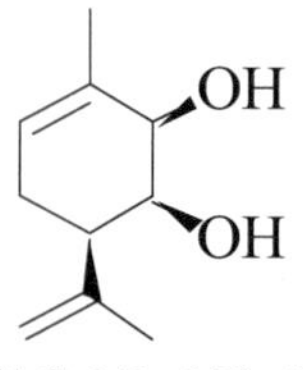

(1*S*,2*R*,6*R*)-**2**

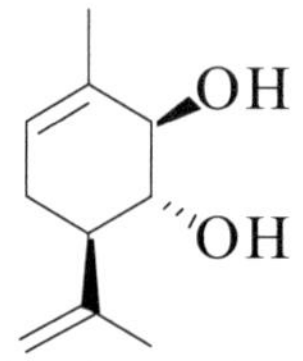

(1*R*,2*R*,6*R*)-**2**

According to the investigation of the antiparkinsonian activity of (1*R*,2*R*,6*S*)-**2** (93% *ee*) isomer, which amounts to 85% of the previously studied (1*R*,2*R*,6*S*)-**2** (70% *ee*), the compound is characterized by high activity and restores the locomotor and exploratory activities almost completely to the rates of the saline group (except for the number of the explored holes). The minor (1*S*,2*S*,6*R*)-**2** isomer demonstrated an unreliable, although visible, antiparkinsonian activity.

The inversion of the configuration of the allylic hydroxy group in position 1 during the transfer from (1*R*,2*R*,6*S*)-**2** to (1*S*,2*R*,6*S*)-**2** resulted in a complete disappearance of the antiparkinsonian activity. Its optical antipode, (1*R*,2*S*,6*R*)-**2**, however, exhibited a significant activity, although it was slightly less than that of the (1*R*,2*R*,6*S*)-**2** isomer.

An unexpected result was obtained after the configuration of the hydroxy group in position 2 was changed. The transfer to a complete *cis*-isomer of (1*R*,2*S*,6*S*)-**2** led to a sudden and nearly full inversion of activity, namely, to a strong increase in hypokinesia and a decrease in the animals' exploratory activity. Compound (1*S*,2*R*,6*R*)-**2**, the enantiomer of (1*R*,2*S*,6*S*)-**2**, displayed no reliable activity, yet it significantly increased the general locomotor activity.

The (1*S*,2*S*,6*S*)-**2** and (1*R*,2*R*,6*R*)-**2** enantiomer pair produced no reliable effect on the locomotor-orientational activity in these tests, but (1*R*,2*R*,6*R*)-**2** led to a visible decrease in the animals' exploratory activity. Thus, it can be said that the absolute configuration of compound **2** greatly influences the antiparkinsonian activity of the compound in the test with MPTP, from nearly full removal to a sharp increase in the symptoms of the parkinsonian syndrome [132].

ANXIOLYTIC-LIKE EFFECTS

Anxiety is very common in various psychiatric diseases accompanying physiological, emotional and cognitive deficits. Patients with multiple psychological diseases including depression and schizophrenia often experience anxiety-related symptoms, such as anger, shame, guilt, sadness, nervousness, and fear [133]. The treatment of anxiety with the commercially available anxiolytic drugs currently involves such problems as adverse and undesirable effects. Other therapies, such as aromatherapy using EOs, are a possible alternative to standard pharmacological treatment and has been used for several conditions (such as chronic pain, depression and anxiety). Thus, it is reasonable to expect that the monoterpenoid components of essential oils will exhibit the anxiolytic activity [134].

Inhaled linalool (3% but not 1%) is anxiolytic in mice. In the light/dark test, 3% linalool increased the time spent in the lit area, besides no changes were noted in the number of crossings. Such anxiolytic activity of inhaled linalool in these mouse models was comparable to that obtained with diazepam [135].

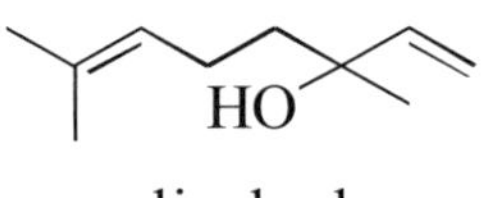

linalool

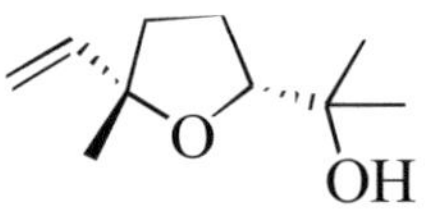

(+)-linalool oxide

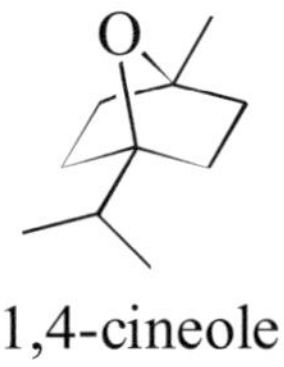

1,4-cineole

Linalool oxide can be found in some herbal EOs, albeit as a minority component. It is a monocyclic alcohol that can be formed from linalool by natural oxidation or may be produced by synthetic processes such as biotransformation of linalool using the fungus *Aspergillus niger* [136]. Linalool oxide (inhalation 0.65%, 2.5% and 5%) exerts an anxiolytic effect on mice without causing motor impairment: linalool oxide inhalations increased the time in the brightly lit chamber and did not appear to cause muscle relaxation or motor coordination deficit, since there was no decrease in the time spent on the bar compared to the control group [134].

1,4-Cineole is one of the minor components of some plant extracts. 1,4-Cineole is a widely-distributed monoterpene ether, which is one of the flavor constituents of lime juice. Its metabolism has been described and metabolites have been isolated from the urine of rabbits [137]. Acute administration of 1,4-cineole presented anxiolytic-like effects in the elevated plusmaze and hole-board tests and this effect was unrelated to benzodiazepine receptors. This effect was also devoid of significant sedative effect as assessed by the open-field test. Parameters observed in the forced swimming, tail suspension and pentobarbital sleeping time tests support the idea that 1,4-cineole possibly presents the depressor activity on the central nervous system [138].

Two new amines **11** and **12** were synthesized by interaction of 2-aminoadamantane and the available monoterpenoid aldehydes citral and (–)-myrtenal. It was established that the amines possess anxiolytic activity in male Balb/C mice in the elevated plus maze test with a single i.p. administration of a dose of 1 mg/kg [139].

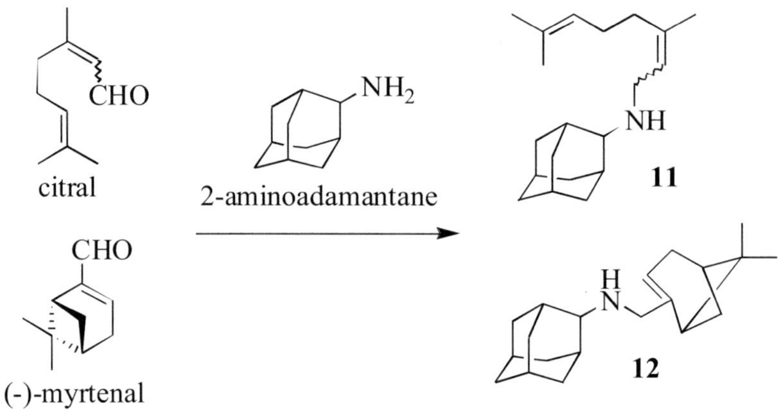

ANTIDEPRESSANT ACTIVITY

Depressive disorder is a common mental disorder associated with a significant negative impact on quality of life, morbidity/mortality, and cognitive function; it affects approximately 10–15% of people over the course of their lives and is expected to become the second leading cause of disability in the world by 2020. Depressive symptoms lead to ill health, increased mortality and have a significant impact on social and occupational functioning [140]. Application of different medicinal plant species for treatment of depression has shown to be effective [141]. Several essential oils obtained from aromatic species of plants are also used in aromatherapy to relieve depression, *e.g.*, *Lavandula spp*, *Jasminum officinale*, *Rosmarinus officinalis*, *Rosa spp* and *Matricaria chamomile* among others [142].

Listea. glaucescens essential oil (100 and 300 mg/kg, i.p.) showed anti-depressant activity in mice in the forced swimming test; furthermore, it did not affect the spontaneous locomotor activity in the open-field test. Two of its constituents, linalool and β-pinene (100 mg/kg intraperitoneally), show antidepressant activity; however, these compounds by themselves have a sedative activity as well [143].

The monoterpenoid lactone (–)-loliolide was isolated from leaves of *Mondia. whitei*. The activity of (–)-loliolide was tested in a serotonin transporter binding assay using [^{3}H]-citalopram as ligand, giving an IC_{50} value of 997 μM. As a non-nitrogenous compound, loliolide might bind to serotonin transporter in a different way compared to the standard nitrogen-containing serotonin reuptake inhibitors [144].

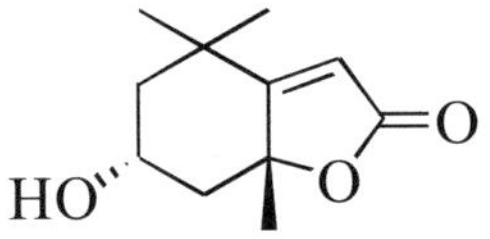

loliolide

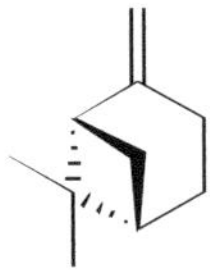
(-)-β-pinene

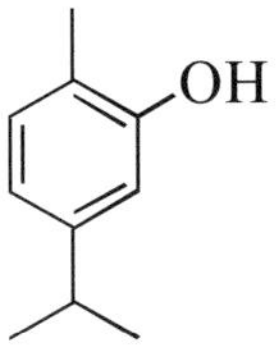
carvacrol

Acute administration of carvacrol (12.5, 25 and 50 mg/kg, oraly) was effective in producing antidepressant effects when assessed in the forced swimming and tail suspension tests. The mechanism of action of carvacrol in these tests is most likely to be dependent on an increase in dopamine level [145].

OTHER TYPES OF ACTIVITY

Citrinae essential oils comprise mainly monoterpenes, aldehydes and alcohols. Among these components, the monoterpene (+)-limonene is the principal component (60–90%) of citrus essential oils. (–)-Limonene isomer occurring in

Lamiáceae family, is also present very sparingly in *citrinae* essential oils. The other monoterpenes in citrus essential oils, γ-terpinene and α- and β-pinenes are known to be the major components of citrus essential oils [146].

Monoterpene compounds in citrus essential oils enhanced monoamine release from rat brain tissue slices. Both (+)- and (–)-limonenes (2.5 and 3 mg/ml) had a significant effect on dopamine release from the rat brain striatum. Moreover, (–)-limonene had a significantly stronger effect than (+)-limonene. In humans, very low concentrations of (–)-linalool, the main component of both *Jasmínum* and *Lavandula*, have a sedative effect on autonomic nerve activity and mood state. In contrast, (+)-linalool, an optical isomer of (–)-linalool, showed an opposite effect [147].

After 1-week administration of (–)-limonene (5, 25 and 50 mg/kg, oraly), GABA contents in the brain increased significantly, while the glutamate concentration decreased significantly. These changes did not affect the basal activity of hypothalamic-pituitary-adrenal, but when rats were given an acute stress, foot shock, (–)-limonene showed a strong ability to attenuate the stress response [148].

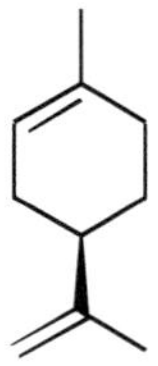
(+)-limonene

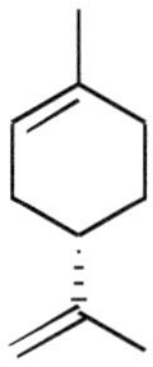
(-)-limonene

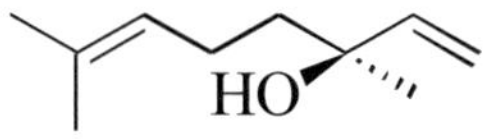

(+)-linalool

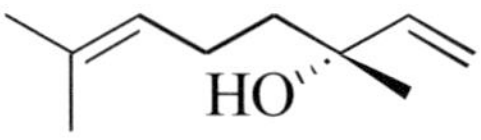

(-)-linalool

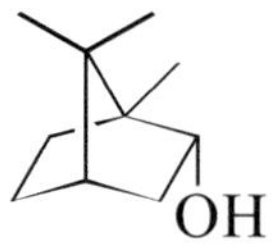

(-)-borneol

Some alcohol monoterpenes can increase propofol concentration by inhibiting propofol metabolism. (–)-Borneol (200 mg/kg, i.p.) increased propofol concentration primarily by inhibiting propofol glucuronidation; whereas (–)-carveol (200 mg/kg, i.p.) and *trans*-sobrerol decreased propofol metabolism by inhibiting oxidation and glucuronidation. It is likely that dietary monoterpene would interact with other drugs [149].

Carvacrol has an estrous-stage specific effect on depressive behaviors and endocrine parameters. The acute administration of carvacrol significantly increased the immobility time during the forced swimming test in female rats, only during the proestrus phase. Carvacrol at a dose of 450 mg/kg, oraly, might have pro-depressive properties in female rats. Together with the reduction of plasma estradiol concentrations in proestrus phase, this natural constituent of essential oils selectively reduced 5-HT (5-hydroxytryptamine) content in the prefrontal cortex and nucleus acumben inducing, in spontaneously cycling female rats, a state of despair which is reversed by a selective inhibition of 5-HT reuptake [150].

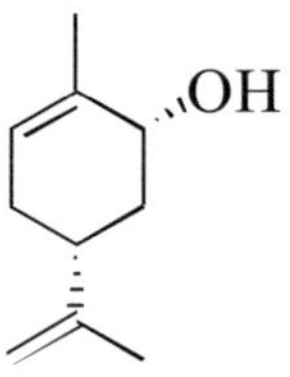

(-)-carveol

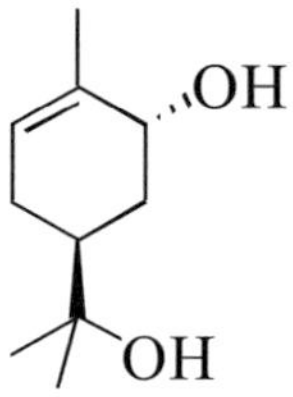

trans-sobrerol

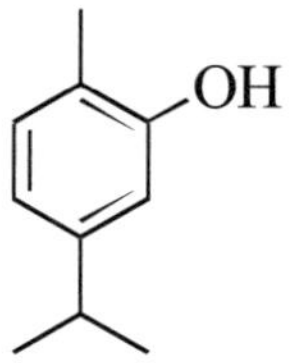

carvacrol

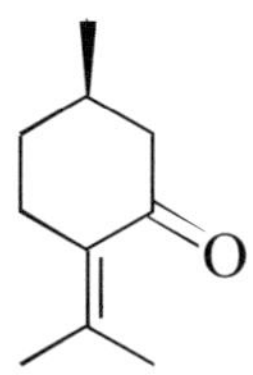

(+)-pulegone

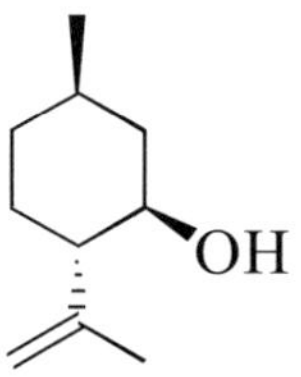

(-)-isopulegol

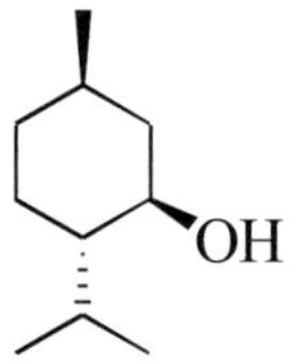

(-)-menthol

(+)-Pulegone at an intraperitoneal dose of 200 mg/kg, i.p., demonstrated a central depressant effect in mice, as observed by a decreased locomotor activity, increased passivity, and sedation 0.5 h after the administration. The CNS-depressant effect of (+)-pulegone was confirmed by an increase in the pentobarbital-induced sleeping time and was observed at both 100 and 200 mg/kg, i.p. [57].

Intraperitoneal treatment with isopulegol (25 and 50 mg/kg, i.p.) did not significantly change the motor activity in mice. Isopulegol, at both doses, was capable of increasing the total time spent in immobility in the forced swimming test, indicating depressant activity, and had no significant effect on the motor coordination of the animals in the rotarod test. Isopulegol at both doses also decreased the sleep latency time in the pentobarbital-induced sleeping test and increased the duration of sleeping, which possibly confirms the previously detected depressant activity [151].

Menthol (100, 200, 400 mg/kg, subcutaneous) normalized the glycine level in cortex and hypothalamus; whereas in hippocampus menthol (200 mg/kg and 400 mg/kg, subcutaneous) showed a significant decrease in concentration of glycine as compared to the control group of young mice. Menthol significantly reversed the amnesia induced by natural aging and β-amyloid protein. Pre-treatment with menthol reversed the amnesia induced in animals upon treatment with β-amyloid on day 10. Menthol improved working memory in aged and young mice. The potentiation of working memory was more profound with menthol at a low dose of 100 mg/kg [152].

It has been shown that inhalation of *Lavandula* oil composed of 25% linalool and 46% linalyl acetate induced anxiolytic (open-field) effects in rats after at least 30 min of inhalation [153]. Linalool (1 and 3%) inhaled for 60 min is clearly sedative, inducing hypothermia, reducing locomotion and increasing pentobarbital-induced sleeping time [154].

(−)-Linalool (50 and 100 mg/kg, i.p.) modulates glutamatergic NMDA receptors, which are directly involved in the learning processes and memory. (−)-Linalool is a glutamatergic receptor antagonist. It can compete with glutamate by binding to the active sites of these receptors, inhibiting the activity they exert. In the open-field test, (−)-linalool reduced exploratory behavior manifested as lower number of rearings only at a dose of 100 mg/kg, i.p. [155].

MECAMYLAMINE

Mecamylamine (Inversine), the first orally available antihypertensive agent launched in the 1950s, is rarely used today for hypertension because of its widespread ganglionic side effects at antihypertensive doses (25–90 mg/day). Mecamylamine is synthesized from monoterpene camphene by various ways [156]. Pharmacologically, mecamylamine has been well characterized as a nonselective and noncompetitive antagonist of nicotinic acetylcholine receptors (nAChRs). Since mecamylamine easily crosses the blood-brain barrier at relatively low doses (2.5–10 mg), it has been used over the past two decades by several research groups investigating the role of central nAChRs in the etiology and treatment of various neuropsychiatric disorders, including addiction disorders, Tourette's syndrome, schizophrenia, and various cognitive and mood disorders [157].

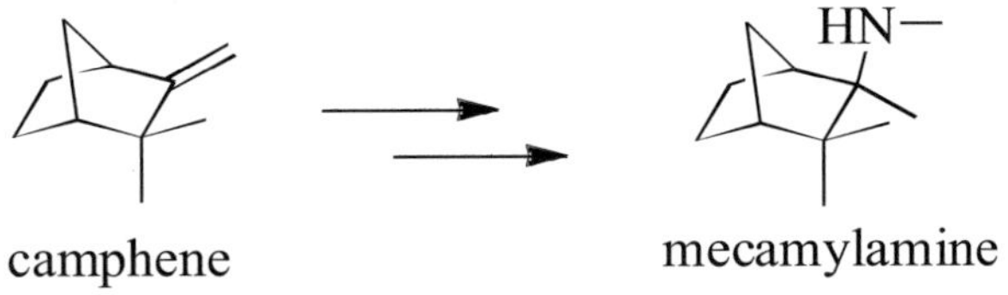

Various doses of mecamylamine had an anxiolytic effect in the elevated plus maze task, light/dark assay, and the social interaction test [158]. Anxiolytic effects of mecamylamine might be associated with brain-derived neurotrophic factor (BDNF) expression. Increased BDNF in the cerebral cortex of rats is closely related to the antianxiety effect of mecamylamine [159]. Mecamylamine at a 0.3 mg/kg dose was capable of inducing the anxiolytic effects in the rats both under the dimly lit and brightly lit conditions in the elevated plus maze test but had no effect under the dimly lit conditions in the social interaction test [13].

The cholinergic theory of depression put forth by Janowsky and colleagues in the 1970s hypothesized that hypercholinergic activity may contribute to depressive symptoms, and more recently it has been hypothesized that antagonism of nAChRs by existing antidepressants and mecamylamine may mediate antidepressant effects [160]. Acute mecamylamine dose-dependently decreases the immobility time in the tail suspension test, a well-characterized behavioral test of antidepressant efficacy. Mecamylamine antagonizes all types of nAChRs with the greatest affinity for α4β2* receptors; however, at higher doses it can also antagonize NMDA receptors [161]. Docking simulations of protonated (*S*)-(+)-mecamylamine and (*R*)-(−)-mecamylamine (in the protonated and neutral forms; data not shown) suggest that they interact with the extracellular edge of the ion channel by forming an ion-pair contact with the acidic residue α4-Glu^{261} at the outer ring [162]. Mecamylamine has a relatively higher specificity for α3β4 AChRs compared to that of the other neuronal AChRs. Thus, these results point out the importance of α3β4 AChRs expressed in the brain, more specifically in the medial habenula, interpeduncular nucleus, ventral tegmental area, dorsolateral tegmentum, basolateral amygdala, locus coeruleus, and hippocampus, for the therapeutic actions of mecamylamine and tricyclic antidepressants, especially considering that some of these brain areas are involved in depression and anxiety [163].

Nicotine is the major addictive component of tobacco, drives to abuse despite the harmful consequences. Nicotine addiction is a complex behavioral phenomenon being dependent on several systems, but the main reinforcing effect of nicotine depends on the activation of the mesolimbic dopaminergic system. Infusion of the nicotine antagonist into the cerebral ventricles or lesions of the mesolimbic dopamine neurons abolishes both locomotor activating and rewarding effect of nicotine. These effects of nicotine are known to be mediated by the nACh receptors located on the dopaminergic neurons [164]. *Via* activation of nAChRs, nicotine stimulates the dopamine neurons in the ventral tegmental area and increases dopamine release in the nucleus accumbens. However, the effects of nicotine on dopamine levels in the nucleus accumbens and on the activity in the ventral tegmental area (known as the mesolimbic pathway of the reward system) are much more modest than those of drugs, such as amphetamines, heroin and cocaine. The transport of nicotine into the brain is diminished by mecamylamine; as a consequence, nicotine binding to nAChRs is reduced [157]. Mecamylamine has been found to potently block the physiological effects of nicotine and to aid in the treatment of smoking cessation, particularly in women [165].

Alcoholism is the third preventable cause of mortality in the world and few therapeutic treatments are available highlighting the importance of understanding the underlying molecular mechanisms of the reinforcing properties of ethanol. Alcohol has multiple actions throughout the central nervous system, including direct or indirect actions on the serotonin, glutamate, $GABA_A$, and dopamine systems. Recent evidence suggests that alcohol may also act through nicotinic acetylcholine receptors, which may in turn affect dopamine function in the ventral tegumental area of the brain [166]. Mecamylamine dose dependently reduced alcohol intake, which also leads to a significant reduction in blood–ethanol concentration suggesting that mecamylamine was not inhibiting the metabolism of ethanol. Sucrose intake, however, was not reduced, indicating specificity for alcohol consumption and not a general effect on reward signaling. Reduction of ethanol intake by mecamylamine was mediated by blockade of neuronal nAChRs expressed in the CNS because the non-specific nAChR antagonist, hexamcthonium, did not significantly alter alcohol consumption [167]. Mecamylamine pretreatment dose dependently decreased ethanol intake in mice by 5–70%. Although ethanol preference was not significantly altered, the highest mecamylamine dose (8 mg/kg) led to a 50% reduction in ethanol preference ratio [14].

Tourette's syndrome is characterized by motor and verbal tics that start before the age of 21; the etiology of this illness is still not understood [168]. Mecamylamine has clinical effects similar to those of nicotine in Tourette's disorder when used at low doses in combination with an antipsychotic drug [169].

Autism is a brain development disorder with unknown etiology characterized by social impairment and repetitive behaviors [170]. Human post-mortem studies show that nAChRs are abnormally depleted in brain regions such as the cerebellum, cortex and thalamus – the brain regions involved in sensory processing and attention [171]. The rationale for using the nAChR antagonist for the treatment of autism is based upon the notion of normalizing cholinergic tone in this disorder. Mecamylamine at a dose of 0.13–0.15 mg/kg/day for 3 months might be useful, although it would appear that resources might be better devoted to a trial of the $\alpha 4\beta 2$ nAChR agonist. As it stands, the use of mecamylamine in children with autism would be off-label and without evidence of efficacy [172].

Mecamylamine can also inhibit neuronal cell death caused by different stimuli through different anti-apoptotic mechanisms. Mecamylamine prevented glutamate-induced neuronal cell death in a concentration-dependent manner. Furthermore, mecamylamine dramatically reversed the condensation of chromatin and the DNA fragmentation [173].

A dose of mecamylamine that is selective for nAChRs (0.3 mg/kg) produced no significant effects on flash-evoked potential (FEP) amplitudes or latencies, body temperature, or behavior in rats. While behavioral, body temperature, and FEP latency effects were observed following administration of the 3.0 mg/kg dose, significant FEP amplitude changes occurred almost entirely following only the 10.0 mg/kg dose of mecamylamine. This is a relatively high dose which may not be selective for nAChRs [174].

CONCLUDING REMARKS

Monoterpenoids are abundant in nature, being the principal components of essential oils. Many native monoterpenoids possess a wide range of biological activities and affect various neuromediatory systems. On one hand, this fact opens possibilities for the development of multi-target drugs; on the other hand, it complicates the attainment of high selectivity of their action, which can result in the emergence of undesired side effects.

Monoterpene functionalization (in particular, one associated with the inclusion of heteroatoms or obtaining heterocyclic monoterpene derivatives) may result in a considerable enhancement of biological activity or increase selectivity of their action. This very promising pathway can presumably be the shortest one in the development of novel CNS-active drugs.

Although a wide variety of the experimental models and the doses used makes direct comparing of the results obtained in different studies more complicated, the available published data allow one to single out the structures that have a potential for the development of new CNS-active drugs.

Let us note that the overwhelming majority of studies devoted to the CNS activity of monoterpenoids have been carried out *in vivo*, which can be to a large extent attributed to the ability of these compounds to simultaneously affect several neuromediatory systems. Furthermore, one should take into account that oxygen-containing monoterpene derivatives resulting from their metabolism can also possess a significant physiological activity. It is very difficult to allow for this fact when planning the *in vitro* experiments.

In the most cases, the absolute configuration of monoterpenoids has the crucial effect on their biological activity. This fact makes it necessary to synthesize (or isolate from the natural sources) all possible stereoisomers of these compounds for serious investigation into their physiological activity.

ACKNOWLEDGMENTS

Authors are grateful to the Russian Ministry of Science and Education (grant 2012-1.3.1-12-000-2009-005, contr. No 8726).

CONFLICT OF INTEREST

The authors state that there is no conflict of interest.

REFERENCES

[1] Koroch, A.R.; Juliani, H.R. Bioactivity of essential oils and their components. In: Flavours and Fragrances; Berger, R.G. Ed.; Springer-Verlag, Berlin, 2007, 87-115.

[2] Dobetsberger, C.; Buchbauer, G. Action of essential oils on the central nervous system: an updated rewie. Flavour and Fragrance J., 2011, 26, 300-316.

[3] Amaral, J.F.; Silva, M.I.G.; Neto, M.R.A.; Neto, P.F.T.; Moura, B.A.; Melo, C.T.V.; Araujo, F.L.O.; Sousa, D.P.; de Vasconcelos, P.F.; de Vasconcelos, S.M.M.; Sousa, F.C.F. Antinociceptive effect of the monoterpene R-(+)-limonene in mice. Biol. Farm. Bull., 2007, 30(7), 1217-1220.

[4] Bonjardim, L.R.; Cunha, E.S.; Guimaraes, A.G.; Santana, M.F.; Oliveira, M.G.B.; Serafini, M.R.; Araujo, A.A.S.; Antoniolli, A.R.; Cavalcanti, S.C.H.; Santos, M.R.V.; Quantans-Junior, L.J. Evaluation of the anti-inflammatory and antinociceptive properties of *p*-cymene in mice. Z. Naturforsch., 2012, 67, 15-21.

[5] Drysdale, A.J.; Platt, B. Cannabinoids: Mechanisms and Therapeutic Applications in the CNS. Current Medicinal Chemistry, 2003, 10, 2719-2732.

[6] de Fonseca, R.F.; Arco, D.I.; Bermudez-Silva, F.J.; Bilbao, A.; Cippitelli, A.; Navarro, M. The endocannabinoid system: physiology and pharmacology. Alcohol. Alcohol, 2005, 40(1), 2-14.

[7] Pacher, P.; Batkai, S.; Kunos, G. The endocannabinoid system as an emerging target of pharmacotherapy. Pharmacol. Rev., 2006, 58, 389-462.

[8] Stern, E.; Lambert, D. Medicinal chemistry endeavors around the phytocannabinoids. Chemistry & Biodiversity, 2007, 4, 1707-1728.

[9] de Bitencourt, R.M.; Pamplona, F.A.; Takahashi, R.N. A current overview of cannabinoids and glucocorticoids in facilitating extinction of aversive memories: Potential extinction enhancers. Neuropharmacology, 2013, 64, 389-395.

[10] Bermudez-Silva, F.J.; Viveros, M.P.; McPartland, J.M.; de Fonseca, F.R. The endocannabinoid system, eating behavior and energy homeostasis: The end or a new beginning? Pharmacology Biochemistry and Behavior, 2010, 95, 375-382.

[11] Hanus, L.O. Pharmacological and therapeutic secrets of plant and brain (Endo)Cannabinoids. Medicinal Research Reviews, 2009, 29(2), 213-271.

[12] Scotter, E.L.; Abood, M.E.; Glass, M. The endocannabinoid system as a target for the treatment of neurodegenerative disease. British Journal of Pharmacology, 2010, 160, 480-498.

[13] Newman, M.B.; Manresa, J.J.; Sanberg, P.R.; Shytle, R.D. Anxiolytic effects of mecamylamine in two animal models of anxiety experimental and clinical. Psychopharmacology, 2002, 10(1), 18-25.
[14] Ford, M.M.; Fretwell, A.M.; Nickel, J.D.; Mark, G.P.; Strong, M.N.; Yoneyama, N.; Finn, D.A. The influence of mecamylamine on ethanol and sucrose self-administration. Neuropharmacology, 2009, 57, 250-258.
[15] Wong, C.; Lau, E.; Palozzi, L.; Campbell, F. Pain management in children: Part 1 — Pain assessment tools and a brief review of nonpharmacological and pharmacological treatment options. Can. Pharm. J., 2012, 145(5), 222-225.
[16] McCurdy, C.R.; Scully, S.S. Analgesic substances derived from natural products (natureceuticals). Life Sciences, 2005, 78, 476-484.
[17] Lima, D.F.; Brandao, M.S.; Moura, J.B.; Leitao, J.M.; Carvalho, F.A.; Miura, L.M.; Leite, J.R.; Sousa, D.P.; Almeida, F.R. Antinociceptive activity of the monoterpene α-phellandrene in rodents: possible mechanisms of action. Journal of Pharmacy and Pharmacology, 2012, 64, 283-292.
[18] Chauhana, R.S.; Kitchlua, S.; Rama, G.; Kaula, M.K.; Aldo Tava. Chemical composition of capillene chemotype of *Artemisia dracunculus* L. from North-West Himalaya, India. Industrial Crops and Products, 2010, 31, 546-549
[19] Vale, T.G.; Furtado, E.C.; Santos, Jr.J.G.; Viana, G.S.B. Central effects of citral, myrcene and limonene, constituents of essential oil chemotypes from Lippia alba (Mill.) N.E. Brown. Phytomedicine, 2002, 9(8), 709-714.
[20] Golshani, S.; Karamkhani, F.; Monsef-Esfehani, H.R.; Abdollahi, M. Antinociceptive effects of the essential oil of Dracocephalum kotschyi in the mouse writhing test. J. Pharm. Pharm. Sci., 2004, 7(1), 76-79.
[21] Him, A.; Ozbek, H.; Turel, I.; Oner, A.C. Antinociceptive activity of alpha-pinene and fenchone. Pharmacologyonline, 2008, 3, 363-369.
[22] Asanova, Zh.K.; Suleimenov, E.M.; Atazhanova, G.A.; Dembitskii, A.D.; Dar A.; Adekenov, S.M. Biological activity of 1,8-cineole from levant wormwood. Pharmaceutical Chemistry J., 2003, 37(1), 28-30.
[23] Siani, A.C.; Garrido, I.S.; Carvalho, E.S.; Ramos, M.F.S. Evaluation of anti-inflammatory-related activity of essential oils from the leaves and resin of species of Protium. J. Ethnopharmacol., 1999, 66, 57-69.
[24] Santana, M.F.; Quantans-Junior, L.J.; Cavalcanti, S.C.H.; Oliveria, M.G.B.; Guimaraes, A.G.; Cunha, E.S.; Melo, M.S.; Santos, M.R.V.; Araujo, A.A.S.; Bonjardim L.R. p-Cymene reduces orofacial nociceptive response in mice. Braz. J. Pharm., 2011, 21(6), 1138-1143.
[25] Rao, V.S.N.; Menezez, A.M.S.; Viana, G.S.B. Effect of myrcene on nociception in mice. J. Pharm. Pharmacol., 1990, 42, 877-878.
[26] Vitalini, S.; Tome, F.; Fico, G. Traditional uses of medicinal plants in Valvestino (Italy). J. Ethnopharmacol., 2009, 121(1), 106-116.
[27] Lima, D.F.; Brandao, M.S.; Moura, J.B.; Leitao, J.M.; Carvalho, F.A.; Miura, L.M.; Leite, J.R.; Sousa, D.P.; Almeida, F.R. Antinociceptive activity of the monoterpene α-phellandrene in rodents: possible mechanisms of action. Journal of Pharmacy and Pharmacology, 2012, 64, 283-292.
[28] Eccles, R. Menthol and and related cooling compounds. J. Pharm. Pharmacol., 1994, 46, 18-630.

[29] Zuker, C.S. Neurobiology: a cool ion channel. Nature, 2002, 416, 27-28.
[30] Tsuzuki, K.; Xing, H.; Ling, J.; Gu, J.G. Menthol-induced Ca^{2+} release from presynaptic Ca^{2+} stores potentiates sensory synaptic transmission. J. Neurosci., 2004, 24, 762-771.
[31] Namer, B.; Seifert, F.; Handwerker, H.O.; Maihofner, C. TRPA1 and TRPM8 activation in humans: effects of cinnamaldehyde and menthol. Neuroreport, 2005, 16, 955-959.
[32] Galeotti, N.; Mannelli, L.; Mazzanti, G. Menthol: a natural analgesic compound. Neuroscience Letters, 2002, 322, 145-148.
[33] Green, B.G.; McAuliffe, B.L. Menthol desensitization of capsaicin irritation. Evidence of a short-term anti-nociceptive effect. Physiol. Behav., 2000, 68(5), 631-639.
[34] Galeotti, N.; Ghelardini, C.; Manelli, L.D.C.; Mazzanti, G.; Baghiroli, L.; Bartolini, A. Local anaesthetic activity of (+) and (–)-menthol. Planta. Med., 2000, 66, 1-2.
[35] Green, B.G. Interactions between chemical and thermal cutaneous stimuli: inhibition (counterirritation) and integration. Somatosens. Mot. Res., 1991, 8(4), 301-312.
[36] Lincka, V.M.; da Silva, A.L.; Figueiro, M.E.; Caramao, B.; Morenof, P.R.H.; Elisabetsky, E. Effects of inhaled Linalool in anxiety, social interaction and aggressive behavior in mice. Phytomedicine, 2010, 17, 679-683.
[37] Peana, A.T.; De Montis, M.G.; Nieddu, E.; Spano, M.T.; D'Aquila, P.S.; Pippia, P. Profile of spinal and supra-spinal antinociception of (–)-linalool. European Journal of Pharmacology, 2004, 485, 165-174.
[38] Letizia, C.S.; Cocchiara, J.; Lalko, J.; Api, A.M. Fragrance material review on linalool. Food Chem. Toxicol., 2003, 41(7), 943-964.
[39] Batista, P.A.; Werner, M.F.P.; Oliveira, E.C.; Burgos, L.; Pereira, P.; Brum, L.F.S.; Story, G.M.; Santos, A.R.S. The Antinociceptive effect of (–)-Linalool in models of chronic inflammatory and neuropathic hypersensitivity in mice. The Journal of Pain, 2010, 11, 1222-1229.
[40] Peana, A.T.; D'Aquila, P.S.; Panin, F.; Serra, G.; Pippia, P.; Moretti, M.D.L. Anti-inflammatory activity of linalool and linalyl acetate constituents of essential oils. Phytomedicine, 2002, 9, 721-726.
[41] Batista, P.A.; Werner, M.F.P.; Oliveira, E.C.; Burgos, L.; Pereira, P.; Brum, L.F.S.; Story, G.M.; Santos, A.R.S. Evidence for the involvement of ionotropic glutamatergic receptors on the antinociceptive effect of (–)-linalool in mice. Neuroscience Letters, 2008, 440, 299-303.
[42] Peana, A.T.; Marzocco, S.; Popolo, A.; Pinto, A. (–)-Linalool inhibits *in vitro* NO formation: Probable involvement in the antinociceptive activity of this monoterpene compound. Life Sciences, 2006, 78, 719-723.
[43] Barocelli, E.; Calcina, F.; Chiavarini, M.; Impicciatore, M.; Bruni, R.; Bianchi, A.; Ballabeni, V. Antinociceptive and gastroprotective effects of inhaled and orally administered Lavandula hybrida Reverchon "Grosso" essential oil. Life Sciences, 2004, 76, 213-223.
[44] de Oliveira, M.G.; Marques, R.B.; de Santana, M.F.; Santos, A.B.; Brito, F.A.; Barreto, E.O.; de Sousa, D.P.; Almeida, F.R.; Badaue-Passos, D.Jr.; Antoniolli, A.R.; Quintans-Junior, L.J. α-Terpineol reduces mechanical hypernociception and inflammatory response. Basic Clin. Pharmacol. Toxicol., 2012, 111(2), 120-125.
[45] Quintans-Junior, L.J.; Oliveira, M.G.; Santana, M.F.; Santana, M.T.; Guimaraes, A.G.; Siqueira, J.S.; de Sousa, D.P.; Almeida, R.N. α-Terpineol reduces nociceptive behavior in mice. Pharm. Biol., 2011, 49(6), 583-586.

[46] Santos, F.A.; Rao, V.S.N. Antiinflammatory and antinociceptive effects of 1,8-cineole a terpenoid oxide present in many plant essential oils. Phytother. Res., 2000, 14, 240-244.

[47] Liapi, C.; Anifantis, G.; Chinou, I.; Kourounakis, A.P.; Theodosopopoulos, S.; Galanopopoulou, P. Antinociceptive properties of 1,8-cineole and β-pinene from the essentisl oil of Eucalyptus camaldulenis leaves, in rodent. Planta. Med., 2007, 73, 1247-1254.

[48] Quintans-Junior, L.J.; Souza, T.T.; Leite, B.S.; Lessa, N.M.N.; Bonjardim, L.R.; Santos, M.R.V.; Alves, P.B.; Blank, A.F.; Antoniolli, A.R. Phytochemical screening and anticonvulsant activity of Cymbopogon winterianus Jowitt (Poaceae) leaf essential oil in rodents. Phytomedicine, 2008, 15, 619-624.

[49] Brito, R.G.; Guimaraes, A.G.; Quintans, J.S.S.; Santos, M.R.V.; De Sousa, D.P.; Badaue-Passos, Jr.D.; Lucca, Jr.W.; Brito, F.A.; Barreto, E.O.; Oliveira, A.P.; Quintans, Jr.L.J. Citronellol, a monoterpene alcohol, reduces nociceptive and inflammatory activities in rodents. J. Nat. Med., 2012, 66, 637-644.

[50] Melo, M.S.; Sena, L.C.S.; Barreto, F.J.N.; Bonjardim, L.R.; Almeida, J.R.G.S.; Lima, J.T.; De Sousa, D.P.; Quintans-Junior, L.J. Antinociceptive effect of citronellal in mice. Pharmaceutical Biology, 2010, 48(4), 411-416.

[51] Nhu-Trang, T.T.; Casabianca, H.; Grenier-Loustalot, M.F. Authenticity control of essential oils containing citronellal and citral by chiral and stable-isotope gas-chromatographic analysis. Anal. Bioanal. Chem., 2006, 386, 2141-2152.

[52] Quantans-Junior, L.J.; Guimaraes, A.G.; Santana, M.T.; Araujo, B.E.S.; Moreira, F.V.; Bonjardim, L.R.; Araujo, A.A.S.; Siqueira, J.S.; Antoniolli, A.R.; Botelho, M.A.; Santos, M.R.V. Citral reduces nociceptive and inflammatory response in rodents. Braz. J. Pharm., 2011, 21(3), 497-502.

[53] Ortiz, M.I.; Ramirez-Montiel, M.L.; Gonzalez-Garcia, M.P.; Ponce-Monter, H.A.; Castaneda-Hernandez, G.; Carino-Cortes, R. The combination of naproxen and citral reduces nociception and gastric damage in rats. Arch. Pharm. Res., 2010, 33(10), 1691-1697.

[54] Ortiz, M.I.; Gonzalez-Garcia, M.P.; Ponce-Monter, H.A.; Castaneda-Hernandez, G.; Aguilar-Robles, P. Synergistic effect of the interaction between naproxen and citral on inflammation in rats. Phytomedicine, 2010, 18, 74-79.

[55] Zhao, D.; Xua, Y.W.; Yanga, G.L.; Husainib, A.M.; Wua, W. Variation of essential oil of *Mentha haplocalyx* Briq. and *Mentha spicata* L. from China. Industrial Crops and Products, 2013, 42, 251-260.

[56] Kocovsky, P.; Turecek, F.; Hajicek, J. Synthesis of natural products: Problems of stereoselectivity. CRC Press: Boca Raton, 1986, p. 186.

[57] de Sousa, D.P.; Nobrega, F.F.F.; Lima, M.R.V.; de Almeida, R.N. Pharmacological activity of (R)-(+)-Pulegone, a chemical constituent of essential oils. Z. Naturforsch, 2011, 66, 353-359.

[58] Il'ina, I.V.; Volcho, K.P.; Korchagina, D.V.; Barkhash, V.A.; Salakhutdinov, N.F. Synthesis of optically active, cyclic α-hydroxy ketones and 1,2-diketones from verbenone epoxide. Helv. Chim. Acta, 2006, 89, 507-514.

[59] Pavlova, A.V.; Tolstikova, T.G.; Morozova, E.A.; Ardashov, O.V.; Il'ina, I.V.; Volcho, K.P.; Salakhutdinov, N.F. Hydroxyketones of *para*-menthane series as promising analgesic. Chemistry for Sustainable Development, 2010, 18, 415-417.

[60] Il'ina, I.V.; Volcho, K.P.; Korchagina, D.V.; Barkhash, V.A.; Salakhutdinov, N.F. Reactions of allyl alcohols of the pinane series and of their epoxides in the presence of montmorillonite clay. Helv. Chim. Acta, 2007, 90(2), 353-368.

[61] Tolstikova, T.G.; Pavlova, A.V.; Dolgikh, M.P.; Il'ina, I.V.; Ardashov, O.V.; Volcho, K.P.; Salakhutdinov, N.F. 3-Methyl-6-(prop-1-en-2-yl)cyclohex-3-en-1,2-diol as analgesic agent. Pat. RU 2409351, 2009.

[62] Il'ina, I.V.; Korchagina, D.V.; Volcho, K.P.; Salakhutdinov, N.F. Reaction of (–)-cis-verbenol epoxide with aromatic aldehydes over montmorillonite K10 clay. Russian Journal of Organic Chemistry, 2010, 46(7), 998-1001.

[63] Tolstikova, T.G.; Pavlova, A.V.; Il'ina, I.V.; Ardashov, O.V.; Volcho, K.P.; Salakhutdinov, N.F. Derivatives of 4,4,7-trimethyl-2-phenyl-4a,5,8,8a-tetrahydro-4H-benz[1,3]dioxine-8-ol – as analgesic agents. Pat RU 2409353, 2009.

[64] Tolstikova, T.G.; Pavlova, A.V.; Morozova, E.A.; Il'ina, I.V.; Volcho, K.P.; Salakhutdinov, N.F. Application of 4,7-dimethyl-2-(prop-1-enyl)-3,4,4a,5,8,8a-heahydro-2h-chromen-4,8-diol as analgesic. Pat. RU 2418578, 2009.

[65] Il'ina, I.V.; Volcho, K.P.; Mikhalchenko, O.S.; Korchagina, D.V.; Salakhutdinov, N.F. Reactions of verbenol epoxide with aromatic aldehydes containing hydroxy or methoxy groups in the presence of montmorillonite clay. Helvetica Chimica Acta, 2011, 94(3), 502-513.

[66] Tolstikova, T.G.; Pavlova, A.V.; Morozova, E.A.; Il'ina, I.V.; Ardashov, O.V.; Korchagina, D.V.; Volcho, K.P.; Salakhutdinov, N.F. 2-(4-Hydroxy-3-metoxyphenyl)-4,7-dimethyl-3,4,4a,5,8,8a-hexahydro-2h-chromen-4,8-diol – novel analgesic agent. Pat. RU 2430100, 2010.

[67] Mackey, C. The anticonvulsants market. Nature Reviews, 2010, 9, 265-266.

[68] Farrant, M.; Nusser, Z. Variations on an inhibitory theme: phasic and tonic activation of $GABA_A$ receptors. Nat. Rev. Neurosci., 2005, 6, 215-229.

[69] Librowski, T.; Czarnecki, R.; Mendyk, A.; Jastrzebska, M. Influence of new monoterpene homologues of GABA on the central nervous system activity in mice. Pol. J. Pharmacol., 2000, 52, 317-321.

[70] Owens, D.F.; Kriegstein, A.R. Is there more to GABA than synaptic inhibition? Nat. Rev. Neurosci., 2002, 3, 715-727.

[71] Sieghart, W. Structure and pharmacology of γ-aminobutyric acid A receptor subtypes. Pharmacol. Rev., 1995, 47, 181-234.

[72] Kubacka, M.; Librowski, T.; Czarnecki, R.; Frackowiak, B.; Lochynski, S. Anticonvulsant and antidepressant activity of the selected terpene GABA derivatives in experimental tests in mice. Pharm. Reports, 2006, 58, 936-943.

[73] Gajcy, K.; Lochynski, S.; Librowski, T. A role of GABA analogues in the treatment of neurological diseases. Current Medicinal Chemistry, 2010, 17, 2338-2347.

[74] de Almeida, R.N.; de Fatima, A.M.; Souto Maior, F.N.; Sousa, D.P. Essential oils and their constituents: anticonvulsant activity. Molecules, 2011, 16, 2726-2742.

[75] Zhang, X.B.; Jiang, P.; Gong, N.; Hu, X.L.; Fei, D.; Xiong, Z.Q.; Xu, L.; Xu, T.L. A-Type GABA receptor as a central target of TRPM8 agonist menthol. PLoS One., 2008, 3(10), e3386.

[76] Watt, E.E.; Betts, B.A.; Kotey, F.O.; Humbert, D.J.; Griffith, T.N.; Kelly, E.W.; Veneskey, K.C.; Gill, N.; Rowan, K.C.; Jenkins, A.; Hall, A.C. Menthol shares general anesthetic

activity and sites of action on the $GABA_A$ receptor with the intravenous agent, propofol. European Journal of Pharmacology, 2008, 590, 120-126.

[77] Corvalan, N.A.; Zygadlo, J.A.; Garcia, D.A. Stereo-selective activity of menthol on $GABA_A$ receptor. Chirality, 2009, 21, 525-530.

[78] Ozek, G.; Ozek, T.; Iscan, G.; Baser, K.H.C.; Hamzaoglu, E.; Duran A. Composition and antimicrobial activity of the essential oil of Tanacetum cadmium (Boiss.) Heywood subsp. orientale Grierson. J. Essent. Oil Res., 2007, 9, 392-395.

[79] de Sousa, D.P.; Nybregab, F.F.F.; de Moraisb Liana, C.S.L.; de Almeida, R.N. Evaluation of the anticonvulsant activity of terpinen-4-ol. Z. Naturforsch, 2009, 64, 1-5.

[80] de Sousa, D.P.; Quantans, L.Jr.; de Almedia, N. Evolution of the anticonvulsant activity of α- terpineol. Pharmaceutical Biology, 2007, 45(1), 69-70.

[81] Silva, M.I.; de Aquino Neto, M.R.; Teixeira Neto, P.F.; Moura, B.A.; do Amaral, J.F.; de Sousa, D.P.; Vasconcelos, S.M.; de Sousa, F.C. Central nervous system activity of acute administration of isopulegol in mice. Pharmacol. Biochem. Behav., 2007, 88(2), 141-147.

[82] Silva, M.I.; Silva, M.A.; de Aquino Neto, M.R.; Moura, B.A.; de Sousa, H.L.; de Lavor, E.P.; de Vasconcelos, P.F.; Macedo, D.S.; de Sousa, D.P.; Vasconcelos, S.M.; de Sousa, F.C. Effects of isopulegol on pentylenetetrazol-induced convulsions in mice: possible involvement of GABAergic system and antioxidant activity. Fitoterapia, 2009, 80(8), 506-513.

[83] Bolkunov, A.V.; Dolgikh, M.P.; Tolstikova, T.G.; Il'ina, I.V.; Volcho, K.P.; Salakhutdinov, N.F. Anticonvulsive medication. Pat. RU 2355390, 2007.

[84] Tolstikova, T.G.; Pavlova, A.V.; Dolgikh, M.P.; Il'ina, I.V.; Ardashov, O.V.; Volcho, K.P.; Salakhutdinov, N.F.; Tolstikov, G.A. (4*S*,5*R*,6*R*)-*para*-Mentha-1,8-dien-5,6-diol is a new highly effective anticonvulsant agent. Doklady Biological Sciences, 2009, 429, 494-496.

[85] Garcia, D.A.; Vendrel, I.; Galofre, M.; Sunol, C. GABA released from cultured cortical neurons influences the modulation of t-[^{35}S]butylbicyclophosphorothionate binding at the $GABA_A$ receptor. Effects of thymol. European Journal of Pharmacology, 2008, 600, 26-31.

[86] Garcia, D.A.; Bujons, J.; Vale, C.; Sunol, C. Allosteric positive interaction of thymol with the $GABA_A$ receptor in primary cultures of mouse cortical neurons. Neuropharmacology, 2006, 50, 25-35.

[87] Goncalves, J.C.; Alves Ade, M.; de Araujo, A.E.; Cruz, J.S.; Araujo, D.A. Distinct effects of carvone analogues on the isolated nerve of rats. European Journal of Pharmacology, 2010, 645, 108-112.

[88] de Sousa, D.P.; de Farias Nobrega, F.F.; de Almeida, R.N. Influence of the chirality of (R)-(–)- and (S)-(+)-carvone in the central nervous system: a comparative study. Chirality, 2007, 19, 264-268.

[89] Costa, D.A.; de Oliveira, G.A.; Lima, T.C.; dos Santos, P.S.; de Sousa, D.P.; de Freitas, R.M. Anticonvulsant and antioxidant effects of cyano-carvone and its action on acetylcholinesterase activity in mice hippocampus. Cell. Mol. Neurobiol., 2012, 32, 633-640.

[90] de Almeida, R.N.; de Sousa, D.P.; Nobrega, F.F.; Claudino, F.S.; Araujo, D.A.; Leite, J.R.; Mattei, R. Anticonvulsant effect of a natural compound α,β-epoxy-carvone and its action on the nerve excitability. Neurosci. Lett., 2008, 443(1), 51-55.

[91] Slamenova, D.; Horvathova, E.; Wsolova, L.; Sramkova, M.; Navarova, J. Investigation of anti-oxidative, cytotoxic, DNA-damaging and DNA-protective effects of plant volatiles

eugenol and borneol in human-derived HepG2, Caco-2 and VH10 cell lines. Mutation Research, 2009, 677, 46-52.
[92] Forster, H.B.; Niklas, H.; Lutz, S. Antispasmodic effects of some medicinal plants. Planta Med., 1980, 40, 309-319.
[93] Ortiz, J.G.; Nieves-Natal, J.; Chavez, P. Effects of Valeriana officinalis extracts on [^{3}H]Flunitrazepam binding, synaptosomal [^{3}H]GABA uptake, and hippocampal [^{3}H]GABA release. Neurochem. Res., 1999, 24, 1373-1378.
[94] Aoshima, H.; Hamamoto, K. Potentiation of $GABA_A$ receptors expressed in Xenopus oocytes by perfume and phytoncid. Biosci. Biotech. Biochem., 1999, 63, 743-748.
[95] Hall, A.C.; Turcotte, C.M.; Betts, B.A.; Yeung, W.-Y.; Agyeman, A.S.; Burk, L.A. Modulation of human $GABA_A$ and glycine receptor currents by menthol and related monoterpenoids. European Journal of Pharmacology, 2004, 506, 9-16.
[96] Granger, R.E.; Campbell, E.L.; Johnson, G.A.R. (+)- And (–)-borneol: efficacious positive modulators of GABA action at human recombinant $\alpha_1\beta_2\gamma_{2L}$ $GABA_A$ receptors. Biochemical Pharmacology, 2005, 69, 1101-1111.
[97] de Sousa, D.P.; Goncalves, J.C.R.; Quantitans-Junior, L.; Crus, J.S.; Araujo, D.A.M.; de Almeida, R.N. Study of anticonvulsant effect of citronellol, a monoterpene alcohol, in rodents. Neuroscience Letters, 2006, 401, 231-235.
[98] Melo, M.S.; de Santana, M.T.; Guimaraes, A.G.; Siqueira, R.S.; de Sousa, D.P.; Santos, M.R.V.; Bonjardim, L.R.; Araujo, A.A.S.; Onofre, A.S.C.; Lima, J.T.; Almeida, J.R.G.S.; Quantans-Junior, L.J. Bioassay-guided evaluation of central nervous system effects of citronellal in rodents. Braz. J. Pharm., 2011, 21(4), 697-703.
[99] Fernandez-Sanchez, L.; Lax, P.; Esquiva, G.; Martin-Nieto, J.; Pinilla, I.; Cuenca, N. Safranal, a saffron constituent, attenuates retinal degeneration in P23H Rats. PLoS One, 2012, 7(8), 1-11.
[100] Tarantilis, P.A.; Tsoupras, G.; Polissiuo, M. Determination of saffron (Crocus sativus L.) components in crude plant extract using high performance liquid chromatography-UV-visible photodiode-array detection-mass spectrometry. J. Chromatogr., 1995, 699, 107-118.
[101] Hosseinzadeh, H.; Sadeghnia, H.R. Protective effect of safranal on pentylenetetrazol-induced seizures in the rat: Involvement of GABAergic and opioid systems. Phytomedicine, 2007, 14, 256-262.
[102] Tolstikova, T.G.; Morozova, E.A.; Pavlova, A.V.; Bolkunov, A.V.; Dolgikh, M.P.; Koneva, E.A.; Volcho, K.P.; Salakhutdinov, N.F.; Tolstikov, G.A. Derivatives of pinane amino acids as new anticonvulsants. Doklady Chemistry, 2008, 422(2), 248-250.
[103] Koneva, E.A.; Volcho K.P.; Salakhutdinov, N.F.; Dolgikh, M.P.; Tolstikova, T.G.; Bolkunov, A.V.; Morozova, E.A.; Pavlova, A.V. Anti-convulsive medicine. Pat. RU 2370260, 2008.
[104] Cang, H.-J.; Kim, H.J.; Chum, H.S. Quantitative structure-activity relationship (QSAR) for neuroprotective activity of terpenoids. Life Sci., 2007, 80, 835-841.
[105] Liu, R.; Zhang, L.; Lan, X.; Li, L.; Zhzng, T.-T.; Sun, J.-H.; Du, G.-H. Protection by borneol on cortical neurons against oxygen-glucose deprivation/reperfusion: involvement of anti-oxidation and anti-inflammation through nuclear transcription factor κB signaling pathway. Neuroscience, 2011, 176, 408-419.
[106] Lin, Z.Z.; Yao, M.C.; Lan, M.X.; Liu, P.Q.; Zhong, G.P.; Pi, R.B. Effects of borneol on distribution of sodium ferulate in plasma and in brain regions of mice. Zhong Cao Yao, 2008, 39, 51-56.

[107] Yan, J.J.; Cho, J.Y.; Kim, H.S.; Kim, K.L.; Jung, J.S.; Huh, S.O.; Suh, H.W.; Kim, Y.H.; Song, D.K. Protection against beta-amyloid peptide toxicity *in vivo* with long-term administration of ferulic acid. Br. J. Pharmacol., 2001, 133(1), 89-96.

[108] Zhao, Z.; Egashira, Y.; Sanada, H. Ferulic acid is quickly absorbed from rat stomach as the free form and then conjugated mainly inliver. J. Nutr., 2004, 134(11), 3083-3088.

[109] Chen, X.H.; Lin, Z.Z.; Liu, A.M.; Ye, J.T.; Luo, Y.; Luo, Y.Y.; Mao, X.X.; Liu, P.Q.; Pi, R.B. The orally combined neuroprotective effects of sodium ferulate and borneol against transient global ischemia in C57BL/6J mice. Journal of Pharmacy and Pharmacology, 2010, 62, 915-923.

[110] Tian, L.L.; Zhou, Z.; Zhang, Q.; Sun, Y-N.; Li, C.-R.; Cheng, C.-H.; Zhong, Z.-Y.; Wang, S.-Q. Protective effect of (±)-isoborneol against 6-OHDA-induced apoptosis in SH-SY5Y cells. Cell. Physiol. Biochem., 2007, 20, 1019-1032.

[111] Ultee, A.; Kets, E.P.; Smid, E.J. Mechanisms of action of carvacrol on the food-borne pathogen Bacillus cereus. Appl. Environ. Microbiol., 1999, 65, 4606-4610.

[112] Yu, H.; Zhang, Z.L.; Chen, J.; Pei, A.; Hua, F.; Qian, X.; He, J.; Liu, C.F.; Xu, X. Carvacrol, a food-additive, provides neuroprotection on focal cerebral ischemia/reperfusion injury in mice. PLoS One, 2012, 7(3), e33584.

[113] Liu, D.Z.; Xie, K.Q.; Ji, X.Q.; Ye, Y.; Jiang, C.L.; Zhu, X.Z. Neuroprotective effect of paeoniflorin on cerebral ischemic rat by activating adenosine A1 receptor in a different manner from its classical agonists. Br. J. Pharmacol., 2005, 146, 604-611.

[114] Liu, H.Q.; Zhang, W.Y.; Luo, X.T.; Ye, Y.; Zhu, X.Z. Paeoniflorin attenuates neuroinflammation and dopaminergic neurodegeneration in the MPTP model of Parkinson's disease by activation of adenosine A1 receptor. Br. J. Pharmacol., 2006, 148(3), 314-325.

[115] Mao, Q.-Q.; Zhong, X.-M.; Li, Z.-Y.; Huang, Z. Paeoniflorin protects against NMDA-induced neurotoxicity in PC12 cells *via* Ca^{2+} antagonism. Phytother. Res., 2011, 25, 681-685.

[116] Mukherjee, P.K.; Kumar, V.; Mal, M.; Houghton, P.J. Acetylcholinesterase inhibitors from plants. Phytomedicine, 2007, 14, 289-300.

[117] Dohi, S.; Terasaki, M.; Makino, M. Acetylcholinesterase inhibitory activity and chemical composition of commercial essential oils. J. Agric. Food Chem., 2009, 57(10), 4313-4318.

[118] Savelev, S.; Okello, E.; Perry, N.S.L.; Wilkins, R.M.; Perry, E.K. Synergistic and antagonistic interactions of anticholinesterase terpenoids in Salvia lavandula efolia essential oil. Pharmacology, Biochemistry and Behavior, 2003, 75, 661-668.

[119] Picollo, M.I.; Toloza, A.C.; Cueto, G.M.; Zygadlo, J.; Zebra, E. Anticholinesterase and pediculicidal activities of monoterpenoids. Fitoterapia, 2008, 79, 271-278.

[120] Kaufmann, D.; Dogra, A.K.; Wink, M. Myrtenal inhibits acetylcholinesterase, a known Alzheimer target. Journal of Pharmacy and Pharmacology, 2011, 63, 1368-1371.

[121] Grundy, D.L.; Still, C.C. Inhibition of acetylcholinesterases by pulegone-1,2-epoxide. Pesticide Biochem. & Physiol., 1985, 23, 383-388.

[122] Miyazawa, M.; Watanabe, H.; Kameoka, H. Ingibition of acetilholinesterase activity by monotrpinoids with a *p*-menthane skeleton. J. Agric. Food Chem., 1997, 45, 677-679.

[123] Miyazawa, M.; Yamafuji, C. Inhibition of acetylcholinesterase activity by bicyclic monoterpenoids. J. Agric. Food Chem., 2005, 53(5), 1765-1768.

[124] Hebert, L.E.; Scherr, P.A.; Bienias, J.L.; Bennett, D.A.; Evans, D.A. Alzheimer disease in the US population: Prevalence estimates using the 2000 census. Arch. Neurol., 2003, 60, 1119-1122.

[125] Williams, P.; Sorribas, A.; Howes, M.J.H. Natural products as a source of Alzheimer's drug leads. Nat. Prod. Rep., 2011, 28, 48-77.
[126] Brum, L.F.S.; Emanuelli, T.; Souza, D.O.; Elisabetsky, E. Effects of linalool on glutamate release and uptake in mouse cortical synaptosomes. Neurochemical Research, 2001, 26(3), 191-194.
[127] Elisabetsky, E.; Marschner, J.; Souza, D.O. Effects of linalool on glutamatergic system in the rat cerebral cortex. Neurochemical Research, 1995, 20(4), 461-465.
[128] Sydow, O. Parkinson's disease: recent development in therapies for advanced disease with a focus on deep brain stimulation (DBS) and duodenal levodopa infusion. FEBS J., 2008, 275, 1370-1376.
[129] Meredith, G.E.; Totterdell, S.; Potashkin, J.A.; Surmeier, D.J. Modeling PD pathogenesis in mice: Advantages of a chronic MPTP protocol. Parkinsonism Related Disorders, 2008, 14, 112-115.
[130] Chuang, C.S.; Su, H.L.; Cheng, F.C.; Hsu, S.; Chuang, C.F. Quantitative evaluation of motor function before and after engraftment of dopaminergic neurons in a rat model of Parkinson's disease. J. Biomed. Sci., 2010, 17(9), 1-11.
[131] Tolstikova, T.G.; Pavlova, A.V.; Morozova, Ye.A.; Ardashov, O.V.; Il'ina, I.V.; Volcho, K.P.; Salakhutdinov, N.F.; Tolstikov, G.A. A highly effective antiparkinsonian drug of a new structural type. Dokl. Biol. Sci., 2010, 435, 398-399.
[132] Ardashov, O.V.; Pavlova, A.V.; Il'ina, I.V.; Morozova, E.A.; Korchagina, D.V.; Karpova, E.V.; Volcho, K.P.; Tolstikova, T.G.; Salakhutdinov, N.F. Highly potent activity of (1*R*,2*R*,6*S*)-3-methyl-6-(prop-1-en-2-yl)cyclohex-3-ene-1,2-diol in animal models of Parkinson's disease. J. Medical Chemistry, 2011, 54, 3866-3874.
[133] Park, D.I.; Kim, H.G.; Jung, W.R.; Shin, M.K.; Kim, K.L. Mecamylamine attenuates dexamethasone-induced anxiety-like behavior in association with brain derived neurotrophic factor upregulation in rat brains. Neuropharmacology, 2011, 61, 276-282.
[134] Souto-Maior, F.N.; de Carvakho, F.L.; de Morais, L.C.S.L.; Netto, S.M.; de Sousa, D.P.; de Almeida, R.N. Anxiolytic-like effects of inhaled linalool oxide in experimental mouse anxiety models. Pharmacology Biochemistry and Behavior, 2011, 100, 259-263.
[135] Linck, V.M.; Silva, A.L.; Figueiro, M.; Caramao, E.B.; Moreno, P.R.H.; Elisabetski, E. Effects of inhaled Linalool in anxiety, social interaction and aggressive behavior in mice. Phytomedicine, 2010, 17, 679-683.
[136] Hilmer, J.M.; Gatfield, I.L. Process for the preparation of linalool oxide or linalool oxide containing mixtures. Patent US 6703218, 2004.
[137] Asakawa, Y.; Toyota, M.; Ishida, T. Biotransformation of 1,4-cineole, a monoterpene ether. Xenobiotica, 1988, 18, 1129-1134.
[138] Gomes, P.B.; Feitosa, M.L.; Silva, M.I.G.; Noronha, E.C.; Moura, B.A.; Venancio, E.T.; Rios, E.R.V.; de Sousa, D.P.; Vasconcelos, S.M.M.; Fonteles, M.M.F.; de Sousa, F.C.F. Anxiolytic-like effect of the monoterpene 1,4-cineole in mice. Pharmacology Biochemistry and Behavior, 2010, 96, 287-293.
[139] Kapitsa, I.G.; Suslov, E.V.; Teplov, G.V.; Korchagina, D.V.; Komarova, N.I.; Volcho, K.P.; Voronina, T.A.; Shevela, A.I.;. Salakhutdinov, N.F. Synthesis and anxiolytic activity of 2-aminoadamantane derivatives containing monoterpene fragments. Pharmaceutical Chemistry Journal, 2012, 46(5), 263-265.

[140] Farmer, C.S.; Farrand, P.; O'Mahen, H. 'I am not a depressed person': How identity conflict affects help-seeking rates for major depressive disorder. BMC Psychiatry, 2012, 12(1), 164.

[141] Sarris, J.; Panossian, A.; Schweitzer, I.; Stough, C.; Schole, A. Herbal medicine for depression, anxiety and insomnia: a review of psychopharmacology and clinical evidence. European Neuropsychopharmacology, 2011, 21, 841-860.

[142] Steflitsch, W.; Steflitsch, M. Clinical aromatherapy. Practising Medicine, 2008, 5, 74-85.

[143] Guzman-Gutierrez, S.L.; Gomez-Cansino, R; Garcıa-Zebadu, J.C.; Jimenez-Perez, N.C.; Reyes-Chilpa, R. Antidepressant activity of Litsea glaucescens essential oil: Identification of β-pinene and linalool as active principles. Journal of Ethnopharmacology, 2012, 143, 673-679.

[144] Neergaard, J.S.; Rasmussen, H.B.; Stafford, G.I.; Van Staden, J.; Jager, A.K. Serotonin transporter affinity of (−)-loliolide, a monoterpene lactone from Mondia whitei. South African Journal of Botany, 2010, 76, 593-596.

[145] Melo, F.H.C.; Moura, B.A.; de Sousa, D.P.; de Vasconcelos, M.M.; Macedo, D.S.; Fonteles, M.M.F.; Viana, G.S.B.; de Sousa, F.C.F. Antidepressant-like effect of carvacrol (5-Isopropyl-2-methylphenol) in mice: involvement of dopaminergic system. Fundamental & Clinical Pharmacology, 2011, 25, 362-367.

[146] Ranganna, S.; Govindarajan, V.S.; Ramana, K.V. Citrus fruits-varieties, chemistry, technology, and quality evaluation part II. Chemistry, technology, and quality evaluation. Crit. Rev. Food. Sci. Nutr., 1983, 18, 313-386.

[147] Fukumoto, S.; Sawasaki, E.; Okuyama, S.; Miyake, Y.; Yokogoshi, H. Flavor components of monoterpenes in citrus essential oils enhance the release of monoamines from rat brain slices. Nutritional Neuroscience, 2006, 9(1/2), 73-80.

[148] Zhou, W.; Yoshioka, M.; Yokogoshi, H. Sub-chronic effects of *S*-limonene on brain neurotransmitter levels and behavior of rats. J. Nutr. Sci. Vitaminol, 2009, 55, 367-373.

[149] Lin, A.L.; Shangari, N.; Chan, T.S.; Remirez, D.; O'Brien, P.J. Herbal monoterpene alcohols inhibit propofol metabolism and prolong anesthesia time. Life Sciences, 2006, 79, 21-29.

[150] Trabace, L.; Zotti, M.; Morgese, M.G.; Tucci, P.; Colaianna, M.; Schiavone, S.; Avato, P.; Cuomo, V. Estrous cycle affects the neurochemical and neurobehavioral profile of carvacrol-treated female rats. Toxicology and Applied Pharmacology, 2011, 255, 169-175.

[151] Silva, M.I.G.; Neto, M.R.A.; Neto, P.F.T.; Moura, B.A.; de Amaral, J.F.; de Sousa, D.P.; Vasconcelos, S.M.M.; de Sousa, F.C.F. Central nervous system activity of acute administration of isopulegol in mice. Pharmacology Biochemistry and Behavior, 2007, 88, 141-147.

[152] Bhadania, M.; Joshi, H.; Patel, P.; Kulkarni, V.H. Protective effect of menthol on β-amyloid peptide induced cognitive deficits in mice. European Journal of Pharmacology, 2012, 681, 50-54.

[153] Shaw, D.; Annett, J.M.; Doherty, B.; Leslie, J.C. Anxiolytic effects of lavender oil inhalation on open-field behavior in rats. Phytomedicine, 2007, 14, 613-620.

[154] Linck, V.M.; Silva, A.L.; Figuero, M.; Piato, A.L.; Herrmann, A.P.; Birck, F.D.; Caramao, E.B.; Nunes, D.S.; Moreno, P.R.H.; Elisabetsky, E. Inhaled linalool-induced sedation in mice. Phytomedicine, 2009, 16, 303-307.

[155] Coelho, V.R.; Gianesini, J.; Borowski, R.V.; Mazzardo-Martins, L.; Martins, D.F.; Picada, J.N.; Santos, A.R.S.; Brum, L.F.S.; Pereira, P. (−)-Linalool, a naturally occurring

monoterpene compound, impairs memory acquisition in the object recognition task, inhibitory avoidance test and habituation to a novel environment in rats. Phytomedicine, 2011, 18, 896- 901.

[156] Stone, C.A.; Torchiana, M.L.; Meckelnberg, K.L.; Stavorski, J.; Sletzinger, M.; Stein, G.A.; Ruyle, W.V.; Reinhold, D.F.; Gaines, W.A.; Arnold, H.; Pfister K. Chemistry and Structure-Activity Relationships of Mecamylamine and Derivatives. J. Med. Chem., 1962, 5, 665-690.

[157] Bacher, I.; Wu, B.; Shytle, D.R.; George, T. Mecamylamine – a nicotinic acetylcholine receptor antagonist with potential for the treatment of neuropsychiatric disorders. Expert Opin. Pharmacother., 2009, 10(16), 2709-2721.

[158] Shytle, R.D.; Silver, A.A.; Sheehan, K.H.; Sheehan, D.V.; Sanberg, P.R. Neuronal nicotinic receptor inhibition for treating mood disorders: preliminary controlled evidence. Depress. Anxiety, 2002, 16(3), 89-92.

[159] Park, D.I.; Kim, H.G.; Jung, W.R.; Shin, M.K.; Kim, K.L. Mecamylamine attenuates dexamethasone-induced anxiety-like behavior in association with brain derived neurotrophic factor upregulation in rat brains. Neuropharmacology, 2011, 61, 276-282.

[160] Janowsky, D.S.; el-Yousef, M.K.; Davis, J.M.; Sekerke, H.J. A cholinergic-adrenergic hypothesis of mania and depression. Lancet., 1972, 2(7778), 632-635

[161] Rabenstein, R.L.; Caldarone, B.J.; Picciotto, M.R. The nicotinic antagonist mecamylamine has antidepressantlike effects in wild-type but not β2- or α7-nicotinic acetylcholine receptor subunit knockout mice. Psychopharmacology, 2006, 189, 395-401.

[162] Arias, H.R.; Rosenberg, A.; Targowska-Duda, K.M.; Feuerbach, D.; Jozwiak, K.; Moaddel, R.; Wainer, I.W. Tricyclic antidepressants and mecamylamine bind to different sites in the human α4β2 nicotinic receptor ion channel. Int. J. Bioch. Cell Biol., 2010, 42, 1007-1018.

[163] Arias, H.R.; Targowska-Duda, K.M.; Feuerbach, D.; Sullivan, C.J.; Maciejewski, R.; Jozwiak, K. Different interaction between tricyclic antidepressants and mecamylamine with the human α3β4 nicotinic acetylcholine receptor ion channel. Neurochemistry International, 2010, 56, 642-649.

[164] Biala, G.; Weglinska, B. Blockade of the expression of mecamylamine-precipitated nicotine withdrawal by calcium channel antagonists. Pharm. Research, 2005, 51(5), 483-488.

[165] Shytle, R.D.; Penny, E.; Silver, A.A.; Goldman, J.; Sanberg, P.R. Mecamylamine (Inversine): an old antihypertensive with new research directions. Journal of Human Hypertension, 2002, 16, 453-457.

[166] Young, E.M.; Mahler, S.; Chi, H.; Wit, H. Mecamylamine and ethanol preference in healthy volunteers. Alcohol Clin. Exp. Res., 2005, 29(1), 58-65.

[167] Hendrickson, L.M.; Zhao-Shea, R.; Tapper, A.R. Modulation of ethanol drinking-in-the-dark by mecamylamine and nicotinic acetylcholine receptor agonists in C57BL/6J mice. Psychopharmacology, 2009, 204, 563-572.

[168] Silver, A.A.; Shytle, R.D.; Sanberg, P.R. Mecamylamine in Tourette's syndrome: a two-year retrospective case study. J. Child. Adolesc. Psychopharmacol., 2000, 10(2), 59-68.

[169] Silver, A.A.; Shytle, R.D.; Sheehan, K.H.; Sheehan, D.V; Ramos, A; Sanberg, P.R. Multicenter, double-blind, placebo-controlled study of mecamylamine monotherapy for Tourette's disorder. J. Am. Acad. Child Adolesc Psychiatry, 2001, 40, 1103-1110.

[170] Martin-Ruiz, C.M.; Lee, M.; Perry, R.H.; Baumann, M.; Court, J.A.; Perry, E.K. Molecular analysis of nicotinic receptor expression in autism. Mol. Brain. Res., 2004, 123(1-2), 81-90.

[171] Lippiello, P.M. Nicotinic cholinergic antagonists: a novel approach for the treatment of autism. Med. Hypotheses, 2006, 66(5), 985-990.

[172] Arnold, L.E.; Aman, M.G.; Hollway, J.; Hurt, E.; Bates, B.; Li, X.; Farmer, C; Anand, R.; Thompson, S.; Ramadan, Y.; Williams, C. Placebo-controlled pilot trial of mecamylamine for treatment of autism spectrum disorders. J. Child. Adolesc. Psychopharmacol., 2012, 22(3), 198-205.

[173] Fu, H.; Dou, J.; Li, W.; Luo, J.; Li, K.C.; Lam, C.S.C.; Lee, N.T.K.; Li, M.; Han, Y. Mecamylamine prevents neuronal apoptosis induced by glutamate and low potassium *via* differential anticholinergic-independent mechanisms. Neuropharmacology, 2008, 54, 755-765.

[174] Hetzler, B.E.; Beckman, E.J. Effects of mecamylamine on flash-evoked potentials, body temperature, and behavior in Long-Evans rats. Pharmacology Biochemistry and Behavior, 2011, 97, 660-668.

Send Orders for Reprints to reprints@benthamscience.net

Frontiers in CNS Drug Discovery, 2013, *2*, 381-406

CHAPTER 11

Use of Zebrafish to Identify New CNS Drugs Acting Through Nicotinic and Dopaminergic Systems

Robert T. Boyd*

Department of Neuroscience, The Ohio State University College of Medicine, Wexner Medical Center, 333 West Tenth Avenue, Columbus Ohio 43210, USA

Abstract: Zebrafish (*Danio rerio*) are a vertebrate animal model with advantages for screening and development of therapeutic agents. The ease of growth and handling and the ability of zebrafish to be treated with compounds in a multi-well format are advantages for high-throughput screening (HTS) work to identify new drugs. Zebrafish have also been used in target confirmation after a lead compound has been identified. *In vivo* structure activity relationship (SAR) studies in zebrafish have also been performed. Indeed, zebrafish can be used at several points in the drug discovery process. Zebrafish are ideal for testing drug toxicity on a large scale, thus saving much time, money and effort to further develop a compound with toxicity in vertebrates. Many behavioral assays developed in other animals, and which are used to assay drugs targeted to several neurological diseases, are available in zebrafish These include assays for locomotion, avoidance behaviors, learning, and conditioned place preference. The use of zebrafish allows one to combine the ability to perform behavioral assays with HTS and thus perform high-throughput *in vivo* drug screening. Many biochemical pathways and genes present in humans are conserved in zebrafish, including those involving the nicotinic cholinergic and dopaminergic systems. Zebrafish is an exciting new system amenable to identification of new drugs to treat disorders due to nicotinic cholinergic and dopaminergic disregulation including nicotine addiction, schizophrenia, Alzheimer's disease and Parkinson's disease.

Keywords: Nicotinic, dopaminergic, zebrafish, *Danio rerio*, cholinergic, high-throughput screening, acetylcholine receptors, pharmacology, drug discovery, *in vivo* screening, behavioral assays, smoking, addiction, schizophrenia, Alzheimer's, Parkinson's.

INTRODUCTION

Zebrafish are a new vertebrate animal model with advantages for screening and development of therapeutic agents. In this chapter I will review the biology of

***Address correspondence to Robert T. Boyd:** Department of Neuroscience, The Ohio State University College of Medicine, Wexner Medical Center, 333 West Tenth Avenue, Columbus Ohio 43210, USA; Tel: 614 292-4391; E-mails: Robert.Boyd@osumc.edu, boyd.16@osu.edu

Atta-ur-Rahman & M. Iqbal Choudhary (Eds.)

zebrafish and how their use can be exploited to complement existing cell culture and mouse studies to test and develop new therapeutic compounds. I will focus on the nicotinic cholinergic and the dopaminergic systems, given their importance in addiction, and in many significant neurological disorders ranging from Alzheimer's disease to Parkinson's disease. I will summarize some of the behavioral assays used in zebrafish which may be used to identify drugs for treating neurological disorders. I will also review some studies which have used zebrafish in high throughput screening (HTS) development and testing of compounds targeted to cholinergic and dopaminergic systems can take advantage of the use of zebrafish for HTS identification of new drugs.

BIOLOGY OF ZEBRAFISH

Since 1930s, zebrafish (*Danio rerio*) have been used to study vertebrate development and basic embryology. The biology of zebrafish makes them an ideal model that can be used to complement studies done in mice or rats. Indeed, zebrafish have a number of advantages over other prominent vertebrate animal models. Similar to mice, numerous wild-type strains are in use and a large number of mutant strains have also been developed. Zebrafish are raised in relatively inexpensive aquatic systems in which thousands of fish can be kept in a modest facility. The feeding and maintenance costs are low compared to other vertebrate animals. Adult zebrafish are about 3-4 cm long and raised ideally at 28.5 C. under a 14/10 or 12/12 light/dark photoperiod. However, embryonic and larval fish which can be used in drug screening are much smaller with dozens able to fit in a 60mm Petri dish. The small size of zebrafish makes them ideal for use in 96 or 384 well plates Zebrafish are prolific with 100-300 embryos per mating or "clutch" [1]. Breeding can be done daily by rotating fish (females can lay eggs weekly), thus providing a plentiful supply of embryos on a continuous basis. Zebrafish embryos develop rapidly and externally (the first somite appears at about 10 hours of development compared to 9-10 days in the rat). Embryogenesis is complete at about 72 hours post fertlization (hpf) and most organs are fully developed between 3-5 days post fertilization (dpf) [2-3]. Zebrafish proceed through a larval stage from 3 dpf to about 29 dpf, a juvenile stage from 30-89 dpf and are reproductively mature adults at about 90 dpf. [4] with an average life span of 3-5 years [5]. The fish are free swimming at all stages and can be used for drug screening efforts at any of these stages, although as noted the smaller size of embryos and larvae make them especially suitable for HTS. Another advantage is that zebrafish are transparent through about 14 dpf. A transparent strain of zebrafish designated Casper [6] is transparent into adulthood and can be used to express reporter genes encoding fluorescent proteins in adults as well as in early naturally transparent embryos and larvae.

Zebrafish neural development occurs in a well characterized pattern and well-defined molecular markers (antibodies, DNA probes) are available to help identify specific cells and brain regions. Many basic cellular and molecular processes are highly conserved in zebrafish. Much of the genome has been sequenced (http: //www.sanger.ac.uk) and consists of approximately 1.45 gigabases on 25 chromosomes. Zebrafish contain the full repertoire of vertebrate genes and in many cases there is a high degree of sequence similarity and synteny between zebrafish and human genes [7-8]. The sequence similarities between zebrafish and human nicotinic acetylcholine receptor (nAChR) and dopamine receptor genes are also quite high [9-11]. The advantages of zebrafish biology and these genetic similarities supports the use of zebrafish in HTS efforts directed at drugs which affect nicotinic and dopaminergic systems.

The biology of zebrafish makes possible the use of a number of genetic tools that are easily applied to invertebrates, but are usually more difficult in vertebrates such as mice. Transgenic zebrafish have been developed which express GFP in specific cells [12] and allow for the activity of specific neurons to be monitored *in vivo* [13]. Zebrafish strains are now available which express fluorescent proteins specifically in a wide variety of cells, at specific points in development, or in response to specific molecules. A large array of mutants has been generated insufficient expression of numerous genes with human orthologs. Gene expression can also be transiently knocked down in zebrafish by the use of antisense morpholino oligonucleotides. Zinc finger nuclease (ZFN) mediated recombination can be used to produce "knock out" zebrafish [14]. Advanced forward and reverse genetic techniques have been applied to zebrafish to identify specific disease genes which produce phenotypes similar to human conditions and to produce model organisms [5,15]. A few of these zebrafish models include Alzheimer's disease, hearing disorders, muscular dystrophy, spinal muscular atrophy (SMA), holoprosencephaly, changes in cocaine sensitivity, responsiveness to nicotine and disruptions in cognitive behavior [5]. Zebrafish models allow for easier observation of disease progression than in other vertebrates, and open the possibility of their use in identifying drugs for therapeutic intervention. These models are ripe for use in HTS screening paradigms.

The zebrafish CNS has many similarities to the human CNS and some differences. Zebrafish have forebrain, midbrain and hindbrain which includes diencephalon, telencephalon, and cerebellum. However the zebrafish telencephalon has only a basic cortex. The motor, sensory, enteric and autonomic nervous systems are comparable. Zebrafish also demonstrate numerous higher functions such as memory, social behaviors, addiction and conditioned responses. However, these behavioral responses may be less complex in humans [16-18]. Overall, the biology of zebrafish make them an excellent resource for use in HTS for drugs that might act similarly in humans.

NICOTINIC ACETYLCHOLINE RECEPTORS AND THE ZEBRAFISH CHOLINERGIC SYSTEM

Acetylcholine is a major neurotransmitter in the vertebrate and invertebrate nervous systems. Classically acetylcholine acts as an excitatory transmitter mediating fast synaptic transmission through nicotinic acetylcholine receptors (nAChRs) or mediates slower signal transduction using G-protein coupled mechanisms *via* muscarinic acetylcholine receptors (mAChRs). We will focus on nAChRs due to their importance in a number of human diseases [19] and their value as potential targets for CNS drug screening efforts in zebrafish.

Neuronal nAChRs mediate synaptic transmission in many parts of the vertebrate central nervous system, as well as in autonomic ganglia, retina and adrenal medulla. nAChRs can be located presynaptically, or postsynaptically, or even in more diffuse patterns on the neuronal soma. Signaling through nAChRs also modulates the release of other neurotransmitters such as dopamine, GABA, glutamate and norepinephrine [20-21]. nAChR signaling is important to several CNS functions including memory, cognition, addiction, sleep, anxiety and neuronal survival [22]. nAChRs are expressed at the neuromuscular junction as well. These receptors are structurally similar to neuronal nAChRs and any drug developed to modify neuronal nAChR function will have to be examined for off-target effects on muscle nAChRs. nAChRs are also widely expressed outside the nervous system in non-neural tissues such as lung, skin, adipose tissue and various immune cells [23-26]. Thus, nAChRs mediate non-neural signaling by acetylcholine in number of different cell types besides neurons and regulate a number of functions and pathways in autocrine and paracrine signaling [25]. Some of these pathways involve differentiation, migration, cell adhesion, proliferation, angiogenesis and apoptosis in normal cells.

Neuronal nAChRs are pentameric molecules [27-28] which function as ligand-gated ion channels (ionotropic) and are composed of multiple α and β subunits, each of which contributes to the ligand binding site. The channels open in the presence of the endogenous ligand acetylcholine or exogenous ligands such as nicotine. The channels can exist in open, closed, or desensitized states. The pentameric receptor forms a transmembrane channel through which Na^+, K^+, and Ca^{2+} pass when the channel is in an open state. In addition to depolarization due to Na^+ influx, there is evidence in neurons that signaling through nAChRs stimulates a number of Ca^{2+}-dependent processes such as activation of PKC, PKA, PI3K, CAM kinase II and ERKs. Binding of agonist opens the channel by an allosteric interaction producing a conformational change in the nAChR [29-30]. Nine neuronal nAChR α subunit genes (α2-α10) and three nAChR β subunit genes (β2-β4) have been identified [21, 31-45]. nAChR subtypes are designated as homo- or hetero-pentameric, depending on the subunit composition. Heteromeric receptors contain both α and β subunits with the α4β2 receptor being the most prominent heteromer in the brain. Agonist binding occurs at α/β interfaces, except in homomeric receptors. Heteromeric nAChRs generally have two agonist binding sites. Homomeric receptors are comprised of only α subunits, and have five agonist binding sites, with the α7 nAChR being the primary homomer. Each of the nAChR α and β genes encodes a protein with an amino-terminal extracellular domain of about 200 amino acids, four hydrophobic transmembrane (TM) domains designated TM1-TM4, a large cytoplasmic loop between TM3 and TM4, and an extracellular carboxy terminal domain. The TM2 domains from each subunit form the ion channel. The agonist and competitive antagonist binding sites are located on the N-terminal regions of the α and β subunits [46-48]. The homology of all neuronal nAChR genes is very high in TM1-TM4, but the length and sequence of the cytoplasmic domain between TM3 and TM4 varies greatly between different nAChR subunits, even in the same species. The biophysical and pharmacological properties of neuronal nAChRs are determined by the subunit combination (receptor subtype) with a number of subtypes having been identified, each with a specific combination of subunits. The number of subtypes present naturally *in vivo* is not known, but multiple subtypes exist (*i.e.*, α4β2, α2β2, α4β4, α7, α3β4, α3β4α5, α3β2, α3β2β4, α3β2β4α5, α3β2α5, α4β2α5, α6β2β3, α4α6β2β3). Multiple subtypes may be present in an individual cell. Many heteromeric nAChRs have 3 α and 2 β subunits, but some α4β2 subunit have 2 α and 3 β subunits. These α4β2 subtypes differ in sensitivity to nicotine [49]. Some nAChRs possess multiple α and multiple β subunits in the same receptor (see above) adding up to five. Thus the diversity of nAChRs subtypes is extensive. Different combinations of α and β subunits produce channels which vary in ion selectivity, conductance, mean channel open time, permeability to Ca^{2+}, and desensitization rate. Each neuronal nAChR subtype also has a distinct pharmacology with both the α and β subunits determining the sensitivity to agonists and antagonists [47, 50-51]. Some nAChR subtypes such as α4β2 and α7 are distributed widely in the brain, while others have a more much more restricted pattern of expression [22,52]. The expression patterns of nAChR subtypes are correlated with CNS regions thought to be involved in specific pathologies with a nicotinic component [19].

Neuronal nAChRs are involved in a large number of neurological processes including pain sensation, locomotion, body temperature regulation, cognition, and reward and addiction [19,52]. nAChR function is involved in several disorders including Alzheimer's disease, Parkinson's disease, schizophrenia, lung cancer, epilepsy, ADHD, Tourette's and of course nicotine addiction [19,52]. Specific subtypes are associated with each of these processes, sometimes more than one.

Neuronal nAChRs are a rich target for CNS drug discovery efforts. Millions of people around the world are addicted to nicotine and most with a desire to stop are unable to do so [52]. There are several cholinergic drugs used to treat nicotine addiction including varenicline (Chantix) which is an α4β2 partial agonist derived from cytisine and mecamylamine, a noncompetitive antagonist. However none of these have been very successful. New therapeutic agents are needed which are nAChR subtypc selective.

Research on treatments of these disorders has focused on identifying drugs which can modify nicotinic signaling, but very few selective ligands for any specific subtype are available. Most efforts until recently have targeted the orthosteric or ligand binding site present at the α/β interface. A number of agonists have been used such as epibatidine, cytisine 1,1-dimethyl-4-phenylpiperazinium (DMPP) in addition to nicotine and of course acetylcholine. Most have little nAChR subtype selectivity, but vary in affinity for different nAChR subtypes. In addition, antagonists are available including mecamylamine, dihydro-β-erythroidine (DHβE, α4β2), methyllycaconitine (MLA, α3, α6, α7, muscle), and α-bungarotoxin (α7) with some subtype selectivity noted in parentheses. More recently small peptides purified from the *Conus* snails have been characterized as antagonists of various nAChR subtypes with varying degrees of selectivity [53]. Many of these agonists and antagonists can't be used as part of treatments in humans due to their pharmacology or biochemical properties, although mecamylamine has been used in combination with nicotine in smoking cessation therapy [54].

The structure of the orthosteric binding pocket is highly conserved among various nAChR subtypes and thus hasn't been a good target for identification of subtype-specific drugs. More recent studies have involved development of positive or negative allosteric modulators (PAMs or NAMs) which work though the allosteric sites, and don't compete with agonists or antagonists at the orthosteric site. Modulators don't activate the receptors by themselves, but enhance (PAM) or inhibit (NAM) receptor activity. By modulating activity, allosteric modulators can enhance or reduce signaling through nAChRs. Since these allosteric sites are unique, more nAChR subtype specificity can be obtained. PAMs and NAMS have been developed which display some nAChR subtype selectivity [55-58]. Some NAMS can block nicotine reinforcement and may be effective as smoking cessation agents [59-60]. PAMs with activity at α7 nAChRs may be useful to treat Alzheimer's disease or schizophrenia and are under development [55]. Zebrafish may be a suitable model to use in HTS for new drugs which regulate nAChR activity, either at the orthosteric or allosteric sites.

An advantage of using zebrafish as a model for CNS drug discovery is that there is a high degree of homology between zebrafish receptor genes and those in humans for many neurotransmitter receptors [11, 61]. Nine zebrafish neuronal nAChR genes as well as the muscle nAChR genes have been cloned [9-10, 62, RT Boyd unpublished]. Many of the zebrafish nAChR protein sequences are between 65-85% identical to their human orthologues. The zebrafish genome contains an array of nAChR genes similar to that present in other species [1,11]. These nAChR subunit sequence similarities are highest in the extracellular domains (ECD) which form the ligand binding region and in TM region 2, the region from each subunit which together form the ion channel. Epibatidine binds to several nAChRs subtypes with high-affinity. We have shown that zebrafish also express high-affinity epibatidine binding at 2 dpf and 5 dpf with affinities comparable to those of human nAChRs [9]. The expression patterns of several zebrafish nAChR subunits have been determined including α2, α4, α6, α7, β2, and β3 [9-10, 63]. There is a significant degree of conservation of anatomical expression between zebrafish and human nAChRs.

The CNS cholinergic system has been mapped in adult zebrafish using antibodies to choline acetyltransferase (ChAT) and acetylcholinesterase (AChE) [64-65]. AChE expressing cells in developing zebrafish embryos have been shown to be necessary for normal neuromuscular and neuronal development [66-67]. The location of cholinergic cells in olfactory bulb, telencephalon, tegmentum, cerebellum, retina, cranial motor nuclei and spinal are similar to the expression patterns seen in other vertebrates [64]. It has been proposed that the zebrafish ventral telencephalic population is a homologue of at least some of the mammalian cholinergic basal forebrain system and that the isthmic superior reticular cell population is a homologue of the mammalian pedunculopon-tine/laterodorsal tegmental system [65].

ZEBRAFISH nAChR PHARMACOLOGY

Given the sequence similarities in zebrafish nAChRs to those of mammals, it might be predicted that the function and pharmacology of many of the zebrafish nAChR subtypes would be similar to those of human nAChRs. The pharmacology of some zebrafish nAChR subtypes has recently been characterized and indeed this is the case, but there are some differences [68]. Three nAChR subtypes expressed in the CNS were characterized, α2β2 α4β2, and α7. In humans the α4β2* (* indicates that other subunits might also be present) nAChR forms the highest affinity nicotine binding sites and are widely expressed in the brain, α2β2* nAChRs have a more restricted expression pattern, but are also expressed in a region potentially important for addiction, the habenulo-interpeduncular pathway [69]. The α7 homomeric receptors are highly expressed in the brain and involved in numerous signaling pathways. α3β4 nAChRs were also characterized; this subtype is predominant in PNS and is often a subtype involved in any potential off-target effects of nicotinic drugs. Zebrafish muscle type nAChRs were also examined since any CNS drugs which severely affect muscle receptors would have little therapeutic use. Understanding any differences in the pharmacology of these subtypes between human and zebrafish is important for any drug development efforts using zebrafish.

All of the zebrafish nAChR subtypes responded to at least 3 μm ACh with the highest potency for α4β2 and the lowest for α3β4 [68]. The potencies of ACh for zebrafish α7 and muscle nAChRs were intermediate between these. Zebrafish α4β2 nAChRs had smaller currents than seen for mammalian α4β2 nAChRs. The kinetics of the responses were similar to mammalian nAChRs and all heteromeric subtypes showed concentration-dependent ACh evoked responses. Zebrafish α7 nAChRs displayed the same pattern of concentration-dependent desensitization as seen with α7 nAChRs in other species [68]. Nicotine was a partial agonist compared to ACh for α4β2, α2β2, and α3β4 nAChRs, but was a full agonist for zebrafish α7 nAChRs. Nicotine displayed the highest potency and efficacy at α4β2 nAChRs and the least for muscle. The effects of cytisine on zebrafish nAChRs were also examined. Cytisine has been used as a lead molecule in the development of smoking cessation drugs such as varenicline (Chantix). Any drug discovery effort in zebrafish aimed at nAChRs will need to understand the effects of cytisine on zebrafish nAChRs. Cytisine is a full agonist for zebrafish α7 nAChRs as it is for mammalian receptors. However is was a weak partial agonist for zebrafish α3β4 nAChRs, in contrast to being a full agonist for mammalian α3β4 nAChRs [68]. Another difference between zebrafish and mammalian nAChRs was that cytisine had the highest potency for α4β2 nAChRs compared to α2β2, α3β4, and muscle nAChRs and a higher efficacy than is seen in α4β2 mammalian receptors. Cytisine is a weak partial agonist for β2-containing nAChRs in other species. Since cytisine is efficacious for human, mouse and rat α3β4 nAChRs, off-target effects at ganglionic nAChRs are a concern in testing cytisine as a smoking cessation medication. Since cytisine has a lower efficacy at zebrafish α3β4 (ganglionic) nAChRs, caution should be exercised in concluding that a drug modeled after cytisine identified in a zebrafish screen would have no ganglionic effects in humans.

α7 nAChRs are thought to be drug targets for therapeutic intervention in schizophrenia and Alzheimer's disease [19]. Several molecules have been tested in mammals as structural motifs for designing α7 selective agonists including choline, 4OH-GTS-21 and tropane [70]. These drugs were not α7 selective agonists in zebrafish, indicating that testing compounds based on these structures may not be advisable in zebrafish.

Many studies in humans and other mammals use mecamylamine in CNS drug studies and behavioral assays because it is an antagonist with higher activity at neuronal than at muscle nAChRs. In zebrafish, as in mammals, mecamylamine was most potent at α3β4 nAChRs with a rank order of potency of α3β4>muscle>α2β2>α4β2>α7 [68]. Mecamylamine also inhibited muscle receptors with an EC_{50} which is similar to that of mouse muscle [71]. CNS subtypes (β2-containing) have mecamylamine sensitivities similar to that of muscle nAChRs. Blockage of α3β4, α7 and muscle nAChRs by mecamylamine was easily reversible. This is different from rat studies in that rat α3β4 nAChRs had a 60% residual inhibition [72]. β2-containing nAChRs experienced long-term inhibition after co-application of ACh and mecamylamine, while muscle activity was reversible, indicating that drug studies in zebrafish could be consistent with studies in other species. Mecamylamine will likely work in drug screening efforts as in other model systems. while keeping in mind these pharmacological studies. However, work with zebrafish [68] demonstrates that mecamylamine is not a selective antagonist for zebrafish CNS neuronal nAChRs.

ZEBRAFISH DOPAMINERGIC SYSTEM

Dopamine is the major neurotransmitter involved in mammalian reward pathways from the ventral tegmental area (VTA) to the nucleus accumbans (NAcc). The dopaminergic system involves dopamine transporters (DAT), receptors, biosynthetic enzymes such as tyrosine hydroxylase (TH) and dopamine beta-hydroxlyase (DBH) and degradative enzymes such as monoamine oxidase (MAO) and catechol-O-methyltransferase (COMT) [73]. Elements of this system such as specific dopamine receptors and DATs are involved in addiction. Zebrafish may be a good model to use in identifying new molecules that affect addiction and reward since zebrafish have orthologues of all four dopamine receptor genes present in humans, as well as orthologues of TH, DBH and some DATs [11]. The protein identities between the human and zebrafish genes are approximately 68% [11]. Phylogenetic analysis matches each zebrafish homolog with its human counterpart.

Zebrafish dopamine receptor genes has been localized with high expression in the diencephalon or tegmentum. The drd1 and dr2 genes are expressed in a pattern very similar to that seen in analogous regions of mammals. One of the zebrafish dopamine transporter genes, slc6a3, is co-expressed in 13 dopamine neuron clusters with TH [74]. Two TH genes are present with th1 widely expressed while the th2 gene is expressed in the pretectum and hypothalamus [11, 75]. Zebrafish however appear to lack mesencephalic dopaminergic neurons [75]. Dopaminergic neurons are present in ventral telencephalon, pretectum, ventral diencephalon, retina, and hypothalamus [76]. A complicated ventral dopaminergic system is however present in zebrafish [75]. Thus many of the molecular components are present. While the location of dopaminergic pathways is not identical in zebrafish and mammals, it may still be possible to identify behaviors mediated by dopaminergic systems in zebrafish and use these behaviors to screen for drugs.

Zebrafish larval movement is mediated by dopaminergic systems. Effects of dopaminergic agonists and antagonists as well as the effects of 1-methyl-4-phenylpyridinium (MPP+) on spontaneous movement of 3-9 dpf zebrafish larvae has been examined in a potential high-throughput assay [77]. Treatment of larvae with the neurotoxin MPP+ reduced the number of dopaminergic neurons and reduced dopamine content. Larvae treated with the agonists apomorphine and ropinirole and antagonists haloperidol and chlorpromazine had different reproducible effects on the pattern of movement. MPP+ treated larvae displayed reduced initiation of spontaneous movement [77]. The locomotor assays had Z scores ranging from 0.13 to 0.42 indicating that these assays were robust enough to be used for screening. Since these assays were performed in 96-well plates and the data collected by video, this work indicates that it could be used to screen for drugs which affect the locomotor pathways and perhaps identify drugs which could be used to treat Parkinson's disease using larval zebrafish,

1-methyl-4-phenyl-1,2,3,6-tetrahydropyridine (MPTP) has been used to induce Parkinson's disease symptoms in several experimental animals including primates and mice. MPTP also produces neurotoxic effects in dopaminergic neurons in larval zebrafish as well [78]. The MPTP-induced neurodegeneration was blocked by a MAO-B or DAT inhibitors or by knockdown of DAT. Since the mechanism of damage is conserved, zebrafish larvae could be used to screen for new compounds which ameliorate the degeneration or effects on swimming behavior and locomotor response produced by MPTP. Zebrafish models of parkinsonism have also been created [79]. These may also be used for screening potential therapeutic compounds. There is great potential to develop zebrafish disease models and behavioral assays which can be used in HTS for drugs which affect dopaminergic pharmacology.

HIGH THROUGHPUT *IN VIVO* SCREENING IN ZEBRAFISH

Typical drug discovery efforts extend for many years using *in vitro* assays with cells and molecular approaches. Eventually this work moves to animals and then human studies, with the process taking 10 years or more to complete. Very few drugs are actually brought to market, although millions of dollars are spent on each failed drug [80]. Problems with drug development often come when a compound doesn't exhibit acceptable ADMET properties (absorption, distribution, metabolism, excretion or toxicity) when tested in animals. The use of zebrafish for high throughput *in vivo* screens may uncover or reveal these problems at an earlier stage in the drug pipeline and result in significant saving. While a zebrafish is not a human, rat or mouse, there is striking conservation of a number of biochemical pathways that make zebrafish a viable model for use in CNS drug development, because of its amenability to *in vivo* screening.

Whole animal screens have been done in fruit fly (*D. melanogaster*) and worms (*C. elegans*). However zebrafish have the advantage of being a vertebrate with genetics, cell biology and physiology much more similar to humans [3]. Many biological compounds which have activity in humans also have similar targets in zebrafish, making it an ideal system for *in vivo* HTS. Many groups and companies are using zebrafish for drug discovery, toxicological screens (*in vivo* screen rather than using cell lines), drug reprofiling, target validation, and testing drug efficacy in whole animal systems. Work can be focused on specific molecular targets, organs or the whole animal. These methodologies can be applied to search for compounds affecting nicotinic and dopaminergic systems.

Zebrafish can be easily arrayed in 96- or 384-well plates. Embryos can then be allowed to develop until the desired age for use in testing. Embryos and larvae don't need feeding up until about 6 dpf. Drugs can be delivered to zebrafish in a manner similar to that done for cells using robotic handling systems or multichannel pipettes. Zebrafish are not affected by up to 1% DMSO so drugs can be dissolved in it as is done in cell based systems. Drugs can be easily delivered to zebrafish in the culture water and absorbed into the fish through skin, mouth or gills [3].

Zebrafish can be used at many steps in the drug discovery process. Toxicology screens are an effective use of zebrafish. Drugs often fail due to off-target effects and zebrafish can be used to identify these in whole animal screens at an early stage in the process and thus save time and money. Zebrafish have been heavily used in environmental toxicology studies, but are certainly amenable to screening of potential lead compounds for toxic effects on numerous organs systems including the CNS. Larval zebrafish possess similar genetic, biochemical, physiological and xenobiotic responses as are present in mammalian systems [3]. Comparison of toxicological profiles of known compounds in humans *versus* zebrafish revealed that most responses were similar, although some differences were noted.

Zebrafish have been used for target confirmation. Target genes can be transiently knocked down using antisense morpholino oligonucleotides or knocked out using zinc-finger nucleases (ZFN) [14, 81] and these fish can be used in HTS protocols. Drug mechanisms of action can also be dissected using these models that will provide new potential targets. Many biochemical or gene-targeted assays can be done using a multi-well format. Transgenic fish expressing fluorescently tagged molecules can be scored for effects on gene or protein expression in a high-throughput manner. Thus drugs affecting nicotinic or dopaminergic system receptors or enzymes can be monitored in real time in live animals and provide a high-throughput *in vivo* screening method.

SAR (structure-activity relationship) studies are commonly used with a lead compound to generate new drugs which may have enhanced potency, efficacy or reduced side effects. SAR studies are often done in cells or other *in vitro* systems. Zebrafish are being used in a growing number of SAR studies to provide an *in vivo* system to test and refine lead compounds. *In vivo* SAR has been used in zebrafish to identify inhibitors of bone morphogenetic protein and VEGF signaling [82]. Zebrafish can be used in high-throughput SAR studies to optimize drugs that modulate nicotinic or dopaminergic systems.

Zebrafish also provide an excellent vertebrate system for high-throughput small molecule screens. Zebrafish have been used in high throughput small molecule screens examining blood cell growth, cancer, heart rhythms, cell cycle regulation, and others [83]. Wild type or mutant fish have been used. Many small scale screens have already been done and have shown the utility and versatility of the system. Imaging and computational analysis of movement or cell changes brought about by drug exposure can be automated to allow for high throughput analysis of complex phenotypes. This is of particular importance in CNS pharmacology since *in vitro* systems can't model the complex behavior of the brain.

Zebrafish can be used for targeted *in vivo* screens also [3]. Recent work has used a target screen for nuclear receptor proteins [84]. Nuclear receptor proteins are important targets as they are involved in a number of cancers, diabetes and neurological disorders, while other target based screens are being developed.

ZEBRAFISH BEHAVIORAL ASSAYS AND USE IN HTS

Clearly larval and adult zebrafish have great utility for identifying problems with toxicology of new compounds and other ADMET properties as well as targeted screens for drugs affecting a large number of individual biochemical and molecular pathways. Given the complexity of many behavioral disorders, it will be necessary to identify molecules that affect complex phenotypes, which means using whole animals to screen for new compounds which affect behaviors. An advantage to drug discovery is the ability to use high throughput small molecule screens. Zebrafish have been used to screen for drugs affecting a number of human disease models, cancer biology, cell cycle regulation, blood vessel growth, heart rhythms, and the expression of numerous genes [83]. To identify drugs which can be used to treat neurological diseases involving the nicotinic and dopaminergic systems, more complex behavioral assays will be required. Zebrafish behavior is amenable to the analysis and automated data acquisition needed to do HTS.

Zebrafish manifest many of the behaviors demonstrated by other animal models such as rat and mice in the presence of neuroactive compounds. Although zebrafish possess a limited telencephalon and no hippocampus, nicotine's effects can be observed in several behavioral paradigms testing cognitive function, stress responses, and locomotor function. Thus many of the behavioral tests used in mice and rats can be used in zebrafish. However zebrafish have not been used until recently for more behavioral based assays looking for drugs to treat CNS disorders or drug abuse and addiction. Small scale studies in larval and adult zebrafish have been used to test the effects of various drugs of abuse including alcohol, cocaine, amphetamine, opiates, LSD, and nicotine [83]. The effects of ethanol has been examined in zebrafish assays quantifying locomotion, tolerance, withdrawal, reward, and aggression. Many of these types of studies have been done in rats or mice, but can now be done in zebrafish. Zebrafish have been used to determine the effects of nicotine on locomotion, conditioned place preference (CPP), and anxiety and to study rewarding effects of cocaine and amphetamines [83, 85-86]. Complex behaviors are exhibited by both larval and adult zebrafish. Adult zebrafish display several types of reward behavior including CPP. A CPP response to several drugs has been elicited in zebrafish including nicotine, cocaine, and amphetamine [85, 87-88]. A number of learning and memory tests have also been applied to adult zebrafish. Although all of the zebrafish circuits associated with learning are not understood, they clearly exhibit this behavior. Tests used include T maze to assess spatial learning, delayed spatial alternation, and active avoidance conditioning [18]. These assays can be high throughput and can be used to screen for drugs which might improve learning. In addition, nicotine and cholinergic signaling are implicated in zebrafish learning [88], demonstrating the relevance of zebrafish behavioral assays to nicotinic drug discovery. Low doses of nicotine (100 mg/l in the water) improved performance in a delayed spatial alternation task, while high doses impaired performance [89]. The "inverted U" pattern of the response is typical when nicotine is used in these paradigms in mammals as well. The antagonist mecamylamine blocked this nicotine-induced improvement in another spatial learning task when given 5 minutes before the task, but not if given 40 minutes prior to the test [90]. Several tests for anxiety have been used in zebrafish including place preference (edge or bottom of tank), tank diving test, locomotor activity, and light/dark preference [18]. A place preference assay was used to test the anxiolytic effects of nicotine in zebrafish [91]. Nicotine was also anxiolytic at 100mg/l and this effect of nicotine was also blocked by 200 mg/l mecamylamine, but only if given with nicotine, not 20 minutes prior. In addition, specific nAChR subtypes were implicated in the anxiolytic effects of nicotine in zebrafish. Both MLA ($\alpha 7$ antagonist) and DHβE ($\alpha 4\beta 2$ antagonist) reversed the anxiolytic effects of nicotine [92]. Thus, the effects of nicotine on learning and anxiety can be examined in zebrafish. Adult zebrafish can also be tested for aggression in several ways including a mirror image test, and observing interactions of two fish [18]. Relevant to nicotinic and dopaminergic systems, various tests of locomotion have been used, some of which might be useful in HTS. Some of these paradigms are mean velocity, total distance moved, and quantification of the number of lines crossed in a grid. Locomotor assays can also be used in screening for Parkinson's drugs which might affect motor activity. Finally, adult assays are available to monitor sleep, mate choice, vision and social preference [18].

Large scale behavioral assays (phenotype-based drug discovery) might be done using larval as well as adult zebrafish. The small size of larval fish makes them easier to use and may be more suitable for HTS efforts. Multi-well plates can be used for behavioral assays. 5-7 dpf larvae are relatively homogenous in structure and physiology, although older larvae can also be used. Larvae are capable of performing simple motor tasks, responding to environmental cues and have functional motor and sensory systems [93]. Larval zebrafish exhibit a wide range of swimming behaviors and other behavioral responses [93-94]. The open field test, a standard test in mice, has been adapted to multi-well plates using larval zebrafish. Various tests of locomotor activity have been applied to larval zebrafish. Larval zebrafish also demonstrate an optomoter response and optokinetic response [95]. Analysis of movement can be automated at a high throughput level. Thus drugs which may affect locomotor behaviors can be screened for. Larval zebrafish also show an acoustic startle response which can be modified by pre pulse inhibition (PPI). Schizophrenics show reduced PPI. Dopaminergic antagonists (antipsychotic drugs) increase PPI in zebrafish [94]. Larval zebrafish might be used to screen for new drugs that increase PPI and thus might be candidate drugs for schizophrenia. Behavioral sleep appears to occur in larval zebrafish [96-97]. Larval zebrafish might also provide a HTS vehicle to look for new compounds which affect sleep. Other larval behaviors may be adapted to HTS to identify drugs affecting learning, and feeding responses [95].

Since the nicotine and dopaminergic systems are intimately involved in drug abuse, identifying new drugs which may aid in smoking cessation or withdrawal from cocaine or amphetamine would be useful. Withdrawal from amphetamine and nicotine can be modeled in rodents [98-99]. Recent work has shown that various drugs of abuse such as amphetamine, and cocaine exhibit reward properties in zebrafish. Nicotine treatment alters CNS gene expression, specifically of some genes involved in addiction pathways [87]. Withdrawal behavior can also be modeled in adult zebrafish [100]. If these assays can be scaled up to at least a moderate throughput level, they might be useful in identifying new lead compounds for treatment of nicotine, amphetamine or cocaine abuse. If this behavior can be modeled in larval zebrafish, HTS may be possible.

Can these behavioral assays be scaled to a high throughput level? In some cases the answer is yes. However it was not until recently that large scale screens for small molecules that affect behavior were done using zebrafish. In work by Rihel *et al.* over 5000 compounds were tested for the ability to modulate behavior in larval zebrafish using a rest/wake protocol [101]. Each compound identified was assigned a behavioral fingerprint and the molecules were then organized into clusters based on fingerprints. This allowed for the analysis of complex behavior in a HTS situation, This approach led to identification of new links between molecules and mechanisms of action and of new pathways [101]. They also showed that drugs which affect neurotransmitter pathways induced effects in zebrafish similar to that seen in mammals. Compounds with shared targets also produced similar behavioral phenotypes.

Neuroactive small molecules have now been identified in a HTS using embryonic zebrafish [102]. They showed that high intensity light produces a series of motor behaviors, which were collectively defined as the photomotor response (PMR). They screened for molecules which affected the PMR. They also used an embryonic touch assay (ETR). It is not clear what behavioral phenotype is being modeling by the PMR but as a proof of principle demonstrates the ability to identify neuroactive molecules in a HTS. Six chemical libraries were screened containing approximately 14,000 compounds. 8-10 embryonic zebrafish were used in each well of 96 well plates. The platform was fully automated. Information was gathered from about 250,000 animals. About 7% of the compounds produced changes in PMR. Known psychoactive drugs affected the PMR in quantifiable ways. Drugs that produced similar effects in the PMR assays could be placed into groups of molecules which produced similar behavioral phenotypes [102]. Behavioral barcodes were used to classify molecules. The barcodes of new molecules could be compared to that of known chemical entities and used to predict mechanisms of action of new compounds [102-103]. During the screen molecules which inhibited AChE were identified. Novel inhibitors of MAO were also found during the screen [102]. This study supports the use of high throughput behavioral screens using embryonic zebrafish for drug discovery. Behavioral assays like PMR could also be used to test for toxicity of chemicals. Identifying dangerous effects early in the discovery process would save time and money. Toxicity testing using embryonic zebrafish in a high throughput manner would be efficient and cost saving.

CPP assays can be used to model reinforcing effects of addictive drugs. CPP has been established in zebrafish A high throughput CPP protocol has now been developed [104]. This assay could be used to screen for nicotine and dopaminergic drugs affecting reward and associative learning. Recently an automated learning and memory task that can be scaled up to 400 fish a day has been developed [105]. Several tests of various types of learning including spatial are being developed in zebrafish. These could be applied to screening for drugs that affect learning, relevant to cognitive impairment observed in Alzheimer's. Behavioral tests of fear and anxiety can also be used with zebrafish [105].

Using zebrafish for identification of new drugs comes with some problems as does any experimental animal. These include dosing regimes, *i.e.*, how do they compare to those in other animals? All ADMET issues must also be addressed. Another is access to the CNS. The zebrafish blood-brain barrier develops at 3 dpf [106], but some behavioral screens have identified psychotropic compounds using zebrafish as old as 7 dpf, indicating that at least some compounds screened will have access at these ages. However, an advantage of using zebrafish is that younger embryonic and larval fish may also be screened. Another concern which will need to be addressed is that zebrafish nAChR and dopaminergic pharmacologies may differ for some compounds which have been tested in mammals. Dopamine D1 receptor agonists produce sedation in larval zebrafish, but arousal in mammals [83]. Given the many similarities in genetics and cell biology of zebrafish and humans, this will hopefully be the exception rather than the rule, but it must be considered. As noted, the pharmacology of some nicotinic compounds in zebrafish have been characterized [68], but others have not. Any new molecules characterized in zebrafish will need to be mapped to the proper receptor or pathways in humans.

SUMMARY

The biology of zebrafish makes it a ideal for use in drug discovery efforts. The ease of growth and handling and the ability of zebrafish to be treated with a compound in multi-well format are advantages for HTS work. Many of the genes and biochemical processes present in mammals are conserved in zebrafish including many elements of the nicotinic cholinergic and dopaminergic systems.

Cell lines have traditionally been used to screen for new compounds, examine cell toxicity, conduct SAR of new compounds and for target validation. Zebrafish have been used in a growing number of studies addressing these same aims. To identify drugs affecting processes or targets involved in many neurological disorders, *in vivo* screening with a vertebrate animal model is desirable. Zebrafish exhibit many of the complex behaviors similar to those seen in rats or mice. Many of these behaviors can be assayed in zebrafish in a low or medium throughput format including locomotion, avoidance behaviors, learning, and CPP. In addition, some can be scaled up for *in vivo* HTS. Zebrafish is an exciting new system amenable to identification of new drugs to treat disorders due to nicotinic cholinergic and dopaminergic disregulation.

ACKNOWLEDGEMENTS

None declared.

CONFLICT OF INTEREST

The authors state that there is no conflict of interest.

REFERENCES

[1] Klee EW, Ebbert JO, Schneider, H, Hurt, RD, Ekker SC. Zebrafish for the study of the biological effects of nicotine. Nicotine and Tobacco Res 2011; 13 (5): 310-312.

[2] Ackermann GE, Paw BH. Zebrafish: a genetic model for vertebrate organogenesis and human disorders. Front Biosci 2003; 8: d1227-53.

[3] Delvecchio C, Tiefenbach J, Krause HM. The zebrafish: a powerful platform for *in vivo*, HTS drug discovery. Assay Drug Dev Technol 2011; 9: 354-61.

[4] Westerfield, M. The zebrafish book. A guide for the laboratory use of zebrafish (Danio rerio). 4th ed., Univ. of Oregon Press, Eugene 2000.

[5] Lieschke, GJ Currie, PD. Animal models of human disease: zebrafish swim into view. Nature Review Genetics 2007; 8 (5): 353-367.

[6] White RM, Sessa A, Burke C, *et al.* Transparent adult zebrafish as a tool for *in vivo* transplantation analysis. Cell Stem Cell 2008; 2 (2): 183-9.

[7] Barbazuk WB, Korf I, Kadavi C, *et al.* The syntenic relationship of the zebrafish and human genomes. Genome Res 2000; 10 (9): 1351-8.

[8] Howe K, Clark MW, Torroja CF, *et al.* The zebrafish reference genome sequence and its relationship to the human genome. Nature 2013; 496 (7446): 498-503

[9} Zirger JM, Beattie CE, McKay DB, Boyd RT. Cloning and expression of zebrafish neuronal nicotinic acetylcholine receptors. Gene Expr Patterns 2003; 3 (6): 747-54.

[10] Ackerman KM, Nakkula R, Zirger JM, Beattie CE, Boyd RT. Cloning and spatiotemporal expression of zebrafish neuronal nicotinic acetylcholine receptor alpha 6 and alpha 4 subunit RNAs. Dev Dyn 2009; 238 (4): 980-92.

[11] Klee EW, Schneider H, Clark KJ, *et al.* Zebrafish: a model for the study of addiction genetics. Hum Genet 2012; 131: 977-1008.

[12] Yoshida T, Mishina M. Neuron-specific gene manipulation in transparent zebrafish embryos, Methods Cell Sci 2003; 25 (1-2): 15-23.

[13] Higashijima S, Masino MA, Mandel G, Fetcho JR. Imaging neuronal activity during zebrafish behavior with a genetically encoded calcium indicator. J Neurophysiol 2003; 90 (6): 3986-97.

[14] Foley JE, Maeder ML, Pearlberg J, Joung JK, Peterson RT, Yeh JR. Targeted mutagenesis in zebrafish using customized zinc-finger nucleases. Nature Protocols 2009; 4 (12): 1855-1868.

[15] Kettleborough RNW, Busch-Nentwich EM, Harvey S, *et al.* A systematic genome-wide analysis of zebrafish protein-coding gene function. Nature 2013; 496 (7446): 494-497.

[16] Dooley K, Zon LI. Zebrafish: a model system for the study of human disease. Current Opinion in Gen and Dev 2000; 10(3): 252-256.

[17] Guo S. Linking genes to brain, behavior and neurological diseases: what can we learn from zebrafish. Genes, Brain, and Behav 2004; 3 (2): 63-74.

[18] Norton W, Bally-Cuif L. Adult zebrafish as a model organism for behavioural genetics. BMC Neurosci. 11: 90

[19] Lloyd GK, Williams M. Neuronal nicotinic acetylcholine receptors as novel drug targets. JPET 2000; 292 (2): 461-467.

[20] Role L, Berg D. Nicotinic receptors in the development and modulation of CNS synapses. Neuron 1996; 16 (6): 1077-85.

[21] Gotti C, Clementi F, Fornari A, *et al.* Structural and functional diversity of native brain neuronal nicotinic receptors. Biochem Pharmacol 2009 78 (7): 703-711.

[22] Gotti C, Zoli M, Clementi F. Brain nicotinic acetylcholine receptors: native subtypes and their relevance. Trends Pharmacol Sci 2006; 27 (9): 482-91.

[23] Sharma G, Vijayaraghavan S. Nicotinic receptor signaling in nonexcitable cells. J Neurobiol 2002; 53 (4): 524-534.

[24] Gahring LC, Rogers SW. Neuronal nicotinic acetylcholine receptor expression and function on nonneuronal cells. The AAPS Journal 2006; 7 (4): E885-E894.

[25] Egleton RD, Brown KC, Dasgupta P. Nicotinic acetylcholine receptors in cancer: multiple roles in proliferation and inhibition of apoptosis. Trends in Pharmacol Sci 2008; 29 (3): 151-158.

[26] Wessler I, Kirkpatrick CJ. Acetylcholine beyond neurons: the non-neuronal cholinergic system in humans. Brit J Pharmacol 2008; 154 (8): 1558-1571.

[27] Cooper E, Couturier S, Ballivet M. Pentameric structure and subunit stoichiometry of a neuronal nicotinic acetylcholine receptor. Nature 1991; 350 (6315): 235-238.

[28] Anand R, Conroy WG, Schoepfer R, Whiting P, Lindstrom J. Neuronal nicotinic acetylcholine receptors expressed in *Xenopus* oocytes have a pentameric quaternary structure. J Biol Chem 1991; 266 (17): 11192-11198.

[29] Lena C, Changeux J-P. Allosteric modulations of the nicotinic acetylcholine receptor. TINS 1993; 16 (5): 181-186.

[30] Unwin N. Refined structure of the nicotinic acetylcholine receptor at 4A resolution. J Mol Biol 2005; 346 (4): 967-989.

[31] Boulter J, Evans K, Goldman D, *et al.* Isolation of a cDNA clone coding for a possible neural nicotinic acetylcholine receptor alpha-subunit. Nature 1986; 319 (6052): 368-374.

[32] Boulter J, O'Shea-Greenfield A, Duvoisin RM, *et al.* $\alpha 3$, $\alpha 5$ and $\beta 4$: Three members of the rat neuronal nicotinic acetylcholine receptor-related gene family form a cluster. J Biol Chem 1990; 265 (8): 4472- 4482.

[33] Couturier S, Bertrand D, Matter J-M, *et al.* A neuronal nicotinic acetylcholine receptor subunit ($\alpha 7$) is developmentally regulated and forms a homo-oligomeric channel blocked by α-Btx. Neuron 1990; 5 (6): 847-856.

[34] Couturier S, Erkman L, Valera S, *et al.* $\alpha 5$, $\alpha 3$, and non-$\alpha 3$: three clustered avian genes encoding neuronal nicotinic acetylcholine receptor-related subunits. J Biol Chem 1990; 265 (29): 17560-17567.

[35] Deneris ES, Connolly J, Boulter, J, *et al.* Primary structure and expression of $\beta 2$: a novel subunit of neuronal nicotinic acetylcholine receptors. Neuron 1988; 1 (1): 45-54.

[36] Deneris ES, Boulter J, Swanson LW, Patrick J, Heinemann S. $\beta 3$: A new member of nicotinic acetylcholine receptor gene family is expressed in brain. J Biol Chem 1989; 264 (11): 6268-6272.

[37] Duvoisin RM, Deneris ES, Patrick J, Heinemann S. The functional diversity of the neuronal nicotinic acetylcholine receptors is increased by a novel subunit: $\beta 4$. Neuron 1989; 3 (4): 487-496.

[38] Goldman D, Deneris ES, Luyton W, Kochhar A, Patrick J, Heinemann S. Members of a nicotinic acetylcholine receptor gene family are expressed in different regions of the mammalian central nervous system. Cell 1987; 48 (6): 965-973.

[39] Nef P, Oneyser C, Alliod C, Couturier S, Ballivet M. Genes expressed in the brain define three distinct neuronal nicotinic acetylcholine receptors. EMBO J 1988; 7 (3): 595-601.

[40] Schoepfer R, Whiting P, Esch F, Blacher R, Shimasaki S, Lindstrom J. cDNA clones coding for the structural subunit of a chicken brain nicotinic acetylcholine receptor. Neuron 1988; 1 (3): 241-248.

[41] Schoepfer R, Conroy WG, Whiting P, Gore M, Lindstrom M. Brain α-bungarotoxin binding protein cDNAs and Mabs reveal subtypes of this branch of the ligand-gated ion channel gene superfamily. Neuron 1990; 5 (1): 35-48.

[42] Seguela P, Wadiche J, Dineley-Miller K, Dani, JA, Patrick JW. Molecular cloning, functional properties, and distribution of rat brain $\alpha 7$: a nicotinic cation channel highly permeable to calcium. J Neurosci 1993; 13 (2): 596-604.

[43] Wada K, Ballivet M, Boulter J, *et al.* Functional expression of a new pharmacological subtype of brain nicotinic acetylcholine receptor. Science 1988; 240 (4850): 330-334.

[44] Elgoyhen AB, Johnson D, Boulter J, Vetter DE, Heinemann S. $\alpha 9$: an acetylcholine receptor with novel pharmacological properties expressed in rat cochlear hair cells. Cell 1994; 79 (4): 705-715.

[45] Elgoyhen AB, Vetter DE, Katz E, Rothlin CV, Heinemann SF, Boulter J. $\alpha 10$: a determinant of nicotinic cholinergic receptor function in mammalian vestibular and cochlear mechanosensory hair cells. Proc Natl Acad Sci USA 2001; 98 (6): 3501-3506.

[46] Luetje CW, Wada K, Rogers S, *et al.* Neurotoxins distinguish between different neuronal acetylcholine receptor subunit combinations. J Neurochem 1990; 55 (2): 632-640.

[47] Luetje CW, Patrick J. Both α- and β- subunits contribute to the agonist sensitivity of neuronal nicotinic acetylcholine receptors. J Neurosci 1991; 11 (3): 837-845.

[48] Luetje CW, Piattoni M, Patrick J. Mapping of ligand binding sites of neuronal nicotinic acetylcholine receptors using chimeric α subunits. Mol Pharmacol 1993; 44 (3): 657-666.

[49] Nelson ME, Kuryatov A, Choi CH, Zhou Y, and Lindstrom J. Alternate stoichiometries of α4β2 nicotinic acetylcholine receptors. Mol Pharmacol 2003; 63 (2): 332-341.

[50] McGehee DS, Role LW. Physiological diversity of nicotinic acetylcholine receptors expressed by vertebrate neurons. Ann Rev Physiol 1995; 57: 521-546.

[51] Harvey SC, Luetje CW. Determinants of competitive antagonist sensitivity on neuronal nicotinic receptor beta subunits. J Neurosci 1996; 16 (12): 3798-3806.

[52] Albuquerque EX, Pereira EFR, Alkondon M, and Rogers SW. Mammalian nicotinic acetylcholine receptors: from structure to function. Physiol Rev 2009; 89 (1): 73-120.

[53] Azam L, McIntosh J M. Alpha-conotoxins as pharmacological probes of nicotinic acetylcholine receptors. Acta Pharmacol Sin 2009; 30 (6): 771.

[54] Rose JE, Westman EC Behm FM. Nicotine/mecamylamine combination treatment for smoking cessation. Drug Dev Res 1996; 38; 243-256.

[55] Williams DK, Wang J, Papke, RL. Positive allosteric modulators as an approach to nicotinic acetylcholine receptor-targeted therapeutics: advantages and limitations. Biochem Pharmacol 2011; 82 (8): 915-930.

[56] Henderson BJ, Pavlovicz RE, Allen, JD, *et al.* Negative allosteric modulators that target human α4β2 neuronal nicotinic receptors. JPET 2010; 334 (3): 761-774.

[57] Henderson BJ, González-Cestari TF, Yi B, *et al.* Defining the structure of a putative binding site of selective antagonist, KAB-18, on human α4β2 neuronal nicotinic receptors using site-directed mutagenesis and structure-activityrelationship studies. ACS Chem Neurosci 2012; 3 (9): 682-692.

[58] Pavlovicz' RE, Henderson' BJ, Bonnell AB, Boyd RT, McKay DB, Li' C-L. Identification of a Novel Negative Allosteric Site on Human α4β2 and α3β4 Neuronal Nicotinic Acetylcholine Receptors. PLoS ONE 2011; 6(9): e24949.

[59] Yoshimura RF, Hogenkamp DJ, Li WY, *et al.* Negative allosteric modulation of nicotinic acetylcholine receptors block nicotine self-administration in rats. JPET 2007; 323 (3): 907-915.

[60] Hall BJ, Pearson LS, Buccafusc JJ. Effects of administration of the nicotinic acetylcholine receptor antagonist BTMPS during nicotine self-administration on lever responding induced by context long after withdrawal. Neuropharmacol 2010; 58 (2): 429-435.

[61] Rico EP, Rosemberg DB, Seibt KJ, Capiotti KM, Da Silva RS, Bonan CD. Zebrafish neurotransmitter systems as potential pharmacological and toxicological targets. Neurotoxicol Teratol 2011; 33 (6): 608-617.

[62] Mongeon R, Walogorsky M, Urban J, Mandel G, Ono F, Brehm P. An acetylcholine receptor lacking both γ and ε subunits mediates transmission in zebrafish slow muscle synapses. J Gen Physiol 2011; 138 (3): 353-66.

[63] Welsh L, Tanguay RL, Svoboda, KR. Uncoupling nicotine mediated motoneuron axonal pathfinding errors and muscle degeneration in zebrafish. Toxicol Appl Pharmacol 2009; 237 (1): 29-40.

[64] Clemente D, Porteros A, Weruaga E, *et al.* Cholinergic elements in the zebrafish central nervous system: Histochemical and immunohistochemical analysis. J Comp Neurol 2004; 474 (1): 75-107.

[65] Mueller T, Vernier P, Wullimann MF. The adult central nervous cholinergic system of a neurogenetic model animal, the zebrafish *Danio rerio*. Brain Res 2004; 1011 (2): 156-169.

[66] Behra M, Cousin X, Bertrand C, *et al*. Acetylcholinesterase is required for neuronal and muscular development in the zebrafish embryo. Nat Neurosci 2002; 5 (2) : 111-8.

[67] Hanneman E, Westerfield M. Early expression of acetylcholinesterase activity in functionally distinct neurons of the zebrafish. J Comp Neurol 1989; 284 (3): 350-61.

[68] Papke RL, Ono F, Stokes C, Urban JM, Boyd RT. The nicotinic acetylcholine receptors of zebrafish and an evaluation of pharmacological tools used for their study. Biochem Pharmacol 2012; 84 (3): 352-65.

[69] Grady SR, Moretti M, Zoli, M, *et al*. Rodent habenulo-interpeduncular pathway expresses a large variety of uncommon nAChR subtypes, but only the $\alpha3\beta4^*$ and $\alpha3\beta3\beta4^*$ subtypes mediate acetylcholine release. J Neurosci 2009; 29 (7): 2272-2282.

[70] Horenstein NA, Leonik FM, Papke RL. Multiple pharmacophores for the selective activation of nicotinic alpha7-type acetylcholine receptors. Mol Pharmacol 2008; 74 (6): 1496-511.

[71] Papke RL, Wecker L, Stitzel JA. Activation and inhibition of mouse muscle and neuronal nicotinic acetylcholine receptors expressed in *Xenopus* oocytes. JPET 2010; 333 (2): 501-18.

[72] Webster JC, Francis MM, Porter JK, *et al*. Antagonist activities of mecamylamine and nicotine show reciprocal dependence on beta subunit sequence in the second transmembrane domain. Br J Pharmacol 1999; 127 (6): 1337-48.

[73] Panula P, Chen Y-C, Priyadarshini M, *et al*. The comparative neuroanatomy and neurochemistry of zebrafish CNS systems of relevance to human neuropsychiatric diseases. Neurobiology of Disease 2010; 40 (1): 46-57.

[74] Holzschuh J, Ryu S, Aberger F, Driever W. Dopamine transporter expression distinguishes dopaminergic neurons from other catecholaminergic neurons in the developing zebrafish embryo. Mech Dev 2001; 101 (1-2): 237–243.

[75] Filippi A, Mahler J, Schweitzer J, Driever W. Expression of the paralogous tyrosine hydroxylase encoding genes th1 and th2 reveals the full complement of dopaminergic and noradreneric neurons in zebrafish larval and juvenile brain. J Comp Neurol 2010; 518 (4): 423-438.

[76] Rink E, Wullimann MF. The teleostean (zebrafish) dopaminergic system ascending to the subpallium (striatum) is located in the basal diencephalon (posterior tuberculum). Brain Res 2001; 889 (1-2): 316-330.

[77] Farrell TC, Cario CL, Milanese C, Vogt A, Jeong J-H, Burton EA. Evaluation of spontaneous propulsive movement as a screening tool to detect rescue of Parkinsonism phenotypes in zebrafish models. Neurobiology of Disease 2011; 44 (1): 9-18.

[78] McKinley ET, Baranowski TC, Blavo DO, Cato C, Doan TN, Rubinstein AL. Neuroprotection of MPTP-induced toxicity. Brain Res Mol Brain Res 2005; 141 (2): 128-37.

[79] Bandmann O, Burton EA. Genetic zebrafish models of neurodegenerative diseases. Neurobiology of Disease 2010; 40 (1): 58-65.

[80] Bowman, TV, Zon LI. Swimming into he future of drug discovery: *in vivo* chemical screens in zebrafish. ACS Chem Biol 2010; 5 (2): 159-161.

[81] Doyon Y, McCammon JM, Miller JC, *et al*. Heritable targeted gene disruption in zebrafish using designed zinc-finger nucleases. Nature Biotechnology 2008; 26 (6): 702-708.

[82] Hao J, Ho J, Lewis, J, *et al. In vivo* structure-activity relationship study of dorsomorphin analogues identifies selective VEGF and BMP inhibitors, ACS Chem Biol 2010; 5(2): 245-253.

[83] Rihel J, Schier AF. Behavioral screening for neuroactive drugs in zebrafish. Developmental Neurobiology 2012; 72 (3): 373-385.

[84] Tiefenbach J, Moll PR, Nelson, MR, *et al.* A live zebrafish-based screening system for human nuclear receptor ligand and cofactor discovery. PLoS ONE 2010; 5 (3): e9797.

[85] Darland T, Dowling JE. Behavioral screening for cocaine sensitivity in mutagenized zebrafish. Proc Natl Acad Sci 2001; 98 (20): 11691-11696.

[86] Webb KJ, Norton WH, Trumbach D, *et al.* Zebrafish reward mutants reveal novel transcripts mediating the behavioral effects of amphetamine. Genome Biol 2009; 10 (7): R81

[87] Kily LJ, Cowe YC, Hussain O, *et al.* Gene expression changes in a zebrafish model of drug dependency suggest conservation of neuro-adaptation pathways. J Exp Biol 2008; 211 (Pt. 10): 1623–1634.

[88] Ninkovic J, Bally-Cuif L. The zebrafish as a model system for assessing the reinforcing properties of drugs of abuse. Methods 2006; 39 (3): 262-274.

[89] Levin ED, Chen E. Nicotinic involvement in memory function in zebrafish. Neurotox and Teratol 2004; 26 (6): 731-735.

[90] Levin ED, Limpuangthip J, Rachakonda T, Peterson M. Timing of nicotine effects on learning in zebrafish. Psychopharmacol 2006; 184 (3-4): 547-552.

[91] Levin ED, Bencan Z, Cerutti DT. Anxiolytic effects of nicotine in zebrafish. Physiol and Behav 2007; 90 (1): 54-58.

[92] Bencan Z, Levin ED. The role of alpha7 and alpha4beta2 nicotinic receptors in the nicotine- induced anxiolytic effect in zebrafish. Physiol and Behav 20081 95 (3): 408-412.

[93] Ali S, Champagne DL, Spaink HP, Richardson, MK. Zebrafish embryos and larvae: a new generation of disease models and drug screens. Birth Defects Res. (Part C) 2011; 93 (2): 115-133.

[94] Fero K, Yokogawa T, Burgess HA. The behavioral repertoire of larval zebrafish. In Kalueff AV, Cachat JM Eds. Zebrafish Models in Neurobehavioral Research, Neuromethods 52 © Springer Science+Business Media, LLC 2011; pp. 249-291

[95] Kokel D, Peterson RT. Chemobehavioural phenomics and behavior-based psychiatric drug discovery in the zebrafish. Briefings in Functional Genomics and Proteomics 2008; 7 (6): 483-490.

[96] Prober DA, Rihel J, Onah AA, Sung RJ, Schier, AF. Hypocretin/orexin overexpression induces an insomnia-like phenotype in zebrafish. J Neurosci 2006; 26 (51): 13400-13410.

[97] Zhdanova IV, Wang SY, Leclair OU, Danilova NP. Melatonin promotes sleep-like state in zebrafish. Brain Res 2001; 903 (1-2): 263-268.

[98] Kokkinidis L, Zacharko RM, Anisman, H. Amphetamine withdrawal: a behavioral evaluation. Life Sci 1986; 38 (17): 1617–23.

[99] Jonkman S, Risbrough VB, Geyer MA, Markou A. A spontaneous nicotine withdrawal potentiates the effects of stress in rats. Neuropsychopharmacology 2008; 33 (9): 2131-2138.

[100] Cachat J, Canavello P, Elegante M, *et al.* Modeling withdrawal syndrome in zebrafish. Behav Brain Res 2010; 208 (2): 371-376.

[101] Rihel J, Prober DA, Arvanite A, *et al.* Zebrafish behavioral profiling links drugs to biological targets and rest/wake regulation. Science 2010; 327 (5963): 348-351.
[102] Kokel D, Bryan J, Laggoner C, *et al.* Rapid behavior-based identification of neuroactive small molecules in zebrafish. Nat Chem Biol 2010; 6 (3): 231-237.
[103] Kokel D, Rennekamp AJ, Shah AH, Liebel U, Peterson RT. Behavorial barcoding in the cloud: embracing data-intensive digital phenotyping in neuropharmacology. Trends in Biotechnology 2012; 30 (8): 421-425.
[104] Mathur P, Lau B, Guo S. Conditioned place preference behavior in zebrafish. Nature Protocols 2011; 6 (3): 338-345.
]105] Gerlai R. High-throughput behavioral screens: the first step towards finding genes involved in vertebrate brain function using zebrafish. Molecules 2010; 15 (4): 2609-2622.
[106] Jeong JY, Kwon HB, Ahn JC, *et al.* Functional and developmental analysis of the blood-brain barrier in zebrafish. Brain Res Bull 2008; 75 (5): 619-628.

INDEX

A

Atta-ur-Rahman & M. Iqbal Choudhary (Eds.)

D

E

F

G

H

M

N

O

P

Q

R

S

T

U

V

Y

Z

Made in the USA
Las Vegas, NV
03 November 2026

57424105R00259